Hearing and Balance in the Elderly

MEDICINE IN OLD AGE

Volumes already published

Bone and joint disease in the elderly
V. Wright, *Editor*
Peripheral vascular disease in the elderly
S.F. McCarthy, *Editor*

Volumes in preparation

Clinical pharmacology and therapeutics
K. O'Malley, *Editor*

Immunology and infection in the elderly
R.A. Fox, *Editor*

Urological problems in the elderly
J.C. Brocklehurst, *Editor*

Gastrointestinal tract disorders in the elderly
J. Hellemans and G. Vantrappen, *Editors*

Arterial disease in the elderly
R.W. Stout, *Editor*

Clinical biochemistry in the elderly
H.M. Hodkinson, *Editor*

Cardiology in the elderly
R.J. Luchi, *Editor*

Prevention of disease in the elderly
J.A. Muir Gray, *Editor*

Blood disorders in the elderly
M.J. Denham and I. Chanarin, *Editors*

Hearing and Balance in the Elderly

Edited by

Ronald Hinchcliffe

MD PhD FRCP DLO

Professor of Audiological Medicine, Institute of Laryngology and Otology,
University of London; Honorary Consultant Neuro-otologist,
Royal National Throat, Nose and Ear Hospital, London

CHURCHILL LIVINGSTONE
EDINBURGH LONDON MELBOURNE AND NEW YORK 1983

CHURCHILL LIVINGSTONE
Medical Division of Longman Group Limited

Distributed in the United States of America by
Churchill Livingstone Inc., 1560 Broadway, New York,
N.Y. 10036, and by associated companies,
branches and representatives throughout
the world.

First published 1983

ISBN   0 443 02075 2

British Library Cataloguing in Publication Data

Hearing and balance in the elderly.—(Medicine
   in old age)
   1. Hearing disorders   2. Geriatrics
   1. Hinchcliffe, R.   II. Series
   618.97'78   RF291.5.A35

Library of Congress Cataloging in Publication Data
Main entry under title:

Hearing and balance in the elderly.
   (Medicine in old age)
   Includes index.
   1. Geriatric otolaryngology. 2. Equilibrium
(Physiology) 3. Aged, Deaf. I. Hinchcliffe, R.
II. Series. [DNLM: 1. Hearing disorders—In old age.
2. Equilibrium—In old age. WV 270 H431] RF 291. 5.
A35H4   1983   618.97'78   82-14787

Printed in Singapore by
Kyodo Shing Loong Printing Industries Pte Ltd.

Introduction

A series of volumes on Medicine in Old Age is necessary and timely. It is not so very long since teaching hospitals in the United Kingdom did not admit patients over the age of 65. Medical students received their entire medical education in teaching hospitals and they were taught by teachers who had done likewise. They rarely saw old people, they were rarely taught about old people and they read text books written by teachers who had not treated old people or undertaken research on them. The scientific knowledge of clinical medicine stopped abrubtly at the age of 65. After that there was something dark, shadowy and threatening called 'senility'.

Medicine has changed radically, and the majority of physicians today deal extensively with elderly ill old patients. Geriatricians too now work in general hospitals with access to diagnostic facilities. As a result a body of knowledge is growing up about the clinical medicine and therapeutics of old age, and is being published in general and specialist journals.

Medicine in old age is complex. Disease is rarely confined to one body system. Coincidental and contributory conditions may be found in many parts of the body, complicating clinical care and management. Psychological, social, epidemiological and resource considerations have to be taken into account. Those working with the old need to be well informed on many aspects of clinical medicine which may not have been recognised when they were students. In addition they must keep up with the new knowledge that must be applied if the elderly patient is to be comprehensively assessed and effectively treated with restoration of independence.

This new series aims to give to doctors working with elderly patients a concise but comprehensive guide to this new knowledge. Each volume in the series will deal with a system of the body or a closely related group of problems; and will return to a topic previously dealt with when the growth of knowledge justifies this. The Editorial Board will select guest editors for each volume whose authority is undoubted and who are able to attract contributions from any country which has contributed to the advance of knowledge. The volumes will stand mid-way between the immediacy of the scientific journal and the urbanity of the standard text book, combining freshness with authority. It is hoped that the profession will find them of value.

Birmingham, 1983   B. Isaacs

Preface

An increasing proportion of our population is now in the older age groups. Older people are particularly afflicted with disorders of hearing and of balance. Over recent years, a considerable body of knowledge has accumulated regarding the extent and nature of the disorders many of which can be remedied. This knowledge has not yet been widely disseminated amongst physicians responsible for the care and management of older people. Moreover much of this knowledge is dispersed amongst a variety of specialist journals. It is hoped that a monograph such as this will help to remedy this deficiency.

London, 1983   R.H.

Contributors

G.R. Barnes PhD
Head of Vestibular Physiology, RAF Institute of Aviation Medicine,
Farnborough, Hampshire, UK

Susan Bellman MA MB BCh FRCS DLO
Senior Registrar in Audiological Medicine, Royal National Throat, Nose and Ear
Hospital, London, UK

Ole Bentzen PhD
Director, Hearing Clinic, University Hospital, Århus, Denmark

Moe Bergman EdD
Professor, School of Communication Disorders, Sackler School of Medicine,
Tel-Aviv University, Tel-Aviv, Israel; Professor Emeritus, Hunter College of the
City University of New York, New York, USA

Adrian Davis BSc MSc
Statistician/Epidemiologist, MRC Institute of Hearing Research,
Nottingham, UK

D. P. Goldstein PhD
Professor, Department of Audiology and Speech Sciences, Purdue University,
West Lafayette, Indiana, USA

Katia Gilholme Herbst MA
Projects and Evaluation Officer, Mental Health Foundation, London, UK

Ronald Hinchcliffe MD PhD FRCP DLO
Professor of Audiological Medicine, Institute of Laryngology and Otology,
University of London; Honorary Consultant Neuro-otologist, Royal National
Throat, Nose and Ear Hospital, London, UK

Bernard Isaacs MD FRCP
Charles Hayward Professor of Geriatric Medicine, University of Birmingham,
Birmingham, UK

Peter Jackson FRCS FRCSE
Consultant Ear, Nose and Throat Surgeon, Bromley and Greenwich Districts;
Honorary Consultant, Royal National Throat, Nose and Ear Hospital,
London, UK

Tapani Jauhiainen MD
Assistant Professor of Audiology, University of Helsinki, Helsinki, Finland

Linda M. Luxon BSc MBBS MRCP
Consultant Physician and Otoneurologist, Institute of Neurology, The National Hospital, London, UK

Geoffrey A. Manley BA MA PhD
Professor and Director, Zoological Institute, Technische Universität, Munich, FRG

C. D. Marsden MSc MBBS FRCP MRCPsych
Professor of Neurology, Institute of Psychiatry and King's College Hospital Medical School, London, UK

Margareta Bjurö Møller MD PhD
Associate Professor of Otolaryngology and Neurological Surgery, University of Pittsburgh School of Medicine, Pittsburgh, USA

J. A. Obeso MD
Research Worker, King's College Hospital Medical School, London, UK

W. J. Oosterveld MD
Professor, Vestibular Department, Academisch Medisch Centrum, Amsterdam, The Netherlands

P. W. Overstall MB MRCP
Consultant in Geriatric Medicine, Hereford General Hospital, Hereford, UK

Sáva Součková MUDr
Senior Registrar in Audiological Medicine, Royal National Throat, Nose and Ear Hospital, London, UK

S. D. G. Stephens BSc MBBS MPhil
Consultant in Audiological Medicine, Royal National Throat, Nose and Ear Hospital, London, UK

M. M. Traub BSc PhD MBBS MRCP
Research Worker, King's College Hospital Medical School, London, UK

Joanna M. C. Zlotnik MB ChB FRCS FRACS
Senior Registrar in Audiological Medicine, Royal National Throat, Nose and Ear Hospital, London, UK

Contents

Hearing

The epidemiology of hearing disorders

INTRODUCTION

There have been several recent pleas and recommendations for more epidemiol-ogical studies of hearing disorders (e.g. Hinchcliffe, 1979; Elliot, 1978; DHSS, 1973; DHSS, 1977). The general methods for the application of epidemiology to audiology have been outlined by Hinchcliffe (1979), while the extent and possible causes of hearing disorders have been listed by Schein and Delk (1974), by Elliott and by Glorig and Gilad (1979a, b). There are many shortcomings in the existing data on hearing disorders in populations, and there are difficulties in interpreting data, both in the scientific and administrative sense, even when they are acceptable as valid. For example, in the specific case of ageing, it is not clear how disability and the consequent handicap resulting from hearing disorders in old age should be assessed and hence what forms of service should be provided in the future. A second problem is that there has been neither a cohesive or testable epidemiological model of the relationship between various causal factors nor an agreed practical framework to guide the medical scientist who wishes to investigate the epidemiol-ogy of hearing disorders.

Age has to be a major variable in any epidemiological study and my focusing on it here does not imply that it has been the primary focus of all the investigations to which I will refer in this chapter. I will examine various types of method for the investigation of hearing disorders and the particular problems they pose in interacting with the variable of age. Some tentative suggestions will be made from studies in which I have been involved in the UK about general methods for epidemiological research in audiology. I shall outline the types of data collected in other studies and the problems associated with that data. Secondly, I shall outline the design and analysis of age-related aspects of data collected in a pilot study of a National Study of Hearing (NSH) in the UK. This study is being conducted over four years (1979–1983) by the Medical Research Council's Institute of Hearing Research (MRC-IHR). Thirdly, I shall discuss age effects in referral for hearing disabilities among series of patients gathered from separate clinics in England and Scotland. The picture of hearing levels and service needs will be rounded out by secondary analysis of data collected in homes for the elderly in South Wales.

General classification of studies of hearing disorders

The various types of epidemiological study to be found in the literature divide according to four major distinctions. The first distinction is between the type of study appropriate to the developed and the developing countries. As Leske (1977) and others have commented, communicative disorders (including hearing) are a common cause of morbidity or chronic impairment in the USA. The implication is that there is a similar concern in most developed countries where basic nutrition and life-threatening communicable disease are no longer the major preoccupation. Most developing countries are not yet able to devote skilled manpower to either assessing or remedying communication disorders. This limits the priority which hearing problems receive and conditions the type of epidemiological data that would be considered relevant, likely to be available, or likely to elucidate the local causes of hearing disorders.

The second major distinction is between studies that have used population-based sampling (or whole population testing) techniques on a large scale, and those using clinical series and small scale samples. The latter generally consists of observations made by otologists or occasionally gerontologists in their clinics. However, there are some very good examples of the use of fairly small samples or populations (n < 1000) to achieve better understanding of a particular question or influence (e.g. Hinchcliffe, 1958; Burns and Robinson, 1970; McKennell, 1963; Herbst and Humphrey, 1981).

The Health Examination Survey 1960–1961 (HES) and the Health and Nutrition Examination Survey 1971–1974 (HANES) (National Center for Health Statistics, 1967; 1970; 1980; Roberts 1979) conducted in the USA have been on a larger scale altogether, and used complex sampling plans. Britain (Wilkins, 1947) and Australia (Upfold and Wilson, 1980) have attempted epidemiological studies on a fairly wide scale too, usually assessing only the prevalence of hearing difficulties and sometimes assumed causes, mainly to assess the need for hearing aids and rehabilitative/preventive programmes. The EEC has also carried out a large scale epidemiological survey (CEC, 1980) of childhood deafness and its assumed causes.

The third distinction concerns the role to which contrasts between circumscribed populations and sub-populations is made to play. There have been several studies of sub-populations in the developing World. Hinchcliffe, (1973) outlines those in Africa and the West Indies, whilst there have been others in such widely different regions as the Arctic (Baxter and Ling, 1974) and India (Pal et al, 1974). To a certain extent these studies have been designed to cast light on local factors in clinically apparent hearing losses but some have been designed to investigate the general nature of hearing decline with age which for many reasons is very difficult to examine in the noise-polluted developed world (e.g. Rosen et al, 1962; Bergman 1966). In the light of possible sex, and racial differences in susceptibility to the same noise levels (Federal Register, 1981), there may be difficulties in such interpretation.

Finally the major variable, age, may be incorporated in one of two ways. All the types of studies so far referred to have been cross-sectional studies; a number of individuals have been examined at a given time (or period of time) and age inferences drawn from the grouping of individuals into age bands. For economic reasons no longitudinal epidemiological studies of hearing have been carried out on a significant scale. Unfortunately it is not possible to make inferences about the individual course or causes of age effects in hearing where only cross-sectional age data are available.

Problems with data

Some of the general shortcomings that may be present in existing data are outlined schematically in Table 1.1. This summary is presented here as part of a practical framework that applies to any audiological research and in particular the epidemiology of hearing. Data are never collected in a perfect fashion. They are always open to distorting influences of a high-level or low-level type. Low-level data distortion, such as digit transportation and transposition, loss of data, wrong or slapdash measurement, are fairly simply recognised and controlled. Higher level factors in distortions due to variation in equipment availability, staff training, motivation of the research teams are not. Further consideration of Table 1.1 is left to the reader who may be interested in interpreting or conducting epidemiological research.

Table 1.1 Some general problems with data collection in epidemiological studies of hearing.

1: Low level problems	(a) Integrity and validity of data
	(b) Missing data and other related problems
	(c) Uniformity of data
	(d) No data base access or portability of data
	(e) Absence of efficient record linkage
	(f) Throwing out raw data
	(g) Type of measurement and calibration available
2: High level problems	(a) Limited generality of the data
	(b) Type of sampling available and used
	(c) Reason and motivation for study
	(d) Staff, availability and training
	(e) Levels of analysis attempted
	(f) Interpretation of data

The interests of four groups of people have also to be considered in designing a study. Firstly, the data should be tailored to the needs of those who commission the study once those 'needs' have been discussed, refined and assessed for practicability in collaboration with the investigators. Next the scale, nature and method of data collection should be consistent with the training and occupational aspirations of the staff collecting it. Thirdly the collection of, and access to, the data should be at least of potential assistance to the individual and not infringe his essential rights to privacy. Finally it should preferably complement, and at least not undermine, the work of health care personnel responsible for the population in the relevant sphere. All these constraints upon investigators mean that the research design has to balance several conflicting needs in any study; this requires checking and piloting to ensure the design can achieve an acceptable proportion of its objectives. For example in the National Study of Hearing (NSH) there are two main classes of objective: to provide prevalence estimates for various degrees and types of hearing loss, and to perform a multi-factorial investigation of hearing disorders; these two objectives are partly in conflict. The overall design, detailed later, was chosen to reconcile the two objectives and balance the interests of groups (1) and (2).

Background studies illustrating problems of definition and methods

The usability of data on the aetiology and severity of hearing disorders provided by a survey depends enormously on the particular aims and objectives of that survey and on the skills of those who carry it out. The sampling design and choice of assessment method (postal questionnaire, interviewer assessment and questionnaire, audiometric assessment, otological assessment—to mention the most commonly used), together with the training and status of the personnel involved, are all critical to the interpretation of the data. As Hinchcliffe (1979) points out, epidemiology today recognises that 'normal' and 'impaired' or 'pathological' states may be considered zones on a continuum. Hence there are many possible definitions of 'disorders'. It is ideal to achieve generality by estimating the complete distribution of people along the entire severity continuum for the disorder concerned, and to a certain extent this approach will be employed in the section on a population-based study (pp. 6–26). However in the practical, clinical world, a tight distinction is sometimes forced between two states 'normal' and 'disordered'. Table 1.2 and the following discussion illustrate the problems

Table 1.2 Percentage of people described as hearing impaired in three separate studies (see text) by seven age groups and sex HES, 1960–62, USA; WILKINS (WIL), 1947, UK; HIS, 1971, USA.

Age group	MALE study HES	WIL	HIS	FEMALE study HES	WIL	HIS	BOTH SEXES study HES	WIL	HIS
18–24	1·2	1·2	{	0·4	0·9	{	0·8	1·0	{
25–34	1·4	1·8	{ 5·1	1·3	1·5	{ 3·4	1·3	1·6	{ 4·2
35–44	3·7	2·1	{	2·2	2·9	{	2·9	2·5	{
45–54	4·1	4·9	{14·0	4·6	4·6	{ 9·0	4·3	4·7	{11·4
55–64	10·6	6·2	{	10·1	6·4	{	10·3	6·4	{
65–74	30·5	12·4	28·0	26·2	12·1	19·0	28·2	12·2	23·1
75–79	48·7	28·0	44·0	47·4	25·0	36·0	48·0	26·0	39·8
18–79	7·6	4·8	8·1	7·1	4·9	6·3	7·3	4·9	7·1

met when (a) different methods are used to assess hearing impairment and (b) different criteria demarcate 'normality' from 'disorder'. Table 1.2 shows the results from three different studies, in terms of the percentage of hearing impaired persons for a given age band and sex.

The Health Examination Survey (HES) was an audiometric survey of about 7000 sampled individuals in the USA. The audiometric survey was conducted in 1960–1962 as part of a larger health survey. Results from a similar survey, the Health and Nutrition Examination Survey (HANES) conducted in 1971–1975 are now becoming available and show some general agreement. The data shown are the percentage, projected to the population, of those with a better ear average hearing level greater than 25 dB HL (averaged over ·5, 1, 2 kHz).

The study labelled WIL was conducted by Wilkins (1947) in the UK, partly as an adjunct to a larger survey being conducted by the Central Office of Information. The aim of the survey was to provide an estimate for the number of National Health Service (NHS) hearing aids that were likely to be needed after the NHS Act came into force in 1948. It was also hoped that information on the incidence and prevalence of 'deafness' could be obtained for the adult (over 16 years) population of England, Scotland and Wales. The sampling was from the civilian population using the maintenance register in force at the time and 31 000 people were sampled. The interviewers used an adapted version of Beasley's (1940) classification scheme. The percentages shown are supposed to reflect a corresponding hearing level of 36 dB HL (ISO, 1964) in the US but this equivalence had not been shown for a British population. As the response categories are not specific about which ear is concerned, only referring to overall 'hearing and understanding', the percentages probably apply to the effective disability as determined chiefly by the better ear hearing levels.

Study HIS, the Health Interview Survey was conducted in 1971 on 134 000 people selected from 44 000 households in the US. The survey used the following checklist 'Does anyone in the family now have deafness in one or both ears? Any trouble hearing with one or both ears? Does anyone in the family use a hearing aid?' The percentages shown in Table 1.2 for the HIS show the pooled prevalence of trouble hearing with one or both ears, and hence probably reflect the hearing disability and the pathology in the worse ear.

There are four points to note from Table 1.2. Firstly, the difference in the methods used and the criteria for impairment do lead to widely discrepant estimates of absolute prevalences. Secondly, there is a strong trend for the percentage with hearing impairment to increase rapidly with increasing age in all studies. The biggest change shown for example in the HES is from 10·3 per cent in the 55 to 64 age group to 28·2 per cent in the 65 to 74 age group. That this figure is not a product of noise exposure in the 1914–1918 War is shown by parallel increases in both male and female volunteers. Thirdly, questionnaire responses may underestimate actual hearing problems. This is partly offset by the fact that the interview surveys have to use a fixed question which was 'calibrated' at a slightly higher level than the audiometric criterion adopted by the HES, and in the under 55 group the figures correspond fairly well. However, fourthly, above 55 years the questionnaire greatly underestimates prevalences. Hence any pegging of questionnaires to audiometric equivalents should be made in an age-dependent fashion (see also Merluzzi and Hinchcliffe, 1972). From knowledge now available it is probable that the 35 dB HL pegging of the Wilkins study, was on average valid having combined two conflicting components, i.e. (a) a more inclusive (i.e. sensitive) criterion of hearing difficulty in church/theatre environments or in group conversation for those under 55 (e.g. about 25 dB HL), and (b) a less inclusive criterion for those over 55 (e.g. about 50 dB HL).

Consideration of these three studies shows some of the consequences of the choice of tests to be used and the criteria adopted for imputing impairment. It is obviously cheaper to perform interviews in large numbers than to do an audiometric assessment on a large random sample. However, as Table 1.2 shows, an audiometric assessment is the minimum for scientific purposes, at least until a well calibrated and reliable set of questions are available for the target population (see Noble, 1978 for a discussion of the merits of the questionnaire approach and its validity). There is a third option available for balancing precision with cost: a combination of questionnaire and audiometric assessment, used with a two-stage sampling procedure (Kish, 1973). This is the approach adopted by the NSH and I shall describe the method and results on pp. 6–27, and make a brief methodological summary on page 6.

A POPULATION-BASED STUDY

No attempt will be made here to review all the pertinent literature on decline of hearing with age or to assess its value by applying the criteria of Table 1.1. This is done by Maurer and Rupp (1979) and by others, including Hinchcliffe (1979), Robinson and Sutton (1979), Roberts (1979), and Elliott (1978). In the last section data obtained on the prevalence of hearing disorders in different age groups was presented to make a methodological point, but also showing the main trends of previous studies. This section will outline a pilot study for the National Study of Hearing which will assess the characteristics and prevalence of hearing disorders for adults in Great Britain, to illustrate general design issues and present new data.

Outline of the pilot study for the NSH

A schematic outline of the stages involved in the planning and execution of the study is shown in Figure 1.1. From 1978–1980, staff were trained in testing procedures on the pilot study and the management procedures for those found to have problems were formulated. There was also a reformulation of the expectations of the official bodies providing the funding (the MRC and the Health Departments of England, Scotland and Wales). The structure, objectives and initial implications of the study have been outlined elsewhere (IHR 1981a, b; Haggard, Gatehouse and Davis, 1981).

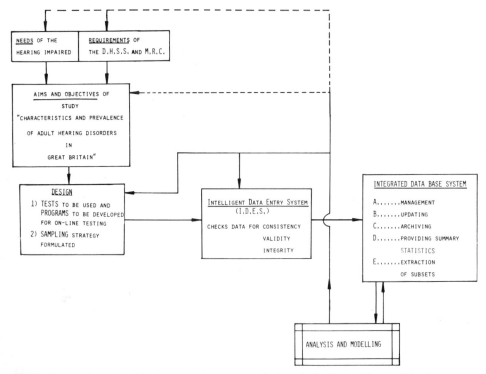

Fig. 1.1 Schematic outline of the data collection and analysis plans for the National Study of Hearing (NSH).

The tests—audiometric, otological, and general medical—were prepared with special attention to uniformity, to their ergonomic requirements and to replicability of procedures and calibration of audiometric equipment. It was predetermined that there would be four test centres, or out-stations, i.e. in Cardiff, Glasgow, Nottingham and Southampton. This meant that only districts near these towns could be sampled for a full audiological assessment; this necessitates a further, national, sample before some of our conclusions can be generalised. Fixed clinical bases meant that a greater depth of audiometric and otological tests could be used. So while the prevalence aspect of the study was of importance, priority was given to the scientific exploitations of the available opportunities in order to characterise the population in terms of combinations of results on a wide range of tests. This would have long term relevance to the needs for different types of hearing aid, provide norms for clinical tests and point out the distributions and clusterings of symptoms in hearing impairment.

All the data collected in this study is entered on-line to the general purpose out-station microcomputer and checked for consistency and validity. Built-in tests for plausibility of values ensure that the data is correctly entered for the right subject and test and any errors can be corrected on the spot. The whole corpus of data is managed by a data base system that should enable easy access and linkage facilities for the records to be collected over the entire study. The pilot study and each of the first two phases of the main study will have influenced some of the tests and data collection procedures in a subsequent phase. A core of tests is kept constant while other aspects of the study can change from phase to phase.

Figure 1.2 shows that the study is organised in two tiers, A and B. Tier A used a postal screening questionnaire (see Appendix A) to ascertain reported hearing disorders, including tinnitus. This was developed from the expanded hearing scale questionnaire of Schein and his colleagues (1970) as used by Ward and his colleagues (1978) in Great Britain. A few biographical questions were also asked, including questions about the possession of hearing aids. Two parallel forms of the hearing questions were used, so that specific biasses could be controlled. Action was taken to combat non-response at both the Tier A and Tier B stages. The numbers shown in Figure 1.2 refer to the pilot study. Over the three-year period 1981–1984 a further 30 000 people will have been contacted at Tier A of whom 2500 progress to Tier B. In addition, a national sample will be contacted and a proportion of these will be audiometrically assessed.

The questionnaire has three main purposes: (1) it gives directly the prevalence of self-reported hearing disorders; (2) it enables us to send further detailed questionnaires to specific groups of interest (e.g. hearing aid users); (3) it provides an efficient stratifying process into Tier B, i.e. it enables us to group individuals systematically on variables which can be shown to account for much of the variance in hearing levels. This stratification is applied to all who return questionnaires, i.e. respondents are grouped on the basis of their reply. A random sample from each group is then selected to proceed to Tier B. Not everyone selected to do so is willing to proceed. So, beside the main planned strata, extra strata are formed by visiting those who have not replied to our invitation or who cannot attend the clinic. The strata for the pilot study were based on the replies to two questions, one of which differed in the two questionnaires. The constant question was the answer

T
I
E
R

A

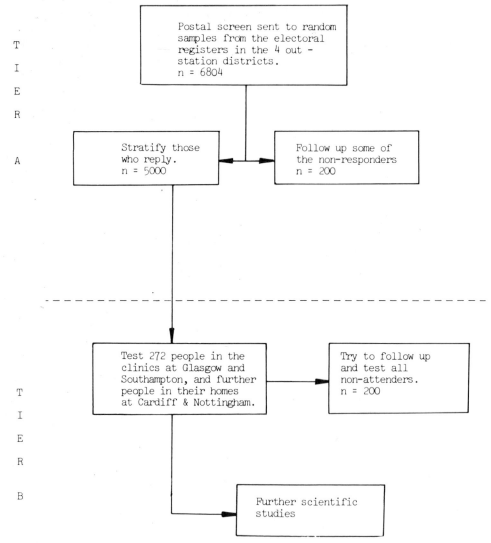

T
I
E
R

B

Fig. 1.2 Simple structure of the NSH pilot study, conducted in 1979–1980. The number who replied to the questionnaire and who have followed up at Tier A and Tier B are approximate, as the fieldwork is continuing.

to the tinnitus question B1 (see Appendix at the end of this chapter). The hearing question was either (a) whether the person could hear and understand a whisper or (b) whether the person had no difficulty hearing a one-to-one conversation with a person on the left and right side separately (see Appendix, Section A, version 1 question 1a and Section B version 2, questions 1 and 2 for details). These versions of the questionnaire are termed 'binaural' and 'monaural' questionnaires respectively.

The tests at Tier B have included the following: pure tone audiometry, air and bone conduction, threshold of uncomfortable loudness (uncomfortable loudness level), acoustic impedance and reflex measures, tone-on-tone masking, standard-ised clinical interview and management, blood tests, sentence-in-noise tests of disability, a shortened version of 'speech audiometry', i.e. identification of monosyllable words in quiet at various intensities, further questionnaires on disability and handicap from hearing disorders including tinnitus, various audio-visual tests, visual acuity tests, and contingent psycho-acoustic measurements of tinnitus. In the results that follow, I shall concentrate on three aspects of the results of the pilot study in relation to age that have not been described in detail elsewhere. These are (a) reported hearing disorders, (b) audiometric hearing levels, and (c) disability as measured by a sentence-in-noise test (SIN).

Reported hearing disorders

A summary to responses to the questionnaires is given in Table 1.3. The results are pooled over the four out-stations and also give an audiometric equivalent for each of the four groups. The averages reported here are over the hearing levels at 0·5, 1, 2 and 4 kHz. The weighted average hearing levels in Table 1.3 are derived

Table 1.3 Percentage of respondents in each of four reported hearing disorders categories. Corresponding audiometric figures are shown in unweighted and weighted form for the better ear. NSH pilot study, 1980.

	% of group in population	BEA of those tested	SD of BEA	Population weighted BEA
No reported hearing disorders (N)	65	11	9	10
Only Tinnitus reported (NT)	9	17	14	27
Only hearing problem reported (HI)	17	26	18	26
Both Tinnitus and hearing problem reported (HIT)	9	40	23	44

by weighting each individual's average according to the prevalence of a group in a particular district (Glasgow or Southampton) for a particular questionnaire (monaural or binaural). The weighted averages show the questionnaire to be fairly efficient in screening for raised hearing levels and emphasise the importance of the tinnitus questions in ascertaining indirectly the present state of a patient's hearing. The increase in variance, as indicated by the standard deviation, over the four groups is significant.

In total, 35 per cent of people reported some kind of hearing disorder, 26 per cent a hearing problem and 18 per cent tinnitus. Of the latter, one half also reported a hearing impairment. The studies detailed in Table 1.2 would lead us to expect a lower figure than obtained even taking discrepancies in criteria for the questionnaires into account. However, the difference is substantiated if an audiometric criterion is applied. Using the 25 dB HL criterion for the better ear average (BEA) at 0·5, 1, 2, 4 kHz and projecting the result into the population, the total percentage with a hearing problem is 19·9 per cent (with a 95 per cent confidence interval of ±4·4 per cent). This should compare fairly directly with the 7·3 per cent found by the HES. The pilot study does not provide enough data to be broken down reliably into the same age bands for each sex as in the HES. Two possible biases in our results are the effect of non-response at Tier A and non-attendance at Tier B. These biases might be additive in that those with no hearing impairment would not co-operate. This is unlikely to account for much of the difference (see IHR, 1981b) as there was no significant difference on the better ear average HL for attenders and non-attenders followed up from the four strata shown in Table 1.3. So an initial prevalence estimate of hearing problems summarised by a BEA >24 dB HL is about 20 per cent. The broad clinical categories of hearing problems is shown in Table 1.4. It is obvious from this that the largest proportion of hearing problems is of a sensorineural origin, particularly in the better ear.

Finally, this section discusses the variation in reported hearing disorders with age. Table 1.5 shows a table similar to Table 1.2 for the two questionnaire types

Table 1.4 Audiometric classification of the population in percentages for better and worse ears. 'Sensorineural' is defined as an AHL > 24 dB HL and an air bone gap <15 dB HL. (Average threshold at 0·5, 1, 2, 4 kHz used for all calculations) NSH pilot study, 1980.

	Normal	Sensorineural	Conductive	Mixed
Better ear	81·0	15·5	1·5	2·0
Worse ear	66·0	20·0	8·0	6·0

Table 1.5 Percentage of people reporting hearing problems, according to two questionnaires, one 'binaural' and the other 'monaural', and percentage reporting tinnitus for seven age groups. NSH pilot study, 1980.

Age group	% hearing problems (Binaural questionnaire)	% hearing problems (Monaural questionnaire)	% Tinnitus report
18–24	13·6	4·0	14·3
25–34	18·9	5·6	14·5
35–44	23·7	7·2	13·8
45–54	26·4	9·6	14·9
55–64	33·4	15·2	19·6
65–74	35·6	25·5	19·9
75 +	47·2	40·0	23·4
All ages	27·6	11·4	18·0

and for reported tinnitus problems. Figure 1.3 summarises the NSH pilot study questionnaire data and contrasts it with studies mentioned above. The monaural (M) and binaural (B) questions were developed from the expanded hearing loss scale questionnaire in the USA (Schein, Gentile and Hasse, 1970). Schein and his colleague, reported that the average hearing level in the better ear was 18 to 22 dB HL and 28 dB HL for the M and B type questionnaires respectively, when the question suggesting the mildest hearing problem was answered in the affirmative. In due time similar equivalent pegging of individual questions will be produced for the UK. Figure 1.4 shows that the M questionnaire gives a higher percentage of 'normal' reports than the B questionnaire. This is contrary to what might have been expected from the inclusive nature of the monaural questions, where the questionnaire is directed towards the worse ear and so should give a lower

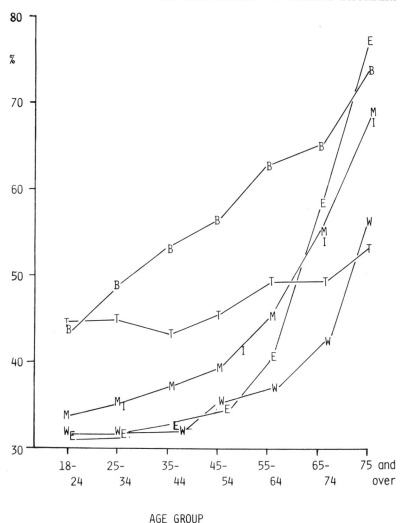

AGE GROUP

Fig. 1.3 Percentage of people in each age group with hearing impairment as defined in the following studies: W—W Wilkins, UK, 1947; I—I the HIS, USA, 1971; E—E the HES, USA, 1960–1962; M—M Monaural questionnaire, UK, NSH Pilot study, 1980; B—B Binaural questionnaire, UK, NSH Pilot study, 1980; T—T Tinnitus questionnaire, UK, (NSH Pilot study, 1980).

prevalence for 'normal' reports. This result may be tentatively rationalised as follows; in order to imagine speech to a single ear the hearing-impaired person probably makes several compensations which increase the imagined clarity and intensity of speech but decrease reverberation and other distorting factors. This would produce less difficulty.

The HIS data plotted in Figure 1.3 can be seen to show good agreement with the monaural questionnaire of this study. The questions used in both of these studies refer to 'one or both ears' and hence both should monitor the worse ear in the population. The appropriate audiometric equivalence to seek for the monaural questionnaire is with the worse ear average (WEA) rather than the BEA.

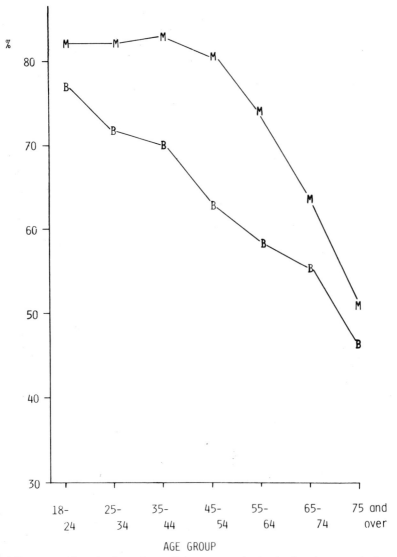

Fig. 1.4 Percentage of people who are 'normal', i.e. not reporting hearing impairment or tinnitus. (NSH pilot study, 1980.)

Nevertheless, comparing the results for the BEA of the HES and the response to both the monaural questions there is good agreement in the pattern of the decline in hearing sensitivity with age for age groups up to 54 years when it is clear that the shape of the results with our own and Wilkins' questionnaire begins to underestimate audiometric hearing losses around 55 and diverges to underestimate both relative and absolute prevalence by as much as 15 per cent at the 75+ age group. The real underestimate is possibly much greater than this, because Table 1.4 shows that in the NSH there are possibly 75 per cent more worse ears than better ears impaired at a given criterion. If this factor is taken into account then the underestimate becomes much larger.

One of the striking aspects of the HES, HIS, and Wilkins studies, and the NSH monaural questionnaire is that they indicate an exponential growth of reported hearing impairment with age (or, as Plomp (1978) suggests, there is a constant doubling time for the prevalence of impairment). The pilot study binaural questionnaire results not only indicate higher prevalence, up to age 74, than other estimates, but there is a fairly linear trend with age. The B and M questions clearly interact differently with age. Whether this is through interpretation of questions or through genuine changes in the determinants of disability remains to be established. This is an issue of some interest in the calibration of questionnaires for use as screening instruments where resources may not extend to full scale audiometry.

Such issues of question phrasing seem even more important with tinnitus. Tinnitus report does seem to be a volatile measure, and depends very much on how the question is phrased, the exclusions made and the context in which it is placed. There is a definite tendency in Figure 1.3 for tinnitus report to increase at older ages, but there does not seem to be a gradual change, more an abrupt shift somewhere between 55 to 64 years of age. Analysis of further questions should shed light on whether this is a shift in response bias (i.e. more false alarms at older age groups) or a phenomenon with a more specific audiological implication.

This discussion indicates that mathematical models should be fitted to reported prevalence data only with utmost circumspection. Nevertheless, besides being the reference grid that ties our audiometric data to the UK population, questions on hearing disorders have been shown to have considerable validity and potential use (a) as screening questions on an individual basis, and (b) as reasonable indicators of hearing disorders in the population, when asked in specific combination and taking age into account.

Distribution of audiometrically obtained hearing levels

It is valuable to know the statistical distribution of hearing levels because this can provide a general criterion-free description of the population. In the first part of this section I will use as an example the mean BEA (0·5, 1, 2 and 4 kHz). From Table 1.4 we can say that the BEA distribution function describes chiefly sensorineural hearing disorders. What follows is therefore applicable to the whole population but is dominated by the sensorineural losses. The cumulative distribution functions (c.d.f.) of BEA and WEA derived from the pilot study are shown in Figure 1.5a. Table 1.3 shows that there is an increase in variance over the four groups (N, NT, HI, HIT) that is almost fivefold. Moreover, it seems that the variance increases with the mean of each group. If this is true of audiometric averages on other groupings with ordered mean values, then a transformation will be necessary to stabilise the variance over the range of measurement. A standard simple technique for equalising variance is to take a logarithmic function of the dependent variable. This is very similar to the model proposed by Hinchcliffe (1962) to describe the psychophysical deterioration of hearing with age. In this case the cumulative distribution function of $\log (BEA + K)$ was taken and is shown in Figure 1.5b for $K = 20$.

It would be ideal to have distributions for a large range of specified subpopulations e.g. women, aged 30–34 years, having no noise exposure. This would require a huge study and the cost of doing this is prohibitive. Even from the NSH

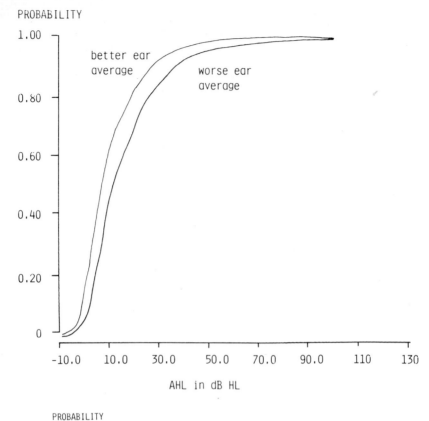

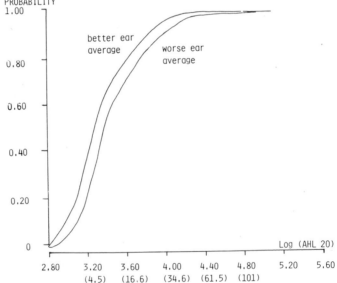

Fig. 1.5a Estimated cumulative distribution functions for Better Ear Average (BEA) and Worse Ear Average (WEA). The average was taken over the four frequencies ·5, 1, 2 and 4 kHz. (NSH pilot study, 1980.)

Fig. 1.5b Estimated cumulative distribution functions for the log functions of BEA and WEA. See text for explanation of function.

(1980–1984) the number of subpopulations that can be reliably described will be fairly small. What can be done, even to some extent from the pilot study, is to present parameter estimates for the distributions. These are presented for better and worse ears in Table 1.6 for five age groups.

Table 1.6 Population projections for the parameters of the distribution of average hearing levels in the better and worse ears, for five age groups. NSH pilot study, 1980.

Age group	Mean	Median	SD	Variance	Skew	Kurtosis
			Better ear			
<39	6·6	5·7	9·2	84	5·1	39·3
40–49	10·5	8·0	9·5	90	2·6	11·9
50–59	15·7	12·0	9·0	81	1·8	4·4
60–69	18·1	15·6	11·9	141	2·3	8·9
>69	26·5	22·7	16·6	277	1·1	2·1
			Worse ear			
<39	9·7	7·0	10·4	109	4·5	31·1
40–49	14·8	11·8	12·7	160	3·0	15·3
50–59	20·9	17·0	11·7	137	2·1	6·0
60–69	24·2	21·1	16·0	254	1·9	6·4
>69	32·6	26·3	21·4	457	1·3	1·8

Note that both mean and median BEA increase with age, and with one exception so does the variance. Skew and kurtosis (the flatness of the distribution) both decrease with age. In other words the distribution becomes more normal, but the variance increases as age increases. Figure 1.6 shows this data in graphic form, giving the normal ranges associated with ±1 SD of the population BEA and the +2 SD upper limit of BEA. The median is always below the mean in this figure, an indication of slight positive skew. This skew is emphasised in Figure 1.7a which plots BEA as a function of age, for all patients who had no missing audiological data. The data in Figure 1.6 refer to the population projection, whereas Figure 1.7 refers to the pooled strata of people actually tested. The high skew and kurtosis of the lower age groups results from a handful of hearing-impaired people in each case. Figure 1.7a shows a tight clustering of BEA at low age levels which becomes less tight, more dispersed, as age increases. When the logarithmic function of hearing level is taken a more even dispersion and a more linear trend emerge as shown in Figure 1.7b. It is worth noting that if a study only has a limited age range then there may be no significant departure from a linear relationship between age and BEA. It is only when a large range is taken, as in this type of study that the transform is desirable. In applying the log transformation, the BEA variable, not age, is transformed (a) because it is the chief dependent variable whose variance we are interested to stabilise and (b) because BEA is a relatively pragmatic derived measure unlike age which is on a physically definable ratio scale.

Table 1.7 shows the fit to four models of how average hearing level (AHL) in better and worse ears can be described as a function of age. Irrespective of whether there was a history of slight noise exposure (about 30 per cent) or otological abnormality (only a small proportion), for both male and females age is a significant factor accounting for a large proportion of the variance. Model 1 states that AHL is a linear function of age, the most parsimonious model. Model 2 is derived from Robinson and Sutton (1979) which states a general power law relation between HL

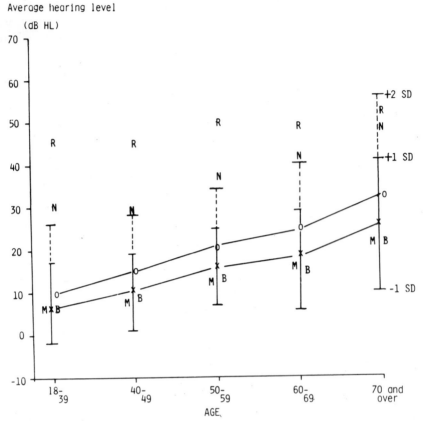

Fig. 1.6 Population weighted mean hearing levels for men and women combined for better ear (x) and worse ear (O), averaged over the frequencies 0·5, 1, 2, and 4 kHz. The ±1SD and the +2SD are marked for the better ear. The median of the better ear is shown as M. The better ear mean average hearing levels over the three frequencies ·5, 1 and 2 kHz are shown as B. The mean BEA for Ballantyne's national sample of ENT clinics is shown as N. The mean BEA for a first issue hearing aid sample from Glasgow Royal Infirmary is shown as R (see p. 7 for an explanation). (NSH pilot study, 1980.)

and age. Model 3 builds in the variance stabilisation transform and is similar to Hinchcliffe's (1962) equation and model 4 is a combination of Models 2 and 3.

The percentage of variance accounted for by each model is a guide to the relative performance of each model. Increasing percentage means a better fit. Model 1 gives a reasonable fit and shows that BEA increases by 5·3 dB per decade, WEA by about 6·5 dB per decade. Progressively better fits are obtained for the four models, but while a large increment comes from using the log transformation model, only a small benefit is obtained using the power law function. So, there seems to be a specific justification for this transform beyond the tidiness of distributions of the AHL. Figure 1.8 presents the BEA and WEA for men and women in seven age groups; it is easier to appreciate the exponential trend of hearing level with age here, where it is consistent in all four conditions, rather than in Figure 1.6 which has only five age groups. I am not interested at this stage in categorically rejecting any model but I will consider what the first three models imply for the progression

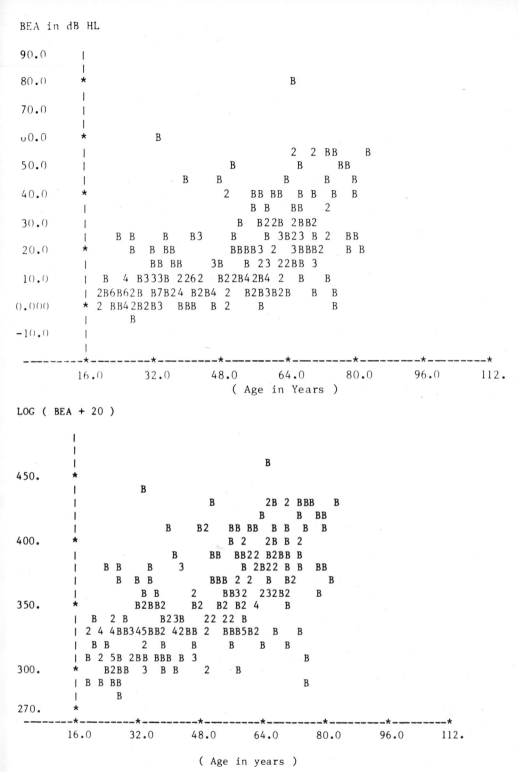

Fig. 1.7a Plot of BEA against age in years. Each point represents an individual (with no missing data) tested as part of the NSH pilot study, 1980. Where a number occurs in the plot, it means that that number of people had the same age and audiometric score.

Fig. 1.7b Plot of log (BEA + 20) against age in years. Each point represents an individual with no missing data tested as part of the NSH pilot study, 1980. Where a number appears in the plot, it means that that number of people had the same age and audiometric score.

Table 1.7 Parameters for four models of the progression of AHL with age, and the percentage of variance accounted for by each of the models. For these models k was taken as 20 dB. The standard error of parameters is shown in brackets. NSH pilot study, 1980.

Model	Better ear			Worse ear		
	a	b	%	a	b	%
1 AHL = b + a (AGE)	·53 (·06)	−7·6 (3·1)	24	·65 (·07)	− 7·1 (3·9)	24
2 AHL = b + a (AGE-18)^2	·0085 (·0009)	7·9 (1·5)	25	·010 (·001)	12·2 (1·9)	25
3 Log(AHL + k) = b + a (Age)	(·013) (·001)	2·9 (·06)	32	·014 (·001)	3·02 (·07)	31
4 Log(AHL + k) = b + a (Age-18)^2	·002 (·0002)	3·3 (·03)	32	·002 (·0002)	3·5 (·03)	32

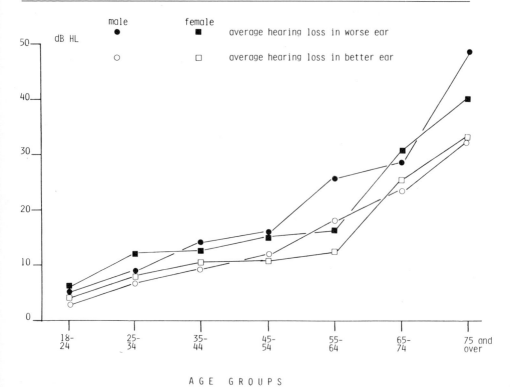

Fig. 1.8 Mean hearing level for seven age groups for men (squares) and women (circles) and for better ear (closed symbols) and worse ear (open symbols).

of hearing levels with age in the population. Table 1.8 shows Model 1 postulates that the progression is constant at about 5 dB per decade. Model 2 postulates that the progression is made up of two components, one due to the age of the person and the other the initial hearing level. Model 3 postulates that it is proportional to an exponential function of the initial hearing level only. Models 2 and 3 carry clear implications for the development of the hearing losses in individuals, or at least for identifiable subgroups. The merit of each of these models may turn out to be different within different subsets of the population.

Table 1.8 Progression of AHL (presumed SNHL) in a period of N years. N1 and N2 are presumed to be the initial and final years of interest. HL1 is the hearing loss in the year N1. Three models are compared and the numbers in the text refer to Table 8, as do the parameters a and k.

Model	Progression of hearing loss in dB/N yrs
1	$\cdot 53\ N$
2	$HL1 + N\ a\ (N1 + N2 - 36)$
3	$(HL1 + k)\ \exp^{a\,N} - k$

Whereas Figure 1.6 showed the BEA over five age groups, Figure 1.9 shows the audiograms of those age groups for left and right ear separately. Progression of hearing level with age is noticeable at all the frequencies reported here. The audiograms are similar to those presented by Maurer and Rupp (1980), using the data of Glorig and Roberts, (1965) and it is apparent that the slope of the audiogram becomes greater with age. That means that any general model for

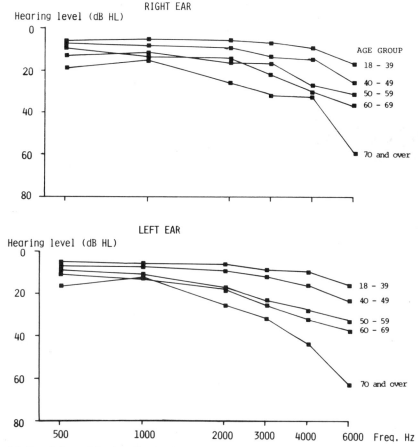

Fig. 1.9 Population weighted median hearing threshold levels, at six frequencies and for five age groups, for right (a) and left (b) ears. (NSH pilot study, 1980.)

hearing level must also take into account a factor relating HL to frequency, and subgroups will be most validly described if this is done.

Sex differences were apparent in the pilot study data (cf IHR 1981b) and indicate that, whilst men have better thresholds at ·5 and 1 kHz, women have better thresholds at 3, 4, 6 and 8 kHz. This difference remains when the effect of age is partialled out. Part of this difference may be due to greater male susceptibility to noise exposure. Likewise part of the aging effect is probably due to cumulative noxious noise exposure. So it would be interesting to further sub-divide the data over these independent variables. In the clinical interview there is an in-depth record made of the noise history and a noise immission rating is made in three separate categories: occupational, social and gunfire. The results of this assessment will be available after the 1981 phase of the study. However question C7 (see Appendix, Section C) asks a general screening question on occupational noise. The population projection for BEA and WEA for the two conditions, noise report and no noise report are shown in Figure 1.10 for the two sexes combined. This suggests that hearing level is an approximately additive function of age, reported noise exposure and better/worse ear.

Figure 1.11 looks at the mean AHL for males and females over the five age groups for the two noise conditions. A fair summary is that noise report adds about 3–5 dB for women at all age groups. However not only is the effect on men much larger but it appears to be multiplicative with age. In these analyses, of course, age and reported noise exposure may confound duration of noise exposure. There is some evidence relating level and duration of noise exposure to effects of noise immission (Burns and Robinson, 1970; Rop and Raber, 1980), which suggests that immission is a logarithmic function of duration of exposure. Thus, where age and duration of noise exposure are confounded, a multiplicative result should be obtained. Two relevant trends are observed here: (1) for men there is a definite confounding of age and duration of noise exposure giving a marked interaction of age and noise on hearing levels, and (2) for the data of Figure 1.10 averaged over men and women, there is little overall confounding and a fairly additive effect of age, noise and ear on hearing levels. The present data are consistent with the log function, if we assume that noise exposure duration is independent of age for women. While qualitatively different effects of noise on women cannot be ruled out (Federal Register, 1981), the trades typically employing women have perhaps lower levels of noise, generally without high levels of impulse noise. Also women are more likely than men to interrupt a working life or hold many different types of job. The NSH is taking more elaborate noise emission ratings so that the assumptions and data presented above can be further tested and more accurately specified.

In summarising this section four points can be made:

(1) The mean, median and variance of average hearing levels increase with age group. Tentative confidence intervals and parameters have been presented for each of five age groups (Table 1.6). Age accounts for more variance in hearing levels in the population than any other variables so far examined in the study, i.e. about 25 to 30 per cent of the variation can be explaind by age alone. Four possible models for the precise form of the relationship and their implications are briefly discussed.

(2) It is desirable to obtain distributions of hearing levels or of some simple

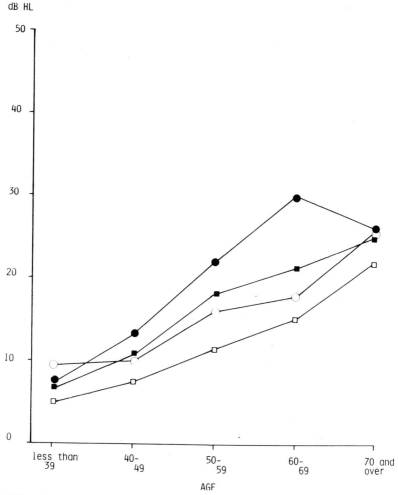

Fig. 1.10 Population weighted median BEA (squares) and WEA (circles) as a function of age and reported noise exposure. The 'no reported noise exposure' groups are the open symbols and the 'reported noise exposure' groups are the closed symbols.

function of hearing level in natural subsets of the population. A logarithmic transformation is recommended with an additive constant of 20 dB on the basis that this function maximises the variance in hearing levels accounted for by age over the whole population. It also helps to stabilise the variance of the dependent variable across our sample group.

(3) The mean population audiograms are presented for each of five age groups (Fig. 1.9). It is concluded that any complete model of the ageing process in hearing requires a term to describe the frequency/age interaction.

(4) The effects of noise report and sex on hearing levels are discussed. In population terms these variables acount for much less variance than age. However, further investigation is likely to enhance both the clinical value of detailed noise history notes by providing norms and our understanding of the processes leading to hearing disorders in the population.

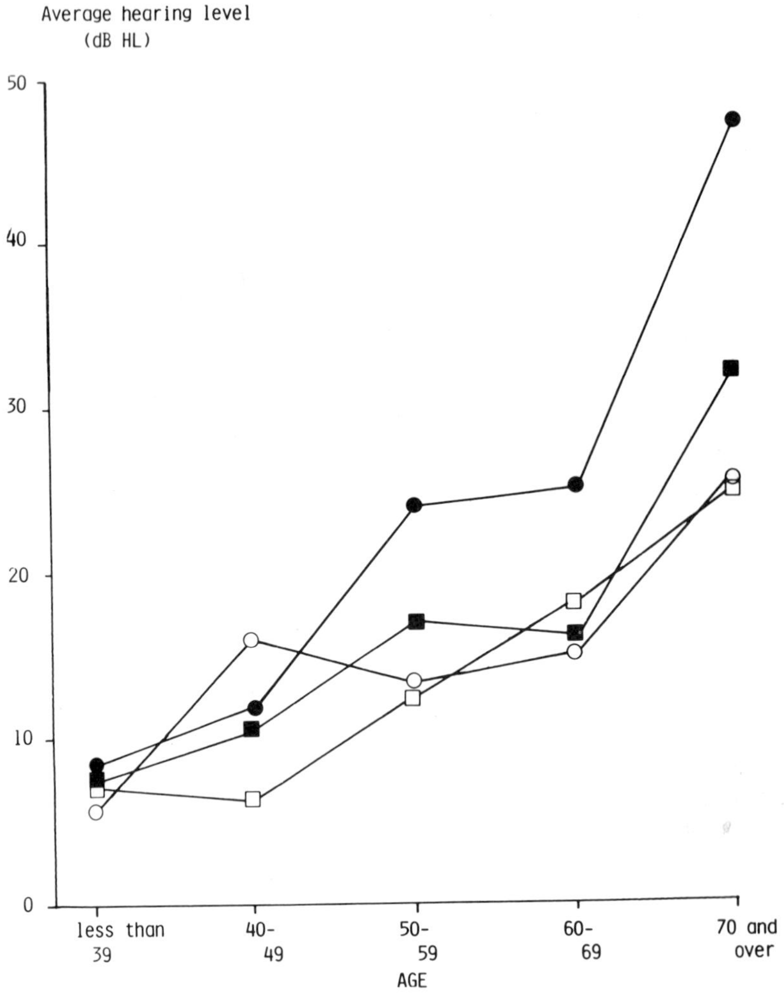

Average hearing level
(dB HL)

Fig. 1.11 Population weighted mean BEA as a function of reported noise exposure for men (circles) and women (squares). The 'no reported noise exposure' groups are the open symbols and the 'reported noise exposure' groups are the closed symbols.

Performance on speech tests

The assessment of hearing by postal questionnaire inevitably focuses on disability rather than either impairment, which is relatively inaccessible to self-judgement, or handicap, which is subject to large biases. The questionnaires that were used in the NSH are concerned with the disability and social handicap that individuals experience because of their hearing. The audiometric assessment of hearing sensitivity is concerned more with the underlying impairment and ultimately the extent of pathology of the individual. Obviously the two are related in a systematic way (Noble, 1978), but there are anomalies, as when someone who expresses an inability to participate in conversation because of his hearing, yet does not have a marked sensorineural hearing loss.

In order to measure disability more directly we used a binaural sentence-in-noise test (SIN). The SIN was developed from the BKB sentence lists (Bamford and Bench, 1979) and is described in more detail by Pearce (1980). There are 50 key items per list. The percentage of correct key items was 98 per cent in quiet (SNO), 68 per cent for intermediate levels (S/N = −7·4 dB) and 40 per cent for an adverse level (S/N = −11·4 dB). On inspection, none of the scores were normally distributed. However the difference between the first two conditions was found to be approximately normally distributed as well as reflecting the specific vulnerability to noise that we wished to measure. This score difference (SCD) was used in the following analyses. Figure 1.12 shows the plot of all subjects having no missing data over the variables SCD and age. Age accounts for more variation in SCD than it does in BEA (Tables 1.7 and 1.8). There is a strong positive correlation between SCD and age, and also SCD and BEA as Figure 1.13 shows. In fact age alone, as Table 1.9 shows, accounts for slightly more variation in SCD than BEA does. The log transformation of BEA does not improve this relationship more than one percentage point.

As the binaural SIN is not a stereophonic, freefield dichotic or specifically spatial test of disability it should be fairly robust to threshold differences between the ears,

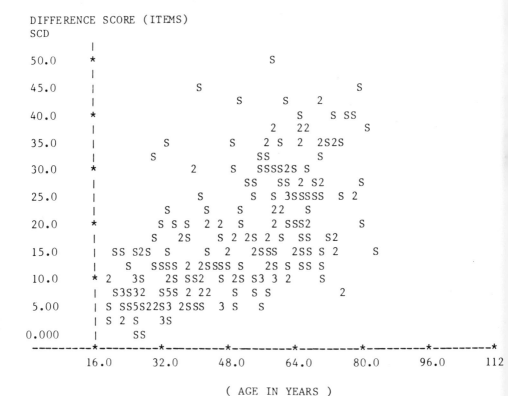

Fig. 1.12 Plot of the derived sentence-in-noise test score (SCD) against age in years. Each point represents an individual with no missing data, tested as part of the NSH pilot study. Where a number appears in the plot, it means that this number of people share values of the independent and dependent variables.

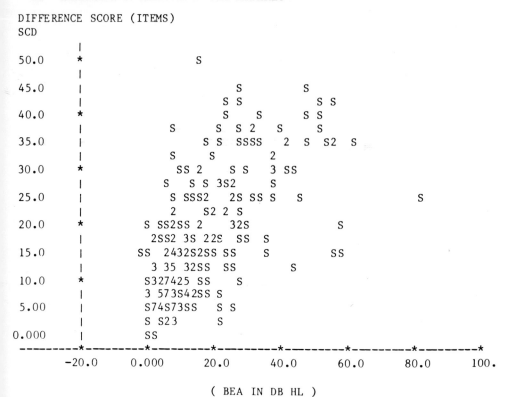

DIFFERENCE SCORE (ITEMS)
SCD

```
        |
50.0    *           S
        |
45.0    |               S           S
        |             S S               S S
40.0    *             S       S     S S
        |       S       S   S 2   S       S
35.0    |           S S   SSSS    2   S  S2  S
        |       S     S         2
30.0    *       SS  2      S S    3 SS
        |       S   S S 3S2       S
25.0    |       S SSS2    2S SS S    S                S
        |       2     S2 2 S
20.0    *     S SS2SS 2      32S              S
        |       2SS2 3S 22S   SS   S
15.0    |    SS   2432S2SS SS     S          SS
        |     3 35 32SS  SS         S
10.0    *    S327425 SS     S
        |    3 573S42SS S
5.00    |    S74S73SS   S S
        |    S S23       S
0.000   |    SS
 --------*--------*--------*--------*--------*--------*--------*
      -20.0    0.000    20.0    40.0    60.0    80.0    100.
```

(BEA IN DB HL)

Fig. 1.13 Plot of the derived sentence-in-noise test score (SCD) against BEA in dB HL. Each point represents an individual with no missing data, tested as part of the National Study of Hearing Pilot study, 1980. Where a number occurs in the plot, it means that this number of people share values of both dependent and independent variables.

Table 1.9 Parameters of the regression of age, BEA and WEA on the difference between performance on two conditions of the Sentence in Noise tests (SNQ and SN-3). Standard errors are shown in brackets. NSH pilot study, 1980.

Model	Intercept	Age coeff	BEA coeff	WEA coeff	% of Variance
Age alone	−1·09 (1·47)	·34 (·03)			38
BEA alone	8·9 (·7)		·46 (·04)		36
Age then BEA	0·4 (1·3)	·22 (·03)	·29 (·05)		49
Age then BEA then WEA	0·1 (1·3)	·22 (·03)	·17 (·07)	·10 (·06)	50

and reflect mainly the better ear. This is in fact the case, the addition of WEA is not significant in the equation. The most parsimonious model of the added difficulty, or disability, in understanding speech in binaural noise is one that fits age first and then BEA, to produce a fit that accounts for about 50 per cent of the variance in SCD scores. This fit can be further improved by adding noise history and sex to the model, but this is not considered further here. This model describes a linear increase in disability with age and also with loss of hearing sensitivity. Its form is essentially different to the model of BEA hearing sensitivity and age (e.g. shown in Figs. 1.7 and 1.8) which shows an exponential decrease in hearing sensitivity with age. In performance terms SCD increases by about 5 per cent every 10 years and about 6 per cent every 10 dB hearing loss.

In summary, it is important to distinguish impairment (e.g. hearing sensitivity) and disability and also to distinguish between the effect of age on each. The SIN fulfils some of the basic requirement for measuring disability and half of the variation in the disability measure SCD is accounted for by age and hearing sensitivity (BEA). The appropriate disability derived measure is shown to be more influenced by age than is hearing impairment. This may help to explain the paradox that younger hearing impaired people often do not seek help, yet older hearing impaired people who seek it do not always derive benefit from the hearing aid received (Hayes and Jerger, 1977; Haggard, 1980). At any rate the present finding underlines the importance of assessing the more central perceptual effects of ageing as well as hearing sensitivity.

Conclusions on ageing from population based studies

Both hearing impairment and auditory ability (understanding speech-in-noise) systematically deteriorate with age. In addition, both the percentage reporting hearing loss and that reporting tinnitus, increase with age, the former in a way predictable from the hearing levels. Age accounts for 25 per cent of the variation in hearing impairment, more in disability score and an appreciable percentage in disability score when the relationship to hearing levels has been taken into account. So far we have isolated no other factor that accounts for even half as much variation as age does over a wide range of otological, audiometric, general medical and biographical variables. A more exhaustive coverage and analysis of these variables in the NSH will identify and quantify more of these sources of variation, and their interactions with age in determining prevalence and magnitudes of hearing impairment in the general population.

Although the method used in the NSH is well known and documented in many text books on survey sampling (e.g. Kish, 1973) it is well worthwhile recapitulating the basic steps considered in the method. First the population of interest to the NSH has been defined as the non-institutionalised population of England, Scotland and Wales. Second a random sample from this population was taken from the most up to date register of electors. Thirdly the respondents are stratified on the basis of some reported characteristics of their hearing or tinnitus. The effectiveness of the particular variables in the stratification should be assessed in analysis of variance of pilot study or preliminary data. Of course the method can be generalised beyond a two stage sampling procedure. The final stage was assessment, experiment, interview and postal questionnaire, combining a number of research objectives. Throughout, care was taken to investigate the effect of non-response in the sampling scheme, so that any biases can be incorporated into the final estimates of key characteristics in the population. The method may also be adapted to give appropriate controls for clinical studies.

SUB-POPULATION STUDIES

Studies on clinic sub-populations

The second traditional focus of epidemiological research is the clinical series, or clinical sample. Such samples have to be used in aetiological studies where prevalence rates are low and are acceptable where effects of service availability or differential referral are *a priori* likely to be small, as when conditions are of universally appreciated seriousness or are subject to legal reporting requirements. The clinic sample is inappropriate for epidemiological work on chronic impairments and disabilities such as hearing disorders. However, for service planning it is valuable to detail the present use of clinics, to characterise those who use them, and see whether the service currently meets the 'real' need in the community. In comparing the whole population with the clinic sub-populations insight is gained into present and future access to the services by groups in the community.

A few preliminary figures from the NSH, as of mid-1981, will provide background to the discussion of two clinic sub-populations. Figure 1.14 shows the percentage of people who responded that they had been to hospital about their hearing or ears. There are significantly more men (13·4 per cent) than women (11·3 per cent) who have consulted, and there is a significant increase with age.

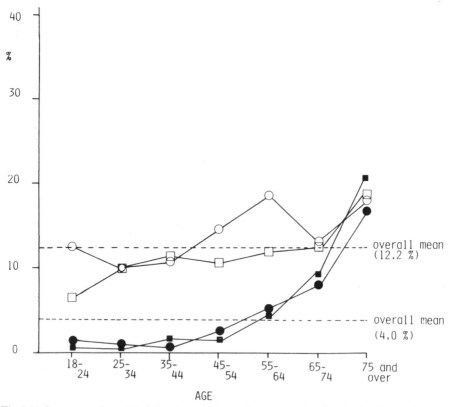

Fig. 1.14 Percentage of men (circles) and women (square) who responded that they had been to hospital about their hearing (open symbols) and who responded that they were in possession of a hearing aid (closed symbols) as a function of age. (National Study of Hearing, 1981.)

A cross-check on validity of the consultation rate lies in the fact in that about 33 per cent of those who currently have difficulty with their hearing in background noise have consulted, whilst only 8 per cent having currently normal hearing have consulted.

The difference in consultation rates between the sexes perhaps stems from a very high rate of consultation in the 45 to 64 year age-range for men. This could arise from the larger number of men likely to seek occupational deafness benefit. Not only are the predominantly male occupations more noisy, but this benefit requires the person to be in the same job for 20 years, less usual for women, and to be under 66 years of age. Figure 1.15 shows the percentage of men and women reporting difficulty with their hearing from the same study, firstly for the hearing difficulty in background noise question (see Appendix, Section A, version 1, question 2e) and secondly for the whisper question (see Appendix, Section A, version 1, question 1a). The whisper question was only asked of half the sample. The same male-female difference is apparent here, arising at similar age groups. This difference can possibly be explained also by the occupational deafness benefit scheme. However the reported hearing difficulty data do not converge so rapidly for the two sexes in the 65 to 74+ age range as do the consultation rates. Reported hearing difficulty increases with age much more rapidly than consultation rate does. So, whilst the difference between men and women is mirrored in both sets of data, the increase with age is seen in the hearing report but not in consultation rates. Thus there would seem to be a uniform shortfall in the access to, or use of, the services by the elderly. Figure 1.14 shows the proportion of people at each age group that possess a hearing aid. This increases exponentially with age, but it is not really until the mid 60s (i.e. around retirement) that the rate of provision of aids catches up with the rate of deterioration of hearing. These results can be used to help interpret studies on clinical populations as they reflect some of the population trends in the use of the Health Service and in the prevalence of hearing disorders.

Ballantyne survey (1975) of ENT clinics

In 1975, consultant otolaryngologists in the UK were requested to provide the audiograms of all adult cases of bilateral sensorineural hearing loss seen in their clinics over a two-week period. The completion rate for our purposes was about 53 per cent of the replies received (i.e. age reported and ·5, 1, 2 and 4 kHz thresholds measured and reported in both ears). The enquiry and its original objectives have been reported by Ballantyne* (1981) while Haggard, Gatehouse and Davis (1981) have used the data to estimate the severity profile of the national clinic population. The results showing BEA and WEA as a function of age are shown here in Figures 1.6 and 1.16. Haggard and his colleagues suggest that the sample may contain a disproportionate number of people in the <49 year age group with mild hearing loss due to disproportionately high return from the Armed Services. Figure 1.16 shows a steady increase with age in both ears. The regression of threshold on age was calculated for the four frequencies (·5, 1, 2, 4 kHz) and for two averages (·5, 1,

---

* This postal enquiry was organised by J. Ballantyne Esq. FRCS with assistance from the DHSS in order to estimate the numbers of people with special needs for rehabilitation. The data were made available to IHR and I am grateful to my colleagues Professor Mark Haggard and Dr Stuart Gatehouse for advice on these data and some of the analyses on which this section is based.

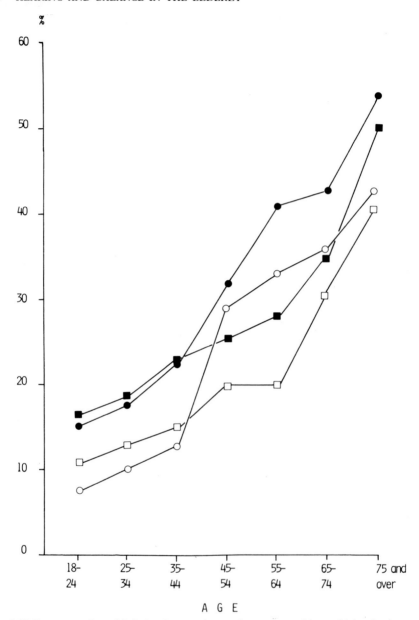

Fig. 1.15 Percentage of men (circles) and women (squares) reporting problems with hearing in different situations as a function of age. (NSH, 1981.)

2, kHz) (B2) and (·5, 1, 2, 4 kHz) (BEA). All the regression coefficients for the slope of the function (shown in Table 1.10) were significant, except for those of the female worse ear at (·5, 1, 2, kHz), separately and for both averages (WEA and W2).

The transformation, log(AHL + k), was tried for all analyses, with k = 20. In all cases the fit was slightly better, but only one or two per cent was added to the

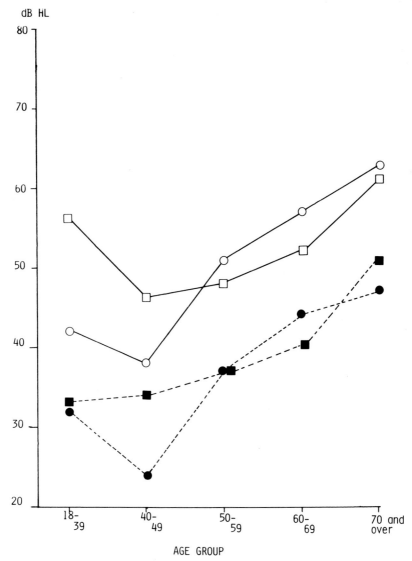

Fig. 1.16 Median BEA (closed symbols) and WEA (open symbols) for men (circles) and women (squares). (Ballantyne national sample of ENT clinics, 1975.)

variance explained. So for simplicity the regressions with the raw data are used here. There are five points to note from Table 1.10:

1. There is a systematic increase in age slopes with increasing frequency, both in men and women, and on both better and worse ears.
2. Compared with the NSH pilot study regression analysis, shown in Table 1.7, much less variance in the BEA is accounted for by age: 6 per cent as opposed to 24 per cent.
3. A similar comparison shows that both the intercept and slope differ between the two samples. There is a higher intercept (33 dB vs −7 dB) and a shallower age

Table 1.10 Regression Coefficient for Hearing Thresholds on Age (Ballantyne Data) BEA is the average over 0·5, 1, 2 and 4 kHz.
B2 is the average over 0·5, 1, and 2 kHz.   %

Freq (kHz)	Slope (dB/yr)	Intercept (dB)	S.E. slope	Variance	Correlation
		Male (n = 306)			
Better Ear					
·5	·16	21	·07	1·7	·13
1	·22	20	·08	2·9	·17
2	·39	19	·08	6·8	·26
4	·48	33	·08	9·6	·31
B2	·26	20	·07	4·0	·20
BEA	·31	23	·07	6·2	·25
Worse Ear					
·5	·35	23	·07	4·4	·21
1	·37	26	·10	4·8	·22
2	·52	25	·09	9·0	·30
4	·51	43	·08	10·9	·33
W2	·41	25	·09	6·8	·26
WEA	·44	29	·08	8·4	·29
		Female (n = 300)			
Better Ear					
·5	·16	30	·06	2·0	·14
1	·24	25	·07	4·0	·2
2	·29	26	·07	5·3	·23
4	·40	30	·07	9·0	·30
B2	·23	27	·06	4·4	·21
BEA	·27	28	·06	5·8	·24
Worse Ear					
·5	·04	51	·09	0·1	·03
1	·07	51	·09	0·1	·03
2	·10	52	·09	0·5	·07
4	·24	54	·09	2·6	·16
W2	·07	51	·09	0·3	·05
WEA	·11	52	·09	0·6	·08

slope (0·29 dB/yr. vs 0·59 dB/yr.) for the clinic population, showing as expected a lesser progression of hearing loss in the clinic group, i.e. and overall high degree of loss that is not largely age determined. Figure 1.6 appears to suggest otherwise, i.e. that the age slopes may be the same in Ballantyne's sample as in the NSH. However, care has to be taken in interpreting this figure, because the two end categories (<39 and 70+) have uncertain means. Thus a line drawn through the points does not necessarily represent the true regression line.

4. The age change for WEA is greater than that for BEA in men.
5. The age change for BEA and WEA in women is very different. In fact for women there is an almost constant WEA intercept at about 52 dB HL, with very little growth with age. This may indicate that referral for women is based upon a relatively fixed worse ear criterion, suggesting a basis in pathology rather than disability or impairment.

An interpretation of these data that is consonant with the NSH 1981 study is as follows. Haggard and his colleagues (1981) suggested that the rise in AHL with age within the clinic sample (Fig. 1.16) indicates a threshold of referral that depends on the distribution of hearing levels for a particular age group; older people accept some hearing loss as 'normal'. This may have to be qualified slightly because less variance is accounted for by age within the clinic than the population sample. This discrepancy has two possible explanations (a) the AHL may be primarily related to aspects of the condition of the patient other than age, within the ENT clinic population, and (b) the magnitude of the average age slope is smaller than in the general population (point 3 above) indicating that the effect spotlighted by Haggard and his colleagues is not quite as large as would be expected if referral occurred for some particular percentile, e.g. the 3 per cent with worst hearing in every age-band. Rather the referral criterion appears to be a compromise between such an extreme age-dependency and the other extreme of a fixed hearing level for initiating referral.

There is a sex difference, characteristic only of the clinic sample that is obscured by the age grouping of Figure 1.16. The men who consult have age-dependent hearing losses in both ears, with the worse ear deteriorating more with age, among women the worse ear is almost constant with only a slight progression of hearing loss in the better ear.

In conclusion, the clinic population is a varied group, containing more specific aetiologies other than age, with more noted as having noise exposure, enhancing what differences between the sexes may exist in the population. The suggestion of differing interactions with age and different referral processes for men and women, is further reinforced by Figure 1.18a which shows the slopes of the audiogram for the Ballantyne sample. This slope summarises the roll-off in the audiogram from low to high frequencies. Despite noise-induced cases providing a high proportion of the new cases among the younger men, this slope increases consistently with age for both ears, presumably reflecting cumulative effects of noise exposure in late referrals. The results for women are less consistent and show a different pattern below 50 years old. These results (Table 1.10, Fig. 1.16 and Fig. 1.18a) tentatively support a difference in the basis of referral for men and women. That referral of men should start at higher losses and that their better ear changes less with age in the clinic group are mutually consistent facts which argue that referral occurs when a man's better ear sinks to a certain value. This suggests that men seek referral more on the basis of inescapable disability than potentially remediable pathology. The overall steeper audiogram slopes indicate that men will present as more disabled than women in the case load.

Hearing aid population—Glasgow Royal Infirmary sample

For health service planning it is necessary to document the use of a clinical sub-population sampling frame further down the system, e.g. at the point where hearing aids are dispensed for the first time to patients at the ENT clinics. This is of interest because, not only does it give us an audiometric snapshot of the hearing aid user, but also enables a comparison between those who were issued aids and those who attended the ENT clinic, who have a sensorineural loss (e.g. as in the Ballantyne survey). In this section the records of a one-in-five sample of first issue hearing aids at Glasgow Royal Infirmary (1973–1979) were interrogated to supply the relevant data. Results for 965 complete records are summarised in Figure 1.17.

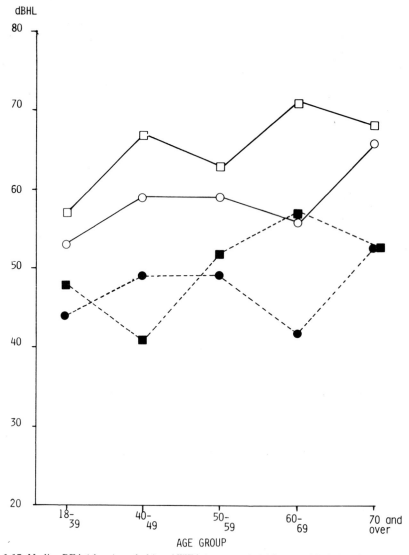

Fig. 1.17 Median BEA (closed symbols) and WEA (open symbols) for men (circles) and women (squares). First issue hearing aid sample at Glasgow Royal Infirmary.

There is an even sharper contrast to the population trends here than in the Ballantyne data because there is no systematic increase of BEA or WEA with age.

Figure 1.6 presents three sets of data: (1) The population study; (2) Ballantyne's national ENT clinic sample (N) and (3) The Glasgow hearing aid sample (R). The slopes of the regression lines are about 5 dB per decade, 3 dB per decade and 1 dB per decade respectively. In fact the regression of AHL on age for the hearing aid sample showed that only for thresholds at 4 kHz for both sexes and for the BEA and WEA of the women was there a statistically significant slope, in the region of 1·5 dB per decade. The intercept was the same for men and women, 42 dB for the better ear and 58 dB for the worse. Figure 1.18b shows that there was an

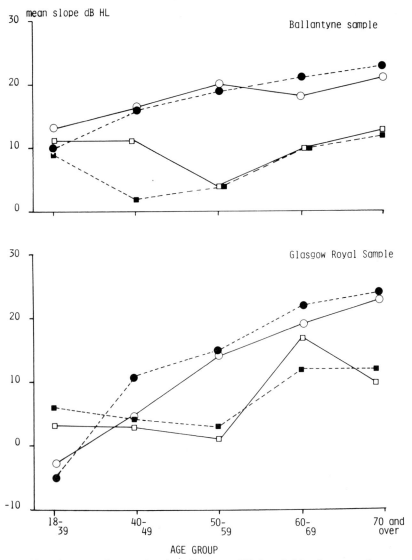

Fig. 1.18 Mean frequency slope as a function of better ear (filled symbols) and worse ear (open symbols) for men (circles) and women (squares) from the Ballantyne sample (a; top) and the Glasgow Royal Infirmary sample (b; bottom). The frequency slope is calculated by the formula
Slope = $((t4K + t2K)-(t1K + t0\cdot5K))/2$, where t4K represent the audiometric threshold at 4 kHz etc.

interaction of age and sex for the audiometric slope index. Insofar as this slope indicates a mix of the disabling noise and age effects, the shift with age to an increase in this mix as the presumed base of referral in men is a gradual one. In the Glasgow hearing aid sample conductive conditions are present and these play more of a role for younger women; this was confirmed in the analysis of the bone conduction audiometric data. In this respect there is a discrete change in the sample composition for women at about 60 years of age, i.e. their retirement age.

Whether any general medical factors, e.g. diet and cardiovascular disease underly this difference over and above the obvious factor of noise remains to be ascertained. The issue of age dependence or independence of the criteria for referral and hearing aid fitting does not appear to be straightforward. There is only a slight increase in hearing level with age within the hearing aid sample yet a distinct trend in the ENT sample. This could be due to the presence of conductive conditions in the hearing aid sample, intentionally absent in the ENT sample and markedly less common in the general population. Alternatively, it could be due to a relatively high threshold for acceptance of aids among the younger population (c.f. p. 10, Fig. 1.14).

The ENT sub-population mean BEA and the general population mean BEA converge with age at the rate of 2 dB per decade. This means that statements concerning variation in service take-up with age have to be carefully worded. For instance 'constant take-up' level may refer either to a constant AHL or to the difference between the population and the hearing aid population, and the referent has to be clearly stated. However, the important question is, does the proportion of the potential candidates for hearing aids in the population who seek help or who are referred, change with age? There is not the precision in the NSH data, so far, to answer this question directly. Evidence of an indirect nature is available from two comparisons. The acceleration in aid ownership (Fig. 1.14) in relation to reported hearing loss (Fig. 1.15) suggests that relative aid acceptance increases markedly with age. The lesser increase in consultation (Fig. 1.14) compared with reported hearing loss suggests that relative help-seeking may decrease with age. This may take the form that if someone has consulted, or been referred, at an early age, for whatever hearing problem, they are more likely to be fitted with an aid subsequently. The limited impairment distributions (Fig. 1.6) support the first trend, but there are no data yet available to lend direct support to the second.

The overlap between the three populations examined here confirms that there must be many more reasons for referral and hearing aid fitting than hearing loss. Nevertheless, age and sex are two variables that influence the pattern of consultation and in a less clear way, the provision and/or acceptance of hearing aids.

Summary and conclusions

I have reported two clinical sub-population studies in the UK. There are many limitations to both sets of data, which restrict the inferences to be drawn, as is typical for this type of study. Only a weak link with age was found in the Glasgow hearing aid data, and a slightly stronger one for the ENT sample. These discrepancies in age effects parallel those between audiometry and self-report found in population studies. We may speculate that the referral criterion depends firstly on the patient's self-perception and secondly on the patient's age, and that there are different patterns in this for men and women. There is a distinct age-dependency in the audiometric slope index among those who consult ENT departments and also in those who are fitted with aids. As slope of the audiogram is a good predictor of disability this suggests that the proportion of referrals due to disabilities that can no longer be hidden or denied increases with age. At the anecdotal level this is hardly a surprising fact. What is important is the interpretation in conjunction with the conservative criterion for referral, and particularly hearing aid acceptance in the younger group. Together these findings provide a more systematic indication than Haggard and his colleagues (1981) did that referrals for the alleviation of auditory disability should in general take place earlier than they do.

A WHOLE POPULATION STUDY

Homes for the elderly in South Glamorgan

The previous two methods, population sampling and clinical sub-population studies have yielded data on the effect of the ageing process upon hearing. The first of these methods excludes people living in institutions and has relatively few people in the age ranges beyond 75 years, leading to an under-representation of this important group. One of the best ways to investigate the hearing of the very old is to test residents in homes for the elderly. Recent studies by Burton (1977), by Martin and Peckford (1977) and by Hart (1980) in the UK and by Alberti (1977) in Canada have used the homes for the elderly as their sampling frame. They have found that 12 per cent of residents actually have hearing aids, agreeing well with the figure for the over 65s in the NSH (1981; see Fig. 1.14) compared with 3 to 4 per cent in the population as a whole (NSH 1980, 1981). However many more would be candidates on the basis of their audiometric results.

Data to throw light on impairment and service needs in the very old were obtained in a collaborative study that the author made with G. Hart and J. A. B. Thomas (see also Hart, 1980). 1132 subjects from 44 homes in South Glamorgan were examined by an otologist and tested audiometrically. The age range of those tested was 63 to 109 years with a mean of about 82 years of age. 11·3 per cent were in possession of a hearing aid. In the following analysis the subjects were split into two groups on the basis of their otological assessment. Any acoustically obstructing wax, scarring of meatus or tympanic membrane, active disease and so on were noted; the presence of any of these in either ear meant the person failed the screen (group OS−). Only 32 per cent of the sample passed the otological screen (group OS+). Table 1.11 shows the BEA, WEA and age in each group for men and women. The four marginal distributions of hearing level are all normal, there being no significant skew or kurtosis. The screened group have an advantage over the unscreened group, but only by about 4 dB in the better ear and 8 dB in the worse ear. These results indicate that 93 per cent of both groups have a BEA worse than 25 dB, and 66 per cent worse than 45 dB.

Table 1.11 BEA and WEA for women and men in two otological groups (Hart, 1980).

	BEA	s.d.	WEA	s.d.	AGE	s.d.	n
			GROUP OS+				
Female	46	18	55	20	81	8	284
Male	44	14	53	19	79	8	121
			GROUP OS−				
Female	50	17	63	20	83	7	526
Male	48	18	62	21	80	8	310

Table 1.12 Regression Coefficients for two Otological Groups (Hart, 1980). (Figures in brackets are standard errors.)

	BEA	WEA	Log(BEA + 20)	Log(WEA + 20)
		GROUP OS+		
Constant	−13·7	2·3	321	350
Age	·75(·12)	·65(·14)	1·14(·21)	·93(·22)
Sex	−·79(1·0)	−·57(2·3)	·26(3·4)	−·15(3·6)
% Variance accounted.	10·4	6·1	8·2	4·8
		GROUP OS−		
Constant	−13·8	0·34	324	359
Age	·78(·08)	·74(·10)	1·17(·12)	·94(·12)
Sex	−·01(1·3)	·90(1·6)	−0·67(2·0)	·51(2·0)
% Variance accounted.	11·1	7·3	11·6	7·3

Table 1.12 gives the regression equations for BEA, WEA and their log counterparts for the two groups OS+ and OS−. Note that the logarithmic functions discussed previously do not perform well here; this is because the distribution is already statistically normal among the elderly, and because the rise in AHL with age is linear within the portion of the age range where most of the individuals are located. Table 1.12 shows that when age is accounted for there is no significant effect of sex in BEA or WEA. The slope of the regression line is about 7·5 dB per decade for BEA and 6·5 dB per decade for WEA in the OS+ group. The better ear progression is now catching up with that in the worse ear. This is the reverse of the result in the general population where it was found that the WEA increased at a faster rate than the BEA (·65 vs ·53 dB/yr) and indicates that symmetrical sensorineural loss now overshadows all other forms.

The results from this study of a whole population have implications for the planned medical and social supervision of homes for the elderly. The absolute figures may not be generalisable to the whole elderly population. However, qualitative insight into the effect of the ageing process on hearing is given in two ways. Firstly, there is a linear deterioration of hearing level in the better ear which is the same for the OS+ and OS− group. The worse ear deteriorates more rapidly for the OS− group. As in the NSH pilot study, the otological status of the groups is relatively unimportant in determining hearing impairment. Unfortunately, no noise history was obtained and therefore it is not possible to investigate the effect of noise. However, as there were no differences in the regression results between men and women, and because women are usually less exposed to noise than men, there is no reason to expect large effects of different noise exposure groups in the age groups studied here. The second point concerns the communicative ability of these elderly people, two thirds of whom had average hearing loss greater than 45 dB. This ability was assessed by a systematic graded rating made by the staff at the homes for each individual. This rating agreed very well with measured BEA, and corroborates the view that the need of the elderly for auditory rehabilitation is not being met by the present services. Hart (1980) notes that only 11 per cent of this population had communicative difficulty that might be attributed to the confusion of senility rather than to hearing difficulty *per se* while 41 per cent had difficulty in communication due to their hearing. This assessment was made on the basis of a graded rating made by the staff at the homes for each individual. This rating agreed very well with measured BEA, and corroborates the view that the need of the elderly for auditory rehabilitation is not being met by the present services.

When experienced audiological staff visited each home after the survey, to provide hearing aids and advice on aural rehabilitation, the percentage of people using aids increased to about 22 per cent i.e. a 100 per cent increase. This still left 32 per cent of the population considered to be able to benefit from a hearing aid as judged by Hart and his colleagues who would not, or could not, use a hearing aid. Much of this must be attributed to the high average age of the population restricting the ability to learn how to control the aid. This suggests that aids should be fitted much earlier to those with hearing problems. If the aids had been fitted some 20 years and 15 dB earlier, some amelioration of what obviously becomes a serious disability and handicap might be possible.

OVERALL SUMMARY AND CONCLUSIONS

The aim of this chapter has been to illustrate the nature of age trends in epidemiological studies of hearing, and their application by referring to some recent studies with which I have been involved. The cost and other overheads of carrying out large scale studies is intrinsically high. If such investigations are to be conducted only every 20 years or so it is important that they investigate as many aspects of hearing as possible on which population based data is required. As there are many clinically known influences on hearing, additive and interactive relationships have to be tested by the use of factorial designs. Multiple stage sampling procedures are required to balance representation of rare sub-groups with a desired level of precision for the prevalence estimates.

An example of how one such study has been planned and designed, together with results from a pilot study were reported on pages 6 to 25. The findings from the pilot study already suggest that the main findings will be of scientific interest and the high prevalence rates mean that the implications will be of administrative importance. The NSH is an ambitious project, designed to meet a multitude of needs both pure and applied. It seeks an overall characterisation of hearing disorders in the population, of which prevalance and incidence are properly seen as but two aspects. The precision of the prevalence estimates has been restricted to the level of which use could be practically made. Previous epidemiological studies which have concentrated more on the restricted public health approach of determining prevalence of defined conditions; we believe that detailed characterisation will enhance the value of the prevalence estimates that the NSH produces by providing a much finer grain of data with clinical and scientific import. Emphasis has been added to disorders of auditory function while retaining the classical documentation of visible organic pathology. The implication for health services already appear to fall more in the functional domains of disability and handicap than in the pathological domain.

The limitations of clinic series and a purely questionnaire approach were shown in the section on sub-population studies (pp. 26 to 34). The amount of population-relevant information that can be gleaned from such sources, must be fairly small. Nevertheless, the data can be useful when assessed from the proper perspective of a population based study. In addition it needs to be emphasised that good statistical advice should be sought first, on what constitutes proper clinical controls, and second on whether the design of the research can actually answer the questions posed, in terms of both collecting the right data and also enough data to give adequate power.

Similar reservations apply to the type of whole population studies reported on pages 35 to 37. There seems to be a resurgence of interest in such studies, and they are useful in focusing attention on a particular section of society that is easy to identify. Whereas the clinic studies are perhaps paradigm-bound, the whole-population study is often equipment-bound; assessment techniques routinely used in the clinic cannot always be used in the home.

Results obtained with these various approaches have been presented and the problems in interpreting the data have been discussed. The major patterns of results are familiar: the amount and severity of hearing disorders increases with age; the age and the sex of a patient to some extent influence the level of impairment at which a user will seek and obtain referral for an ENT appointment, or hearing aid and finally hearing thresholds continue to deteriorate well into the ninth and tenth decade. The chief scientific interest lies in probing beyond this level.

It is important to distinguish conceptually between the pathology, impairment, disability and handicap that are consequent on a particular hearing disorder. Pure tone sensitivity can furnish various derived measures which have greater or lesser relevance to these different domains. Threshold measures in general may be a fairly direct measure of physiological impairment. Certain speech measures on the other hand, when other information is known, may be good clinical indicators of disability. Acknowledging that the patterns shown in the NSH pilot study do not entirely unravel the domains of impairment and disability, there are two types of 'ageing processes' indicated in the data. The first is an increase in physiological impairment with age. It follows an exponential time course. This is shown in the growth of the AHLs with age and in the percentage of people who exceed a given criterion. It is also reflected, to a certain extent in the questionnaire screening data. The second process is a growth of disability (or handicap) which seems to have a more linear time course, if the SIN test results are accepted as a gross measure of disability.

The pattern of hearing aid use with age as shown in Figure 1.14 also seems to follow an exponential path, although not exactly the same one as impairment. While an aid does not offset all aspects of the disability, the total disability makes those aspects that an aid can offset more critical. If disability criteria were used effectively more people would be fitted with aids earlier. Given this greater emphasis on disability and handicap which are partly justified by the results above, the precise needs for, and use of, rehabilitation services should be highlighted in future epidemiological research.

My three main conclusions reflect the methodological, service-geared and scientific elements of this chapter. Firstly, epidemiology should provide a wide-ranging, multi-factorial characterisation of hearing disorders over age. In interpreting the results from any such study the context aims and design of the study, and the audiological definitions and equipment calibration, and pegging of the difficulty level of questionnaire items and tests have to be taken into account.

Whatever the overall or marginal prevalence of 'hearing impairment', several different perspectives on the available data show a short-fall in the number of people receiving rehabilitative assistance. Among the young this is seen as a high criterion relative to the distribution of hearing levels for the group. Among the old there is a lower relative criterion but the large numbers who might come forward still do not. Thirdly, caution must be exercised in the interpretation of age effects from cross-sectional studies. Scientifically we may draw some tentative conclusions about individual ageing processes but they need to be tested longitudinally. From a planning point of view cross-sectional studies are insensitive to the changing needs of the population; some circumspection is required to project either the characterisation or the service needs of the present 45-year-olds 20 years hence from those in the present 65-year-old group.

The elderly are the largest group of people with hearing disorders and they also pose the biggest set of health service problems in an industrialised society. The communication difficulties met in attempting to alleviate these problems are the most professionally evident aspect of the handicap arising from impairment of hearing, which in many cases pervades the rest of their lives.

APPENDIX

Section A Version 1
We are interested in finding out if you have a hearing problem. If you wear a hearing aid, please answer the following questions as if you were not wearing your hearing aid.

1. Can you usually hear and understand what a person says to you in a quiet room
   a. if he whispers to you?   YES   NO
   b. if he speaks normally to you?   YES   NO
   c. if he speaks loudly into your better ear?   YES   NO
2. Do you find it very difficult to follow a conversation if there is a background noise, e.g. TV, radio, children playing?   YES   NO
3. Are you totally deaf in both ears?   YES   NO
4. Can you hear better with your left ear, right ear or are they both the same?

   LEFT   SAME   RIGHT
   BETTER   BETTER

Section A Version 2
We are interested in finding out if you have a hearing problem in either your left ear, right ear or both. If you wear a hearing aid, please answer the questions as if you were not wearing your hearing aid.

1. Indicate how well you hear a person who is talking to you when he is sitting on your *left* hand side in a quiet room.
   a. WITH NO DIFFICULTY
   b. WITH SLIGHT DIFFICULTY

   c. WITH GREAT DIFFICULTY
   d. DO NOT HEAR AT ALL

2. Indicate how well you hear a person who is talking to you when he is sitting on your *right* hand side in a quiet room.
   a. WITH NO DIFFICULTY
   b. WITH SLIGHT DIFFICULTY
   c. WITH GREAT DIFFICULTY
   d. DO NOT HEAR AT ALL

3. Answer this question for *both* ears together.
   Do you find it very difficult to follow a conversation if there is a background noise, e.g. TV, radio, children playing?
   YES   NO

Section B

In this section we are interested in whether you get ringing or buzzing noises in your head or ears. The occasional whistling or ringing in the ears of less than 5 minutes duration should not be counted. Also do not count those times when this happens just after very loud sounds, e.g. discos, shooting, or noise at work.
If you *do not* get noises in your head or ears turn to Section C.

1. Where do you most commonly hear buzzing or ringing in your head or ears?
   a. IN THE LEFT EAR
   b. IN THE RIGHT EAR
   c. IN BOTH EARS
   d. IN THE HEAD

2. Indicate how annoying you find noises in your head or ears.
   a. NOT ANNOYING AT ALL
   b. ANNOYING TO A SLIGHT DEGREE
   c. ANNOYING TO A MODERATE DEGREE
   d. ANNOYING TO A SEVERE DEGREE

3. Indicate to what extent noises in your head or ears affect your ability to lead a normal life.
   a. NOT AT ALL
   b. TO A SLIGHT DEGREE
   c. TO A MODERATE DEGREE
   d. TO A SEVERE DEGREE

4. Do you ever get a buzzing or ringing noise in your head or ears that interferes with your getting to sleep?
   YES   NO

Section C

General Information
The following basic facts would be most useful to us and will allow us to ensure that the replies we get are representative of the population of the country. I would like to stress that this information will be kept strictly confidential.

1. What is your date of birth?   DAY   MONTH   YEAR
2. What is your occupation?   _____
3. If you are married what is your
   wife's or husband's occupation?   _____
4. Do you usually write with your right hand?   YES   NO
5. Were you born a twin?   YES   NO
6. Has anyone in your family ever had difficulty
   with their hearing—
   a. when they were under about 65 years old?   YES   NO
   b. when they were over about 65 years old?   YES   NO
7. Have you ever worked in a place for more than six months
   where you had to raise your voice to be heard?   YES   NO
8. Have you ever had a hearing aid?   YES   NO
9. Do you currently use a hearing aid?   YES   NO
10. Are you registered as a disabled person with your
    Local Authority because of your hearing?   YES   NO

Comments:

Thank you for taking the trouble to fill in the questionnaire. This will be of great help to us.

ACKNOWLEDGEMENTS

Part of the work described was reported at a BSA meeting in July 1980 and at the XVth International Congress of Audiology, 1980.

I am very grateful to Ross Coles, Mark Haggard, Geoff Hart, Anne Sempik, Mark Lutman and Stuart Gatehouse for their comments on earlier drafts of this chapter, and to Karen Heartfield for typing the manuscript.

REFERENCES

Alberti P W 1977 Hearing aids and aural rehabilitation in a geriatric population. Le Journal D'Oto-Rhino-Laryngologie Supplement 4
Ballantyne J 1981 Rehabilitation of the adult deaf: a survey. Paper read at the Royal Society of Medicine, Section of Otology.
Baxter J D, Ling D 1974 Ear disease and hearing loss among the Eskimo population of the Baffin zone. Canadian Journal of Otolaryngology 3 : 110–122
Beasley W C 1940 The general problem of deafness in the population. Laryngoscope September 1940
Bench J, Bamford J 1979 Speech-hearing tests and the spoken language of hearing-impaired children. Academic Press, London
Bergman M 1966 Hearing in the Mabaans. Archives of Otolaryngology 84 : 411–415

Burns W, Robinson D W 1970 Hearing and noise in industry. HMSO, London

Burton D K 1977 Hearing-impaired residents in local authority homes for the elderly. Manchester North Regionl Association for the Deaf (MIMES)

CEC 1979 Childhood deafness in the European Community by Martin J AM and Moore W J. Commission of the European Communities Brussels

DHSS 1973 Deafness: Report of a Departmental enquiry into the promotion of research. Rawson A HMSO Reports on Health and Social Subjects No 4

DHSS 1977 Report of sub-committee appointed to consider the role of social services in the care of the deaf of all ages. Advisory Committee on Services for Hearing-impaired people.

Elliott L L 1978 Epidemiology of hearing-impairment and other communicative disorders. Advances in Neurology 19: 399–420

Federal Register 1981 Occupational noise exposure. Department of Labor, Occupational Safety and Health Administration Friday January 16th 1981 Part III

Gilad O, Glorig A 1979 Presbyacusis: The Ageing Ear Part II. Journal of the American Auditory Society 4: 207–217

Glorig A, Gilad O 1979 Presbyacusis: The Ageing Ear Part I. Journal of the American Auditory Society 4: 195–206

Glorig A, Roberts J 1970 Hearing levels of adults by age and sex: United States 1960–1962. Vital and Health Statistics 1965 Series 11, No 11

Haggard M 1980 Six audiological paradoxes in the provision of hearing aid services. In: Studies in the use of amplification for the hearing-impaired. Excerpta Medica 1980, 1–14

Haggard M, Gatehouse S, Davis A 1981 The High Prevalence of Hearing Disorders and its implications for services in the UK. British Journal of Audiology 15: 241–281

Hart G 1980 The hearing of residents in homes for the elderly (South Glamorgan). University Hospital of Wales

Hayes D, Jerger J 1979 Scandinavian Audiology 8: 53

Herbst K G, Humphrey C 1980 Hearing impairment and mental state in the elderly living at home. British Medical Journal 281: 903–905

Hinchcliffe R 1958 The pattern of the threshold of perception for hearing and other special senses as a function of age. Gerontologia 2: 311–320

Hinchcliffe R 1962 Ageing and sensory thresholds. Journal of Gerontology 17: 45–50

Hinchcliffe R 1972 Some geographical aspects of neuro-otology with particular reference to the African. African Journal of Medical Sciences 3: 137–148

Hinchcliffe R 1979 Epidemiology of hearing. In: Beagley HA Auditory investigation: the scientific and technological basis. Clarendon Press, Oxford

IHR 1981a A population study of hearing disorders in adults. Journal of Royal Society of Medicine 74: 819–827

IHR 1981b Prevalence and causes of hearing disorders: rationale and findings of a pilot population study. In preparation

Kish L 1973 Survey sampling. New York, Wiley

Leske M 1977 Prevalence estimates of communication disorders in the US. Report for the NINCDS communicative disorders panel.

Leske M 1981 Prevalence estimates of communicative disorders in the US Language, Hearing and Vestibular Disorders. ASHA 23: 229–237

Martin D N, Peckford R W 1977 Hearing-impairment in homes for the elderly. North Yorkshire Social Services Department Report

Maurer J F, Rupp R R 1972 Threshold of subjective auditory handicap. Audiology 12: 65–69

Merluzzi F, Hinchcliffe R 1972 Threshold of subjective auditory handicap, Audiology 12: 65–69

National Center for Health Statistics Series 10 No 35 1967 Characteristics of persons with impaired hearing US July1962–June 1963. US Department of Health Education and Welfare

National Center for Health Statistics Series 2 No 37 1970 Development and evaluation of an expanded hearing loss scale questionnaire. US Department of Health Education and Welfare

National Center for Health Statistics Series U No 215 1980 Basic data on hearing-levels of adults 25-74 years US 1971–75. US Department of Health Education and Welfare

Noble W 1978 Assessment of Impaired Hearing: a critique and a new method. Academic Press, London

Pal J, Bhatia M L, Prasad B G, Dayal D, Jath P C 1974 Deafness among the urban community—an epidemiological survey at Lucknow (UP). Indian Journal of Medical Research 62: 857–868

Pearce J L 1980 BKB Sentence lists—contextual analysis and reduction of redundancy by masking. Unpublished MSc thesis. Southampton University

Plomp R 1978 Auditory handicap of hearing-impairment and the limited benefit of hearing-aids. Journal of the Acoustical Society of America 63: 533–549

Roberts J 1979 Hearing levels of adults 25–74 years of age in the general population by sex and race: US 1971–1975 and 1960–1962. 97th meeting of Acoustical Society America

Robinson D W, Sutton G J 1979 Age effect in hearing—a comparative analysis of published threshold data. Audiology 18:320–334

Rop I, Raber A 1980 Application of a linear logistic model to describe hearing-impairment as a function of noise exposure and age. In: Tobias J W (ed) Proceedings of the Third International Congress on noise as a Public Health Problem

Rosen S, Bergman M, Plester D, El Mofty A, Satti M H 1962 Presbyacusis study of a relatively noise-free population in the Sudan. Annals of Otology, Rhinology and Laryngology 71:727–742

Schein J, Delk M 1974 The Deaf Population of the United States. National Association of the Deaf, Maryland

Schein J, Gentile A, Haase K W 1970 Development and evaluation of an expanding hearing loss questionnaire. Vital and Health Statistics Series 2 No 37 1970

Upfold L J, Wilson D A 1980 Hearing-aid distribution and use in Australia. The Australian Bureau of Statistics 1978 Survey. Australian Journal of Audiology 2:31–36

Ward P R, Tucker A M, Tudor C A, Morgan D C 1975 Self assessment of hearing-impairment: test of the expanded hearing ability scales questionnaire on hearing-impaired adults in England. British Society of Audiology, Meeting. 12 Dec

Wilkins L T 1948/49 Survey of the prevalences of deafness in the population of England, Scotland and Wales. Central Office of Information, London

The hearing mechanism

INTRODUCTION

The aim of this chapter is to describe the structure and function of the peripheral auditory system. It should be pointed out at the outset that although the anatomical data is in the main well established and agreed upon, there are still important areas of doubt, disagreement or lack of information. This problem is, however, far more serious for the functional aspects, where it is true to say that crucial gaps in our knowledge still exist and the field of ideas is very much in flux.

The task of the peripheral ear is that of providing an optimum interface between the brain and the stimuli present in the outside world. In the case of the hearing portion of the ear, these stimuli consist of sounds—oscillatory changes in the air pressure with patterns in their frequency, time and intensity—which may be of significance to man. Our understanding of the capabilities of this system are based on increasingly powerful psychoacoustical and, partly, electrophysiological tools. It is, however, useful and important to compare data from other mammals where intensive investigations have been carried out using surgical invasion and more discriminative anatomical and electrophysiological techniques. These data help immensely in our understanding of the ear of man and support, qualify and vastly extend the observations made with the more limited techniques which can be applied in the case of man. The high degree of uniformity observed in the anatomy and physiology of the ears of different mammals make such comparative material of direct interest to the human psychoacoustician.

It is useful at this point to discuss one important general concept in the field of sensory physiology, that of dividing the sense organ into *accessory structures* and the *receptor cells and their nervous innervation*. Such a division is an important aid to understanding the function of the ear and in identifying causes of abnormal function. In this case, accessory structures are those structures through which the stimuli must pass in order to reach and activate the receptor cells. These structures (the outer and middle ears, inner ear fluids, basilar membrane, tectorial membrane and supporting cells of the spiral organ of Corti) in turn *funnel, amplify* and *filter* the sound stimuli and greatly influence the character of the 'window' through which the receptor cells 'see' the outside world. The receptor cells can only react to stimuli which successfully pass the accessory-structures filter. Because these accessory structures are so complex, there exists a variety of pathologies which can exert a profound effect on the functional abilities of the auditory system, although the actual receptor cell system is quite normal.

44

Through the chain of accessory structures, the sound stimulus retains its character of a physical oscillation. The task of the receptor cells and their innervating nerve fibres is to *transform this signal into the standard code of the nervous system*, which can then be transmitted to the brain for further processing. This transformation, within definite limits, allows the encoding of several aspects of the stimulus—frequency, intensity and time patterns. In the brain—through intricate comparisons of information in different nerve fibres of the same ear and between ears—this coded information can be processed in various ways at different brain levels.

THE STRUCTURE AND FUNCTION OF THE OUTER AND MIDDLE EAR

The outer or external ear consists of the auricle (pinna) and external acoustic meatus (Fig. 2.1). In mammals in general, the development and mobility of the auricle make it obvious that its primary function is to provide a directional funnel

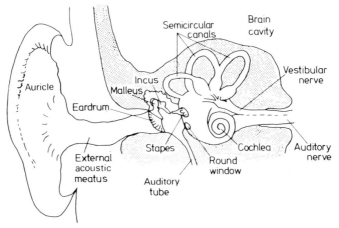

Fig. 2.1 Schematic diagram of the arrangement of the outer, middle and internal ear in man. (Reproduced from Moore, 1977 by kind permission of the publishers).

for sound. Even in man, where the auricle is relatively poorly developed and virtually immoveable, it plays an important role in sound localisation. In combination with the resonance tube created by the external acoustic meatus, it also performs a frequency-dependent amplification on the sound stimulus, which influences the threshold, in man especially amplifying in the range near 4 kHz. One consequence of this is, however, the increased susceptibility of the ear to damage by loud noises in that frequency range (Shaw, 1974).

At the same time, the presence of an outer ear provides significant protection from damage by objects hitting the head. It also increases the travel time of sound between the two ears, which may be significant in sound localisation by small mammals. The middle ear is an *impedance-matching transformer*. Such a device is an essential component of the accessory structures, because the mechanical impedance of the fluids of the internal ear to sound is very much greater than the impedance in air. Without an impedance-matching system, most of the sound energy would simply be reflected from the air/body interface. In order to understand the ways in which the match is achieved, it is necessary to understand the structures involved in concentrating the energy.

The eardrum, or tympanic membrane (TM) which forms the barrier between the outer and the middle ear is a more or less circular, slightly conical, thin membrane. It is tightly attached to the long arm of the malleus, or hammer, the outermost of the three ear ossicles (Fig. 2.2). The attachment reaches from almost

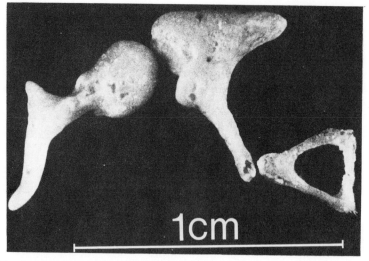

Fig. 2.2 The three middle-ear ossicles of man (compare Fig. 2.1).

the upper border of the TM to its centre. Impinging sound energy induces an oscillating in-and-out motion of the TM and a similar, but smaller, motion of the malleus. This movement of the malleus is greatest at its point of attachment to the centre of the TM, because the point of rotation is at the edge of the TM, where much of the mass of the malleus lies. At this point also, the incus (anvil) attaches to the malleus, so the motion is transmitted to the next ossicle. The incus has also much of its mass at this point of rotation, so the effective mass of the ossicles is very much reduced—so much so that it has been difficult to demonstrate an expected effect of their mass on the ossicular transfer characteristic (Johnstone and Taylor, 1971). The arm of the incus pushes directly on the stapes (stirrup), so the motion is transferred through the stapes base (footplate) in the oval window to the fluids of the cochlea.

The rotation point of the malleus-incus pair forms the fulcrum of a lever system, in which the lever arm of the incus is shorter than that of the malleus (length ratio 1·3 : 1; Békésy, 1960). In this way, more force is exerted on the stapes than moved the malleus initially. More important in man is the fact that the energy-collecting area of the TM is very much larger (ratio 18 : 1 in man; Wever et al, 1948) than the area of the stapes base, thus producing an additional energy concentration (e.g.

Tonndorf and Khanna, 1970). Of course, the entire area of the TM does not move with an equivalent displacement, being stationary at its border and having maximum displacement somewhere between the border and the malleus. It is therefore very difficult to precisely calculate the magnitude of the influence of the area ratio. Additionally, it is possible that the slightly curved, conical form of the TM increases the force applied to the malleus. The total maximum effect of the middle ear produces an increase in sensitivity of the internal ear in the mid-frequency range of about 25 to 30 dB (Wever and Lawrence, 1954). Its influence is, however, frequency dependent. When the velocity of middle-ear structures is compared to the velocity of the driving air particles, the middle ear increases in efficiency up to a few hundred hertz, has then a steady characteristic to relatively high frequencies, falling off rapidly beyond 5 kHz. Figure 2.3 is a schematic diagram of the transfer characteristic of the middle ear.

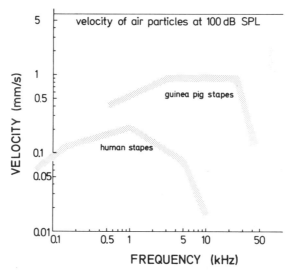

Fig. 2.3 The transfer characteristic of the human middle ear compared to that of the guinea pig, which is more 'typical' of mammals in general in terms of its hearing range. The input to the middle ear at all frequencies is a constant sound pressure level, i.e., a constant velocity of air particles (6 mm.s^{-1} at 100 dB SPL, cf. upper line). The stapes velocity for man in the living state may well be higher than for the cadaver data given here. Human data recalculated from Rubinstein et al, 1966; guinea-pig data from Manley and Johnstone, 1974.

The working point on this transfer characteristic can be changed by an air pressure difference across the TM. This is a phenomenon familiar to all and experienced most frequently during rapid altitude changes. The auditory (Eustachian) tube, connecting the middle ear to the upper throat region, is normally closed, but can be opened by jaw motions or swallowing. It can thus be seen from Figure 2.3 that over a significant frequency range, the middle ear operates highly efficiently, following the air particle motion with an inevitable frictional loss. An additional important influence on the transfer characteristic of the middle ear is that exerted by the two middle-ear muscles. The *tensor tympani* attaches to the malleus and, on contraction, tenses the TM by pulling it further into the middle ear. This makes transmission at low frequencies less efficient.

The *stapedius* muscle connects to the side of the head of the stapes near the incus articulation and when contracted pulls the top of the stapes sideways. This creates a partial disarticulation of the joint and a general loss of efficiency of the ossicular chain. Both of these muscles are part of the mechanisms which act to protect the inner ear from damage due to high sound pressures (Morgan et al, 1978). This sensitivity to damage is an inevitable consequence of the extraordinary sensitivity of the ear.

THE STRUCTURE AND FUNCTION OF THE COCHLEA

Like the receptor cells of the vestibular system, the receptors, or 'hair' cells of the auditory component of the internal ear and their supporting cells are usually considered to be in a cavity filled with endolymph, although it is still uncertain whether the fluid beneath the tectorial membrane is endolymph—or perilymph-like. Endolymph, unlike most other body fluids, has a high concentration of potassium ions. To maintain isotonicity, the concentration of sodium ions is, accordingly, drastically reduced compared to the other cochlear fluid, the perilymph. The perilymph cavity originates during development from the break-down of mesenchyme cells surrounding the cochlear duct, and in adults is connected with the cerebral fluid space. Through this cavity the oscillations of the stapes are transmitted to the endolymph and the receptor-supporting cell complex, the spiral organ. Where the endolymph and the perilymph come into contact, they are separated by two structures, i.e. the vestibular (Reissner's) membrane separates the scalae media and vestibuli, the surface of the spiral organ the scalae media and tympani (Figs. 2.4 and 2.5). The entire system of three scalae is coiled together into a 'cochlea' (Gk : snail).

Pressure changes induced in the scala vestibuli perilymph by motion of the middle ear are equalised either through motions of the cochlear partition (basilar membrane plus spiral organ) and/or through the helicotrema at the cochlear apex, which connects the scala vestibuli with the scala tympani at the apical end. At the basal end of the cochlea, the scala tympani is closed off by the thin round window membrane, which yields easily to pressure and returns some of the sound energy to the middle ear. The vestibular membrane is extremely thin, making it possible to view the scalae vestibuli and media as hydrodynamically one scala.

Although the perilymph-filled scalae are much larger at the base of the cochlea than at the apex, the dimensions of the structures of the endolymph scala, the scala media, tend to be roughly the same or larger at the apex. Thus there is a clear gradient in the width of the basilar membrane, which is about three times wider at the apex. There are corresponding dimensional changes in the size of the spiral organ and the tectorial membrane.

Structure of the spiral organ of Corti

The basilar membrane supports on its upper side a complex but systematically organised group of receptor and supporting cells (Figs. 2.5 and 2.6; Ades and Engström, 1974). Towards the axial side of the spiral organ (of Corti) are found two rows of prominent supporting cells, the pillar cells. These rows are inclined to

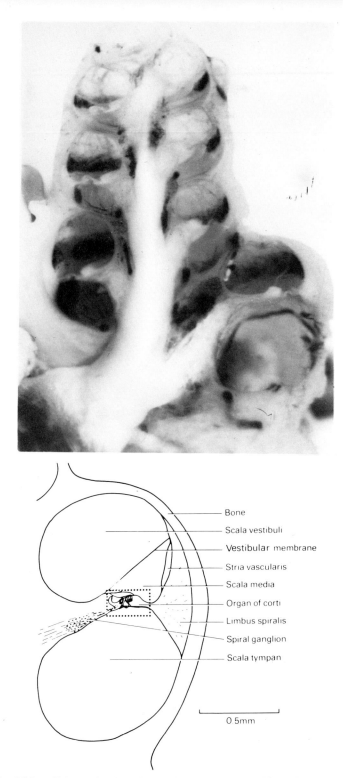

Bone

Scala vestibuli

Vestibular membrane

Stria vascularis

Scala media

Organ of corti

Limbus spiralis

Spiral ganglion

Scala tympani

0 5mm

Fig. 2.4 *Top*: Mid-modiolar section through an entire, unstained decalcified guinea-pig cochlea, illustrating its coiled structure. The auditory nerve appears white. The section through the lower basal turn (bottom right) is schematically enlarged in the bottom part of this figure. The basilar membrane of the guinea pig is about 18·5 cm long. *Bottom*: Enlarged diagram of a section through the upper basal turn of the guinea-pig cochlea. The area in the dotted rectangle is further enlarged in Fig. 2.6. (Reproduced from Zwicker and Manley, 1981 by kind permission of the publishers).

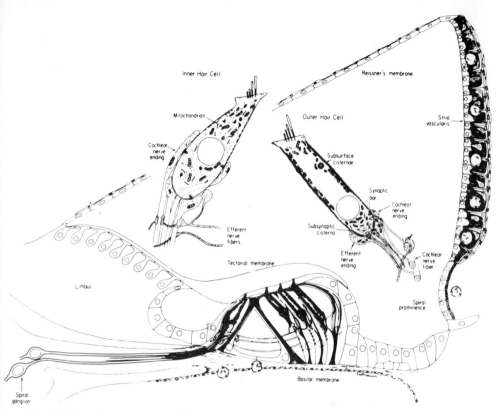

Fig. 2.5 Schematic drawing illustrating the general arrangement of the hair cells and their innervation in the second turn of the guinea-pig cochlea. Inset diagrams show the inner and outer hair cells and their synapses (see text for description). (Reproduced from Smith, 1978 by kind permission of the publishers).

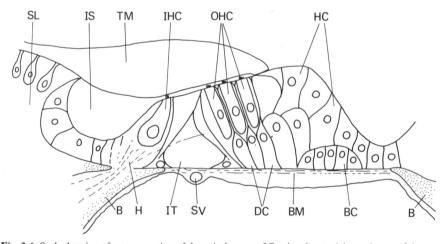

Fig. 2.6 Scale drawing of a cross-section of the spiral organ of Corti and tectorial membrane of the basal turn of the guinea-pig cochlea illustrating the size and placement of the tectorial membrane in life (drawing of Dr. A. Kronester-Frei). SL—spiral limbus; IS—inner spiral sulcus; TM—tectorial membrane; OHC—outer hair cells; HC—Hensen's cells; B—bone; H—habenula; IT—inner tunnel; SV—spiral blood vessel; DC—Deiter's phalangeal cells; BM—basilar membrane; BC—Boettcher's cells; IHC—inner hair cells. The basilar membrane is here 150 μm wide.

each other, building the 'arch of Corti' or inner tunnel. These cells contain many bundles of microfibrils which run the whole length of the cell from the upper surface of the spiral organ (the reticular lamina) to the basilar membrane. The phalanges of the Deiter's cells may also have a similar function. The supporting cells are arranged in such a way as to provide maximum support for the hair cells. On the axial or inner side of the tunnel is found a single row of sensory cells, the inner 'hair' cells, closely surrounded by relatively unspecialised supporting cells.

The inner hair cells (IHC) support on their upper surface several rows of stereocilia, the rows being oriented longitudinally, i.e. along the length of the basilar membrane. The cilia of the most lateral rows are longest (up to 5·7 μm, Lim, 1980). The microtubules of the cilia are deeply rooted in the electron-dense cuticular plate found in the most apical region of the cell. This plate is not complete but has on the outside (i.e. next to the tunnel) an opening in which is found a basal body, the remains of the degenerated fetal kinocilium. The hair cell is in general shaped like a bulbous column, with the cell nucleus more or less central and the normal organelles scattered throughout the cytoplasm. At the base of the IHC are found typical structures (e.g. synaptic bodies, vesicles and membrane thickenings) associated with chemical synapses. Inner hair cells are exclusively or predominantly innervated by afferent nerve fibres (i.e., fibres which transmit information away from the cell towards the brain). It has been demonstrated in other mammals (Spoendlin, 1975, 1979) that *more than 90 per cent of the afferent innervation terminates on IHCs*, apparently with most fibres only making contact with one single hair cell, but with each hair cell receiving many afferent synapses (Fig. 2.7). Efferent fibres transmitting information from the brain seldom show significant synaptic contact with IHCs, but synapse instead with the afferent fibres (axo-dendritic synapses). These efferent fibres to IHC afferents (about 1700 fibres) appear to originate predominantly in the ipsilateral superior olive (Warr, 1978; Warr and Guinan, 1979) (Fig. 2.8). The IHCs are in many respects more similar to

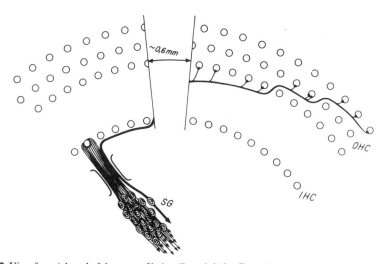

Fig. 2.7 View from 'above' of the rows of hair cells and their afferent innervation to illustrate the difference in pattern and density of innervation of the two hair-cell populations. (Reproduced from Spoendlin, 1978 by kind permission of the publishers).

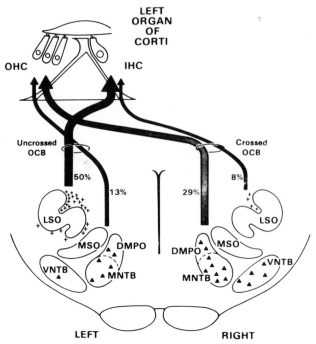

Fig. 2.8 A schema of the origins and terminations of the olivocochlear bundle in the cat. It can be seen that 63 per cent of olivocochlear bundle neurons to one cochlea originate on the ipsilateral side, predominantly innervating IHC afferents. Of the 37 per cent of neurons from the contralateral side, most innervate OHC's. DMPO—dorsomedial periolivary nucleus; IHC—inner hair cells; LSO—lateral superior olivary nucleus; MNTB—medial nucleus of the trapezoid body; MSO—medial superior olivary nucleus; OCB—olivocochlear bundle; OHC—outer hair cells; VNTB ventral nucleus of the trapezoid body. (Reproduced from Warr, 1978 by kind permission of the publishers).

the typical, primitive vertebrate hair cell type than the outer hair cells (OHCs). These OHCs form three or four parallel rows on the outer side of the tunnel, separated from each other by the narrow processes of the Deiter's cells. They possess a cuticular plate with embedded stereocilia, but the stereocilia are arranged in a 'W'-formation, with the site of the basal body of the kinocilium in the notch of the 'W'. Unlike the IHCs, which are closely surrounded by supporting cells, the OHCs are surrounded by fluid spaces, being attached at the top to the reticular lamina and at the bottom to the nerve fibres (Fig. 2.5). The OHCs are tall cylinders, more or less divided into an upper and lower region by the nucleus. In the upper region, there is a specialised arrangement of endoplasmic reticulum and mitochondria next to the cell membrane. The endoplasmic reticulum is complex and connected by electron-dense bridges to the cell membrane, which in this region is thicker and less dense than usual. In the lower region of the cell, there are many mitochondria and synaptic connections with both afferent and efferent nerve fibres (Smith, 1978). Only 10 per cent of the total afferent complement of the auditory nerve makes contact with OHCs (Spoendlin, 1978). These nerve fibres enter the spiral organ with all others, through the habenula perforata of the osseous spiral lamina, run beneath the IHCs, cross the tunnel, turn basalward for about 500 μm and then innervate OHCs of all three rows (Fig. 2.7). Thus the sparse afferent bundle is spread over all OHCs, each fibre innervating 10 to 20 receptor cells. The actual synapses are, however, not quite 'normal' in their structure when compared to other chemical synapses and to the afferent synapses of the IHCs (see Manley, 1978 for refs.). The efferent complement to the OHCs (about 700 fibres) comes predominantly from the contralateral superior olive and trapezoid body (Warr, 1978), each fibre forming large synapses on many OHCs (Fig. 2.8). The entire upper surface of the spiral organ forms the reticular lamina, a rigid layer consisting of the upper surfaces of the hair cells and supporting cells.

During development, the spiral organ begins as a less-well-defined mass of cells overlaid by extracellular material secreted mainly by cells of the Kölliker's organ but also partly by cells on the limbus (Hinojosa, 1977). As development continues, the spiral organ differentiates out into its specialised cell types and a group of cells between the limbus and the IHCs (the Kölliker's organ) sink away from the extracellular material (the tectorial membrane, t.m.) to form the inner sulcus. The other cells also pull away from the t.m. to some extent (Lim, 1977). The result for the hair cells appears to be that the IHC stereocilia have no or only a weak connection to the t.m., whereas the OHC stereocilia have a firmer contact (see Manley, 1978 for refs). Beyond the OHCs, the t.m. retains a close contact with the supporting cells of the spiral organ (Fig. 2.6), forming a sub-tectorial space with no direct fluid pathway to the scala media proper (Kronester-Frei, 1979). The tectorial membrane consists of a protofibril gel with two intermingled types of protofibrils (Kronester-Frei, 1978). Uncertainty remains as to their exact nature, but there is evidence for both protein and acid mucopolysaccharide content (e.g. Steel, 1980).

All the epithelial cells surrounding the scala media, including the vestibular membrane, are joined to their neighbours by occluding tight junctions between cell membranes (Smith, 1978). Such junctions strongly impede ion flow through the interstitial spaces, so that the cells themselves retain a high degree of control over the ion fluxes. This provides on the one hand a mechanism to prevent large losses of potassium ions from the scala media or gain of sodium ions from all around. It also, on the other hand, provides a mechanism for channelling ion fluxes to those cells which alter their resistance to ion flow during stimulation (exclusively or mostly the hair cells). The normal small leaks of ions and the ion exchange which occurs during sound stimulation are dealt with by selective ion pumps in the cells of the stria vascularis, a richly vascularised area of specialised cells in the outer wall of the scala media (Fig. 2.5). These cells are highly active and maintain, by their selective pump activity, not only the high potassium content but a high positive DC potential relative to the rest of the body's extracellular spaces, of 80 to 100 mV. Shutting off the oxygen supply to these cells results within two minutes in a loss of this *endocochlear potential* or EP. After two minutes, a negative EP is measurable, which appears to be referable to the expected potassium diffusion potential, as the potassium leaks out of the scala media (Johnstone and Sellick, 1972).

The function of the spiral organ
Stated simply, the function of the spiral organ is to transform the oscillations in the cochlear fluids into a neural code. Although strictly speaking this is the function of the hair cells and their synapses, there is convincing evidence that the accessory

structures of the spiral organ exert a profound influence on the realisation and pattern of this transformation. When one considers, however, the bewildering variety of ideas and models currently being discussed as to how this transformation occurs, one can get the impression that we have made little progress in the last 10 years. This impression is, however, false. While it is true to say that certain very basic aspects are not understood (e.g. the actual function of the outer hair cells!), a wealth of data makes it possible at least to place profound limits on the possible explanations of the mechanisms. These limits will be discussed historically for the one aspect which has been most intensively investigated, frequency selectivity.

Since the early investigations of Helmholtz (see Békésy, 1960) it has been known that the human ear has an impressive ability to discriminate between sounds which have similar frequencies of oscillation. Helmholtz' ideas concerning a piano-string-like vibration of tiny strips of the basilar membrane (developed for the then-conceived air-filled cochlea) provided an explanation which remained unchallenged until George von Békésy's superb and exhaustive work on the cochlea (collected in Békésy, 1960). In this case, Békésy investigated the fluid-filled cochlea of human and animal cadavers and developed a method for observing the tiny motions of the vestibular membrane (assuming the scala media to move as a unit) and the basilar membrane using stroboscopic light reflected from minute silver particles added to the fluid. Although it was necessary for him to use non-physiological sound pressures (120 to 140dB SPL) to actually observe motion, his findings are still considered basically valid, at least for the low-frequency areas he could investigate with this technique.

The following key findings came out of Békésy's work. He demonstrated the existence, not of standing resonances, but of *travelling waves*. By various manipulations, he also demonstrated that the travelling wave did not operate like that in a long rope which is whipped at one end—i.e., the energy did not travel along the basilar membrane itself. The velocity of the travelling waves was orders of magnitude slower than the velocity of sound in fluids. Thus, the sound energy in a short click is applied virtually simultaneously along the entire basilar membrane and is dissipated from the round window within a couple of microseconds, before the basilar membrane begins to move. The stiffer, more basal, parts of the basilar membrane have a shorter response latency than the more apical parts, and begin to move first. Thus the progression of response latencies leads to the setting up of a travelling wave which appears to move from base to apex. Where the wave has its displacement maximum depends on the frequency content of the original stimulus. High frequencies reach a peak near the stapes, low frequencies near the apex of the cochlea. This provides the basis for the *tonotopic arrangement* of frequency responses of nerve fibres in the cochlea (Fig. 2.9). The actual distribution of peak locations is approximately logarithmic (frequency against distance). The character of the travelling wave is illustrated in Figure 2.10. From the cochlear base, the wave gradually builds up in displacement, but drops off rapidly on the apical side of the peak. For loud, low-frequency stimuli, a large area of the basilar membrane is set in motion.

This latter fact somewhat disturbed Békésy, for it was not immediately obvious how a broad stimulation of the sensory organ could be reconciled with the fine discrimination ability of the ear. Impressed by the then new data concerning the

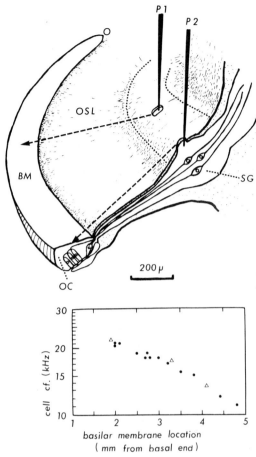

Fig. 2.9 Diagram illustrating the experimental verification of the tonotopic arrangement of the spiral organ of Corti responses. The upper drawing illustrates the technique of recording from the spiral ganglion (SG) in Rosenthal's canal of the cochlea. Fibres from these locations (P 1, P 2) can be traced across the osseous spiral lamina (OSL) to the basilar membrane (BM) and the spiral organ of Corti (OC). The innervation site can then be located by its distance (in mm) from the basal end of the cochlea. In the lower graph are given by dots the most sensitive frequencies (CF's—between 11 and 22 kHz) of neurons innervating BM regions from 2 to 4·8 mm. Triangles indicate the displacement maxima of those locations on the basilar membrane. (Reproduced from Robertson and Manley, 1974 by kind permission of the publishers).

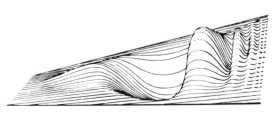

Fig. 2.10 Three-dimensional diagram to illustrate the general form of the travelling wave on the basilar membrane, frozen in one instant of time. The vertical dimension is highly exaggerated. (Reproduced from Tonndorf, 1960 by kind permission of the publishers).

evidence for *lateral inhibition* phenomena in receptors of the visual system of *Limulus*, the horseshoe crab (Hartline and Ratliff, 1957), Békésy carried out a series of studies of lateral inhibitory phenomena. For this, he used the skin of the forearm as a model for the spiral organ, and applied comparable stimuli through blown-up models of the cochlea. Here, he was able to demonstrate a lateral inhibition which led to a 'sharpening' of the sensation—i.e., the subjects' impression was of a vibration much more limited in extent than was in fact the case. Békésy extended these studies to the visual system and pursued these until his death. The very magnitude of Békésy's pioneering contributions led to the fact that his ideas on lateral inhibitory phenomena dominated the discussion of auditory sharpening mechanisms for too long. Neurophysiological recordings from single auditory nerve fibres rapidly confirmed one fact—the output of the cochlea, despite the broadly tuned response of the basilar membrane, consists of single nerve fibre responses which are themselves very sharply 'tuned' (Fig. 2.11). At low intensities, they respond only to a very limited bandwidth of frequencies, this bandwidth growing with increasing sound pressure. Other findings were to be expected from Békésy's data. Different nerve fibres were found with characteristic (or most sensitive) frequencies (CF) throughout the whole of the species' audible range. These were later (see, e.g. Fig. 2.9) demonstrated to be exquisitely tonotopically arranged. Also, the 'tuning' slope of the threshold sensitivity or tuning curve was higher on the high frequency side of the CF than on the low frequency side. This was generally to be expected from the basilar membrane

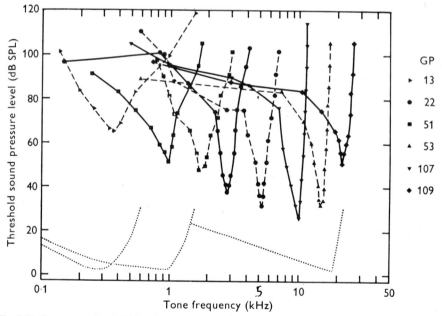

Fig. 2.11 Frequency-threshold ('tuning') curves of eight cochlear nerve fibres in the guinea-pig. Each cell responds most sensitively to a narrow frequency range. The dotted curves below are analogous curves for the displacement sensitivity of different locations on the basilar membrane. They are arbitrarily positioned on the SPL scale and illustrate the broadness of most measures of basilar-membrane tuning. (Reproduced from Evans, 1972, by kind permission of the publishers).

excitatory displacement pattern demonstrated by Békésy (Kiang et al, 1965; Evans, 1972).

True lateral inhibition required synaptic interaction between nerve fibres. Feedback from the brain via the efferent system was rapidly ruled out as an intermediary, due to the long times necessary. Another obvious possibility which received much attention was an influence of the afferent nerve fibres of the OHCs on the afferents of the IHCs. Various models were developed, some of which can now be eliminated due to our better understanding of the anatomy of the nerve fibre innervation (Spoendlin, 1978). Data rapidly accumulated to modify and finally *eliminate* true (i.e. synaptic) lateral inhibition as a possible explanation of the sharpening mechanism in the spiral organ. For example, it was clearly demonstrated that there are no synapses between IHC and OHC afferents (Spoendlin, 1975). In addition, physiological investigations demonstrated that the tuning properties of the afferents did not require time (e.g. 500 μs for a chemical synapse delay) to develop (see e.g. de Boer, 1969; Evans and Wilson, 1973). Some authors favoured a non-classical (electrical?) interaction as the fibres passed together through the habenula (e.g. Evans, 1974; Evans and Wilson 1973; Lynn and Sayers, 1970). Curiously, it had proven impossible to demonstrate clearly the existence of two populations of afferent fibres from the physiological data (see e.g. Robertson and Manley, 1974). For some reason, the 10 per cent of afferents from the OHCs (Spoendlin, 1975) were either not active or were not to be easily separated in physiological data from those of the IHCs. The latter conclusion seemed on anatomical and functional grounds unacceptable, i.e. a large functional difference was expected.

Accumulated evidence indicated that the *OHC's* and *IHC's* almost certainly had very *diverse functions*. *First*, their innervation was not only totally separate, but also quite different in its pattern (Fig. 2.7). *Secondly*, the OHC's dominated the production of extracellular electrical potentials in the cochlear fluids out of all proportion to their relative number (Dallos et al, 1972a and b). *Thirdly*, the OHC stereocilia appear to be firmly attached to the tectorial membrane, whereas those of IHCs may not be attached at all (see Manley, 1978 for refs). *Fourthly*, the efferent systems synapse quite differently with the two sets of receptors (Warr, 1978). *Lastly*, the IHC and OHC organelles show conspicuous differences in size, arrangement and distribution (the afferent synapses of IHC and OHC differ, and there are conspicuous metabolic differences between IHC and OHC dendrites; Manley, 1978; Smith, 1978; Spoendlin, 1975). It thus became an acceptable conclusion (in the mid-1970s) that an interaction between OHC- and IHC- 'systems' occurred not between afferent fibres, but *in the spiral organ itself* (e.g. Manley, 1978). Thus, earlier evidence for an interaction (e.g. the apparent need for a 'sharpening' mechanism; the effects of 'selective' destruction of OHC with ototoxic drugs; the inhibitory effect on all afferent fibres of stimulating efferents which only or predominantly innervate OHCs, e.g. Wiederhold and Kiang, 1970) could be reinterpreted, with the mechanisms confined to the spiral organ. Such considerations received an important new foundation and impetus from the work of Russell and Sellick (1977a and b) and Sellick and Russell (1978). These authors provided, for the first time, convincing intracellular recordings from IHCs. These data demonstrated clearly that the receptor potentials of the IHCs (i.e. preceding

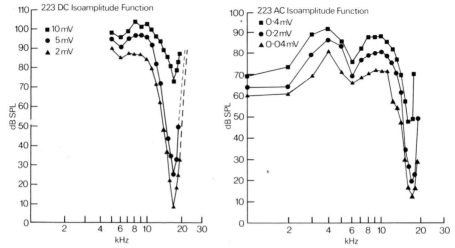

Fig. 2.12 Analogous frequency-isoamplitude curves for a guinea-pig inner hair cell, to be compared to Fig. 2.11. When low intracellular response criteria are used (left direct-current response; right alternating-current response at the stimulus frequency), the tuning is highly selective. (Reproduced from Sellick and Russell 1978 by kind permission of the publishers).

the nervous activity) were just as sharply tuned as the threshold curves of the nerve fibres (Fig. 2.12). To date, there are no extensive and convincing intracellular data from OHCs.

The fact that the frequency selectivity of the auditory nerve fibres is thus already established at the periphery of the auditory pathway and that the function of the OHC's appeared to be confined to the spiral organ itself (indeed, a recent suggestion is that the OHC afferents do not reach the brain, Spoendlin, 1979), naturally led to considerations of ways in which OHCs could interact with IHCs. This interaction must precede or be concurrent with the building of the IHC receptor potentials. The interaction could be chemical (unlikely, although the diffusion distances are small), electrical, mechanical or electro-mechanical. The fact that the spiral organ is in some respects a mechano-electrical transducer, and that such transducers can operate in the reversed mode (e.g. motor/generator) makes an electro-mechanical explanation attractive. This notion recently received a strong new impetus from a somewhat unexpected direction. Kemp (1978, 1980) demonstrated the presence of *acoustical 'echos'* in the external ear canal following the presentation to the ear of, say, a short click (Fig. 2.13). These were relatively long-latency echos (>5ms) whose frequency content was correlated with known points of sensitivity and insensitivity in the subject's audiogram. One of the most interesting aspects from the point of view of our discussion, is that the total amount of energy emitted by the cochlea via the middle ear is often as large as that in the original stimulus. This can only be true where the energy in the echo, or part of it, is being generated in the cochlea. This implies that *the spiral organ can emit mechanical energy*, presumably as a result of the generation of electrical events in the hair cells resulting directly—or indirectly—from the original stimulus. Models of such phenomena can provide a feedback system in which OHCs affect the character or magnitude of the IHC stimulus (e.g. Zwicker, 1979).

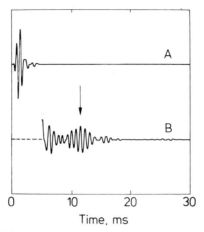

Fig. 2.13 Top: Waveform of short stimulus used to elicit 'echos' in the ear canal. Bottom: Recorded trace magnified 36 dB relative to the top trace. The arrow indicates the peak of the 1·3 kHz echo, which occurs about 10 ms after stimulus onset. For clarity, both traces were filtered with an octave-band filter set at 1·4 kHz. Unpublished data of Prof. E. Zwicker; used by permission.

This exciting possibility may help solve one of the prevailing problems in cochlear physiology. The problem revolves around the fact that Rhode (1973) found in the squirrel monkey cochlea that the basilar membrane behaved non-linearly at high intensities. This non-linearity was a compressive one such that if extrapolated to threshold sound pressure levels the displacement curve of the basilar membrane would have been very sharp indeed—equivalent to those of single nerve fibres (Fig. 2.14). This non-linearity was not found in the guinea pig (Johnstone et al, 1970; Wilson and Johnstone, 1975), then later found, but weak (LePage and Johnstone, 1980). Near-simultaneous measurements in the cat cochlea of basilar membrane motion and nerve fibre tuning (Evans and Wilson, 1975) seemed to support the idea that the basilar membrane was indeed more poorly tuned than the nerve fibres and that a 'second filter', i.e. beyond the filter of the basilar membrane, was necessary to produce sharp frequency tuning. The perimortem studies of Rhode (1973) showed, however, a profound change in the motion of the basilar membrane of the squirrel monkey within a few minutes after death—i.e. within a time period of anoxia from which the cochlea is known to recover after re-administration of oxygen. That the change could be due to changes in basilar membrane fibres seemed highly unlikely—it seemed then possible tentatively to conclude that the collapse of normal functioning of the spiral organ altered the motion of the basilar membrane.

The new evidence from cochlear echos of active mechanical output from the spiral organ makes this conclusion now much more attractive. This extra contribution from the spiral organ may vary in its magnitude from place to place in the cochlea, may vary with species and may in some species not be easily reflected in the basilar membrane motion as customarily measured. That such an effect is not easy to detect in the guinea pig may reflect this species' sensitivity to damage and/or a difference between an 18 kHz region of the cochlea and the 7 kHz region measured by Rhode. Recent data strengthen the idea that the motion pattern of the basilar membrane is physiologically vulnerable (LePage and Johnstone, 1980), a

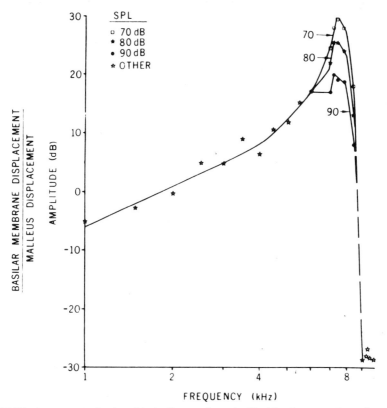

Fig. 2.14 Displacement amplitudes of the basilar membrane in dB with reference to the malleus displacement at different frequencies for three sound pressure levels (70, 80 and 90 dB SPL), for an approximately 7 kHz location in the squirrel monkey cochlea. The fact that the three curves do not overlap at the peak indicates the response is non-linear at the peak frequencies. (Reproduced from Rhode, 1970, by kind permission of the publishers).

vulnerability which may depend largely on the integrity of the outer hair cells (LePage et al, 1980). In addition, it has been shown (Mountain, 1980) that stimulation of the efferent pathways running predominantly to the OHCs in the cat produces a decrease in the magnitude of (nonlinear) distortion products measurable in the cochlear echo in the external ear canal. Thus, as suggested by Kim et al (1980), it may be reasonable to conclude that at threshold sound pressure levels the basilar membrane/spiral organ complex is as sharply tuned as cochlear nerve fibres. It may also be suggested that this sharp tuning is at least partly due to *active mechanical responses involving the OHCs*. (It should be noted here that if this is true, the distinction made between the 'accessory structures' and 'receptor cells' breaks down, as OHCs would then be part of the accessory structures of the IHC's). Any active response must, of course, have a built-in feedback system in order to control the magnitude of the oscillation. Thus mechanisms may exist to feed energy into the motion of the basilar membrane—spiral organ complex, to control the oscillation and to protect the delicate mechanisms once the mechanical motion is so large as to require no active support or, indeed, to be of damaging magnitude. These ideas, of course, indicate that the sharp 'tip' of the neural tuning curve results from an addition of active input, rather than a suppression of side-bands (e.g. Manley, 1978).

To isolate these mechanisms at a cellular level is, however, very difficult. This results both from a lack of detailed information on the real anatomical arrangement and of the properties of the constituents of the spiral organ, and from the fact that the spiral organ, being an exquisitely sensitive mechano-receptive structure, is a difficult experimental subject. Progress on these experimental fronts is being made, e.g. in our understanding of the nature of the tectorial membrane (Kronester-Frei, 1978, 1979), and in the development of techniques for closer investigation of the spiral organ itself (e.g. Manley and Kronester-Frei, 1980a and b) (Fig. 2.15). Until the experimental data are extended and improved, it will not be possible to discriminate between the wealth of theoretical models available today. Thus, due to the perseverance of a large group of workers, our concept of the function of the spiral organ has undergone a gradual evolution over the last 40 years, punctuated occasionally by important new advances. The 1980s will certainly be as productive and exciting and could perhaps bring a more complete understanding of cochlear function, without which considerations of pathology and healing lack a firm substrate.

SOME ADDITIONAL ASPECTS

Of course, the cochlea processes information other than that concerned purely with the frequency aspect. Thus, the *time structure* and *pattern of sound pressure level* are also encoded and transmitted to the brain. It may be worthwhile here to point out that a filter system which is highly selective for frequency will represent the time structure of the stimulus poorly, due to the long time constant of sharp frequency filters. The time discriminatory ability of the human ear is, however, more than adequate to deal with the individual components of, say, human speech.

The coding of sound pressure level

Sound-pressure-level coding requires a consideration of threshold and supra-threshold aspects. Threshold for the human ear varies, of course, with frequency, but for the healthy young ear lies, by definition, near 0 dB SPL (about 20 μPa). That the ear can be so sensitive is due to a number of factors. *First* must be cited the good impedance match provided by the middle ear, so that as much sound energy as possible reaches the internal ear. *Secondly*, the area of basilar membrane which moves is (especially at high frequencies) smaller than the area of the stapes foot-plate, so the displacement amplitude of the basilar membrane is up to 50 times larger than that of the stapes (Johnstone et al, 1970). Even so, at high sound levels the displacement is only several hundred Ångström units. At threshold, the motion is 100 dB less, or a few thousandths of an Ångström, if we can assume the motion of the basilar membrane to be linear. *Thirdly*, the bio-electrical potentials of the hair cells and cochlea provide powerful 'batteries' which presumably raise the sensitivity level of the spiral organ to small motions (Davis, 1960). *Fourthly*, the hair cell/afferent-neuron synapses are 'noisy'; that is, spontaneous activity can be measured constantly in the afferent fibres (e.g., Manley and Robertson, 1976). This spontaneous activity consists of more or less randomly occurring action potentials, whose overall rate of occurrence ranges from 0 to over 100 per second.

This system is highly energy-consuming but does make it possible, within a small group of hair cell synapses to be sure that at a given moment in time there is always one neuron on the brink of firing an action potential. This probability of firing can be influenced by small stimuli. Thus a stimulus does not actually have to bring the cell from resting potential to threshold potential and beyond, for the synapses

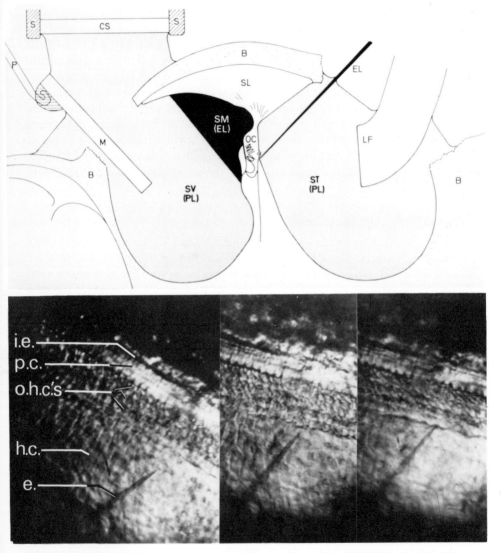

Fig. 2.15 *Top*: Diagram illustrating an optical technique to observe the path of a glass electrode (EL) during a penetration through the spiral organ of Corti (OC). Light from a light fibre (LF) in scala tympani (ST) shines through the spiral organ and scala media (SM) filled with endolymph (EL) and is reflected by a mirror (M) in the perilymph (PL) of scala vestibuli (SV) up to a cover slip (CS) of a microscope. B—bone; P—support pin; S—cover slip suspension; SL—spiral lamina. *Bottom*: Photographs through the microscope illustrating a glass electrode (e) in the spiral organ in three locations about 10 μm apart, in Hensen's cells (h.c.) and approaching the outer hair cell rows (o.h.c.'s) p.c.—pillar cells of the inner tunnel; i.e.—inner edge of the basilar membrane. (Reproduced from Manley and Kronester-Frei, 1980a, by kind permission of the publishers).

themselves are constantly oscillating about the action-potential firing level. To detect a stimulus, a simultaneous rate or pattern change in several fibres is probably necessary, but the system with spontaneous activity is still more sensitive than one without. *Lastly*, it is possible that the active feedback mechanisms in the spiral organ, as mentioned above, play a role in raising the hair cell's sensitivity, but our knowledge is as yet insufficient to define any such role.

The coding of sounds of different intensity requires the cooperation of many individual nerve fibres, at least to cover the codable range of 100 dB. Individual nerve fibres possess a dynamic range of the order of 40 dB (Fig. 2.16; Sachs and Abbas, 1974). Thus, within 40 dB of sound pressure increase above the level at which that single neuron raises its firing rate above the spontaneous level (the threshold), the level is reached at which the neuron is firing at its maximum rate. Several mechanisms operate, however, to extend this individual limit for the whole cochlea. For example, many cells alter their firing *pattern* (but not rate) to very low level stimuli, adding 10 to 20 dB to the dynamic range covered by the firing rate increase. In addition, not all fibres of the same or similar CF have the same threshold, but vary up to 20 dB. Thus some fibres will be near their saturation firing rate when another fibre is just above its threshold rate. In actual fact, the saturation rate at 40 dB above threshold for rate increase is also, for perhaps half the neuron population, not a firm saturation plateau, but a prominent decrease in the rate of increase of firing rate. Thus, above this slope-change point, the cell does in fact continue to slowly increase its rate (Fig. 2.16). The area of displacement of the basilar membrane also changes with sound pressure level, so that the displacement envelope covers a larger number of cells at higher intensities. These cells are recruited into the coding network, so that at very high sound levels it is possible that a change in sound pressure is detected partly by cells on the periphery of the excitation pattern. Taken together, these factors are probably adequate to explain the ear's ability to code an *enormous dynamic range*. Whether single hair cells themselves are ever exposed to such a dynamic range is, however, open to question. Non-linear behaviour of some sort is detectable in basilar-membrane motion and non-linear phenomena are so common and prominent in the electrical and neural response of the spiral organ cells (Zwicker and Manley, 1981) that it is possible that some of the non-linearity is mechanical in nature in the motion of the spiral organ and tectorial membrane. Békésy showed, for example, that the electrical potentials produced by the hair cells were largest where a motion produced in the tectorial membrane induced a radial shear between the spiral organ and the tectorial membrane (Békésy, 1960). If this is true in the living, intact cochlea, then it is likely that the transformation from an up-and-down motion of the basilar membrane to radial shear at the surface of the spiral organ is a *non-linear* process.

Phase locking to the stimulus

It has been known for some time (e.g. Rose et al, 1968) that auditory nerve fibre discharges show phase-locking behaviour—that is, the probability that the nerve fibre will produce an action potential is greatest during a certain phase of the stimulating sine wave. Thus at low frequencies, where the number of cycles of the stimulus per second is lower than or near the maximum discharge rate of the fibre,

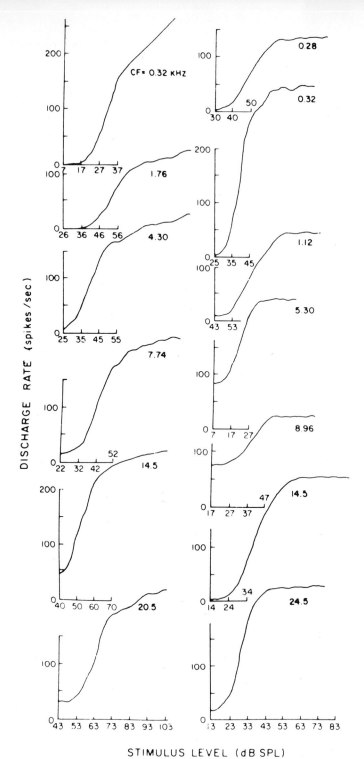

Fig. 2.16 Discharge rate (spikes/s) plotted versus stimulus level (dB SPL) for 13 cat auditory-nerve fibres. CF (characteristic frequency) is indicated in each case and was used as the stimulus. Units on the left do not show a plateau in the discharge rate at higher SPL. (Reproduced from Sachs and Abbas, 1974, by kind permission of the publishers).

the neuron discharge pattern often strongly reflects the waveform of the stimulus (Fig. 2.17). As the stimulus frequency rises, this behaviour becomes weaker, although when the stimulus frequency exceeds the maximum discharge rate of the neuron, the neuron simply skips cycles and discharges every second, third, etc. wave. At about 4 kHz, this behaviour tends to vanish and not be detectable, at least in single neurons (Fig. 2.17). Similar behaviour has been observed in high CF

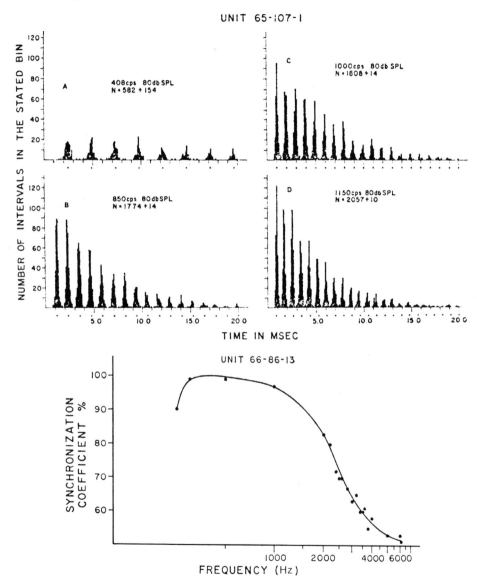

Fig. 2.17 *Top*: Inter-spike-interval histograms for an auditory-nerve fibre to four different pure tones (408–1150 Hz), at 80 dB SPL. N = number of sampled intervals. The periodic nature of the response indicates intervals appropriate for phase locking to the different waveforms. *Bottom*: For a different fibre (CF: 6 kHz), the relation between the coefficient of synchronization (100 per cent = perfect phase locking) and the stimulus frequency. Above 4–5 kHz, phase locking is virtually absent. (Reproduced from Rose et al, 1968 by kind permission of the publishers).

IHCs by intracellular recording (Sellick and Russell, 1978). Here, the AC component of the receptor potential is larger than the DC at low frequencies, becoming gradually relatively smaller as the frequency increases. At higher frequencies it is presumably too small to significantly affect the time pattern of transmitter output at the synapse.

Whether such phase-locked neuron discharges are used or usable by the brain centres for distinguishing different *frequencies* of the stimulus is an open question— it is possible that at low frequencies such information is useful in addition to that provided by the location of the stimulus on the basilar membrane (place-principle) which, at low frequencies, is not highly selective. The phase information preserved in neuron discharges is, however, certainly used by the brain for *sound localisation*. Here, the relative time of arrival of phase-locked action potentials from the two ears (presumably at the superior olive) can be used to determine the ear at which the stimulus arrived first and hence contribute to the localisation of the sound source.

Cochlear potentials

It may have surprised some readers that the various cochlear potentials, which have been so extensively investigated in the past, have so far hardly been mentioned. This reflects in part a real change which has occurred in the research carried out in this field and in part a realisation that a detailed understanding of these potentials no longer forms a necessary preliminary to a discussion on internal ear function. In order to integrate important previous work, however, they do need to be briefly discussed (see also Dallos, 1973; 1978).

The *endocochlear potential* (EP) has been mentioned previously. It is a positive potential of some 80 to 100 mV in scala media whose generation depends on an intact supply of oxygenated blood to the stria vascularis. A lack of oxygen leads to the scala media dropping to a potential of -30 to -40 mV in a few minutes, this potential being close to a diffusion potential expected to be set up by the potassium ions in scala media (in high concentration) diffusing out. Classically, the endo-lymph and thus the EP, has been considered to be in contact with the surface of the spiral organ (e.g. Davis, 1960) so that the EP would form a battery helping to drive K^+ ions through the hair cells, thus sensitising them to mechanical stimuli. This classical view may be incorrect (Lawrence et al, 1973; Manley and Kronester-Frei, 1980b) and the EP may have a different function, or (an) additional function(s).

Another steady potential, this time a negative one, was often stated to be present in the spiral organ (the 'organ of Corti potential'). This has repeatedly been shown to be an artefact (e.g. Manley and Kronester-Frei, 1980b).

Two other important cochlear potentials, both stimulus-related, are the *summating potential* (SP) and the *cochlear microphonic* (CM). Both of these can be recorded from almost anywhere in or near the cochlea, but their sign and/or magnitude depend on the location of the recording electrode(s) and the frequency and intensity of the stimulus. Several useful reviews can be consulted for details of these factors. It will be sufficient here to mention some basic findings. It appears that these potentials are wholly or almost wholly generated by the hair cells. Large electrodes pick up potentials generated by large numbers of hair cells, and the interpretation of these potentials is complicated by the fact that it is not possible to define the area from which they originate with any degree of accuracy. In addition, the various generators are not necessarily operating in phase or with the same output strength. The OHCs seem to dominate the production of these potentials (Dallos et al, 1972 a and b) even more than one would expect from their dominant numbers. This has led to the idea that the OHCs shunt more current than IHCs, which is probably directly or indirectly related to the mechanisms of hair-cell interactions discussed above. Thus the CM, which is an AC signal with the same frequency as the stimulus, and the SP, which is a DC shift in the magnitude of the EP and attributable to the presence of the stimulus, are regarded as reflecting hair-cell activity in a general way. Their interpretation is, however, not easy, so that as soon as intracellular hair-cell recordings were available, with intracellular AC and DC receptor potentials, the tendency was to concentrate on the latter as being more easily interpreted. The cochlear potentials do have the great advantage of ease of recording and have provided and still provide useful measures of cochlear function.

The last important cochlear potential is that generated by the summed activity of the responding nerve fibres, the *compound action potential* (CAP) (Fig. 2.18). Again, the actual determination of the origin of the electrical activity giving rise to the recorded potential is not straight-forward, and requires highly defined and refined stimuli. The ease of recording this signal, however, makes it a useful clinical tool for attempting to define sites of hair cell damage, etc. Recently there have been many investigations of the extent to which these CAPs can be used as a diagnostic tool, and attempts to understand their origin (see e.g. Eldredge, 1978; Antoli-Candela and Kiang, 1978).

The processing of auditory information in the brain

The great majority of the approximately 30 000 afferent auditory nerve fibres from one cochlea in man connect the IHCs with second-order neurons of the cochlear nuclei. These fibres form a large array spread out in space in the cochlea and innervating regions of the spiral organ which differ in their preferred frequency of stimulation. It has been shown repeatedly that the afferent fibres from the cochlea project *systematically* to the brain and, indeed, that central pathways and nuclei are organised in clear geometrical arrangements. Thus the peripheral distribution of frequencies achieved by the response properties of the basilar membrane—spiral organ complex is preserved to a great extent (at least in some parts of the pathway) all the way up to the auditory cortex. This representation of frequency according to the place of stimulation or the location of certain cells in an array is called a *tonotopic organisation.*

Ignoring the effects of the auricle (pinna) on an acoustic stimulus, it can be said that the information in the auditory nerve of one side contains no information as to the *location of the stimulus in space.* Thus, as compared to the visual system, it is necessary in the auditory system for there to be an extensive exchange of information between the two sides of the brain in order to extract information concerning source location through a comparison of sound intensity, phase and latency. This interaction occurs first between third-order neurons in the superior olivary complex in the brainstem (Fig. 2.19) and at higher brain levels.

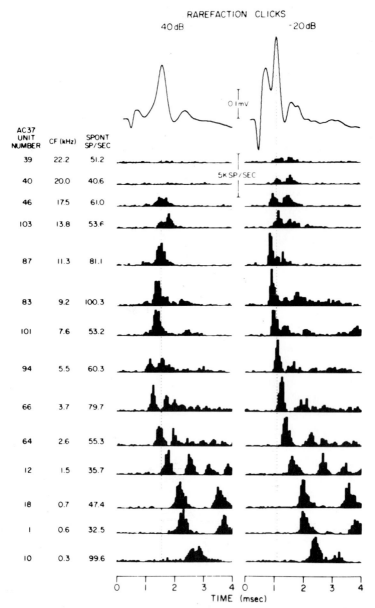

Fig. 2.18 Post-stimulus-time histograms for 14 units in the cat auditory nerve to rarefaction click stimuli at two levels (−40 dB and −20 dB from maximum output). Characteristic frequencies range from 0·3 to 22·2 kHz. Compound action potential (CAP) responses to the same stimuli are shown at the top. It can be seen that mid-and high-frequency units contribute prominently to the CAP. (Reproduced from Antoli-Candela and Kiang, 1978 by permission of the publishers).

Most investigations of the activity of auditory neurons in the brain have failed to produce the *full documentation* of responses to steady and dynamic, complex stimuli necessary for a good understanding of information processing (Webster and Aitkin, 1975). There has been a tendency to concentrate on looking at responses to pure tone stimuli presented by a fixed sound source to one ear only. While this

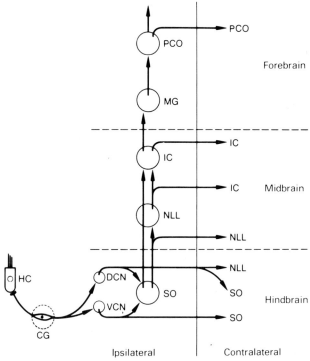

Fig. 2.19 Highly simplified diagram of the main afferent pathways of the auditory brain. HC—hair cell; CG—cochlear ganglion; DCN—dorsal cochlear nucleus; VCN—ventral cochlear nucleus; SO—superior olive; MTB—medial nucleus of the trapezoid body; NLL—nucleus of the lateral lemniscus; IC—inferior colliculus; MG—medial geniculate; PCO—primary cortex.

approach may be justified for studying the peripheral organ and auditory nerve, it produces a totally inadequate and probably misleading picture of the auditory pathway. To make matters worse, most early data was collected in *anaesthetised preparations*. It is now known that anaesthesia has a dramatic effect on the resting and response activity of cells in the auditory pathway, even at levels as low as the cochlear nucleus (Brugge and Geisler, 1978; Webster and Aitkin, 1975). For these reasons, our present understanding of information processing in the auditory brain is somewhat confused and inadequate.

The principal nuclei of the main auditory pathway are shown schematically with their main connections in Figure 2.19. All information in the primary afferents is received and recoded in the *cochlear nuclear complex*. The primary fibres bifurcate, sending an ascending branch to the anteroventral cochlear nucleus (AVCN) and a descending branch to both the posteroventral cochlear nucleus (PVCN) and the dorsal cochlear nucleus (DCN). These three main divisions have been recognised anatomically in many mammals, including man, and can be sub-divided into numerous smaller cell groups. The tonotopic organisation is complete and orderly and isofrequency sheets of cells are found. The diversity in the morphology of the cells and their terminals is reflected in the variety of their response properties. While many cells of the AVCN respond in a similar fashion to auditory nerve fibres, many PVCN cells are excited by some tones and only inhibited by others.

Inhibitory influences are most pronounced in the diverse and complex response activity of DCN cells. These cells apparently also receive second-order input from the AVCN. These cells often not only show excitation to some frequencies and inhibition to others, but also have a complex time course of activity, with 'on' and/or 'off' activity at the beginning and end of the stimulus respectively. It is often not possible to predict a cell's response to a complex sound, such as white noise, from a knowledge of its responses to simpler sounds. Some cells do not even respond to pure tones presented alone.

Neurons of the *superior olivary complex* are found in a number of subdivisions, and receive input from both cochlear nuclear complexes. It is suspected that the cells receiving this binaural input play an important role in extracting, for example, information related to the location of a sound source. Some cells seem to have their activity primarily determined by the average binaural intensity level. Other cells, in contrast, are sensitive to interaural intensity changes. Yet other cells are sensitive to differences in the time of arrival of the stimuli at the two ears, individual cells often to a preferred delay time (Brugge and Geisler, 1978).

At higher levels of the auditory pathway, such as the *inferior colliculus*, *medial geniculate* and *primary auditory cortex*, the cell responses become increasingly complex. An earlier notion that frequency selectivity became greater at higher levels of the brain has been superseded by the finding that cells in higher centres show a greater variety of selectivity. Although some cells are indeed more sharply tuned, others are much broader than primary fibres, having sometimes W-shaped 'tuning curves'. Again, responses to single tones often show enormous variety in the frequency, time and intensity domains. In general, cells seem able to select out certain specific stimulus configurations and their response specificity cannot usually be predicted from a knowledge of their responses to simple stimuli. At these levels also, the state of arousal or attentiveness of the organism plays an important role, via influences from centrifugal fibres; that is, the 'significance' of the stimulus seems to be important. There is also often a sensitivity only to complex sounds originating in a certain defined location in space.

It is tempting, in observing the highly individualistic responses of, say, cortical neurons and their selective responses to specific vocalisations to suggest the presence of *feature detectors* which respond only to certain highly complex and significant stimuli. However, before such speculations can have a firm foundation, it is necessary to study the responses of such neurons much more extensively. Thus we are still a long way away from understanding the neurophysiological basis of speech analysis.

ACKNOWLEDGEMENTS

Thanks are due to Professor Eberhard Zwicker and Dr Karen Steel for very valuable discussions and comments on an early version of the manuscript.

REFERENCES

Ades H W, Engström H 1974 Anatomy of the inner ear. Handbook of sensory physiology, V/1, auditory system. Springer Verlag, Berlin, Ch 5 p 125–158
Aitkin L 1979 The auditory midbrain. Trends in neurosciences 2: 308–310

Antoli-Candela F Jr, Kiang N Y S 1978 Unit activity underlying the N_1 potential. In: Naunton R F Fernández C (eds) Evoked electrical activity in the auditory nervous system. Academic Press, New York, pp 165–191

Békésy G von 1960 Experiments in hearing. Trans Wever E G. McGraw-Hill, New York

Boer E de 1969 Reverse correlation II: initiation of nerve impulses in the inner ear. Koninkl. Nederl. Akademie van Wetenschappen, Proceedings, Series C, 72, 129–151

Brugge J F, Geisler C D 1978 Auditory mechanisms of the lower brainstem. Annual Review of Neuroscience I : 363–394

Dallos P, Billone M C, Durrant J D, Wang C-Y, Raynor S 1972a. Cochlear inner and outer hair cells: functional differences Science 177 : 356–358

Dallos P, Schoeny Z G, Cheatham M A 1972b Cochlear summating potentials: descriptive aspects. Acta Oto-Laryngologica, Suppl. 302

Dallos P 1973 The auditory periphery—biophysics and physiology. Academic Press, New York

Dallos P 1975 Electrical correlates of mechanical events in the cochlea. Audiology 14 : 408–418

Dallos P 1978 Cochlear electrophysiology. In: Naunton R F Fernández C (eds) Evoked electrical activity in the auditory nervous system. Academic Press, New York, pp 141–150

Davis H 1960 Mechanism of excitation of auditory nerve impulses. In: Rasmussen G L, Windle W (eds) Neural mechanisms of the auditory and vestibular systems. Thomas, Springfield, Ill. Ch. 2 pp 21–39

Davis H 1968 Mechanisms of the inner ear. Annals of Otology, Rhinology and Laryngology 77 : 644–655

Eldredge D H 1978 Interpretation of evoked neural responses: facts and illusions related to the methods for recording whole-nerve action potentials. In: Naunton R F, Fernández C (eds) Evoked electrical activity in the auditory nervous system. Academic Press, New York, pp 151–164

Evans E F 1972 The frequency response and other properties of single fibres in the guinea pig cochlear nerve. Journal of Physiology 226 : 263–287

Evans E F 1974 Auditory frequency selectivity and the cochlear nerve. In: Zwicker E, Terhardt E (eds) Facts and models in hearing. Springer Verlag, New York, pp 118–129

Evans E F 1975 Normal and abnormal functioning of the cochlear nerve. Symposia of the Zoological Society of London 37 : 133–165

Evans E F, Wilson J P 1973 The frequency selectivity of the cochlea. In: Møller A R (ed). Basic mechanisms in Hearing. Academic Press, New York, pp 519–551

Evans E F, Wilson J P 1975 Cochlear tuning properties: concurrent basilar membrane and single nerve fiber measurements. Science 190 : 1218–1221

Hartline H K, Ratliff F 1957 Inhibitory interaction of receptor units in the eye of limulus. Journal of General Physiology 40 : 1357–1376

Hinojosa R 1977 A note on the development of Corti's organ. Acta Otolaryngologica 84 : 238–251

Johnstone B M, Taylor K J, Boyle A J 1970 Mechanics of the guinea pig cochlea. The Journal of the Acoustical Society of America 47 : 504–509

Johnstone B M, Taylor K J 1971 Physiology of the middle ear transmission system. Journal of the Oto-Laryngological Society of Australia 3 : 226–228

Johnstone B M, Sellick P M 1972 The peripheral auditory apparatus. Quarterly Reviews of Biophysics 5 : 1–57

Kemp D T 1978 Stimulated acoustic emissions from within the human auditory system. The Journal of the Acoustical Society of America 64 : 1386–1391

Kemp D T, Chum R A 1980 Observations on the generator mechanism of stimulus frequency acoustic emissions—two tone suppression. In: Van den Brink G, Bilsen F A (eds) Psychophysical, physiological and behavioural studies in hearing. Delft University Press

Kiang N Y-S, Watanabe T, Thomas E C, Clark L F 1965 Discharge patterns of single fibres in the cat's auditory nerve. Research Monograph No. 35. The MIT Press, Cambridge, Mass

Kim D O, Neely S T, Molnar C E, Matthews J W 1980 An active cochlear model with negative damping in the partition: comparison with Rhode's ante- and post-mortem observations. In: Von den Brink G, Bilsen F A (eds). Psychophysical, physiological and behavioural studies in hearing. Delft University Press

Kronester-Frei A 1978 Ultrastructure of the different zones of the tectorial membrane. Cell and Tissue Research 193 : 11–23

Kronester-Frei A 1979 Localisation of the Marginal Zone of the Tectorial Membrane in Situ, Unfixed, and with in Vivo-like Ionic Milieu. Archives of Oto-Rhino-Laryngology 224 : 3–9

Lawrence M, Nuttall A L, Clapper M P 1973 Electrical potentials and fluid boundaries within the organ of Corti. The Journal of the Acoustical Society of America 55 : 122–138

LePage E L, Johnstone B M 1980 Basilar membrane mechanics in the guinea pig cochlea—details of nonlinear frequency response characteristics. The Journal of the Acoustical Society of America 67, Suppl. 1, S 45

LePage E L, Johnstone B M, Roberston D 1980 Basilar membrane mechanics in the guinea pig cochlea—comparison of normals with kanamycin-treated animals. The Journal of the Acoustical Society of America 67, Suppl. 1, S 46

Lim D J 1972 Fine morphology of the tectorial membrane—its relationship to the organ of Corti. Archives of Otolaryngology 96:199–215

Lim D J 1980 Cochlear anatomy related to cochlear mechanics. A review. The Journal of the Acoustical Society of America 67:1686–1695

Lynn P A, Sayers B McA 1970 Cochlear innervation, signal processing and their relation to auditory time-intensity effects. The Journal of the Acoustical Society of America 47:525–533

Manley G A 1978 Cochlear frequency sharpening—a new synthesis. Acta Oto-Laryngologica 85:167–176

Manley G A, Robertson D 1976 Analysis of spontaneous activity of auditory neurons in the spiral ganglion of the guinea pig cochlea. Journal of Physiology 258:323–336

Manley G A, Kronester-Frei A 1980a Organ of Corti: observation technique in the living animal. Hearing Research 2:87–91

Manley G A, Kronester-Frei A 1980b The electrophysiological profile of the organ of Corti. In: Van den Brink G, Bilsen F A (eds) Psychophysical, physiological and behavioural studies in hearing. Delft University Press

Moore B C J 1977 Introduction to the psychology of hearing. McMillan, London

Morgan D E, Dirks D D, Kamm C 1977 The influence of middle-ear muscle contraction on auditory threshold for selected pure tones. The Journal of the Acoustical Society of America 63:1896–1903

Mountain D C 1980 COCB Stimulation alters cochlear mechanics as reflected in ear-canal pressure measurements. The Journal of the Acoustical Society of America 67, Suppl. 1, S 89

Rhode W S 1971 Observations of the vibration of the basilar membrane in squirrel monkeys using the Mössbauer technique. The Journal of the Acoustical Society of America 49:1218–1231

Rhode W S 1973 An investigation of post-mortem cochlear mechanics using the Mössbauer effect. In: Møller A R (ed) Basic mechanisms in hearing. Academic Press, New York, pp 49–67

Robertson D, Manley G A 1974 Manipulation of frequency analysis in the cochlear ganglion of the guinea pig. Journal of Comparative Physiology 91:363–375

Rose J E, Brugge J F, Anderson D J, Hind J E 1968 Patterns of activity in single auditory-nerve fibres of the squirrel monkey. In: Reuck A V S, Knight J (eds) Hearing mechanisms in vertebrates. Ciba Foundation Symposium. Churchill, London

Rubinstein M, Feldman B, Fischler H, Frei E H, Spira D 1966 Measurement of stapedial-footplate displacements during transmission of sound through the middle ear. Journal of the Acoustical Society of America 40:1420–1426

Russell I J, Sellick P M 1977a, Tuning properties of cochlear hair cells. Nature 267:858–860

Russell I J, Sellick P 1977b The tuning properties of cochlear hair cells and Addendum. In: Evans E F, Wilson J P (eds) Psychophysics and physiology of hearing. Academic Press, London, pp 71–84

Sachs M B, Abbas P J 1974 Rate versus level functions for auditory-nerve fibres in cats: tone-burst stimuli. The Journal of the Acoustical Society of America 56:1835–1847

Sellick P M, Russell I J 1978 Intracellular studies of cochlear hair cells: filling the gap between basilar membrane mechanics and neural excitation. In: Naunton R F, Fernández C (eds) Evoked electrical activity in the auditory nervous system. Academic Press, New York, pp 113–139

Shaw E A G 1974 Transformation of sound pressure level from the free field to the eardrum in the horizontal plane. The Journal of the Acoustical Society of America 56:1848–1861

Smith C A 1978 Structure of the cochlear duct. In: Naunton R F, Fernández C (eds) Evoked electrical activity in the auditory nervous system. Academic Press, New York, pp 3–19

Spoendlin H 1975 Neuroanatomical basis of cochlear coding mechanisms. Audiology 14:383–407

Spoendlin H 1978 The afferent innervation of the cochlea. In: Naunton R F, Fernández C (eds) Evoked electrical activity in the auditory nervous system. Academic Press, New York, pp 21–41

Spoendlin H 1979 Neural connections of the outer hair-cell system. Acta Oto-Laryngologica 87:381–387

Steel K 1980 The proteins of normal and abnormal tectorial membranes. Acta Oto-Laryngologica 89:27–32

Tonndorf J 1960 Shearing motion in scale media of cochlear models. Journal of the Acoustical Society of America 32:238–244

Tonndorf J, Khanna S M 1970 The role of the tympanic membrane in middle ear transmission. Annals of Otology, Rhinology and Laryngology 79:743–753

Warr W B 1978 The olivocochlear bundle: its origins and terminations in the cat. In: Naunton R F, Fernández C (eds) Evoked electrical activity in the auditory nervous system. Academic Press, New York, pp 43–65

Warr W B, Guinan J J Jr 1979 Efferent innervation of the organ of corti: two separate systems. Brain Research 173:152–155

Webster W R, Aitkin L M 1975 Central auditory processing. In: Gazzaniga M S, Blakemore C (eds) Handbook of psychobiology. Academic Press, New York, pp 325–364

Wever E G, Lawrence M 1954 Physiological acoustics. Princeton University Press, Princeton, p 69–114

Wiederhold M L, Kiang N Y-S 1970 Effects of electrical stimulation of the crossed olivo-cochlear bundle on single auditory-nerve fibres in the cat. Journal of the Acoustical Society of America 48 : 950–965

Wilson J P, Johnstone J R 1975 Basilar membrane and middle-ear vibration in guinea pig measured by capacitance probe. Journal of the Acoustical Society of America 57 : 705–723

Zwicker E 1979 A model describing nonlinearities in hearing by active processes with saturation at 40 dB. Biological Cybernetics 35 : 243–250

Zwicker E, Manley G A 1982 The Auditory system of mammals and man. In: Hoppe W, Lohmann W, Markl H, Ziegler H (eds) Biophysics. Springer Verlag, New York

Investigation of disorders of hearing

INTRODUCTION

Hearing disorders are caused by various pathological processes located in different parts of the ear, the vestibulocochlear (eighth cranial) nerve and the parts of the central nervous system which subserve receptive acoustic communication. At the present time we have a rather detailed knowledge of how pathologic processes of different aetiologies affect functioning of the outer and middle ear. Internal ear pathophysiology is less well understood and we have but a very limited knowledge of pathological mechanisms involving central neural pathways and nuclei. The outer and middle ears are easily accessible for observation, surgery, and investigations by histological and microbiological methods. The internal ear and intracranial organs can be observed visually, or specimens taken from them, only at surgery or post-mortem. In addition, physiological mechanisms concerned with the coding and decoding functions of the internal ear and neural pathways are less well known compared to sound conduction by the outer and middle ears.

The disorders of hearing are usually classified from the functional point of view (Davis, 1962) as:

1. Those affecting sound conduction to the cochlea, i.e. conductive hearing disorders
2. Those affecting signal transformation from the mechanical to bioelectrical phenomena in the cochlea, in its sensory and neural units as well as further signal information processing along the cochlear nerve and central pathways and centres, i.e. sensorineural hearing disorders.

Conductive hearing loss implies attenuation of the incoming acoustical signal, although the degree of attenuation can differ at different frequencies, whereas sensorineural disorders include additional auditory malfunctions in complex acoustic signal processing (Davis, 1962). The latter group is thus rather heterogenous because the site of a pathological process ranges from the cochlea to the cerebral cortex, thus affecting various stages of signal analysis.

Sensorineural hearing disorders are classified into the following subgroups:

1. Cochlear.
2. Neural.
3. Central disorders.

The third group can be further subdivided into brain stem and cortical disorders.

The term 'retrocochlear' has been used to encompass both subgroups 2 and 3.

In clinical diagnostic work differentation of the sensorineural subgroups is not always easy or even possible, because our knowledge of the type and extent of the pathology involved is not detailed enough. For example ageing presumably affects different structures and to varying degrees in the cochlear and neural elements (Saxén, 1937; Schuknecht, 1964; 1974).

When facing the task of investigating disorders of hearing the aim is twofold: allocation of the disorder in question to one of the main groups and subgroups outlined above; and, if possible, making an aetiologic diagnosis of the disorder in question.

The first step must, of course, be taken before the second step of specific diagnosis is possible. The latter cannot, or probably even need not, always be made with a high degree of probability. Even the first classification and a lower probability concerning aetiological diagnosis is sometimes a sufficient programme for a patient. Take advanced age as an example. A symmetrical sensorineural hearing impairment falling off at an increasing rate towards higher frequencies is usually enough to furnish a diagnosis of presbyacusis. It is difficult to make a more definite diagnosis as to its metabolic, circulatory or degenerative aetiology. Or consider a sudden sensorineural hearing loss as another example. A pure tone audiometric sensorineural curve with a sharp fall off to high frequencies and a history of sudden onset is often as far as we can get. Whether the aetiology is infective, toxic, metabolic, circulatory or even traumatic remains usually obscure even by the methods of investigation currently available.

The methods used for investigation of disorders of hearing include:

1. Anamnesis (case history).
2. Ear examination with otoscopy.
3. Examination of the function of the auditory (Eustachian) tube.
4. Hearing tests employing psychoacoustic methods using different aspects and attributes of audition.
5. Measurements of the acoustic impedence of the ear under different conditions.
6. Electrophysiological measurements of bioelectric potentials which are presumed to arise in the ear and along the neural auditory pathways and other parts of the central nervous systems.
7. Radiologic examination of the temporal bone and of intracranial structures, perhaps employing contrast media and computer techniques.
8. Examination of the function of the vestibular organ of the labyrinth.
9. Histological, microbiological and biochemical examinations of specimens obtained during otoscopy or surgery.
10. Diagnostic explorative surgery or diagnostic medication (available in certain cases).
11. Follow-up of the disorder over a period of time.

ANAMNESIS

Probably the most valuable information for the diagnosis of disorders of hearing is the case history. It includes not only the time and type of onset of the hearing loss, its time course and different qualitative aspects of it, but even other symptoms associated with the hearing loss such as pain and discomfort of the ear, sense of fullness and pressure in the ear, secretion, its quality, quantity and smell, vertigo or dizziness or other features of balance problems, tinnitus, headache and symptoms from other cranial nerves as well as from various regions of the central nervous system (Hinchcliffe, 1979).

Type of onset
It is important to record the type of onset of the hearing loss. Cases of abrupt hearing loss are referred to either as acute hearing loss, acute auditory failure or sudden deafness; terms often used as a diagnosis although the aetiological background includes a number of different pathologies (Saunders, 1972). The moment the hearing loss occurs may be so distinct that the patient is able to give the exact time of it. Sometimes it developes during a period of a few minutes or a few hours. Abrupt onset is, of course, often the case with traumatic hearing loss, where the aetiology, although not the pathology is also obvious. An abrupt onset is dramatically experienced by the patient even when it is question of only a moderate loss.

The majority of the hearing disorders, however, have a gradual onset which is not assignable to a specific day, week or even month. In presbyacusis the onset is so gradual that the patient himself may not be aware of the hearing disorder until it has progressed to a severe degree. It is often the relatives, who first point out that the person is 'hard-of-hearing'. Likewise otosclerosis has a gradual onset.

Time course
The time course of the disorder should also be noted. Presbyacusis typically progresses gradually (Hinchcliffe, 1959; Spoor and Passchier-Vermeer, 1969). The rate can vary, depending on the general health of the elderly patient. Rapid progression, indicating risk for complete deafness in the near future, is an alarming sign; any previous aetiological diagnosis should be reconsidered. In traumatic hearing loss and cases of acute hearing loss (sudden deafness) spontaneous improvement, or improvement following treatment can occur and it usually takes a few weeks before a steady state in hearing threshold is reached. In some cases there is no measurable threshold improvement but the patient learns to use the disordered hearing better for auditory communication.

Fluctuation of hearing
An important symptom of a hearing disorder is the fluctuation of hearing. It occurs typically in Ménière's disease, usually as a variation of the low frequency thresholds. In that disease fluctuations coincide with variations in the tinnitus and are associated with attacks of vertigo. Other fluctuating hearing disorders occur on other aetiological bases.

Perception of speech
Information from the patient regarding perception of speech and other acoustic signals in the environment can give an indication of the relative threshold losses for the different frequencies. Typically high frequency hearing loss results in difficul-

ties in the detection of signals from the door bell and the telephone as well as inability to hear environmental sounds such as those from birds and grasshoppers. Typically, too, a high frequency hearing loss is a greater handicap in noisy surroundings arising from either industrial or traffic noise or competing speech, such as in parties and larger groups of people (Aniansson, 1973). Similarly reverberation in halls with poor acoustic absorption in particular impairs the auditory communication ability of patients with a high frequency hearing loss. The reason is that the effect of masking* by low frequency sounds in environmental noise and competing speech (Miller, 1947; Kryter, 1950) spreads to the high frequencies. Patients themselves even report spontaneously that, in noise, they hear but are unable to discriminate speech. In certain disorders of hearing, especially presbyacusis, speech discrimination in noise is particularly sensitive to masking (Palva, 1955a; Jokinen, 1973).

Asymmetry of symptoms
The history of the hearing disorder recorded from the patient naturally includes information on the degree of asymmetry of the symptoms. Some types of hearing disorders, for example, presbyacusis, are typically symmetrical, whereas others are mainly unilateral, e.g. acute hearing losses and vestibulocochlear nerve schwannomas. Thus asymmetrical sensorineural hearing disorders cannot be considered to be presbyacusis only; a tumour of the vestibulocochlear nerve should be suspected unless proven otherwise (Palva et al, 1978).

The quality and quantity of the valuable information which the patient can provide by his case history depends greatly on the conditions under which the patient is living and communicating. Patients who are active in certain occupations (musicians, teachers, service occupations, etc) need more perfect hearing to fulfil their duties successfully than do elderly retired patients mainly communicating in quiet conditions at home.

Discomfort
Attention should also be paid to other auditory signs such as discomfort experienced from loud sounds and diplacusis. This is experienced by everyone provided that the sound pressure level is high enough, but certain cases discomfort is already reached at lower stimulus levels, a symptom usually associated with a phenomenon termed loudness recruitment. In some cases it may be very irritating for the patient and can occur also without any measurable hearing loss. Diplacusis refers to a phenomenon whereby a single sound stimulus gives rise to the perception of two sounds. These two sounds may be in the same ear (monaural diplacusis) or in different ears (binaural diplacusis). Both types of diplacusis are associated with cochlear hearing disorders.

Tinnitus
Tinnitus is the perception of a sound that cannot be related to a specific external sound source. It often causes annoyance and concern to the patient. Its onset, quality, intensity and time course are often recorded. Such information seldom

* The ability of one sound (simple or complex) to raise the threshold of audibility of another sound.

gives direct evidence for a specific pathology. Tinnitus can occur in connection with any kind of hearing disorder (Fowler, 1940; Nodar, 1978). It sometimes occurs even in patients without any measurable hearing loss (Heller and Bergman, 1953). Sometimes tinnitus is objectively audible to the examiner on auscultation. It may then be due to vascular malformations in the region of the ear or to spontaneous contractions of the muscles of the middle ear or of the auditory tube. In the majority of cases tinnitus is, however, only subjective and we have no verified explanation of its pathological mechanism. The subject of tinnitus is of such importance that a separate chapter (Ch. 7) is allocated to it.

As stated above, all other symptoms from the ear and other organs surrounding the ear should be considered and recorded in the case history. Attention should be paid to the temporal relations between other symptoms and the hearing disorder itself. The correlation of the onset of the hearing loss with infections, use of drugs, exposure to trauma or to noise, affliction with cardiovascular and neurological diseases, physical and psychological stress, and pregnancy occuring prior to, or concurrent with, abnormal hearing may give valuable indications of a possible aetiology. Finally, other risk factors should be sought such as a family history of hearing disorders. Hereditary factors are of importance even when the onset of the hearing disorder is in adult or advanced age.

AUDIOMETRY

After acquisition of the case history various hearing measurements by psycho-acoustic methods constitute the bases for the investigation of disorders of hearing. The central role is played by the threshold of hearing for pure tones, but it should always be born in mind that it portrays only one, and a limited, aspect of audition. Suprathreshold measures are sometimes of equal importance and the audiometric tests are by no means complete without them.

Threshold tonal audiometry
The threshold of hearing for pure tones is recorded for both air and bone conduction signals by conventional audiometric methods. Air conduction measurements must be obtained using earphones placed properly on the external ear with headbands (Figs. 3.1 to 3.3).

Bone conduction thresholds are measured by bone conduction receivers placed on the mastoid or forehead (Hulka, 1941; Lierle and Reger, 1946; Rainville, 1955; Naunton, 1957; Palva, 1958.) Using appropriate masking of the opposite ear (Zwislocki, 1951; 1953; 1960; Lidén et al, 1959; Naunton, 1960; Studebaker, 1962; Lidén, 1971), the investigation provides reliable pure tone thresholds even in severe hearing disorders.

Threshold is defined as the signal level giving rise to an auditory sensation in more than 50 per cent of presentations (Carhart and Jerger, 1959). The reader is refered to textbooks in audiology and other papers on threshold determination and on guidelines for masking (Hirsh, 1952; Hinchcliffe and Littler, 1958; Ventry et al, 1971).

The difference between pure tone air and bone conduction thresholds, frequently referred to as the 'air-bone gap', usually differentiates between a conduc-

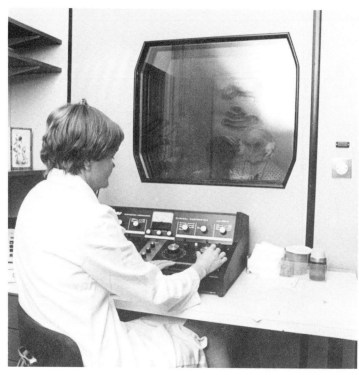

Fig. 3.1 Pure tone threshold audiometry being conducted on an elderly patient seated in an audiometric booth. The audiometer is being operated by an audiometrician and the pure tone threshold of hearing is recorded on a chart which is termed an audiogram.

tive and a sensorineural hearing disorder. In conductive disorders, air conduction thresholds (as referred to the international standard value used for the calibration of audiometers) are elevated, whereas bone conduction thresholds are within normal limits. In conductive disorders, outer or middle ear pathology implies attenuation for the input sound signal. In sensorineural disorders, air and bone conduction values overlap since the conductive middle ear mechanism is working normally. In combined cases (mixed hearing loss) air conduction thresholds are poorer than bone conduction thresholds.

Psychoacoustic audiometry requires cooperation by the patient, understanding of instructions and alertness. Problems arise in cases of exaggeration of losses, reduced intelligence, reduced alertness and senility. In psychoacoustic measurements the criteria used by aged subjects can differ from those used by younger adults, the elderly being more cautious (Potash and Jones, 1977). In every case where the reliability of responses is suspect the results should be checked by other means, both clinical (including the use of tuning forks and voice tests) and audiometric (other threshold determinations) (Fletcher, 1929). The Rinne test and sound lateralisation in asymmetrical cases measured by the Weber test provide information which can be used to confirm the outcome of a pure tone audiometric threshold determination (Groen, 1962). Conductive hearing loss is associated with a true negative Rinne response and, in the Weber test, sound lateralisation towards the ear with conductive impairment. With the use of tuning forks, however, it may

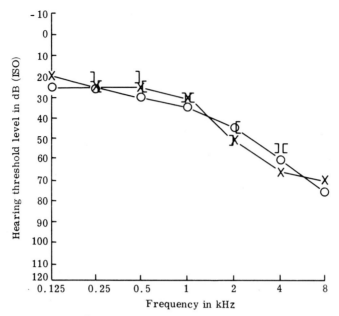

Fig. 3.2 Pure tone audiogram of a patient with a sensorineural hearing loss. The audiogram slopes towards the higher frequencies, as in presbycusis. The air- and bone-conduction threshold values coincide in sensorineural hearing loss.
Symbols: o air conduction, right
             x air conduction, left
             [bone conduction, right
             ] bone conduction, left.

be difficult to obtain exact and reliable quantitative date on the degree of hearing loss at different frequencies although previous generations of audiologists succeeded in doing so. Every audiogram must in addition be evaluated in the light of the findings from otoscopy, including testing the mobility of the tympanic membrane and the existence of an aerated tympanic cavity using a pneumatic speculum. Obstruction by cerumen and collapse of the ear canal resulting from connective tissue degeneration in the elderly must be excluded as erroneous sources of air-bone gap (Ventry et al, 1961; Hildyard and Valentine, 1962).

When a conductive hearing disorder has been detected, verified and quantified, further investigation by other methods should be directed at a more detailed diagnosis of the type of pathology. From a functional point of view patients with purely conductive hearing disorders are able to use their suprathreshold hearing for communication without difficulties provided the conductive air-bone gap is compensated by adequate amplification. This implies that these individuals demonstrate normal results in other suprathreshold auditory tests (see later). Sometimes, however, in spite of a conductive loss, patients exhibit signs of recruitment (Anderson and Barr, 1960). This can be the case, for example in otosclerosis (Palva et al, 1975). Likewise a lower threshold of uncomfortable loudness can be measured among the elderly which is out of proportion to the conductive gap at threshold level.

If pure tone threshold audiometry indicates a sensorineural hearing disorder and it is compatible with the findings from the otoscopic examination, further

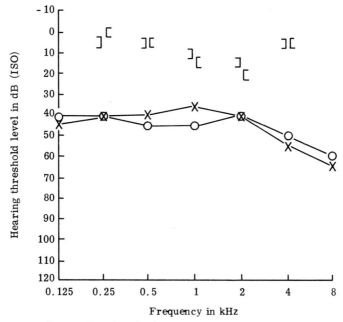

Fig. 3.3 Pure tone audiogram of a patient showing separation of the air- and bone-conduction thresholds, indicating conductive hearing loss. The slight (20 dB HL) notch at 2 kHz on the bone conduction audiogram is commonly found in conductive hearing loss. It is referred to as Carhart's notch and it does not indicate a sensorineural hearing loss. It is mechanical in origin and due to the exclusion of the normal effects of middle ear resonance on auditory acuity as measured by bone conduction audiometry. See caption of Fig. 3.2 for key to symbols.

psycho-acoustic measurements can be carried out for defining the subgroup of sensorineural disorders in question. For this purpose several measurements are employed which characterise hearing at suprathreshold levels, viz:

1. Speech perception.
2. Loudness recruitment.[*]
3. Auditory adaptation.
4. Differential intensity and/or frequency sensitivity.
5. Comfortable and uncomfortable levels of hearing.
6. Directional hearing.
7. A number of other features of loudness and pitch perception mon- or binaurally measured.

Speech audiometry
Speech is certainly the most important of the complex acoustic signals to which man attends. Speech perception depends upon several features of speech stimuli, which contribute to extrinsic redundancy, as well as upon linguistic parameters of the test material, which contribute to intrinsic redundancy (Teatini, 1970; Jauhiainen, 1976). Both sets of variables can be manipulated seperately in order to obtain a speech discrimination test suitable to the audiologic diagnostic problem in

---

[*] The growth of loudness (the subjective magnitude of sound intensity) more rapidly than normal.

question. Conventionally, a performance intensity function is constructed, with the test word sound level as the stimulus measure and the percentage of correct items indentified as the response measure. The stimulus measure is plotted on the horizontal axis, and the response measure on the vertical axis of a graph termed a speech audiogram. Usually a sigmoid function results where the stimulus level corresponding to 50 per cent correct identification is called the speech reception threshold (SRT). The point of maximal discrimination is recorded usually some 30 dB above the speech reception threshold (Hudgins et al, 1947; Egan, 1948; Hirsh, 1952; Hahlbrock, 1970) (Fig. 3.4).

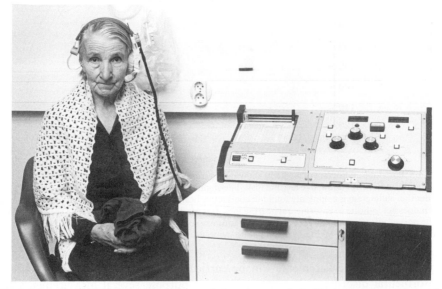

Fig. 3.4 An elderly patient being tested by acoustic impedance methods. She is wearing a headset with a probe for the measurement of the acoustic impedance in the right ear; an earphone is applied to the left ear. A plotter, on the left hand side of the equipment, records impedance changes.

Conventional speech audiometry employs two types of word lists. Disyllabic spondee words with higher intrinsic redundancy provide a performance intensity function which runs steeply in the region of 50 per cent discrimination resulting in only a small variation of the speech reception threshold. For the measurement of maximal discrimination, monosyllabic test words, usually constituting phonetically balanced lists, are used. These possess less internal redundancy and thus result, even in cases with normal hearing, in a maximal word discrimination score of somewhat less than 100 per cent (French and Steinberg, 1947). This kind of material is thus more sensitive to speech discrimination loss than the more redundant bisyllabic test word material. The degree of redundancy varies in different language domains.

A multitude of other types of speech material is also sometimes used for routine speech audiometry. For special purposes, numerals, sentences, either natural or synthetic, nonsense words and logatomes have been used (Teatini, 1970).

The speech reception threshold bears a distinct relation to the mean pure tone threshold, usually expressed as the average of thresholds recorded at 0·5, 1 and

2 kHz (Fletcher, 1929; Carhart, 1946). Thus the speech reception threshold can be used for authentication of the pure tone threshold audiogram. This is useful in cases such as suspected malingering or functional hearing loss.

The percentage of maximal speech discrimination provides more diagnostic information. A lot of evidence shows that a notable discrimination loss is encountered specifically in retrocochlear disorders (Walsh and Goodman, 1955). However, the speech discrimination loss also depends on the degree of the average pure tone loss even in cochlear disorders and on the type of audiogram as well as the age of the patient (Gaeth, 1948; Bergman et al, 1976). Steeply sloping high frequency losses usually result in a low discrimination score even in the absence of a retrocochlear pathology (Aniansson, 1973).

Manipulation of the extrinsic redundancy of speech audiometric test word material is achieved by such means as:

1. Decreasing the signal-to-noise ratio or the signal level (Jauhianen and Nuutila, 1977).
2. Frequency filtering, frequency distortion (Bocca et al, 1954, Hirsh et al, 1954; Palva, 1965; Palva and Jokinen, 1970).
3. Time compression (Calearo and Lazzaroni, 1957; Garvey, 1953; Bocca and Calearo, 1963; de Quiros, 1964).
4. Interruption (Miller and Licklider, 1950; Bocca and Calearo, 1963).
5. Amplitude compression (Lynn and Carhart, 1963; Hohansson, 1973).
6. Frequency transposition (Johansson, 1966).
7. Employing competing speech signals (Jerger, 1964).

Various dichotic and binaural modifications (Cherry and Taylor, 1954; Bocca, 1955; Matzker, 1958; 1962; Linden, 1964) may be used for the purpose of investigating different central phenomena concerned with complex acousticolinguistic signal detection and the influence of central lesions on this analysis. Verified lesions in the temporal lobe of the cerebral cortex, in the auditory projection of the brain as well as in the brain stem have been demonstrated to result in abnormal findings in speech tests of low extrinsic redundancy (Korsan-Bengtsen 1968; 1973).

Suprathreshold tonal audiometry

In subjects with normal hearing the growth of loudness from threshold follows a specific psychophysical power function with a definite slope (Stevens, 1957; 1959). In sensorineural hearing disorders the slope of this function can vary. A steeper slope indicates that new sensory- or neural units are recruited faster with increasing stimulus level (Pohlman and Kranz, 1924; Fowler, 1928; 1936; Denes and Naunton, 1950). Thus a point along the loudness function is reached where equal loudness is obtained in normal and in sensorineurally impaired ears with equal stimulus sound pressure level.

The measurement of loudness function in unilateral cases can be performed with Fowler's (1928) alternate binaural loudness matching method. In bilaterally symmetrical cases, Reger's (1936) monaural bifrequency loudness matching method can be applied. The former method presents, alternatively, pure tone stimuli of the same frequency to the different ears until equal loudness is reported at equal stimulus intensities as an indicator of loudness recruitment. The latter method employs two different frequencies alternatively in the same ear; tones at those two frequencies are matched for loudness. It is usually considered, as suggested by Dix, Hallpike and Hood (1948), that loudness recruitment refers to cochlear pathology and is absent in retrocochlear pathology (Denes and Naunton, 1950; Palva, 1957; Hallpike and Hood, 1959). However, verification of a cochlear versus retrocochlear lesion cannot be done by this method.

One of the suprathreshold psychoacoustical phenomena which has been exploited in clinical investigations of hearing disorders is differential sensitivity to loudness. In subjects with normal hearing this is a function of sensation level so that differential sensitivity is poor near threshold but improves at higher sensation levels (Denes and Naunton, 1950). In cases with sensorineural hearing loss good differential sensitivity is considered to indicate recruitment (Lüscher and Zwislocki, 1947, Lidén and Nilsson, 1953; König, 1962). However, the tests of differential sensitivity of loudness, such as the SISI-test (Jerger et al, 1959), give widely overlapping values in different kinds of sensorineural pathology (Hirsh et al, 1954; Rahko, 1975). Sometimes differential sensitivity to frequency is also used in clinical audiology (Leshowitz et al, 1975). The method of noise audiometry (Langenbeck, 1951; Palva et al, 1953), measurement of the critical band (de Boer, 1959; Scharf and Hellman, 1966) and psychophysical tuning curves (Zwicker and Schorn, 1978) are further attempts to feature aspects of frequency coding and its disorders in the cochlea.

Close to the saturation level of the loudness function lies the threshold of uncomfortable loudness (loudness discomfort level). This occurs before complete saturation is obtained at the threshold of pain. The phenomenon of recruitment implies a reduced dynamic range of hearing, i.e. reduced difference between the threshold of hearing and the saturation level. This can be measured by what Hood and Poole (1966) and Schmitz (1969) term the loudness discomfort level. In the majority of disorders of conductive type there is no reduction of the dynamic range of hearing whether measured by conventional methods or loudness recruitment or by the threshold of uncomfortable loudness. However, sometimes recruitment can be obtained even in conductive disorders (Andersson and Barr, 1960).

Measurement of auditory adaptation
A further feature of hearing impairment is the degree of auditory adaptation occurring during the course of sustained acoustic stimulation. Various methods, using different sensation levels and different durations, are employed to measure the degree of adaptation. In subjects with normal hearing, slight degrees of auditory adaptation may be recorded (Schubert, 1944; Denes and Naunton, 1950; Hood, 1950; 1956; Palva, 1955b; Carhart, 1957; Karja and Palva, 1970). Extensive adaptation is usually attributed to retrocochlear pathology, whereas in cochlear disorders moderate adaptation may be obtained (Hallpike and Hood, 1951; Lierle and Reger, 1955; Palva, 1964; Palva et al, 1967). Adaptation is also a function of the frequency.

Békésy audiometry
One of the methods often used for the measurement of adaptation is a modification of automatic *Békésy-audiometry* (Békésy, 1947) using interrupted and con-

tinuous test tone tracings (Reger and Kos, 1952; Jerger, 1960). An elevation of the threshold of the continuous tone compared to that of the interrupted tone is an indication of the occurrence of adaptation. Forward and reversed continuous tracings are also used for this purpose (Karja and Palva, 1970; Palva and Jauhiainen, 1976). A diminution in the excursion width of Békésy-audiograms is additionally considered to indicate the presence of recruitment, possibly featuring differential sensitivity at threshold (Lundborg, 1952; Palva, 1956).

The above main groups of psycho-acoustic audiometry are applied clinically with various modifications. Several other methods may also be used, among them directional hearing tests (Sanchez-Longo and Forster, 1958; Nordlung, 1963; Groen, 1969). Not all laboratories include all possible methods in their routine battery of tests, but a careful selection is used for differentiating between various types of sensorineural disorders. The ultimate success in differentiation and diagnosis is something less than 100 per cent. Definite correlations between the observed pathology at different sites and the results of psychoacoustic tests still wait for confirmation (Parker et al, 1962). In statistical terms, however, cochlear pathology is characterised by recruitment, absence of, or a moderate degree of, auditory adaptation and good or moderate discrimination of speech.

ACOUSTIC IMPEDANCE STUDIES

In the past two or three decades, psychoacoustic methods to obtain information on the function of the organ of hearing have been supplemented with measurements of the acoustic impedance of the ear. This method provides information on the functional integrity of the ear which is not influenced by the patient's motivation criteria of judgement and which does not require his active cooperation (Fig. 3.5). As a matter of fact, the amount of information available from impedance measurements is so extensive that it is becoming a method applied most frequently next to conventional pure tone threshold audiometry.

The modern equipment used for the measurement of the acoustic impedance of the ear has developed to such a degree of automation and reliability that the method commends itself to routine clinical use. Acoustic impedance is usually measured using a probe tone of 220, 660 or 800 Hz. So-called static impedance which is measured under atmospheric pressure (Zwislocki, 1957) is of less importance because of the rather great inter-individual variability. Relative impedance changes, either due to air pressure changes in the ear (tympanometry) or changes evoked by middle ear muscle reflexes, presumably primarily the stapedius reflex, are most frequently exploited for diagnostic purposes.

Tympanometry refers to the recording of compliance (inverse of acoustic capacitive reactance) as a function of the pressure artificially regulated in the outer ear canal. A tympanometric recording (Fig. 3.6) (tympanogram) primarily reflects the properties of the tympanic membrane, the ossicles and the ventilation of the tympanic cavity. The method is widely used in addition to an otoscopic examination and other conventional means to study the function of the auditory tube and can give further verification and diagnostic information on conductive disorders such as those due to fluid in the middle ear, and tubal occlusion which result in a decreased pressure in the middle ear (Metz, 1946; Terkildsen and Thomsen, 1959;

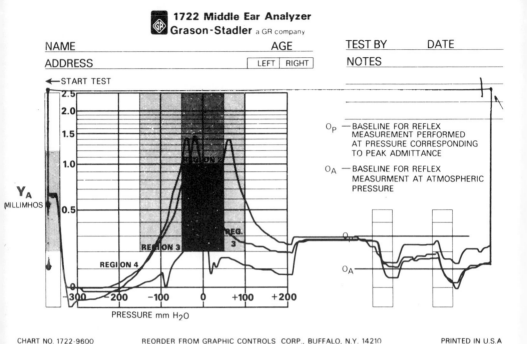

Fig. 3.5 Automatic tympanogram recorded on an otologically normal subject. The middle of the three peaked curves was the first to be recorded; it shows a slight negative middle ear pressure (this is normal) and an admittance of 1·4 siemens (milimhos); the peaked curve to the left was recorded after swallowing with the nose pinched (this aspirates some air from the middle ear cleft); the curve to the right, which shows a peak at about +600 Pa (labelled' +60 mm H_2O' on the graph) has been produced after a Valsalva manoeuvre; this inflates the middle ear cleft and slightly increases the middle ear pressure. The continuation of the tympanograms to the right produces two successive depressions in the tracing; These are two consecutive recordings of the ipsilateral acoustic stapedius reflex (after Hinchcliffe, 1979).

Brooks, 1968; Lidén et al, 1970). However, certain limitations exist, especially in judging conductive disorders postoperatively, the audiometrically measured air-bone-gap does not always accord with abnormal tympanograms and vice versa (Sorri, 1979). In the aged, tympanosclerosis and atrophic changes in the drum membrane may give low or abnormal high compliance values respectively. The use of impedance audiometry to register and measure the stapedius reflex is more valuable for clinical diagnostic purposes than tympanometry alone. Since the whole reflex arc is being studied, the method can be used in the assessment of:

1. The reduced dynamic range of the ear which is stimulated to elicit the reflex. For this purpose the reflex threshold for the stimulated ear is recorded and compared with the hearing threshold of that ear. Conclusions can then be drawn on the dynamic range of the ear and its implications for loundness recruitment (Metz, 1946; Thomsen, 1955; Klockhoff, 1961).
2. The decay of the reflex during sustained stimulation; this is presumed to indicate adaptation of the afferent part ot the reflex arc.

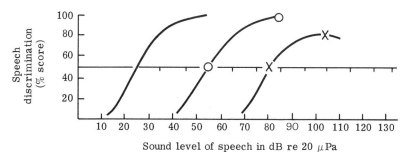

Fig. 3.6 A speech audiogram showing speech discrimination in per cent (per cent of speech items correctly repeated) as a function of sound level of test material. The curve on the left is a normal curve, the middle one shows a speech reception threshold of 30 dB and a maximal discrimination score of 100 per cent. The curve on the right shows a speech reception threshold of 55 dB and a maximal speech discrimination score of 80 per cent.

3. Brain stem pathology, where disruption of the crossing neural pathways may abolish a contralateral reflex leaving the ipsilateral one intact.
4. The function of the facial nerve which innervates the stapedius muscle.
5. Existence of a conductive disorder if equivocal as judged on pure tone air- and bone-conduction audiometry.

Provided that there is no conductive hearing loss or facial nerve palsy on the side where the acoustic impedance is being measured, the stapedius reflex threshold is widely considered as an objective and valid method for measuring the reduced dynamic range of hearing associated with loudness recruitment. For example in bilateral symmetrical losses or with subjects unable to cope with psychoacoustic measurements. A number of studies show elevated reflex thresholds in retrocochlear disorders, where also lack of recruitment or decruitment can be demonstrated (Lidén and Korsan-Bengtsen, 1973). Likewise, objective data on adaptation demonstrated by the reflex decay test points to the possibility of a retrocochlear process (Anderson et al, 1969; 1970).

The advantage of impedance is its objectivity. In addition it is a rather rapid and reproducible procedure. Since even minor conductive disorders can completely abolish an impedance change, the presence of middle ear pathology limits its application for stapedius reflex threshold and decay measurements.

ELECTROPHYSIOLOGICAL INVESTIGATIONS

The past two decades have also seen the introduction of another group of objective methods for investigating the function of the ear and the neural structures involved in audition. The development of electrophysiological techniques: electrodes, amplifiers, filters, and, above all, electronic averaging and other computerised methods of bioelectic signal analysis, has provided equipment for recording minute bioelectric potentials elicited by acoustic stimuli from the background of random neural (or muscular) bioelectric activity arising in various stations along the auditory pathway. With appropriate methods nearly all stations along the auditory pathway from the cochlea to the cortex are now accessible for measurement with noninvasive techniques and with the benefit of obtaining objective recordings. The following groups of potentials are becoming more widely used for clinical diagnostic purposes:

1. Bioelectrical potential of the cochlea, referred to as electrocochleography (Portman et al, 1967; Sohmer and Feinmesser, 1967; Yoshie et al, 1967; Elberling, 1971; Aran and Portman, 1976).
2. Brain stem potentials (Jewett and Williston, 1971; Terkildsen et al, 1973).
3. Slow cortical potentials (Keidel and Spreng, 1963; Davis and Zerlin, 1966).

From the clinical point of view, these methods, designated together as electric response audiometry (ERA), are used in order to:

1. Give information on the hearing level in cases where conventional psychoacoustic methods are not applicable, or are not giving valid results.
2. Give topodiagnostic information on sensorineural disorders, such as cochlear, vestibulocochlear nerve, brain stem or cortical pathology.
3. Give prognostic information in certain cases of sensorineural pathology.

In addition the methods are now being applied to other problems in neurology, especially for the evaluation of brain stem disorders (Robinson and Rudge, 1977).

Threshold determinations by methods of electric response audiometry are applied to cases where conventional psychoacoustic measurements are not successful such as with malingering and mental retardation. Sometimes patients of advanced age are unable to give dependable responses to pure tone audiometry. These patients may be conveniently investigated with brain stem and slow cortical responses. Adults usually give sufficient passive cooperation and the background EEG activity is sufficiently low for valid and reproducible results to be obtained (Beagley and Kellogg, 1969).

Over recent years, ERA-methods have provided increasing topodiagnostic information. Labyrinthine hydrops exhibits a high amplitude negative summation potential which can be used to verify the diagnosis (Schmidt et al, 1974; Eggermont, 1976; Gibson et al, 1977). Abolition of brain stem responses beyond three milliseconds, a greater than normal delay in the Jewett V wave or prolonged conduction time between waves II and V seem to be correlated with cerebellopontine angle lesions causing a retrocochlear disorder (Setters and Branckmann, 1977). In addition, various processes, whether isolated, multiple or diffuse, in the brain stem can abolish or prolong latencies of different wave complexes originating probably in the cochlear, olivary or collicular nuclei of the auditory pathway. Prognostic information may be obtained in cases of acute hearing loss. The amount of information obtained from, and experience derived from, these methods used with verified lesions up till now is still limited to assess the role of these methods in the future.

The benefit of ERA-methods is the objectivity concerning the subject himself, whereas interpretation of the results does not always fulfil the requirements of strict objectivity on the part of the audiologist (Gibson, 1978).

AUDITORY TUBAL FUNCTION MEASUREMENTS

The assessment of the function of the auditory tube is included when the nature and aetiology of conductive hearing disorders is being studied and diagnosed.

Inflammatory pathological processes often involve the tube. This produces morphological changes in the mucous membrane and disorders of function in terms of suppressed ventilation of the tympanic cavity, decreased air pressure in the tympanic cavity, retraction of the tympanic membrane, attenuation of sound conduction through the middle ear and further morphological changes in the structures of the middle ear.

Tubal function can be studied by air flow and air pressure measurements or by acoustic techniques. In addition to conventional clinical methods such as the valsalva (forced expiration against closed mouth and nostrils) or toynbee (swallowing with nostrils and mouth closed) manoeuvres, instrumental methods have been developed. One of them is tympanometry as outlined above (Holmquist, 1969). Tubal occlusion results in abnormal tympanograms. This method, however, is applicable only when the tympanic membrane is intact. Pressure equalisation procedures which introduce either positive or negative pressures into the ear canal and record possible pressure equalisation during swallowing, can give some information (Flisberg et al, 1963; Miller, 1965; Siedentop et al, 1968). However, pressure techniques are not physiological and do not always correlate with, for example, postoperative findings for aerated middle ear cavities.

Acoustic measurement, called sonotubometry i.e. recording changes in sound conduction through the auditory tube, provides more physiological, and thus clinically more valid, information on tubal function in pre- and postoperative evaluations (Virtanen, 1977; Virtanen et al, 1980). This method is also available for the measurement of the patulous tube, a disorder sometimes giving troubling symptoms from the ear without measurable hearing loss.

OTHER INVESTIGATIONS

Although the main emphasis in this chapter is devoted to audiometric methods for investigating disorders of hearing other methods should equally be applied when needed to study the type and location of the pathology causing the hearing disorder.

Radiological investigations

Radiological examination of the ear is of paramount importance. In cases of conductive disorders, such as chronic otitis and its sequelae, as well as suspected middle ear malformations, it is important to define the nature and extent of the pathologic process. Experienced radiodiagnosticians can provide valuable diagnostic information to the clinician. Roentgenograms of the internal acoustic meatus, with and without contrast media, are usually needed before the diagnosis of a suspected cerebellopontine angle process can be made with certainty. Neuroradiography with angiography, pneumoencephalography and computerised axial tomography may also be needed.

Investigation of the vestibular system

Investigations into function and integrity of the vestibular system, especially of the labyrinth, are valuable for diagnosis. Several disorders also involve receptors in the vestibular system of the labyrinth. Quantitative evaluation of the function of the horizontal semicircular canal is possible by caloric stimulation and electro-nystagmographic recordings (Fitzgerald and Hallpike, 1942; Jongkees and Philips-zoon, 1964). Patients with disorders of the labyrinth involving both cochlear and vestibular receptors may or may not have subjective symptoms of vertigo and dizziness, depending on the time course of development of the disorder.

Biochemical microbiological and histological investigations

These give further valuable information for making an aetiological diagnosis. Outer and middle ear pathologic processes are accessible for taking specimens for microscopic observation and microbiological examinations. Information from these investigations is used primarily for outlining the management of the disorders by operative or chemotherapeutic means. The internal ear and the vestibulocochlear nerve, as well as more central neural structures, are accessible for specimens obtained only in connection with operative procedures, or post mortem, for the verification of the pathologic process involved and its location.

Biochemical studies can be done, when effusion, secretion, internal ear fluid or cerebrospinal fluid is available for chemical analysis. However, since we should not forget systemic diseases in search for an aetiology, other biochemical or immuno-logical methods should be used for the following purposes: Antibodies for rubella, syphilis, mumps, blood lipids (Booth, 1977), blood clotting mechanisms (Ruben et al, 1969), determination of endocrine hormones and tests of endocrine function (Jorgensen and Buch, 1961; Quick et al, 1973; Taylor and Irwin, 1978) and other tests for systemic diseases (Lindsay and Zuidema, 1950). In addition, clinical pharmacology may provide methods for the analysis of blood, cerebrospinal fluid or even cochlear fluids for ototoxic drugs or other chemicals, when these are suspected to be of aetiological importance. However, a definite conclusion of the relationship between a systemic or generalised disease and the occurrence of a hearing disorder is difficult to draw since a number of individuals with a systemic disease have no symptoms of any disorder of the hearing mechanism (Drettner et al, 1975).

Even when all available methods have been employed for diagnosing a hearing disorder, there are cases where the probability of correct diagnosis still remains rather low. The clinician must, however, take some decision in order to plan therapeutic procedures. In some cases he may wish to apply diagnostic surgery, if an unknown conductive disorder waits for diagnosis. Explorative tympanotomy permits the diagnosis of such cases as congenital anomalous ossicles, adhesions and labyrinthine fistula. The surgeon has, of course, the possibility to proceed to reconstruction in the same operation.

Diagnostic medication is also a method which may be used for confirmation of the suspected diagnosis. A typical example of this is the glycerol test for Ménière's disease. This is used not only for verifying labyrinthine hydrops but also for demonstrating the therapeutic effect of diuretics (Klockhoff and Lind-blom, 1966). In other sensorineural cases of unknown aetiology, diagnostic medication may be prescribed. For example vasodilators may be prescribed if an ischaemic disorder is suspected, or antiepileptic medication in the treatment of severe tinnitus.

Finally, attention should be paid to the role of follow up of the hearing disorder for confirmation of the suspected aetiology. The further development of the hearing disorder in terms of rate of progression, change in symptoms, probable fluctuation or even spontaneous improvement can give information for arriving at a more probable diagnosis for the case in question.

CONCLUSIONS

The investigation of disorders of hearing, particularly sensorineural cases, constitutes a difficult problem. A specific aetiological diagnosis can be given with accuracy in less than 100 per cent of cases. In particular, the task of differentiating the various sensorineural disorders requires a battery of audiometric tests, since no one single test provides enough information. The different methods included in the battery of tests are those discussed in the preceding paragraphs. Modifications to these tests, and even other methods, may be found in various clinics and centres. Even if a wide range of tests are employed, there is never complete certainty of the diagnosis which can be obtained by them (Lundborg, 1952; Schuknecht and Woellner, 1955; Johnson, 1968; Palva and Jauhiainen, 1976).

In the examination of a patient with a hearing disorder one needs to consider what is the required degree of probability of correct diagnosis and to what extent time-consuming and costly procedures are justified. This decision depends on the likelihood that the patient has a neoplastic disease and of the possibilities available for curative medical treatment. However, the possibilities to offer patients with sensorineural hearing disorders definite cure with improvement of hearing or even an end of expected progression are very limited. Thus in many centres one of the main purposes of extensive audiological and other investigations of sensorineural disorders is to exclude the possibility of a cerebellopontine angle process, particularly a vestibulocochlear schwannoma, or other intracranial space occupying lesion, as a cause of a unilateral sensorineural hearing disorder. If the risk of such a disorder is very small the clinician is often content with getting enough information the type of sensorineural hearing loss needed for rehabilitative measures, usually the dynamic area of the available hearing and the available speech discrimination with amplification. This is often the case when a symmetrical sensorineural hearing impairment is sloping to high frequencies in a patient with advancing age, where the diagnosis of presbyacusis can be made and is completely adequate for the situation even though subgrouping to sensorineural, metabolic etc., cannot, or need not, be made.

Correlations between the type, extent and location of the morphological pathology and the results of psychoacoustic, acoustic impedance and electrophysiological tests is as yet a problem partially unsolved. Even if a definite macroscopic morphological pathology can be localised strictly to a certain site, microscopic morphological or at least functional disorders can extend beyond it and possibly explain the audiometric findings. In post-mortem studies different changes in the cochlea and the vestibulocochlear nerve may be observed, but we lack the correlation between the type and degree of audiometric hearing loss on the one hand and, on the other hand, aetiology and pathogenesis.

REFERENCES

Anderson H, Barr B 1960 Conductive recruitment. Acta Otolaryngologica 62:171–184
Anderson H, Barr B, Wedenberg E 1969 Early diagnosis of 8th nerve tumours by acoustic reflex tests. Acta Otolaryngologica Suppl. 263:232–237
Anderson H, Barr B, Wedenberg E 1970 The early detection of acoustic tumours by the stapedius reflex test. Ciba Symposium, Stockholm
Aniansson G 1973 Binaural disrcimination of 'everyday' speech. Acta Otolaryngologica 75:334–336
Aran J -M, Portmann M 1976 Applied cochlear electrophysiology. In: Hinchcliffe R, Harrison D F N (eds) Scientific foundations of otolaryngology. Heinemann, London
Beagley H A, Kellogg S E 1969 A comparison of evoked response and subjective auditory thresholds. International Audiology 8:345–353
Békésy G V 1947 A new audiometer. Acta Otolaryngologica 35:411–422
Bergman M, Blumenfeld V G, Gascardo D 1976 Age-related decrement in hearing for speech. Sampling and longitudinal studies. Journal of Gerontology 31:533–538
Bocca E 1955 Binaural hearing: Another approach. Laryngoscope 65:1164–1171
Bocca E, Calearo C 1963 Central hearing processes. In Jerger J (ed) Modern developments in audiology. Academic Press, New York
Bocca E, Calearo C, Cassinari V 1954 A new method for testing hearing in temporal lobe tumours. Acta Otolaryngologics 44:219–221
Boer E de 1959 Measurement of the critical bandwidth in cases of perception deafness. Proceedings III International Congress of Acoustics, Elsevier, Amsterdam
Booth J B 1977 Hyperlipidaemia and deafness: A preliminary survey, Proceedings of the Royal Society of Medicine 70:642–646
Brooks D 1968 Use of the acoustic impedance meter. Sound 2:40
Calearo C, Lazzaroni A 1957 Speech intelligibility in relation to the speed of the message. Laryngoscope 67:410–419
Carhart R 1946 Speech reception in relation to pattern of pure tone loss. Journal of Speech and Hearing Disorders 11:97–108
Carhart R 1957 Clinical determination of abnormal auditory adaptation. Archives of Otolaryngology 65:32–39
Carhart R, Jerger J 1959 Preferred method for clinical determination of pure tone thresholds. Journal of Speech and Hearing Disorders 24:330–353
Cherry E C, Taylor W K 1954 Some further experiments upon the recognition of speech with one and with two ears. Journal of Acoustical Society of America 26:554–559
Davis H 1962 A functional classification of auditory defects. Annals of Otology Rhinology and Laryngology 71:693–704
Davis H, Zelin S 1966 Acoustic relations of the human vertex potential. Journal of the Accoustical Society of America 39:109–116
Denes P, Naunton R S 1950 The clinical detection of auditory recruitment. Journal of Laryngology 64:375–398
Dix M R, Hallpike C S, Hood J D 1948 Observations upon the loudness recruitment phenomenon, with special reference to the differential diagnosis of disorders of the internal ear and eighth nerve. Proceedings of the Royal Society of Medicine 41:516–526
Drettner B, Hedstrand H, Klockhoff I, Svedberg A 1975 Cardiovascular risk factors and hearing loss. Acta Otolaryngologica 79:366–371
Egan J P 1948 Articulation testing methods. Laryngoscope 58:955–991
Eggermont S S 1976 Summating potentials in electro-cochlegraphy. Relation to hearing pathology. In Ruben R J, Salomon G, Eberling C (eds) Proceedings of the Symposium on Electrocochleography, University park press, Baltimore, Md
Elberling C, Salomon G 1971 Electrical potentials from the inner ear in man in response to prominent sounds generated in a closed acoustic system. Revue de Lanyngolergie Supplement 691–762
Fitzgerald G, Hallpike C S 1942 Studies in human vestibular function. Brain 65:115–131
Fletcher H 1929 Speech and Hearing. Van Nostrand, New York, NY
Fletcher H 1940 Auditory patterns. Reviews of modern Physics 12:47–65
Flisberg K, Ingelstedt S, Örtengren U 1963 Controlled "ear aspiration" of air. A "physiological" test of the tubal function. Acta Otolaryngologica Suppl. 182:35–38
Fowler E P 1928 Marked deafened areas in normal ears. Archives of Otolaryngology 8:151–155
Fowler E P 1936 A method for the early detection of otosclerosis. Archives of Otolaryngology 24:731–741
Fowler E P 1940 Head noises. Archives of Otolaryngology 32:903–914
Fowler E P 1950 Sudden deafness. Annals of Otology, Rhinology and Laryngology 59:980–987

French N R, Steinberg: J C 1947 Factors governing the intelligibility of speech sounds. Journal of the Acoustical Society of America 19:90–119

Gaeth J H 1948 A study of phonemic regression in relation to hearing loss. Thesis, Northwestern University, Chicago III

Garvey W D 1953 The intelligibility of speeded speech. Journal of Experimental Psychology 45:102–108

Gibson W P R 1978 Essentials of clinical electric response audiometry. Churchill Livingstone, London

Gibson W P R, Moffat D A, Ramsden R T 1977 Clinical electrocochleography in the diagnosis and management of Méniere's disorder. Audiology 16:389–401

Groen J J 1962 The value of the Weber test in Schuknecht H F (eds) International Symposium on Otosclerosis. Little Brown & Co., Boston

Groen J J 1969 Diagnostic value of lateralization ability for dichotic time difference. Acta Otolaryngologica 67:326–332

Hahlbrock K -H 1970 Sprachaudiometrie. G. Thieme Verlag, Stuttgart

Hallpike C S, Hood J D 1951 Some recent work on auditory adaptation and its relationship to the loudness recruitment phenomenon. Journal of the Acoustical Society of America 23:270–274

Hallpike C S, Hood J D 1959 Observations upon the neurological mechanism of the loudness recruitment phenomenon. Acta Otolaryngologica 50:472–486

Heller M E, Bergman M 1953 Tinnitus aurium in normally hearing persons. Annals of Otology, Rhinology and Laryngology 62:73–83

Hildyard V H, Valentine M A 1962 Collapse of the ear canal during audiometry. Archives of Otolaryngology 75:422–423

Hinchcliffe R 1959 The threshold of hearing as a function of age. Acustica 9:303–308

Hinchcliffe R 1979 Audiology In: Maran A G D, Stell P M (eds) Clinical Otolaryngology, Blackwell, Oxford

Hinchcliffe R, Littler T 1958 Methodology of air conduction audiometry for hearing survey. Annals of Occupational Hygien 1:114–133

Hirsh I J 1952 The measurement of hearing. McGraw Hill, New York

Hirsh I J, Palva T, Goodman A 1954 Difference limen and recruitment. Archives of Otolaryngology 60:525–540

Hirsh I J, Reymonds E G, Joseph M 1954 Intelligibility of different speech materials. Journal of the Acoustical Society of America 26:530–538

Holmquist J 1969 Eustachian tube function assessed with tympanometry. Acta Otolaryngologica 68:501–508

Hood J D 1950 Studies in auditory fatiue and adaptation. Acta Otolaryngologica Suppl, 92:1–56

Hood J D 1956 Fatigue and adaptation of hearing. British Medical Bulletin 12:125–130

Hood J D 1960 Principles and practice of bone conduction audiometry. Laryngoscope 70:1211–1228

Hood J D, Poole J P 1966 Tolerable limit of loudness. Journal of the Acoustical Society of America 40:47–53

Hudgins C V, Hawkins J E, Karlin J E, Stevens S S 1947 The development of recorded auditory tests for measuring hearing loss for speech. Laryngoscope 57, 57–89

Hulka J H 1941 Bone conduction changes in acute otitis media. Archives of Otolaryngology, 33:333–350

Jauhiainen T 1976 Some factors affecting auditory word discrimination. Scandinavian Audiology 5:79–82

Jauhiainen T, Nutila A 1977 Auditory perception of speech and speech sounds in recent and recovered cases of aphasia. Brain and Language 4:572–579

Jerger J 1960 Békésy audiometry in analysis of auditory disorders. Journal of Speech and Hearing Research 3:275–287

Jerger J 1964 Auditory tests for disorders of the central auditory mechanism in Field W, Alford B (eds) Neurological aspects of auditory and vestibular disorders. Charles C Thomas, Springfield

Jerger J, Shedd J, Harford E 1959 On the detection of extremely small changes in sound intensity. Archives of Otolaryngology 69:200–211

Jewett D L, Williston S S 1971 Auditory evoked far field averaged from the scalp of humans. Brain 94:681–696

Johansson B 1966 The use of transposer for the management of the deaf child. International Audiology 5:362–372

Johansson B 1973 The hearing aid as a technical audiological problem Scandinavian Audiology Suppl 3:55–76

Johnson E W 1968 Auditory findings in 200 cases of acoustic neuromas. Archives of Otolaryngology 88, 598–603

Jokinen K 1973 Presbyacusis VI Masking of speech. Acta Otolaryngologica 76:426–430

Jongkees L B W, Philipszoon A J 1964 Electronystagmography. Acta Otolaryngologica Suppl. 189
Jorgensen M B, Buch N H 1961 Studies on inner-ear function and cranial nerves in diabetics. Acta Otolaryngologica 53 : 350–364
Kärjä J 1974 Perstimulatory supra-threshold adaptation III. Sensorineural deafness. Acta Otolaryngologica 78 : 73–80
Kärjä J, Palva A 1970 Reverse frequency-sweep Békésy audiometry. Acta Otolaryngologica Suppl 263 : 225–228
Katz J 1962 The use of staggered spondaic words for assessing the integrity of the central nervous system. Journal of Auditory Research 2 : 327–337
Keidel W D, Spreng M 1963 Elektronisch gemittelte langsame Rindenpotentiale des Menschen bei akustische Reizung. Acta Otolaryngologica 56 : 318–328
Klockhoff I 1961 Middle ear muscle reflex in man. Acta Otolaryngologica Suppl. 164
Klockhoff I, Lindblom U 1966 Endolymphatic hydrops revealed by glycerol test. Acta Otolaryngologica 61 : 458–462
König E 1962 Difference limen for intensity. International Audiology 1 : 198–202
Korsan-Bengtsen M 1968 The diagnosis of hearing loss in old people in Lidén G (ed) Geriatric Audiology, Almqvist & Wiksell, Stockholm
Korsan-Bengtsen M 1973 Distorted speech audiometry. Acta Otolaryngologica Suppl, 310
Kryter K D 1950 The effects of noise on man. Journal of Speech and Hearing Disorders Monogr. 1
Langenbeck B 1951 Neues zur Praxis und Theorie der Geräuschaudiometrie. Zeitschrift für Laryngologie, Rhinologie und Otologie 30 : 423–441
Leshowitz B, Lindström R Z, Zurek P 1975 Measurements of frequency selectivity of listeners with sensorineural hearing loss. Journal of the Acoustical Society of America 59, 2–3
Lidén G 1971 The use and limitations of the masking noise in pure tone and speech audiometry. Audiology 10, 115–128
Lidén G, Nilsson G 1953 Differential audiometry. Acta Otolaryngologica 38 : 521–527
Lidén G, Nilsson G, Anderson H 1959 Masking in clinical audiometry. Acta Otolaryngologica 50 : 125–136
Lidén G, Petersen J L, Björkman G 1970 Tympanometry. Acta Otolaryngologica Suppl. 263 : 218–224
Lidén G, Korsan-Bengtsen M 1973 Audiometric manifestations of retrocochlear lesions. Advances in Otorhinolaryngology 20 : 271–287
Lierle D M, Reger S N 1946 Correlations between bone and air conduction acuity measurements over wide frequency ranges in different types of hearing impairments. Larynsgocope 56 : 187–224
Lierle D M, Reger S N 1955 Experimentally induced temporary threshold shifts in ears with impaired hearing. Annals of Otology, Rhinology and Laryngology 64 : 263–277
Linden A 1964 Distorted speech and binaural speech resynthesis test. Acta Otolaryngologica 58 : 32–48
Lindsay J R, Zuidema J S 1950 Inner ear deafness of sudden onset. Laryngoscope 60 : 238–263
Lundborg T 1952 Diagnostic problems concerning acoustic tumours. Acta Otolaryngologica Suppl. 99
Lüscher E, Zwislocki J 1947 A simple method for indirect monaural determination of the recruitment phenomenon. Acta Otolaryngologica Suppl. 78 : 156–168
Lynn G, Carhart R 1963 Influence of attack and release in compression amplification on understanding speech by hypoacusis. Journal of Speech and Hearing Disorders 28 : 124–140
Matzker J 1958 Ein binaurale Hörsynthese-Test zum Nachweis zerebraler Hörstörungen. Georg Thieme Verlag, Stuttgart
Matzker J 1962 The binaural test. International Audiology 1 : 209–211
Metz O 1946 The acoustic impedance measured on normal and pathological ears. Acta Otolaryngologica Suppl. 63
Metz O 1952 Threshold of reflex contractions of muscles of the middle ear and recruitment of loudness. Archives of Otolaryngology 55 : 536–543
Miller G A 1947 The masking of speech. Psychological Bulletin 44 : 105–129
Miller G A, Licklider J C R 1950 The intelligibility of interrupted speech. Journal of the Acoustical Society of America 22 : 167–173
Miller G F 1965 Eustachian tube function in normal and diseased ears. Archives of Otolaryngology 81 : 41–48
Naunton R F 1957 Clinical bone-conduction audiometry. Archives of Otolaryngology 66 : 281–298
Naunton R F 1960 A masking dilemma in bilateral conductive deafness. Archives of Otolaryngology, 72 : 753–757
Nodar R H 1978 Tinnitus aurium: An approach to classification. Otolaryngology 86 : 40–46
Nordlund B 1963 Directional audiometry. Acta Otolaryngologica 57 : 1–18
Palva A 1965 Filtered speech audiometry. Acta Otolaryngologica Suppl. 210
Palva A, Jokinen K 1970 Presbyacusis V: Filtered speech test. Acta Otolaryngologica 70 : 232–241
Palva T 1955a Studies of hearing for pure tones and speech in noise. Acta Otolaryngologica 45 : 231–243

Changes in hearing measures with increasing age

INTRODUCTION

That there is a decline in hearing threshold with increasing age has been known for many years. As early as 1899, Zwaardemaker showed that it was the high frequency range of hearing that was affected first by age. Presbyacusis is thus characterised by a lowering of the highest frequency that can be perceived. Zwaardemaker found that there was such a close relationship between the upper frequency of hearing and a person's age that he later made use of this relationship to estimate the ages of the patients in his practice. He used a Galton pipe to produce test sounds which were nearly pure tones and which could be varied in frequency up to 16 kHz.

As it does in young people with normal hearing, the threshold in people with presbyacusis increases very rapidly with increasing frequency as long as the upper frequency limit of hearing is above 10 kHz. When presbyacusis has progressed to affect frequencies below 10 kHz, the slope of the hearing threshold also diminishes. Thus below 10 kHz the hearing threshold increases less steeply than it does at frequencies above 10 kHz.

Since clinical audiometers cover only the frequency range up to 8 kHz, threshold elevations that occur between 8 kHz and 20 kHz are not detected in routine testing. Hearing loss due to age or other factors is, therefore, usually not detected before it reaches such a degree that frequencies at or below 8 kHz are also affected. This limitation of modern clinical audiometers in testing upper frequency hearing levels is of importance in evaluating the results of population studies. The nature of the hearing loss related to age is better characterised by a decline in the upper frequency limit of hearing than by a certain hearing loss at particular frequencies such as is usually determined by conventional audiometry. The Galton pipe that Zwaardemaker used to measure the upper frequency limit of hearing would thus identify more characteristic properties of age-related hearing loss than would present-day audiometry. It may be noted that, before audiometers became standardised, at least one audiometer widely used in Scandinavia could determine the 'upper frequency limit of hearing' by continuously varying the frequency while the intensity remained fixed. The frequency at which the subject could no longer hear the tone was called the upper frequency limit of hearing.

Presbyacusis in the ordinary audiometric frequency range manifests itself as a smooth 'ski slope' curve. Age-related hearing loss can, therefore, usually be distinguished from a noise-induced hearing loss by the fact that the latter more often affects frequencies at 4 kHz more than those at 8 kHz. However, it is usually not possible with any certainty to distinguish the effect of age on pure tone thresholds from the effects of such things as ototoxic drugs, diuretics, head trauma, or vascular disorders. In addition, certain hearing disorders related to heredity are difficult to distinguish audiometrically from the effects of ageing.

CROSS-SECTIONAL STUDIES OF PURE TONE THRESHOLDS AS A FUNCTION OF AGE

An abundance of studies designed to describe changes in pure tone thresholds as a function of age have been published (Bunch and Raiford, 1931; Beasley, 1940; Steinberg et al, 1940; Johansen, 1943; Leisti, 1949; Webster et al, 1950; Glorig, 1954; Sataloff and Menduke, 1957; Hinchcliffe, 1959a; Hinchcliffe and Jones, 1968; Jatho and Heck, 1959; Glorig and Davis, 1961; Glorig and Nixon, 1962; Corso, 1963; Kell et al, 1970; Berger et al, 1977). In most of these studies the subjects were selected in one way or another. Most authors chose to exclude subjects with various middle ear disorders, internal ear diseases, a history of noise exposure, dizziness, a difference in threshold between the ears greater than certain values, a low frequency hearing loss, etc. In other studies no such definite selection criteria were applied, but since many of these studies made use of volunteers, they in fact selected their subjects since use of volunteers in itself implies a selection process. Studies using totally randomly selected subjects are rare.

In order to obtain the most representative data on age-related hearing loss, Spoor (1967) compiled the results of eight different publications on hearing level as a function of age for men and women. The studies he selected were performed between 1938 and 1963 and included a total of 7617 ears of male subjects and 5990 ears of women (Table 4.1). The mean or median pure tone threshold values (air conduction), in the audiometric frequency range of 125 to 8000 Hz, as a function of age obtained in these eight studies are shown separately for men and women in Figures 4.1 and 4. 2. The threshold at age 25 was used as a reference and the average hearing loss is shown relative to the hearing level at age 25. A great discrepancy may be noted among the results of the different studies. For instance, at 4 kHz the mean or median threshold at the age of 75 varied from 37 to 61 dB among these eight studies (Fig. 4.3). It should be mentioned that very few sub-

Table 4.1 Summary of values obtained for hearing thresholds in eight studies.

Author	Number of ears		Value given
	men	women	
Beasley, 1938	2002	2660	mean
Johansen, 1943	155	155	mean
Glorig, 1957	1724	1741	median
ASA Report, 1954	—	—	mean
Hinchcliffe, 1959	326	319	median
Jatho and Heck, 1959	399	361	mean
Glorig and Nixon, 1962	2518(R)	—	median
Corso, 1963	493	754	median
	7617	5990	

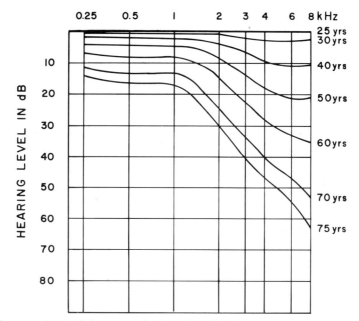

Fig. 4.1 Pure tone thresholds for men as a function of age (from Spoor, 1967).

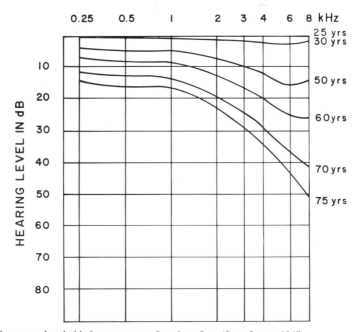

Fig. 4.2 Pure tone thresholds for women as a function of age (from Spoor, 1967).

jects from higher age groups were included in any of these studies. Hinchcliffe (1959a) studied one of the largest groups of ears from elderly persons and reported on 47 ears of people of each sex aged 65 to 74 years. Glorig and Nixon (1962), in their study of 2518 male ears, present audiometric data on only 54 ears with a mean

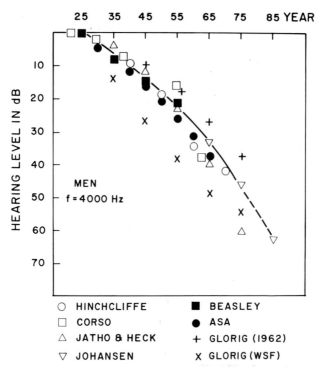

Fig. 4.3 Hearing level at 4 kHz as a function of age—results from eight population studies (Table 4.1).

age of 74·5 years. Corso (1963) tested 154 ears of subjects aged 59 to 65 years. Johansen (1943), whose individual data are closest to Spoor's compiled data, tested 20 men and 20 women in each decade, the oldest group having a mean age of 82·5 years for men and 84·3 years for women.

Using the hearing threshold at 25 years of age as a reference, Spoor (1967) concluded that the eight studies he reviewed indicated that the threshold elevation is higher for men than it is for women, most obviously in the higher age groups (Figs. 4.1 and 4.2). None of the results of these studies, however, prove that the difference in hearing threshold for men and women is really sex-related because men and women presumably have been exposed to noise differently. Thus, the differences in hearing thresholds of men and women could either be the result of more frequent noise exposure in men or it could be sex-related. The fact that in Spoor's compiled data men show a higher degree of hearing loss at 8 kHz, however, might point to a true sex difference. It is worth noting that the difference between the thresholds of men and women in these data is only apparent above 2 kHz. Hinchcliffe (1959a) also reported results which showed a difference in hearing threshold between women and men, but the difference he noted decreased with increasing age. In addition, he did not discuss these findings in detail, and it is not clear whether they are the result of a real change in threshold with age or the result of population selection.

Robinson and Sutton (1979) arrived at results similar to those of Spoor (1967), also compiling data from eight population studies, four of which were the same as those evaluated by Spoor (1967). However, Robinson and Sutton used hearing at age 18 as the reference level for their study, rather than hearing at age 25.

In another study of hearing thresholds in a suburban Jamaican population, Hinchcliffe and Jones (1968) found that, on the average, women had poorer hearing at 500 to 2000 Hz than did men. They explained this sex difference as being due to a sex-linked sensorineural hearing loss among the Jamaican females, as men and women in this population had not suffered different noise exposure.

Similar findings were obtained by Kell and his colleagues (1970), who determined the pure tone thresholds of residents of the island of Westray in Northern Scotland. The women had a more pronounced hearing loss in the low frequency range than did the men, but, at 8 kHz, the decrease in hearing as a function of age was the same for both sexes. Unfortunately, this island population is as likely as the Jamaican population to have been genetically influenced by isolation.

In reviewing the results of the cross-sectional studies included in Spoor's (1967) paper, it is important to note that only mean or median values of hearing loss are given. There is thus no information available about the shape of the distribution of hearing loss among the subjects. This is also the case for most other studies of hearing threshold as a function of age. It cannot be assumed that the hearing threshold values as a function of age have a normal (Gaussian) distribution; in fact the distribution is likely to be skewed. The threshold distribution function may even be bimodal, particularly for higher frequencies, which would indicate that two groups of people were involved, one with better hearing than the other. The mean or median values of the whole group of subjects may therefore not be adequate descriptors of the change in hearing threshold with age. Also, the difference in hearing in men and women included in the study is different at different ages; this may also affect the results.

There has been much discussion as to whether the commonly seen decline in hearing with age is a result of a normal ageing process or a result of exogenous factors related to our industrialised environment. Studies of the hearing threshold as a function of age in a non-industrialised society are few, and the results of these studies have not resolved this question. The study by Rosen and his colleagues (1962) of the hearing threshold as a function of age in members of the Mabaan tribe in Sudan is the only generally known research on hearing threshold as a function of age in a non-industrialised society. Rosen and his colleagues (1962) determined the threshold of hearing on 541 randomly selected subjects from the Mabaan tribe with ages ranging from 10 to over 90 years. These people were characterised by not having been exposed to noise in their environment. Also, they had significantly lower blood pressure than is generally accepted as 'normal' in the industrialised Western world. These investigators found that the decline in hearing in all age groups was much smaller than the mean hearing loss in people of the same age in Western societies described in the studies discussed above. Interestingly, they also found a difference in hearing threshold between men and women of the same age, women having a higher threshold than men from 50 years of age onward at 6 kHz. This difference between men and women increased with increasing age up to age 69, after which the difference became less pronounced. Rosen et al did not discuss this part of their results, perhaps because of the fact that rather few people in the study were in the higher age groups, and only a few of these were tested—20 male ears and 10 female ears, aged 70 to 79. In addition, members of the Mabaan tribe usually did not know their age, and if they did so, were liable to give a higher age than their real age because being old in their society conferred upon them a more honorable status. Therefore, Rosen et al used certain external signs such as dentition and puberty to estimate the ages of their subjects. These difficulties in estimating the ages of the members of the Mabaan tribe contribute to the uncertainty of the results in general and make it difficult to compare these results with those of studies using subjects from the Western world.

In contrast to the results of Rosen and his colleagues (1967), the results of Leisti (1949) show that the differences between the hearing thresholds of men and those of women in an industrialised country (Finland) are not statistically significant. Any differences observed were ascribed to external factors, such as noise. However, Sataloff and Menduke (1957) found poorer hearing in men than in women at age 65, although at the age of 90 there was no observed difference between the hearing of men and that of women in the frequency range 250 to 4000 Hz. These latter authors found such a low correlation between age and degree of hearing loss that they stated that 'past the age of 65, a person's age gives little information concerning his expected hearing loss' (Sataloff and Menduke, 1957). However, these data are not totally conclusive since the subjects, particularly the women, tended to understate their age by as much as 15 years!

There are very few studies of the pure tone hearing threshold in randomly selected populations of elderly people. One such study, done by Milne and his colleagues (1971) and Milne and Lauder (1975) in Edinburgh, included a random sample of 748 people, of whom 65 per cent (215 men and 272 women) aged 62 years and over were studied. The subjects were drawn from the census of 26 903 persons who qualified for inclusion in the population study, but the proportion of women in the study was significantly smaller than that in the census. The subjects underwent a broad clinical examination at a hospital during 1968 and 1969, as well as a number of special examinations including pure tone audiometry. The participants were retested one and five years later (see p. 109).

The median pure tone thresholds for two age groups in this Edinburgh study, 62 to 69 years and 70 to 90 years, showed a greater hearing loss in men than in women. In the 'younger' group, the difference between men and women at 8 kHz was 15 dB, while in the 'older' group this difference was only 7 dB. Also, the women in both age groups had a more pronounced hearing loss below 1 kHz than did the men. However, only the results on the better ear for each person were reported.

In a study performed by Møller (1981) the pure tone hearing thresholds were determined on 70-year-old people selected randomly from the population of a medium-sized industrial city in Sweden (Gothenburg). The population study (Rinder et al, 1975) comprised 1148 men and women, born on days ending with 2, 5, and 8, from July 1, 1901, to June 30, 1902, and corresponding to almost one-third of all 70-year-old people in the city. Great efforts were devoted to keeping the response rate as high as possible, and 973 (or 85 per cent) of those selected participated in the population study. Two-fifths of the participants comprised a subsample of 197 women and 179 men (752 ears) whose hearing was tested. The mean pure tone hearing losses for men and women in this study are shown in Figures 4.4 and 4.5. As these figures show, the hearing thresholds for men and

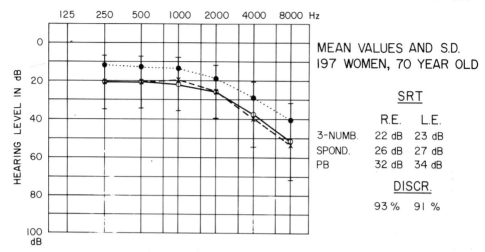

Fig. 4.4 Mean values obtained by pure tone and speech audiometry in 197 women, 70 years old (from Møller, 1981). Dotted line = Spoor's (1967) data on 70-year-old women.

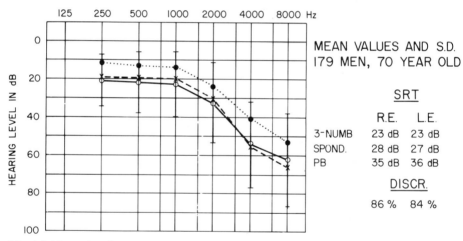

Fig. 4.5 Mean values for pure tone and speech audiometry in 179 men, 70 years old (from Møller, 1981). Dotted line = Spoor's (1967) data on 70-year-old men.

women are very similar between 250 and 1000 Hz. Above 1000 Hz the mean hearing loss in men is greater than that in women and the difference reaches values of about 10 dB at 8 kHz and 15 dB at 4 kHz. The difference in hearing loss in men and women may be explained on the basis of noise exposure in men as very few of these women born in 1901 and 1902 had been exposed to industrial noise.

The distribution of hearing thresholds at 1, 4, and 8 kHz for men and women in Møller's (1981) study are shown in Figures 4.6 to 4.8. Non-measurable hearing at maximum output of the audiometer was listed as 99 dB HTL. The distribution at 1000 Hz is skewed, as is typical for thresholds, but the distribution is nearly identical for men and women. At 4 kHz, the thresholds have bimodal distribution for men but are almost symmetrically distributed for women. The bimodal

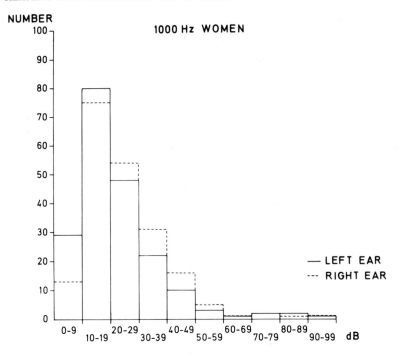

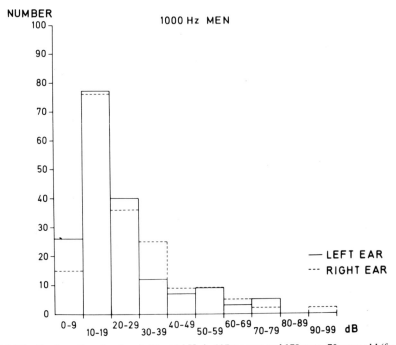

Fig. 4.6 Distribution of hearing thresholds at 1 kHz in 197 women and 179 men, 70 years old (from Møller, 1981).

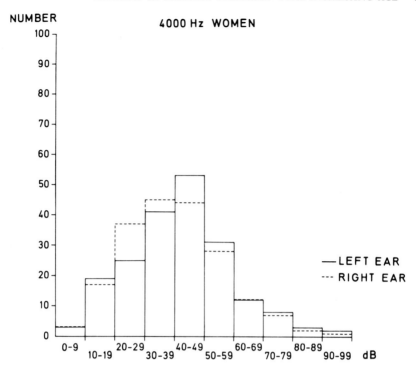

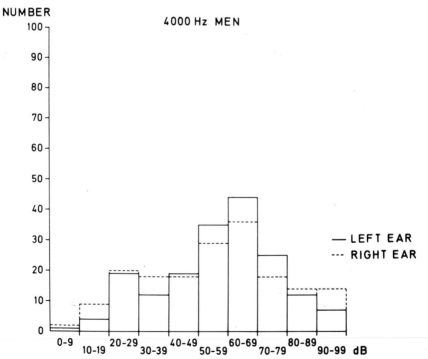

Fig. 4.7 Distribution of hearing thresholds at 4 kHz in 197 women and 179 men, 70 years old (from Møller, 1981).

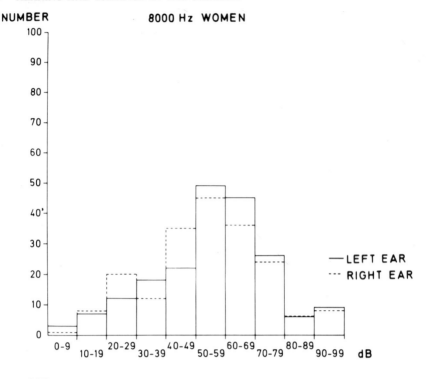

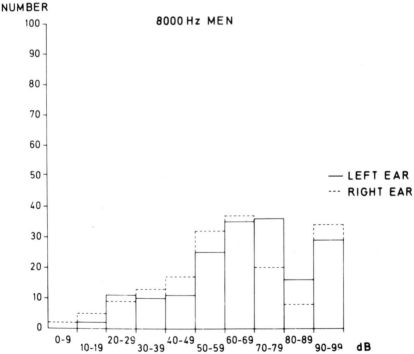

Fig. 4.8 Distribution of hearing thresholds at 8 kHz in 197 women and 179 men, 70 years old (from Møller, 1981).

distribution might indicate one noise-exposed and one non noise-exposed group of men. At 8 kHz more men than women have a hearing loss greater than 90 dB. It is also worth noting that 17 female ears and 12 male ears of these 70-year-old people have a hearing threshold that is 20 dB or better over the entire frequency range from 250 Hz to 8 kHz.

The threshold values obtained in Møller's (1981) study of 70-year-old people indicate somewhat larger hearing losses than the eight selected studies described by Spoor (1967). This is to be expected because the 70-year-old people in Møller's (1981) study were not selected and, therefore, people with various types of conductive hearing disorders, uni- and bilateral internal ear disorders, Ménière's disease, etc. as well as people who were exposed to industrial noise, were included. In addition, the latter study included nine totally deaf ears.

It should be noticed from the results of this study that the mean hearing loss is greater for the left ear than for the right ear above 2 kHz, both for men and women. Such a difference between right and left ears was first observed in men by Glorig (1957), and later also by Hinchcliffe (1959b). Hinchcliffe ascribed the difference in sensitivity to pure tones as being the result of the individual concerned firing a rifle. However, as this difference also exists in the ears of women, who presumably have not fired as many rifles as men, another reason for this difference should be sought. It is interesting to note that the left vertebral artery is more elongated by age than is the right vertebral artery (Jannetta 1981, personal communication); this might cause a reduction in the blood supply to the left internal ear which would subsequently affect the hearing threshold in that ear.

The results of the cross-sectional studies discussed above do not enable us to distinguish whether the sex difference in hearing loss as a function of age is a real difference or is the result of external factors that influence men and women differently. The most important such external factor is probably exposure to noise, but there may be other factors of importance such as a difference in the use of alcohol and in smoking. One way in which this apparent difference between the hearing of men and of women might be resolved is through longitudinal studies.

The effect of noise on the progress of hearing loss is complex and cannot be described in any simple way. It depends on such factors as the intensity and character of the noise, length of exposure to the noise, and, very likely, hereditary predisposition to such a hearing loss. Nevertheless, one can make a few generalisations about noise-induced hearing loss. It is generally found that the hearing loss caused by heavy noise progresses relatively rapidly at first and then reaches a more or less constant and stable value, whereas exposure to noise of moderate levels may result in a decline in hearing threshold that progresses more steadily over a longer time. The effect of noise exposure on pure tone thresholds is illustrated in Figure 4.9. It is obvious that the hearing loss increases with increasing exposure time, and that, after long-term noise exposure, frequencies below 4 kHz also show threshold elevations. In addition, it is obvious that the combination of presbyacusis and the effects of noise exposure may result in a very complex time course of decline in the hearing threshold.

To complicate matters further, it is not only industrial noise that is of importance in inducing hearing loss. The daily wear and tear on the ear produced by the noises from motors, machines and leisure equipment (often referred to as

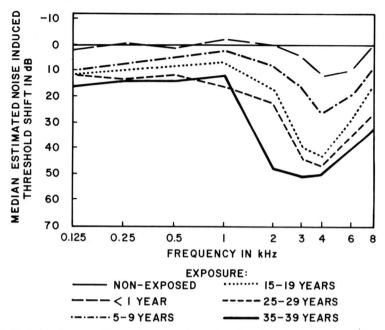

Fig. 4.9 Typical audiograms obtained from ears after various durations of noise exposure (Source: US Department of Health, Education and Welfare, Occupational Exposure to Noise, Health Services and Mental Health Administration, National Institute for Occupational Safety and Health, 1972).

'socioacusis') has been claimed to likewise lead to hearing loss. At this time, it may not be possible to predict the precise course of a 'noise-induced hearing loss'.

Presbyacusis is generally accepted as a sensorineural hearing loss: a hearing loss due to damage to hair cells and/or neural elements in the auditory nerve and ascending auditory pathways. The hearing loss is characterised audiometrically by similar values for air and bone conduction, although some authors (Glorig and Davis, 1961; Rosen et al, 1964) have reported an air-bone gap, mainly in the high frequency range, from individuals with presbyacusis. This air-bone gap has been attributed to changes in the middle ear that come with increasing age: stiffening of the tympanic membrane and changes in the articulations of the ossicular chain. However, it is more likely that the air-bone gap measured is due to ear canal collapse or, more often, to the use of an earphone with a hard cushion which has a poor fit to the auricle. Also, the fact that subcutaneous tissue is often reduced in the elderly and that there may be changes in the properties of the mastoid bone in elderly, could equally well cause an apparent air-bone gap.

LONGITUDINAL STUDIES OF PURE TONE THRESHOLDS AS A FUNCTION OF AGE

The progression of hearing loss with age can be estimated only indirectly from cross-sectional studies. Longitudinal studies in which hearing thresholds have been compared on the same people over many years should provide more valid information regarding age-related hearing loss. However, the results of only a very few such studies have been published. A longitudinal study by Milne and Chopin (1975) and Milne (1977) documented a decline in hearing threshold over a five-year period in two groups of subjects, one group between the ages of 62 and 69 years and another group between 70 and 90 years of age when entering the study. The original study comprised 215 men and 272 women, of whom 113 men and 148 women were retested after five years (78 men and 60 women had died, and 24 men and 64 women could not be re-examined for various other reasons). Milne (1977) found that 66 per cent of the men aged 62 to 69 years when entering the study five years later had a decrease in hearing threshold at 8 kHz greater than 5 dB, while of the men in the 70-to-90-year group only 31 per cent had the same amount of threshold shift. In women, 56 and 48 per cent, respectively, showed a similar change in the high frequency threshold. These findings might be interpreted as showing that the hearing acuity of women deteriorates continuously while that of men does not. However, as there is no way to compare the hearing thresholds of those who died or were not available for the five-year follow-up study to those of the individuals originally tested, no sure conclusions can be made. Also, the age variation in the older group (those 70 to 90 years old) is too large to allow any detailed conclusions about threshold changes due to age to be made. Milne did conclude from his longitudinal study that the greater the hearing loss was at the time of the original examination, the smaller was the change in hearing threshold after five years, and he also found that, at 1 kHz only, age had an effect on the hearing threshold in men, but not in women.

The study by Møller (1981) of hearing in 70-year-old people included a follow-up study five years later of the same randomly selected people. Of the 376 subjects whose hearing was tested at age 70, 261 were tested again at age 75. Thirty men and 27 women had died, and 25 men and 33 women (18 per cent) did not come for a second hearing test. The results of this study are shown in Figures 4.10 and 4.11, which give the mean hearing loss for men and women separately. It may be seen that, whereas the men showed only a 3 to 5 dB decrease in hearing threshold,

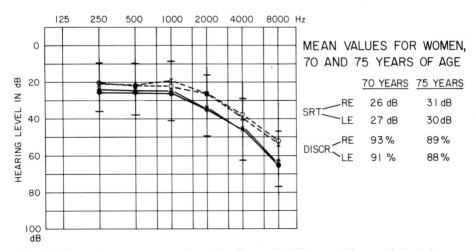

Fig. 4.10 Mean values on pure tone and speech audiometry in 137 women, 75 years old. Dashed lines = pure tone thresholds at age 70 (from Møller, 1981).

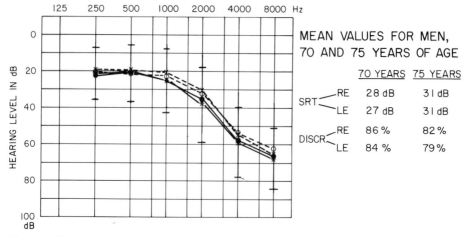

Fig. 4.11 Mean values for pure tone and speech audiometry in 124 men, 75 years old. Dashed lines = pure tone thresholds at age 70 (from Møller, 1981).

women had as much as a 15 dB decline in hearing threshold at 8 kHz. Perhaps the most surprising finding is that the hearing threshold in women declined not only at the higher frequencies but also at the lower frequencies during the five-year interval. Analysis of the pure tone thresholds for those men and women who had died before the age of 75 or who had not come for the second testing showed no difference compared to the mean pure tone threshold at the age of 70; this was true for both men alone and women alone. Although the decrease in hearing between the ages of 70 and 75 years in men may be affected by earlier noise exposure, the deterioration in the hearing in women between the ages of 70 and 75 can be considered to reflect a true decrease in the hearing function with increasing age.

SPEECH AUDIOMETRY

The perception of speech is usually only affected by a threshold elevation which includes the frequency range 300 to 3000 Hz. Since frequencies at and above 4 kHz are of minor importance for perception of speech, a hearing loss due to age must have progressed to a certain degree before it affects speech discrimination. When the hearing loss affects frequencies below 4 kHz, the speech perception can be impaired, but how much depends on many factors. The perception of novel words is more affected than that of everyday or connected speech and comprehension of speech in a noisy background is more affected than listening to speech in quiet. This is true of almost all types of sensorineural hearing loss in which mainly the high frequencies are impaired.

It is worth noting that almost all our knowledge about the relationship between sensorineural hearing loss and speech discrimination is based on studies in which the speech sounds are presented through earphones and in a noise-free environment. In the natural situation where speech reaches both ears and where there is almost always interference from background noise, speech perception may be quite different. In fact, practical experience as well as research reveals that background noise impairs speech perception, particularly in people with presbyacusis. Another factor of importance is that speech tests make use of one- or two-syllable words, whereas most normal conversation includes words of many syllables and the syntax of the language in itself provides information to the listener.

Although it is relatively well known how the results of structured speech tests can be interpreted for people with normal hearing, little is known about what a certain decrease in discrimination measured by such a test means in terms of reduction in the ability to understand connected speech in a noisy background. It is somewhat surprising how little actually is known about the perception of connected speech in background noise and its relation to the degree of hearing loss as reflected in the tone audiogram.

Relationship between speech discrimination and sensorineural hearing loss
The relationship between threshold elevation for pure tones in people with sensorineural hearing losses of various aetiologies and the discrimination scores (per cent correctly heard phonetically balanced words, or PB-words) for one-syllable words presented through earphones in quiet is shown in Figure 4.12. It is

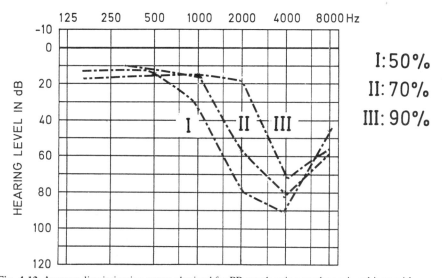

Fig. 4.12 Average discrimination scores obtained for PB-words using earphones in subjects with varying degrees of high-frequency hearing loss (from Lidén, 1954).

obvious from these data that the hearing loss must affect frequencies at or below 2 kHz in order for the discrimination score to be noticeably reduced. When the hearing loss involves frequencies below 2000 Hz, the discrimination scores decrease rapidly. It needs to be emphasised that these values are average values and there is naturally a certain variation among different subjects, since many factors play an important role in the discrimination of speech, among others, age.

When the same speech material, i.e. PB-words, is presented together with background noise, the discrimination scores are substantially reduced. Aniansson (1974) tested the ability of subjects to discriminate PB-words when they were presented mixed with background noises with different signal-to-noise ratios and also when they were presented with competing sounds from radio and from one to three male voices. He found that, in subjects with normal hearing, the discrimination scores were reduced by 30 per cent on all tests in which the PB-words were presented with competing background sounds. Test subjects with a hearing loss of 50 dB in the frequency range of 2000 to 6000 Hz had average discrimination scores of 5 to 25 per cent under the same listening conditions. Those with normal hearing at 2000 Hz, but with a threshold elevation of 50 dB at 3000 to 6000 Hz, had an average discrimination score of 88 per cent in a quiet environment and scores of 26 to 62 per cent listening for the same words with different competing sounds in the background (see Fig. 4.13). It needs to be emphasised that the results he

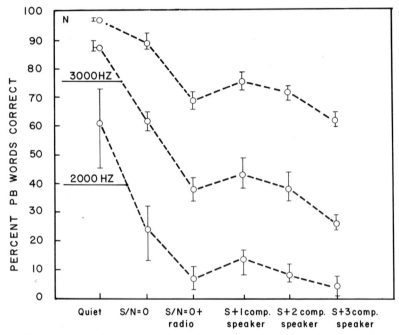

Fig. 4.13 Mean discrimination scores for PB-words presented with competing background sounds to normal ears and ears with different degrees of high-frequency hearing loss (from Aniansson, 1974).

reported were obtained from young listeners (25 to 49 years old), and that their hearing losses were due to exposure to noise. However, there is no reason to doubt that similar results would be obtained from elderly people with the same degree of hearing loss in the high frequency range.

Plomp and Mimpen (1979) studied the influence of noise on speech perception. They found that the hearing handicap of the elderly manifests itself primarily in noisy environments. In contrast to previously reported studies, which used various types of monosyllabic words, these investigators used sentences as test material. They found that female listeners on the average did worse than men. In experiments using various levels of background noise they showed that the allowable background noise levels were 8 to 10 dB lower in the elderly than in young people with normal hearing. Aniansson's (1974) and Plomp and Mimpen's

(1979) results thus clearly show that background or, more correctly, competing sounds severely hamper the ability of people with high frequency hearing losses to perceive speech.

Relationship between speech perception and presbyacusis

Speech perception in ears with presbyacusis cannot be predicted on the basis of our knowledge about the relationship between the pure tone audiogram and speech discrimination in young ears. Several studies have been performed to establish the relationship between pure tone thresholds and speech discrimination in the elderly. However, most of these studies are highly selected as the tests were performed on patients who came to centres for speech and hearing. In one such study, Pestalozza and Shore (1955) evaluated the relationship between pure tone and speech reception thresholds and discrimination scores in 185 elderly people, aged 60 to 90 years, selected from 1500 patients who had been tested at the Central Institute for the Deaf (CID), St. Louis, Missouri, during a two-year period. They found a close relationship between pure tone hearing loss in the frequency range of 500 to 2000 Hz and loss of discrimination. The discrimination loss was always severe and became more severe as the hearing loss as recorded by the pure tone audiogram increased.

It is commonly found that speech discrimination scores are lower in the elderly than would be expected on the basis of their pure tone audiograms. This is referred to as 'phonemic regression', first described by Gaeth (1948) who assumed that the reduced speech perception was a result of changes in the central auditory system that occur with increasing age. In order to estimate the effect of age on speech perception, Pestalozza and Shore (1955) compared the discrimination scores of 25 subjects 40 years of age or less with the discrimination scores of elderly people with the same audiometric profile: a gradually increasing sensorineural loss in the high frequency range. As can be seen from Figure 4.14, the young ears had better discrimination scores than did the ears of the elderly, despite the fact that individuals in both age groups had the same degree of hearing loss as measured by tone audiometry. The authors ascribe this difference in speech perception to 'phonemic regression' and state that 'in old individuals discrimination for speech is very poor even in the presence of a mild hearing loss' (Pestalozza and Shore, 1955). The authors did, however, emphasise that patients were selected to participate in the study as they presented to CID for treatment of hearing problems. A similar phenomenon was described by Goetzinger and Rousey (1959), who studied elderly people referred to a speech and hearing clinic. Goetzinger and Rousey reported an average discrimination score of 76 per cent in men and women in the age group 70 to 79 years, while in the age group 80 to 91 years (24 subjects), the mean discrimination score was 70 per cent. Similar findings were reported by Klotz and Kilbane (1962), who studied 170 members of a senior citizen center, 81 of whom were in the age group 71 to 80 years. The discrimination score in this group was 84 per cent.

In an unselected group of old people, the findings are rather different. Thus, Møller (1981) found in a randomly selected population of 70-year-old people that the mean discrimination score was 93 per cent in women and 86 per cent in men

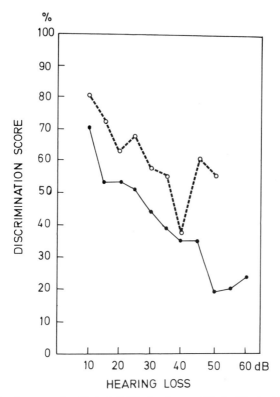

Fig. 4.14 Discrimination scores for elderly (solid line) and young (Dashed line) subjects with the same degrees of hearing loss as tested by pure tone audiometry (from Pestalozza and Shore, 1955).

(see Figs. 4.4 and 4.5). These discrimination scores are much higher than those reported by earlier investigators, but are in good agreement with what should be expected on the basis of the pure tone audiograms when compared with those of young people with a similar degree of sensorineural hearing loss. The discrepancy between the results of the latter study (Møller, 1981) and earlier studies is most likely due to the fact that the earlier studies were based on populations which were selected in one way or another.

The study by Møller (1981) involved 376 70-year-old people who were a sub-sample of a cross-section of the population used to study medical and social conditions in this age group (Rinder et al, 1975). 197 women and 179 men had hearing tests, including pure tone audiometry (see p. 103); in addition, their speech reception thresholds (SRT) and discrimination scores were obtained.

When the discrimination scores were studied in detail, it emerged that, at the age of 70 years, 75 per cent of the women had a discrimination score that was equal to or better than 92 per cent, and only 8 per cent had a discrimination score below 76 per cent. The distribution of the discrimination scores is illustrated in Figure 4.15. The discrimination scores for 70-year-old men were, as expected, slightly lower than those for women, but as many as 50 per cent of the men had a discrimination score that was equal to or better than 92 per cent and only 18 per cent had a discrimination score below 76 per cent (Fig. 4.16). In reviewing these results it

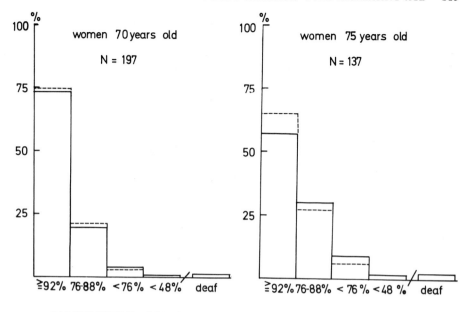

DISCRIMINATION SCORES IN WOMEN,   70 and 75 years old

Fig. 4.15 Discrimination scores for women tested at ages 70 and 75 years (from Møller, 1981).

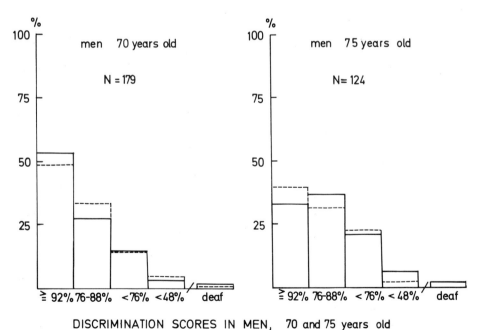

DISCRIMINATION SCORES IN MEN,   70 and 75 years old

Fig. 4.16 Discrimination scores of men tested at ages 70 and 75 years (from Møller, 1981).

must be emphasised that an unselected group of 70-year-old people was studied. Consequently, a number of the participants had conductive hearing losses due to various causes, unilateral sensorineural hearing losses, or an ear that was totally deaf (this last condition was present in nine individuals).

It can, therefore, be concluded from this study that speech discrimination in the elderly in general is not reduced noticeably more than it is in young people with the same degree of pure tone hearing loss.

At age 75 years, 137 of the women and 124 of the men in Møller's (1981) study were tested again with the same type of speech tests. It was found that pure tone hearing thresholds had deteriorated more in the women than they had in the men. However, the mean speech discrimination scores were reduced by nearly the same amount (4 to 5 per cent) in both men and women. The distribution of speech discrimination scores is shown in Figures 4.15 and 4.16. From these figures it may be seen that while the distribution of scores in women is nearly the same as it was at the age of 70, the distribution of scores for the 75-year-old men is nearly flat, with 35 per cent of them having a discrimination score equal to or better than 92 per cent. There is no clear difference between right and left ears, but there is a slight tendency for the left ears to have a lower speech discrimination score than the right ears.

It is obvious that when the speech tests are performed by traditional methods using earphones and quiet test booths, the elderly in general have very good speech perception. This is also obvious in daily life—very few elderly people have difficulty hearing ordinary conversational speech, and, if they have, it is usually when they are in an environment where there is background noise.

The term 'phonemic regression' has, over the years, been widely used to describe the finding that the speech discrimination scores of the elderly are lower than would be expected on the basis of their pure tone audiogram. However, Møller's (1981) data provide little support for the idea that central auditory disturbances dominate the picture of hearing in the elderly. Naturally there exist, in all age groups, people who have well-preserved hearing when tested with pure tone audiometry but who have severely reduced speech discrimination scores. However, these people are rare, and in many cases the findings can be ascribed to poor testing procedures (inadequate instructions), language problems, reduced mental ability and, in a few cases, the presence of bilateral lesions of the central auditory pathways and auditory cortex.

It is important to note that the results of Møller (1981), as well as those referred to earlier (Pestalozza and Shore, 1955; Goetzinger and Rowsey, 1959; Klotz and Kilbane, 1962), were obtained using earphones and monaural listening in quiet. The advantage of binaural hearing is, thus, not included. Probably more importantly, the influence of normal background noise is not taken into account in these studies.

In discussing the ability to understand speech, either in quiet or under normal circumstances, it is important to emphasise the large variations which occur between individuals. Thus, individuals with the same pure tone thresholds or the same speech reception thresholds do not necessarily have the same speech discrimination scores. Plomp and Mimpen (1979) found, in testing people between the ages of 20 and 89 years, that the most important source of variance in speech discrimination was the background noise. The next most important factor was variations between individuals and not the person's age as such.

LOW-REDUNDANCY SPEECH TESTS FOR EVALUATION OF CENTRAL AUDITORY DISORDERS IN THE ELDERLY

Ordinary speech contains much more information than is actually necessary for normal communication. This redundancy makes speech intelligible even to listeners with functional impairment of the peripheral hearing organ and auditory pathways. In addition, since each auditory cortex receives input from both ears, the auditory system itself is intrinsically redundant. Because of this extrinsic and intrinsic redundancy, ordinary speech tests generally fail to reveal lesions in the central auditory pathways and auditory cortex. In fact, Bunch (1928) showed that a whisper was heard equally well in both ears in a patient who had undergone total right-sided hemispherectomy. Nylén (1939), Bocca and his colleagues (1954), Bocca (1963), Berlin and Lowe (1972), and Korsan-Bengtsen (1973), among others, have provided evidence that normal speech can be perceived despite lesions in the central auditory pathways and auditory cortex.

Lesions in the central auditory pathways and cortex cannot be diagnosed by ordinary speech tests because of the high redundancy in speech material. Bocca and his colleagues were the first to show that lowpass filtered speech gave a reduced discrimination score in the ear contralateral to a lesion in the auditory cortex while the ipsilateral ear showed normal perception of the speech material low in redundancy. In a series of excellent experiments, Bocca and his group systematically varied the redundancy of speech messages using, besides frequency distorted speech, speech with an accelerated rate or speech that was periodically interrupted as well as 'competing speech' in which two speech messages were presented simultaneously, one to each ear. Using these different low-redundant, or distorted, speech tests, Bocca's group showed that, in patients with unilateral lesions of the central auditory pathways and cortex, the discrimination score was significantly reduced in the ear opposite to the lesion while in the other ear normal scores were obtained. Since these observations were made, numerous investigations have been performed to evaluate central auditory lesions by means of distorted speech tests (Matzker, 1959; Katz et al, 1963; Feldmann, 1964; Jerger, 1964; Kirikae et al, 1964; Lindén, 1964; Antonelli, 1968, 1970b; Korsan-Bengtsen and Møller, 1973), and Bocca's original findings have been shown to be valid.

It is assumed that presbyacusis is caused not only by loss of hair cells in the internal ear, but also by degeneration in the central auditory pathways and auditory cortex. Low-redundant speech tests have, therefore, been used to diagnose central auditory lesions in the elderly.

That speech perception in the elderly frequently is much poorer than would be expected from their pure tone thresholds has, as was mentioned earlier, been attributed not only to functional changes in the internal ear but also to degenerative changes in the ascending auditory pathways and auditory cortex. Saxén (1937) reported two types of degenerative changes, namely atrophy of the spiral ganglion and angiosclerotic changes of the internal ear. Schuknecht (1964) described four types of presbyacusis, one of which was called neural and was considered to be due to a reduced number of spiral ganglion cells, and probably also to pathological changes in the higher auditory pathways. (However, most of his results were based on histological examination of cat ears. Only one human was studied in this series.)

Kirikae and his colleagues (1964) performed histopathological studies of eleven brains, selected at random from autopsies on 500 persons aged 68 to 87 years. They found uniform atrophy as well as degeneration in all major nuclei of the central auditory pathways, both below and above the decussation of the auditory nerve fibres at the base of the fourth ventricle. The same histopathological changes were found by Hansen and Reske-Nielsen (1965) during autopsy examination of 12 patients, most of them above 80 years of age.

Calearo and Lazzaroni (1957) tested the intelligibility of accelerated speech to six elderly subjects 70 to 85 years old. All of the elderly had a hearing loss that was considered to be within the 'physiological' range. Calearo and Lazzaroni found that the discrimination of accelerated speech with a rate of 350 words per minute was 40 per cent in the elderly, compared to 100 per cent in young ears. These results were ascribed to degenerative changes in the central nervous system with lengthening of the time required to identify the speech message.

In a further study, Antonelli (1970a) tested 50 elderly subjects in the age group 60 to 70 years with an average age of 63 years. Pure tone audiometry showed a mild high frequency hearing loss in all subjects and the average discrimination score for normal speech was 100 per cent. When these elderly were tested with low-redundancy speech tests, including frequency-distorted speech, accelerated or time-compressed speech and interrupted speech with various rates of interruption, the elderly had an average of 30 to 50 per cent lower scores on these tests compared to young, normal adults. Similar findings were obtained by Kirikae and his colleagues (1964) using frequency-distorted speech and interrupted speech with monaural and binaural presentations. The difference in performance again was ascribed mainly to degenerative changes in the central auditory systems of the elderly subjects.

Similar types of distorted speech, i.e. periodically interrupted speech with 10, 7, or 4 interruptions per second, accelerated speech with a speech rate of 300 words per minute, and lowpass filtered speech, were used by Korsan-Bengtsen (1973) to evaluate the performances of normal test subjects of different ages as well as of 25 ears of individuals with sensorineural losses due to cochlear lesions. Twenty test-subjects aged 50 to 60 years showed an average reduction in discrimination on these tests of 6 to 24 per cent compared to the results from young, normal listeners (see Fig. 4.17). Korsan-Bengtsen showed that the performances of patients with congenital sensorineural losses on these tests did not differ from those of young, normal listeners. On the other hand, patients with acquired sensorineural losses had severely reduced discrimination scores when tested with a low-redundancy speech test.

Using the same distorted speech test, Møller (1981) tested a randomly selected group of 70-year-old people. The subjects involved in this study were part of a new population study in Gothenburg, Sweden, comprising 474 men and 562 women born in 1906 and 1907 (Svanborg et al, 1981). Two fifths of the participants comprised a subsample of 219 women and 170 men who had hearing tests including pure tone and speech audiometry. One third of these participants of the

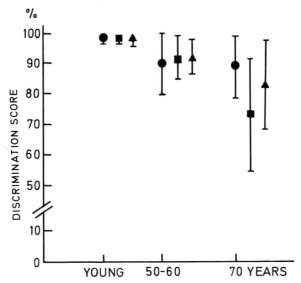

Fig. 4.17 Mean discrimination scores obtained on three different types of low-redundancy speech tests in young subjects, 50- to 60-year-old subjects, and 70-year-old men and women. ● = interrupted speech, 10 interruptions per second; ■ = interrupted speech, 7 interruptions per second; ▲ = accelerated speech, 300 words per minute (Møller, 1981).

study were also tested with distorted-speech audiometry in order to evaluate the degree of central auditory dysfunction in this age group. Those 70-year-old people selected for distorted speech audiometry had to have symmetrical sensorineural hearing losses.

Fifty men and 89 women were thus tested with accelerated speech with a rate of 300 words per minute. The mean score for men was 82 per cent and for women 83 per cent for the right ear (Fig. 4.17). These scores are only 15 per cent lower than those obtained in young, normal ears with the same speech material (Korsan-Bengtsen, 1973). The standard deviation was, as expected, very large, which indicates that, in an unselected group of 70-year-old people, there are those with well-preserved central auditory functions as well as those with presumable lesions in the auditory cortex and central auditory pathway.

Twenty-five men and 35 women were also tested with interrupted speech with 10 interruptions per second. As seen from Figure 4.17, the mean score for men was 87 per cent and that for women was 91 per cent, for the right ears. These values are unexpectedly high in view of earlier findings by Antonelli (1970a), who also tested the hearing of elderly subjects. It was originally planned that the 70-year-old people should be tested with three different types of low-redundancy speech tests. When it was found that the discrimination scores on interrupted speech with 10 interruptions per second were so high, this test was abandoned and only accelerated speech and interrupted speech with seven interruptions per second were used. On the more difficult test with seven interruptions per second, 35 men had a mean discrimination score of 73 per cent and 63 women had a mean discrimination score of 65 per cent, for the right ear, as is seen from Figure 4.17.

It would thus seem that, from the results of distorted-speech audiometry, there exists a certain degree of central auditory dysfunction in these men and women in an unselected population of 70-year-old people tested with interrupted speech with seven interruptions per second.

Still, the values obtained by Møller (1981) are an average of 15 to 20 per cent better than those obtained by Antonelli (1970a). Although there is no obvious explanation for the difference between Møller's (1981) and Antonelli's (1970a) results, the test methods were somewhat different, and the languages used were different (Italian versus Swedish) in these two studies. In addition, as shown by Korsan-Bengtsen (1973), practice with the testing procedures has an effect on the results of distorted-speech audiometry. Because distorted-speech messages sound unfamilar to an untrained listener, each test was always preceded by a short training period in the study by Møller (1981). This might account for the higher scores obtained by subjects in this study compared to those of subjects in the study by Antonelli (1970a).

An interesting observation is, however, that the right ears (the ears contralateral to the dominant hemisphere for speech) gave somewhat higher scores than the left ears on all tests in the studies by Møller (1981). This was not observed in young, normal subjects nor in the group of 50-to-60-year-old people studied by Korsan-Bengtsen (1973). As right and left ears were tested first randomly, the observed difference between the ears cannot be explained as a training effect, but might represent differences between the left and right auditory cortex that is related to age.

CONCLUSION

It follows from the discussion in this chapter that our knowledge about the *normal* deterioration of the hearing sense with age is limited despite much effort and many studies. Most of these studies on changes in hearing as a function of age are cross-sectional studies, where the selection of what is regarded as 'normal' has been a significant obstacle. Many groups studied have not been random samples. The results that are available show that hearing is, on average, well-preserved into the beginning of the seventh decade. These results should, however, be viewed as they are, namely, mean values. The individual variation is large and many people will in their seventies suffer a disabling hearing loss without it being possible to identify a direct cause of the hearing loss except age. When the hearing loss as a function of age is considered, it is only the elevation of the pure tone threshold that is considered in the majority of the studies. Whether or not the same relationship between hearing loss for pure tones and speech discrimination under normal listening conditions is the same for the elderly as it is for young people with sensorineural hearing loss is not known.

REFERENCES

Aniansson G 1974 Methods for assessing high frequency hearing loss in every-day listening situations. Acta Oto-Laryngologica (Stockh.) Suppl. 320
Antonelli A R 1968 Further investigations on cortical deafness. Acta Oto-Laryngologica (Stockh.) 66:97–100
Antonelli A R 1970a Sensitized speech tests in aged people. In: Rojskjaer C (ed) Speech audiometry, Second Danavox Symposium, Odense, p 66–79

Antonelli A R 1970b Sensitized speech tests: Results in lesions of the brain. In: Rojskjaer C (ed) Speech audiometry. Second Danavox Symposium, Odense, pp 176–183

ASA Report Z-24-X2 1954 The relation of hearing loss to noise exposure

Beasley W 1940 The general problem of deafness in the population. Laryngoscope 50 : 856–905

Berger E H, Royster L H, Thomas W G 1977. Hearing levels of non-industrial noise exposed subjects. Journal of Occupational Medicine 19: 664–670

Berlin C I, Lowe S S 1972 Temporal and dichotic factors in central auditory testing. In: Katz J (ed) Handbook of clinical audiology. Williams and Wilkins, Baltimore pp 280–312

Bocca E, Calearo C, Cassinari V 1954 A new method for testing hearing in temporal lobe tumours. Acta Oto-Laryngologica (Stockh.) 44 : 219–221

Bocca E 1967 Distorted speech tests. In: Graham B A (ed) Sensory-neural hearing processes and disorders, Little Brown, Boston, pp 359–370

Bunch C C 1928 Auditory acuity after removal of the entire right hemisphere. Journal of the American Medical Association 90 : 2102

Bunch C C 1929 Age variations in auditory acuity. Archives of Otolaryngology 9 : 625–636

Bunch C C, Raiford T S 1931 Race and sex variations in auditory acuity. Archives of Otolaryngology 13 : 423–434

Calearo C, Lazzaroni A 1957 Speech intelligibility in relation to the speed of the message. Laryngoscope 67 : 410–419

Corso J F 1963 Age and sex differences in pure-tone thresholds. Archives of Otolaryngology 77 : 385–405

Feldmann H 1964 Dichotischer Diskriminationstest, eine neue Methode zur Diagnostik zentraler Horstörungen. Archiv für Ohren-, Nasen- und Kehlkopfheilkunde 184 : 294–329

Gaeth J H 1948 Study of phonemic regression in relation to hearing loss. Thesis, Chicago, Northwestern University

Glorig A 1957 et al, Wisconsin State Fair Hearing Survey, American Academy of Ophthalmology and Otolaryngology

Glorig A, Davis H 1961 Age, noise and hearing loss. Annals of Otolaryngology 70 : 556–571

Glorig A, Nixon J 1962 Hearing loss as a function of age. Laryngoscope 72 : 1596–1610

Goetzinger C P, Rousey C L 1959 Hearing problems later in life. Medical Times 87 : 771–780

Hansen C C, Reske-Nielsen E 1965 Pathological studies in presbycusis. Archives of Otolaryngology 82 : 115–132

Hinchcliffe R 1959a The threshold of hearing as a function of age. Acoustica 9 : 303–308

Hinchcliffe R 1959b The threshold of hearing of a random sample rural population. Acta Oto-Laryngologica (Stockh.) 50 : 411–422

Hinchcliffe R, Jones W I 1968 Hearing levels of a suburban Jamaican population. International Audiology 7 : 239–258

Jannetta P J 1981 Personal communication

Jatho V K, Heck K H 1959 Schwellenaudiometrische Untersuchungen über die Progredienz und Charakteristik der Alterschwerhörigkeit in den verschiedenen Lebansabschnitten (zugleich ein Beitrag zur Pathogenese der Presbyakusis). Laryngology Rhinology and Otology (Stuttg.) 38: 72–88

Jerger J F 1964 Auditory tests for disorders of the central auditory mechanism. In: Fields W S, Alford B R (eds) Neurological aspects of auditory and vestibular disorders. Thomas, Springfield, Illinois, pp 77–93

Johansen H 1943 Undersgelser over den Aldersbetingede Tunghrhed. Munksgaard, Kobenhavn

Katz J, Basil R H, Smith J N 1963 A staggered spondaic word test for detecting central auditory lesions. Annals of Otology 72 : 908–917

Kell R L, Pearson J C G, Taylor W 1970 Hearing thresholds of an island population in north Scotland. International Audiology 9 : 334–349

Kelley N 1939 A study in presbycusis. Archives of Otolaryngology 29 : 506–513

Kirikae J, Sato T, Shitara T 1964 A study of hearing in advanced age. Laryngoscope 74 : 205–220

Klotz R E, Kilbane M 1962 Hearing in an aging population. New England Journal of Medicine 266 : 277–280

Korsan-Bengtsen M (Møller B M) 1973 Distorted speech audiometry. Acta Oto-Laryngologica Stockh.) Suppl. 310

Leisti T J 1949 Audiometric studies of presbycusis. Acta Oto-Laryngologica (Stockh.) 37 : 555–562

Lidén G 1954 Speech audiometry. Acta Oto-Laryngologica (Stockh.) Suppl. 114

Lindén A 1964 Distorted speech and binaural speech resynthesis tests. Acta Oto-Laryngologica (Stockh.) 58 : 32–48

Matzker J 1959 Two new methods for the assessment of central auditory functions in cases of brain disease. Annals of Otology 68 : 1185–1197 ·

Miller M H, Ort R G 1965 Hearing problems in a home for the aged. Acta Oto-Laryngologica (Stockh.)
    59:33–44
Milne J S, Maule M M, Williamssen J 1971 Method of sampling in a study of older people with a
    comparison of respondents and non-respondents. British Journal of Pres. Medicine 25:37–41
Milne J S, Chopin J M 1975 Reviews after one and five years in a longitudinal study of ageing persons.
    Age and Ageing 4:152–160
Milne J S, Lauder I J 1975 Pure tone audiometry in older people. British Journal of Audiology 9:50–58
Milne J S 1977 A longitudinal study of hearing loss in older people. British Journal of Audiology
    11:7–14
Møller A R 1975 Noise as a health hazard. Ambio 4:6–13
Møller B M 1981 Hearing in 70 and 75 year old people: Results from a cross sectional and longitudinal
    population study. American Journal of Otolaryngology 2:22–29
Nylén C O 1939 The otoneurological diagnosis of tumours of the brain. Acta Oto-Laryngologica
    (Stockh.) Suppl. 33
Pestalozza G, Shore J 1955 Clinical evaluation of presbycusis on the basis of different tests of auditory
    function. Laryngoscope 65:1136–1163
Plomp R, Mimpen A M 1979 Speech-reception threshold for sentences as a function of age and noise
    level. Journal of the Acoustic Society of America 66:1333–1342
Rinder L, Roupe S, Steen B, Svanborg A 1975 Seventy-year-old people in Gothenburg. A population
    study in an industrialised Swedish city. Acta Medica Scandinavica 98:397–407
Robinson D W, Sutton G J 1979 Age effect in hearing—a comparative analysis of published threshold
    data. Audiology 18:320–334
Rosen S, Bergman M, Plester D, El-Mofty A, Sath M 1962 Presbycusis study of a relative noise-free
    population in the Sudan. Annals of Otology, Rhinology and Laryngology 71:727–743
Rosen S, Plester D, El-Mofty A, Rosen H V 1964 High frequency audiometry in presbycusis: a
    comparative study of the Mabaan tribe in the Sudan with urban propulations. Archives of
    Otolaryngology 79:18–32
Sataloff J, Menduke H 1957 Presbycusis. Archives of Otolaryngology 66:271–274
Saxén A 1937 Pathologie und Klinik der Altersschwerhörigkeit. Acta Oto-Laryngologica (Stockh.)
    Suppl. 23
Schuknecht H F 1964 Further observations on the pathology of presbycusis. Archives of
    Otolaryngology 80:369–382
Spoor A 1967 Presbycusis values in relation to noise-induced hearing loss. International Audiology
    6:48–57
Steinberg J C, Montgomery H C, Gardner M B 1940 Results of the World's Fair hearing tests. Journal
    of the Acoustic Society of America 12:291–301
Svanborg A et al 1981. To be published.
Webster J C, Himes H W, Lichtenstein M 1950 San Diego County Fair Hearing Survey. Journal of the
    Acoustic Society of America 22:473–483
Zwaardemaker H 1899 Der Verlust am hohen Tonen mit zunehmendem Alter: ein neues Gesetz.
    Archiv für Ohrenheilkunde 47

Disorders of hearing in the elderly

INTRODUCTION

People over the age of 65 years who have hearing problems constitute two groups: persons in whom deterioration of the hearing function starts at that period of their life, and those persons with some degree of hearing loss before their sixty-fifth birthday. In Denmark the second group consists of one third of the whole population of hearing impaired over the age of 65 years. This proportion is based upon knowledge gained over some 30 years of work in the rehabilitation of hard-of-hearing and of deaf individuals which began in 1951. On 27 January 1950, an Act was passed by the Danish Parliament which dealt with the provision of hearing aids and batteries as well as the repair of aids. Expenses in connection with the operation of the Act are met by the State. During 1951 and the first months of 1952, three State Hearing Centres (in Copenhagen, Odense and Århus) were established with an otologist trained in audiology in charge of each centre. A uniform procedure was agreed upon as well as uniform case sheets for the whole country, which has a population of 4 million, with a view to subsequent statistical studies of the work done.

Useful statistics were reported in the book *Danish Audiology 1951–1976*, which was printed on the 25th anniversary of the launching of the scheme. The book has the subtitle *Report from the Laboratory Denmark*. In this chapter, data and other information will be quoted from this report for which we are indebted to the many patients with hearing defects. The group over 65 years of age represented about 50 per cent of the total group.

SIZE AND NATURE OF THE PROBLEM

Prevalence of hearing disorders in elderly persons
The prevalence of impaired hearing in Denmark was studied by Bentzen and Jelnes (1955) who examined a representative sample of the Danish population. The investigation was based on information obtained by inquiries as to the 'condition of hearing' of each member of a number of households. By questioning 1569 hospitalised patients information was collected on 5000 persons whose distribution for age, sex, residence and occupation was shown to be identical to that of the general population of Denmark. In this representative sample of the entire population it was noted that 407 persons suffered from a social handicap due to defective hearing.

Of these, 369 (91 per cent) presented for a clinical audiological examination. This showed that 301 individuals satisfied the criteria set up for a social handicap due to permanently impaired hearing. The prevalence of impaired hearing in the population was thus found to be 6 per cent. Of the 301 persons under consideration, 55 showed impaired hearing in one ear only.

The proportion of hearing handicapped persons increased with increasing age. In the age group under 20 years the prevalence was 1·2 per cent, between 20 and 60 years 4·9 per cent and over 60 years 27·1 per cent. A diagnosis of presbyacusis made in 35 per cent, followed by chronic otitis media in 33 per cent. Hearing defects due to noise occurred in 11 per cent, and due to otosclerosis in 7 per cent. The severity of the hearing loss was classified according to Beasley (1940), viz. Stage 1: 'The individual has difficulties in understanding speech in church, at the theatre or in group conversation, but can hear speech at close range', Stage 2: 'The individual has difficulty in understanding ordinary direct conversation at close range, but can hear satisfactorily over the telephone or can hear loudly spoken speech'. Stage 3: poorer hearing.

Of the 109 persons with presbyacusis, 35 per cent of the individuals represented Stage 1, the rest either Stage 2 or poorer hearing. It is the latter which would need assistance from the State Hearing Centre which was just to be established.

Now, 30 years later, it is interesting to recall the great scepticism which the 6 per cent prevalence of hearing-defective individuals in Denmark aroused. Today, the total of 14 audiological clinics spread all over the map of Denmark have in the 29 years of their existence treated 180 000 persons with hearing aids.

Prevalence of elderly persons asking for assistance from the audiological clinics

Since 1976, the three State Hearing Centres have been supplemented with eleven County Municipal Audiological Clinics. These 14 institutions annually examine and treat over 53 000 patients, half of whom are rehabilitation patients and half are hospital patients referred for diagnostic evaluation.

At the clinic in Århus a survey was made during the first three months of 1979 of all patients presenting for examination. The clinic provides audiological services for a population of 570 000. The age distribution of the general population compared to that of the patients seen in the audiological clinic is shown in Table 5.1.

The proportion of patients who are under 19 years of age is the same as that of

Table 5.1 Age distribution of the patients seen at the Århus audiological clinic during three months of 1979, compared with the age distribution of the general population.

Age group (years)	Frequency distribution of general population (569 011 inhabitants)	Frequency distribution of patients at the audiological clinic (525 patients)
0–6	11%	15%
7–19	19%	12%
20–64	57%	32%
over 65	13%	41%

the general population who are in this age range. For persons over 65 years of age, the proportion seen in the audiological clinic is three times greater than their representation in the general population.

For all groups mentioned, the audiological activity was analysed, being divided into investigation and audiological treatment. Among the 525 patients, 107 were investigated for suspected hearing defects; 80 per cent of these were under the age of 19 years. Of the 418 patients who were treated audiologically, 49 per cent were over the age of 65 years of age, and 36 per cent were between 20 and 64 years of age.

This survey was made in order to obtain a statistical background for the different types of skill groups needed in the overall audiological service in order to establish that optimal care which a particular hearing-defective person would be demanding. This will be dealt with later.

The degree of hearing loss in persons over 65 years of age asking for audiological examination and treatment was investigated among the 233 persons in that age group. In 217 cases the hearing loss was symmetrical, in the remaining 15 cases asymmetrical. Table 5.2 shows the distribution of hearing loss for the group with symmetrical losses.

Table 5.2 The distribution of hearing loss in 217 patients over the age of 65 years with symmetrical hearing loss and requesting examination and treatment at the audiological clinic. The hearing loss is given as the average for the frequencies 0·5, 1 and 2 kHz.

Age group (years)	Average hearing loss (db HL)					Total
	0–15	16–30	31–60	61–80	Over 81	
65–74	14	43	39	2	2	100
75–84	2	34	44	8	3	91
85–89	1	9	5	1	1	17
Over 90	1	3	4	1	0	9
Total	18	89	92	12	6	217
Percentage	8	41	42	6	3	

The distribution of hearing loss, is 83 per cent with slight (16 to 30 dB) or moderate (31–60 dB) hearing loss, 8 per cent with very slight (0 to 15 dB) and 9 per cent very severe (over 61 dB) hearing loss. These data demonstrated by hearing-defective elderly persons turning up for audiological assistance indicate the good prospect of treatment with hearing aids. In general, a hearing aid will lift a hearing defect at the 31 to 60 dB level to the next step, i.e. 16 to 30 dB HL.

The presumed effect of the audiological treatment in the 217 elderly persons, after a period of time with training, supported by assistance from various skill groups, would be about 50 per cent obtaining an aided hearing loss of less than 30 dB, about 40 per cent with an aided hearing loss of 31 to 60 dB, and the remaining 10 per cent still having severe hearing difficulties in spite of systematic use of aids. These good results of the audiological treatment in the majority of the elderly are also a consequence of the fact that so few (in this series 15 out of 217 persons, i.e. 7 per cent) demonstrate asymmetrical hearing loss. This type of hearing loss will always cause some trouble in treatment with binaural aids.

The distribution of the hearing loss in these 15 patients is shown in Table 5.3.

Table 5.3 The distribution of the asymmetrical hearing loss in 15 patients over the age of 65 years presenting for examination and treatment at the audiological clinic.

| 10–25 dB/60–75 dB | One ear/the other ear | 45 dB/100 dB | 60 dB/105 dB |
	30–40 dB/80–90 dB		
65 years	65 years, 66 years	85 years	72 years
71 —	68 — 74 —		
72 —	75 — 76 —		
77 —	78 — 81 —		
	82 —		
(4)	(9)	(1)	(1)

Extent of need

An investigation of a random sample of elderly persons showed need for audiological treatment in 15 to 20 per cent of the sample.

Kronholm (1965) studied 117 persons in an old people's home. Ages ranged from 64 to 94 years (average 82 years). Wax formation was found to be a problem in one or both ears in 43 people. Audiometry showed the hearing loss in the better ear to be 31 to 60 dB (57 subjects), 61 to 80 dB (41 subjects), and over 81 dB (11 subjects). Hearing aids were in use by 19 individuals and were prescribed for another 49 individuals. The 40 per cent prevalence of cerumen and the need for hearing aids in 60 per cent of cases emphasises the need for audiological services among the elderly placed in special institutions.

An investigation made in 1965 in the county of Arhus of 575 persons over 65 years of age, all living in institutions, showed the number of patients in an old people's home who required audiological treatment. At the first visit of the team from the Hearing Centre, 20 per cent were already being treated with hearing aids. The otological and audiological examination revealed an additional 57 hard-of-hearing individuals in need of hearing aids. A total of 30 per cent were thus in need of hearing aids.

Among the 575 persons examined, 369 (65 per cent) were 80 years of age or over. A hearing loss of 31 to 60 dB was found in 47 per cent; over 60 dB in 7 per cent, of the whole group.

AETIOLOGY

Hearing disorders in the elderly may be divided principally into presbyacusis which developed in individuals with previously normal hearing and presbyacusis developing in individuals who were hard-of-hearing or deaf from childhood, adolescence or adulthood. These two groups will be dealt with separately.

PRESBYACUSIS IN PERSONS WITH NO PRE-EXISTING HEARING DEFECT

In the following, the definition, the pathology, the clinical picture and the treatment of presbyacusis will be discussed.

Definition

The term 'presbyacusis' implies a hearing loss caused by degenerative changes due to ageing (Schuknecht, 1974).

The State Hearing Centres of Denmark have defined presbyacusis as a hearing defect occurring after the age of 65 years after the exclusion of any other cause.

Pathology

Since Zwaardemaker first described the clinical manifestations of high-tone hearing loss from ageing in 1899, there have been many reports on this condition. Today pathologists identify four types of presbyacusis-dependent on the selective atrophy of different morphological structures in the cochlea. The hearing losses are usually symmetrical in the two ears and slowly progressive. Based on Schuknecht's (1974) classification, the types are:

1. *Sensory presbyacusis*
   Audiometry: High-tone loss not affecting hearing for speech frequencies—the condition progresses very slowly.
   Pathology: Light-microscopy studies show atrophy of both supporting cells and hair cells with a concomitant loss of cochlear neurons.

2. *Neural presbyacusis*
   Audiometry: Loss of speech discrimination relatively more severe than the hearing for pure tones. Elderly patients with rapidly progressive neural presbyacusis often demonstrate associated diffuse degenerative changes in the central nervous system. Because of poor discrimination these patients find amplification to be of limited value.
   Pathology: The temporal bones of these individuals reveal a loss in the population of cochlear neurons often involving the entire cochlea, but consistently more severe at the basal turn. Involvement of the apical region causes poor speech discrimination.

3. *Strial presbyacusis*
   Audiometry: The clinical feature is the flat audiometric pattern usually associated with an excellent speech discrimination score until the loss exceeds 50 dB. Affected individuals respond well to the use of hearing aids.
   Pathology: Patchy atrophy of the stria vascularis in the middle and apical turns of the cochlea is typical. The guinea pig is the only animal other than man which has been found to show strial atrophy. The stria vascularis appears to be the source of the positive 80 mV dc potential of the scala media. It is also thought to be the site of endolymph formation. The content of oxidative enzymes in the stria is considered to be essential to the production of energy to support cochlear function. It would thus seem reasonable for the atrophy of the stria vascularis to lead to hearing loss.

4. *Cochlear conductive presbyacusis*
   Audiometry: Bilaterally symmetrical threshold losses with straight-line descending audiometric curves beginning at 1 kHz or 2 kHz. The speech discrimination scores are inversely related to the steepness of the audiometric curve which in a great part determines the effectiveness of treatment with hearing aids.

Pathology: Microscopic studies of the cochlea exhibiting descending threshold patterns usually fail to reveal morphological changes in the sensory or neural structures. It is proposed, therefore, that hearing loss is due to a disorder in the motion mechanism of the cochlear duct (The notion that hearing loss in these patients might be due to a disorder of the brain or auditory nerve is untenable) Schuknecht (1974) added that the audiograms showing bilateral sensorineural hearing loss for frequencies over 1 kHz–2 kHz occur in ears with chronic suppurative diseases as well as in otosclerosis, diseases which cause an acceleration of the atrophic changes normally occurring in the supporting tissue.

Presbyacusis may thus be a result of degenerative defects in the peripheral part of the hearing organ, the cochlea and the central pathways. In the aforementioned four different types of cochlear presbyacusis quoted from Schuknecth, he states that Type 2 (Neural presbyacusis) is often associated with diffuse degenerative changes in the central nervous system exhibited by motor weakness and lack of coordination, tremors, irritability, loss of memory and intellectual deterioration.

In respect of Type 4 (cochlear conductive presbyacusis), it is to be noted that many clinicians consider otosclerosis to cause sensorineural hearing loss.

The pathology of age related hearing loss has been studied by Jørgensen (1961) in a series derived from the collection of temporal bones compiled by Kristensen and lodged in the ENT Department of the University Hospital, Copenhagen. The material comprised 25 temporal bones from patients ranging in age from 2 months to 84 years. Apart from the well-known loss of ganglion cells in the basal part of the cochlea which progresses with age, there was also, in PAS-stained preparations, thickening of the capillary walls of the stria vascularis. This latter change also progressed with age and was related to arteriosclerosis.

The relationship between generalised arteriosclerosis and arteriosclerosis localised in the cochlea is relevant to the observation that hearing loss is the second most common disease in elderly persons.

In the Pathological Institute of the University of Århus, Hansen and Reske-Nielsen (1965) examined the histopathological changes found in the temporal bones as well as in the central pathways and centres of 21 patients. Apart from two patients aged 60 years and 69 years, all the subjects were more than 80 years of age. Of these subjects, six had been examined and treated with hearing aids at the State Hearing Centre, Arhus. These patients had had a symmetrical hearing loss for high frequencies with the exception of two patients who had an additional unilateral conductive loss and one patient who had a total loss of hearing on one side. Low-frequency hearing losses varied from 10 to 60 dB HL (averaged over the frequencies 250 500 and 1000 Hz).

In ten patients, histological examination showed alterations in the basal cochlear turn as well as in the central auditory pathways which the authors state can explain the hearing loss for high tones, whereas the hearing loss for low frequencies was assumed to be exclusively centrally determined. In one patient with a normal cochlea, the cause of the hearing loss was presumably localised to the cochlear nerve as well as in the central pathways. In another patient, the hearing loss on one side was most likely caused by peripheral as well as by central pathological alterations.

These studies of the central auditory pathways and centres in patients from the State Hearing Centre began when Bentzen (1961), for four years, audiometrically followed a progressive lesion of the first and second cochlear neurons in a 56-year-old man with an astrocytoma localised to the pons.

Cortical hearing loss in a patient with a glioblastoma has been studied by Hansen and Reske-Nielsen (1963). There was a high-frequency hearing loss but with no discoverable damage to the peripheral auditory organ. Post-mortem examination showed right temporal-lobe destruction and post operative diffuse brain oedema partially blocking the function of the left temporal lobe.

Clinical picture

A systematic audiological study of presbyacusis started in Denmark in 1951 when the free medical examination and provision of hearing aids gave all groups of deaf and hard-of-hearing persons a chance of audiological rehabilitation.

In the course of the first year after the passing of the Act, 7000 applications were received from persons desiring audiological examination and treatment.

In the first two to three years, cases of otosclerosis and of the sequelae of otitis media were commonly found.

The clinical and audiometric examinations were structured in accordance with the experiences gained at the military audiological clinics in the USA and the UK. Speech audiometry in the Danish language was developed by Røjskjær (1952), using phonetically balanced words for measuring speech intelligibility and determining the speech discrimination score.

For the examination of elderly people it very soon became apparent that the speech intelligibility test had to be changed from words to the more easily understandable numbers. Apart from this no special test has been used in the evaluation of hearing-aid candidates among the elderly.

A test procedure which seemed to be of special value (at least as far as the topographical diagnosis is concerned) was the crossed and uncrossed acoustic stapedius-reflex threshold determination (Quaranta, Cassano and Amoros, 1980). This test was used in order to verify whether ageing produces brain-stem auditory lesions.

The examination showed in 55 per cent of the presbyacusis cases a brain-stem disorder characterised by the absence of one, several or all the acoustic reflexes; very often there was an abnormal difference between crossed and uncrossed acoustic reflex thresholds.

All hearing-defective patients (without regard to age) have been prescribed hearing aids. Using information gained by the Danish system of paedo-audiology, early adult hearing-aid users, especially the elderly, have been given a trial period with the aid at home in daily life situations.

This trial period of about three months encompasses experience, observation and training. It is regarded as an essential part of the whole medical and audiological examination. The fact that the aids are the property of the State— since 1978 of the County Municipality—makes it possible to return, if necessary, the aid after a period of time without any economic consequences for the patient in question.

Since 1965, the Danish rehabilitation programme for elderly persons with hearing disorders has received invaluable support through the establishment of what have been termed hearing welfare assistants.

For these elderly persons living in institutions examination of the hearing often has to be made with a portable audiometer. The impressions for the ear moulds are taken by the technician in the team, and a trial with the aids is started when the ear mould is ready.

This need for audiological services in these institutions for the elderly was met by the establishment of an audiological service supported by the hearing welfare assistants.

Our experience demonstrated the importance of trying hearing aids, even in otherwise handicapped elderly persons. Experience has shown that an apparently senile person may change completely when his hearing defect is compensated by the use of aids and supported by the personnel at the institution or by a visiting teacher for the hearing impaired in the patient's home.

Treatment

Hearing aids
During the lifetime of the Danish audiological service, there has been a marked development in the electro-acoustic equipment available to the audiological clinic. The original body-worn aids have given way to ear-level aids, i.e. hearing spectacles (1955) and ear hangers (1957), with an associated considerable increase in therapeutic possibilities.

Since 1960, the technical basis for stereophonic binaural audiological treatment has been provided by our hearing centre. Since 1963, this has been the standard method, irrespective of the age of the patient. The experiences gained since then concerning hearing aid treatment of bilateral hearing defects can be summarised: 'When we fit a monaural aid on an individual with a bilateral hearing loss, we are trading one handicap for another (Bentzen, 1980). In the district comprising a population of about 570 000 served by this clinic the educational service is performed by one full-time senior instructor, three full-time instructors and 22 hearing welfare assistants. This part of audiological work which is concerned with the after-care of the patients renders it possible for us to prescribe binaural aids as a routine. With this safety net provided by the pedagogical service we have been able to study the possibilities of accomplishing binaural treatment on a large scale.

In our clinic, Tonning (1973), in his thesis on directional hearing with hearing aids, has studied binaural hearing-aid treatment from an experimental viewpoint. The largest follow-up study, involving 1147 persons (731 over the age of 60 years) was performed by Jordan, Greisen and Bentzen (1967). By questionnaires supplemented by a clinical examination, the effect of binaural treatment was followed by observation periods from six months to three years (average 14 months). Table 5.4 shows the use of binaural aids related to the ages of the patients.

The period of using two aids was designated 'full-time' where they were in use every day and all day; for the rest of the users the designation was 'part-time'. In 92 per cent of the cases the binaural treatment was carried out with ear-level aids. The follow-up of the total series of 1147 persons showed that 78 per cent used two aids,

Table 5.4 Follow-up of the use of binaural hearing aids in 1147 patients over 15 years of age.

Age in years	%	Full-time use %	Part-time use %	Not used %
15–59	37	36	43	22
60–69	28 ⎫			
70–79	27 ⎬	27	49	22
80 and over	8 ⎭			
Total		32	47	22

Table 5.5 Distribution of types of hearing aids used in binaural treatment of 1147 patients.

| Age | Ear-level aid | | Body-worn aids | |
	Ear hanger	Hearing spectacles	Pocket aid	combination
15–59 years	318	63	20	15
Over 60 years	616	61	29	25
Total (1147)	934 (81%)	124 (11%)	49 (4%)	40 (3%)

19 per cent used one aid and 3 per cent had laid their aids aside. The types of hearing aids which were issued to 731 persons over 60 years of age who received binaural treatment are indicated in Table 5.5.

The influence of binaural hearing aids for the improvement of the discrimination ability of hard-of-hearing patients over 65 years of age was examined by Bentzen and Hastrup (1966). These authors reported a study on 50 persons with ages ranging from 65 to 85 years (average 73 years) treated with binaural hearing aids. The auditory discrimination test developed by Kirsten and Kurt Kristensen (1967) for children was used. The patients were examined with both one and two aids. A drawing corresponding to each test was used to indicate the correct response. In 48 cases, the use of two aids gave an average error of 5·8, compared with 11·4 errors when using only one hearing aid. In one case, better discrimination occurred with the use of one hearing aid. This test has been shown to be especially suitable for elderly patients. This examination has also provided the opportunity to judge the patient's reactions, including his confidence; these are better when using binaural hearing aids. Under the condition of the examination procedure, both the patient and his relatives who are present have had the opportunity to observe directly any improvement in hearing. In these cases, such improvement is due to improved discrimination ability through the use of both the right and the left ears. This is a positive incentive to both the patient and his relative to continue the treatment. This demonstration indicates that binaural hearing-aid treatment of the elderly reduces discrimination losses quite significantly in the great majority of cases. This suggests that this treatment should be instituted whenever possible, using the discrimination test as a therapeutic yard-stick. During the last 15 years the work of the instructors in paedo-audiology has been supported by the hearing welfare assistants.

The hearing welfare assistants

An important factor in the accomplishment of hearing-aid treatment is the motivation for sound amplification especially in the elderly. The need for amplification depends on the patient's general somatic and psychological health, his family, social and working situations. These conditions require that a simple statement of the hearing capacity determined by pure-tone and speech audiometry must be supplemented by an interview and analyses of the whole situation of the elderly in question. By visiting the patient's home the hearing welfare assistant can contribute very much to the correct programming of the total rehabilitation which the hard-of-hearing needs.

This domiciliary service started in the Municipality of Århus in 1965 and has been extended to cover work in hospitals, in nursing homes and in old people's homes. The welfare assistant is a woman without pedagogical training who works as an assistant instructor in collaboration with senior or regional instructors, teachers with special education in paedo-audiology. In accordance with the Social Welfare Act the hearing welfare assistant is responsible to the welfare departments of the local authorities. According to the Danish experience one hearing welfare assistant is required for every 20 000 inhabitants (Brandsborg and Frost, 1976).

The work of these welfare assistants involves the implementation of the treatment already prescribed and in ensuring that the hearing impaired use the hearing aids with which they have been provided. These assistants can also be of use in many small matters which are nevertheless important to the patient, e.g. cleaning the earmould, changing batteries or cords, and obtaining other items required for auditory rehabilitation.

An important part of this service entails visits to the patient's home, and in accompanying patients who are in especially difficult situations on visits to the hearing centre, to the ophthalmologist, to the optician or to the otologist. Apart from the development of the mini-aids required for binaural ear-level hearing, the establishment of the service of hearing welfare assistants was the most important step in the provision of optimal audiological treatment for presbyacusis.

Care for the elderly with presbyacusis
Optimal medical care in hospital depends very much on the welfare assistants who, on their daily round to all departments, endeavour to solve the problems of hearing-impaired patients which may or may not be related directly to hearing aids. These assistants thereby support the nurses in their responsibilities for these patients (Fig. 5.1).

Elderly patients with aphasia also often obtain appreciable help from the use of hearing aids (even in cases of slight hearing defect) when under the care of a speech therapist, and between lessons, for picking up the bombardment of language from anyone in the ward.

PRESBYACUSIS IN ELDERLY PERSONS WITH A PRE-EXISTING HEARING DEFECT

An individual who is deaf or hard-of-hearing from birth, childhood, youth or adulthood, will, in advanced age, develop additionally an age-related hearing loss. This physiological phenomenon will, together with his possibly progressive hearing defect from early life, result in a deterioration of his total hearing capacity.

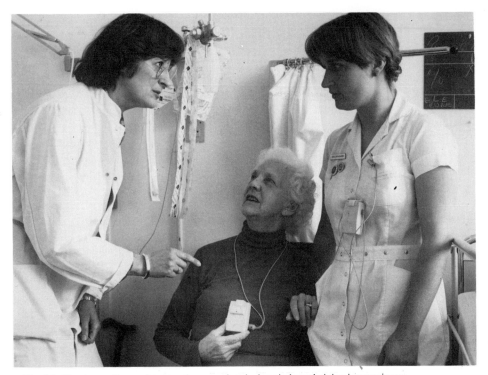

Fig. 5.1 Hearing welfare assistant on her round at the hospital ward giving instruction to hard-of-hearing patient and her nurse.

The nature of the pre-presbyacusis situation concerning the causes of hearing defects in earlier life can be obtained from an analysis of the main diagnoses in patients of all age groups treated at the Hearing Centre, Arhus, in one year from April 1974 to March 1975.

Among 2288 main diagnoses, 2200 refer to chronic hearing disorders, of which 53 per cent were diagnosed as presbyacusis. Nearly all the remaining main diagnoses were in patients younger than 65 years. Table 5.6 shows the diagnoses in

Table 5.6 Diagnoses made in chronic hearing disorders in patients younger than 65 years and the distribution and the severity of hearing loss.

Main diagnosis	0–30 dB	31–60 dB	61 dB and over	Total	%
Unknown	210	177	12	399	37
Sequelae of otitis media	110	81	8	199	20
Occupational	113	47	1	151	15
Conductive otosclerosis	43	25	5	100	10
Cochlear otosclerosis	8	15	2	100	10
Post-traumatic	51	9		60	5
Congenital	35	19	6	60	5
Hereditary	22	15		37	4
Miscellaneous	24	14	2	40	4
Total				1046	

decreasing order of frequency. The pre-presbyacusis situation for patients treated over many years at the audiological clinic is thus illustrated in that Table.

Sensorineural defects caused by trauma or explosions and 25 per cent of the patients with hearing defects arising from chronic otitis media show essentially no progression in their hearing loss. 15 per cent of the patients with noise-induced hearing loss show progression, and 10 per cent with conductive losses or cochlear otosclerosis experience slight or severe progression of their hearing loss before the age of 65 years.

The largest group of sensorineural hearing defects was that where a diagnosis had not been made. This group seems to include a large number of cases of cochlear otosclerosis. A considerable number of patients with this diagnosis experience some progression during their lifetime.

This problem of cochlear otosclerosis was examined by Sindrason, Eriksen and Halaburt (1979) in 102 patients with a sensorineural hearing defect. In collaboration with the X-ray Department and the Hearing Clinic of the University Hospital, Arhus, the patients were examined by the polytome semiaxial and axial pyramidal projections. Thirty of them had no X-ray changes around the oval window or in the otic capsule, while 72 patients had radiological changes in one or both ears which were indistinguishable from those of otosclerosis. Among the 72 X-ray positive patients, 32 had previously been reported to be undiagnosed. In the same series, 33 patients had previously been diagnosed as occupational hearing loss; in 30 patients, the tomography appeared to be positive. This series also included 15 cases of 'senile' hearing loss in which 12 patients were X-ray positive (see below).

Hearing aids

The problem of hearing-aid treatment in this group of elderly persons differs in some ways from that of the patients with 'pure' presbyacusis. For persons over 65 years, who at that age turned up for the first time at the audiological clinic with a chronic non-discharging otitis media in both ears as well as presbyacusis, the treatment is easily established. The high discrimination score associated with the conductive part of the hearing loss enables these patients to be fitted with binaural ear-level aids immediately. In a short time they become accustomed to these aids.

Individuals who have experienced bilateral sensorineural hearing defect as a result of many years of occupational noise exposure now ask for treatment as soon as they reach retirement. The change in their daily life and the desire to attend courses in some leisure activity makes them motivated for treatment with hearing aids. The combination of presbyacusis with their noise trauma may, as a result of the loudness recruitment caused by the noise damage, produce difficulties in the tolerance of amplified sound. This can be ameliorated by using hearing aids with compression which, according to our experience, is used in about 40 per cent of all cases of hearing defects in the elderly (at least at the start of using hearing aids).

Patients with conductive and/or cochlear otosclerosis who for many years have been treated with hearing aids which they have fully accepted as part of their appearance, present another problem after the age of 65 years. In consequence of the progressive deterioration of their hearing there is the problem of obtaining hearing aids which are powerful enough to produce adequate amplification. Once being accustomed to ear-level hearing aids, they very much resist the idea of using a body aid, even if such a model is the only one adequate for them. In such cases, operation for otosclerosis may be appropriate for patients over 65 years of age. In a survey of 446 stapedectomies, Andersen and Warrer (1966) reported the results of this operation in 23 cases performed on 18 patients over the age of 65 years (13 unilateral and five bilateral operations). The indication for the operation was either to obtain hearing good enough to be able to skip the aid or, in the patient with a very severe hearing loss, to obtain a result which post-operatively enabled him to use hearing aids. In four patients with a very severe hearing loss the hearing after the operation came within range for a hearing aid. The authors concluded that patients over 65 years of age have the chance of a hearing gain equal to that in an operation for otosclerosis in younger age groups, and that the operative risk has not been demonstrated to be any higher in elderly patients.

This statement concerning operation for otosclerosis in the elderly is fully in agreement with the overall view of hearing disorders in elderly patients. They must have the full impact of the modern development of the electro-acoustic industry as well as the development of medicine here represented with microscopic surgery. These are developments which have taken place at the time when they were working in that part of the population which is responsible for the future of mankind. The following will deal with the influence which progress in industry and medicine could have on their years to come after they have passed into the elderly group.

THE EXTENT OF ELECTRO-ACOUSTIC HELP

The need for modern electro-acoustics in elderly individuals

Hearing aids are the fundamental equipment used to eliminate the problems of communication caused by hearing disorders. Apart from simple electro-acoustic devices such as a powerful doorbell and telecoil for the television, no further, more sophisticated, secondary devices should be installed before the patient has been accustomed to his daily life with his new hearing for a period of at least three months. This procedure supports the attempt performed by the patient himself, the hearing instructor and the hearing welfare assistant in re-establishing a hearing world around the former hard-of-hearing person. The telecoil for TV enables him through his hearing aids to follow the performances in this very important news and amusement instrument. Often this establishment of optimal contact with the radio and TV is in high contrast with his ability to understand his old and ill wife with her faint voice. This problem can only be solved through tele-acoustics. This term covers the devices shown in Figure 5.2. The 102-year-old, hard-of-hearing man in the picture is using a radio receiver attached to his hearing aids. His wife, sitting on the sofa, is using the microphone of a radio transmitter which the hearing welfare assistant during her visit to the home is instructing the couple to handle. This electro-acoustic equipment helps the man to hear his wife as her voice now seems to be quite close to the entrance of his external ear canals.

This system which has been used in schools for the education of hard-of-hearing and deaf children has a far greater field of application. This system has to follow the hearing-defective child home where the members of the family by using the microphone and transmitter will be in close contact even if placed in different

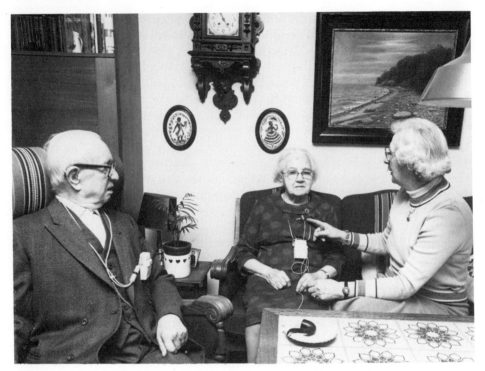

Fig. 5.2 A 102-year-old, hard-of-hearing man using hearing aids and receiver visited by the hearing welfare assistant instructing his wife in talking with him through her microphone and transmitter.

rooms. Experience gained by this system has proved to be of great value in securing small deaf children optimal language bombardment from their parents and siblings at home. The use of this form of tele-acoustics will in the future be of great help to elderly persons with hearing disorders.

The tele-acoustic device is produced in several types using different systems, such as infrared light, radio short waves and magnetic induction-field systems. The last system was constructed by an Australian electronic engineer in his attempt to help his deaf wife to overcome her hearing problems in daily life. The demonstration of the capabilities of the ·magnetic induction-field transmission which I observed in their home gave an immense impression of the extent to which a deaf person's own problems can inspire the development of modern electro-acoustic equipment.

Radio-alarm-system for elderly persons in their homes

The development of modern electro-acoustic equipment has made it possible to decentralise the supervision of elderly persons, healthy or ill, staying alone in their own home. The person within this system uses a portable transmitter in order to bring it into function if she comes into troubles, such as slipping on the floor of the bathroom, unable to help herself. The radio signal from her transmitter is received at the central receiver placed at the fire station. The man on duty calls the nearest home nurse over the telephone in her car, asking for assistance. When this contact is established, he presses the button for the return call to the woman in trouble in her bathroom. She receives his message through a loudspeaker placed in the drawing room and shortly after the home nurse is on the spot to help her. This system is in use in some municipalities in Denmark. It was first introduced in Viborg which has 40 000 inhabitants. Through its effective and fast operation it has demonstrably decentralised the supervision of elderly persons. Their need for being placed under day and night care at an institution has been minimised. The radio alarm system is considerably more economic.

This solution of a very important practical problem in their life is only one aspect of the total care for the elderly.

'AT RISK' INDIVIDUALS

Elderly persons at risk

The identification of risk or high-risk individuals at birth, or early in life is difficult. By that time there has been no (or minimal) observation period. For elderly persons who have had a life of 65 to 70 years or more, this problem is solved. But it is still not generally accepted that the reaction of a particular individual in question as a result of his somatic construction (the internal milieu) will enable us to characterise his degree of risk in the years to come. It is desirable to forecast his situation before illness and/or trauma has caught him.

The problem of the elderly person at risk can be illustrated by reference to the peripheral hearing organ, viz. the middle and, especially, the internal ear. Remember the statement by Békésy: 'the ear is our biggest skin organ'. A woman of 58 years of age turned up at our hearing clinic with bilateral tinnitus and symmetrical severe high-tone loss due to an explosion eight days previously as she left a New Year's party. Descending the staircase and coming down to the front door, she was suddenly exposed to a great 'bang'. She was deafened from a small explosive thrown down the middle of the room. She was very astonished (and so were we) at the degree of damage to her internal ears. We took a biopsy of the skin. The pathologist told us that the light microscopic examination showed metachromasia of the ground substance and degenerative changes in the elastic and collagen fibres (Bentzen and Stadil, 1971). Exactly the same picture had been found (Bentzen, 1961) in patients with clinical and audiometric otosclerosis and in patients with osteogenesis imperfecta (Stadil, 1961).

Otosclerosis a universal disease

As mentioned earlier, in the first years after its start in 1952, our clinic was visited by a large number of patients with otosclerosis. Having examined 500 to 600 cases up to 1957, it was from a clinical point of view quite evident that these patients have a particular somatic structure. The systematic manifestation of their somatic abnormalities in hair, nails and skin, with a tendency to subcutaneous bleedings and to looseness in the joints, indicated that otosclerosis may be only one manifestation of a universal defect in the connective tissues. Therefore in 1960 biopsy of the skin was taken in 18 cases of otosclerosis. All showed the abnormalities mentioned in relation to the woman with lesions in the internal ear caused by fireworks explosions. These findings were later supplemented by a questionnaire to women with otosclerosis about the birth weight of their children.

Table 5.7 The distribution of birth weight in neonates of otosclerotic mothers, compared with Statistics of the Newborn, 1964, Århus, Denmark.

Birth weight	Normal population	Mothers with otosclerosis
More than 4·5 kg	2·2 %	9·7 %
Under 2·6 kg	6·4 %	8·4 %
Number of children	1369	675

Table 5.7 shows the result. Children of whom the father and/or the mother had diabetes were excluded.

Corneometry was later introduced into the examination of these patients. In collaboration with Niels Ehlers, head of the Ophthalmological Department of the University Hospital, Århus, measurement of the thickness of the cornea by an optical method was introduced. The results are plotted on a corneogram (Fig. 5.3).

In the discussion of X-ray positive tomography in patients with sensorineural hearing disorders, Sindrason and his colleague (1979) mentioned that corneometry performed in this group of X-ray positive individuals could be relevant to the problem of 'Elderly persons at risk'. As mentioned before, 72 patients showed different degrees of sclerotic abnormalities on tomography performed with axial and semiaxial views. Later, 38 patients (19 women and 19 men from this series) all X-ray positive, were called upon for corneometry. In all, two thirds were cornea-positive, i.e. either a too thin or a too thick cornea was found in 16 women and 7 men, the highest frequency of cornea-positive individuals in any group of patients examined so far (Bentzen, 1979).

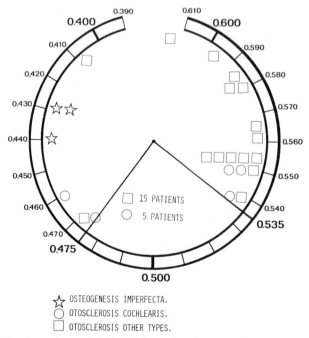

Fig. 5.3 The results of corneometry (corneal thickness given in mm) performed on patients with different types of otosclerosis and plotted on a corneogram.

An analysis was made of ten women with sensorineural hearing loss in whom X-ray studies and corneometry were both positive in order to draw a picture of their total numbers of pregnancies and children (Bentzen and Hartvig Jensen, 1980). The pregnancies and births in these ten women, not primarily selected for the purpose of analysing their outcome, are shown in Table 5.8.

Table 5.8 Pregnancies and births in a series of 10 women all cornea-positive with X-ray-positive cochlear otosclerosis, indicating insufficiency of the organ of connective tissue.

Pregnancies
Total: 32 — Abortion: 1 — Extra-uterine: 2 (same mother)

Births	Under 2·6 kg	2·6 – 4·5 kg	Over 4·5 kg	Girls	Boys
29 cases					
Single (28)	1	26	1	17	11
Multiple (1)	1	1			

Postpartum complications	
Severe haemorrhage	4 cases (same mother)
Defective children	3
Rubella embryopathy	1 girl
Unilateral deafness	1 boy (twin)
Micrognathia, etc.	1 girl (twin)

The connective tissue organ in persons at risk

Studies of clinical symptoms and histological defects of the skin in patients with otosclerosis have demonstrated that this disease is a universal one. Corneometry (objective measurement of the thickness of the cornea) often shows abnormal thickness in otosclerosis, especially in the X-ray positive cochlear otosclerosis. In collaboration with a medical group in the Danish army, corneometry has been performed on soldiers who have sustained noise trauma to the internal ear as a result of shooting. This pilot study indicated that corneometry may be of some value in the pretraumatic evaluation of noise-sensitive persons at risk.

Studies of hearing-impaired persons have provided the starting point for the information quoted so far acquired. Supplementary studies have shown that positive corneometry in patients with microscopic abnormalities of the skin is present in other groups of patients. This combination of abnormalities was found in a group of patients operated on for spontaneous retinal detachment, in the Opthalmological Department of the University Hospital, Århus (Hansen, Ehlers, Bentzen and Søgaard, 1971). This suggests a universal abnormality of constitution, possibly as a predisposition to the development of retinal detachment.

In collaboration with the clinic of internal medicine at the hospital, our Eye department has examined the thickness of the cornea in patients with *diabetes mellitus*. Eighty-one insulin-dependent juvenile diabetic out-patients with a mean diabetes duration of 15 years were examined. The mean corneal thickness was higher in the diabetic patients than in the controls in the same age range. Moreover, the corneal thickness in those patients with proliferative retinopathy was higher than in those without these changes (Olsen, Busted and Schmitz, 1980).

A 48-year-old woman and her three daughters and one son, all with normal hearing, were examined by corneometry and skin biopsy. The patient (HCA 63·107) had suffered from an acute optic neuritis on one side, followed three months later by involvement of the other eye. Clinical examination showed silky hair, brittle nails, tendency to subcutaneous bleedings and hyperflexibility of the finger nails. Corneometry showed the thickness of the cornea to be 605 μm. Light-microscopic examination of the skin showed atrophy of the epidermis and degenerative changes in the collagen and elastic fibres. The corneal thickness was also abnormal (In her four children the measurements were 600, 585, 565 and 545 μm). Examination of the skin in all four children showed mild degenerative abnormalities in the collagen tissue (Bentzen, 1980).

Ongoing examinations of patients with Reiter's disease indicate a high incidence of cornea-positive individuals with tissue type B27. Corneometry in patients with chromosome abnormalities (Henriksen, Ehlers and Bentzen, 1976) and in mongoloid children and their parents (Bentzen, 1980) failed to demonstrate any relation between the chromosomal condition and corneal thickness. In conclusion, corneometry is of value in the diagnosis of insufficient somatic constitution which characterises individuals as belonging to the group of persons at risk.

Elderly persons at risk: examples

The hearing disorders in elderly persons may reflect their somatic structure as a whole. It is a common observation that presbyacusis occurs early and develops rapidly in some families; other families show the opposite picture. Any interview of an elderly individual asking for assistance from the hearing clinic should concentrate not only on the hearing problem, but also extend to take into account all illnesses in the past. Female patients should be asked about their pregnancies and birth histories. Both sexes should be asked about diseases in their children.

Some case histories will illustrate this problem:

HCS 24·355, born in 1901 into a healthy family. At age 18 years, appendectomy with hernia repair. At 32 years, 40 years and 44 years, rheumatic fever. At 45 years of age, operated on for polypi ventriculi; at 50 years of age, iridocyclitis right eye. Genital prolapse operated on at 56 years of age, cholelithiasis operated on at 63 years; during the operation diverticuli coli diagnosed. Since 76 years of age treated for pernicious anaemia. Since 60 years of age treated with hearing aids for cochlear otosclerosis.

Examination of hearing: Bilateral sensorineural hearing defect (average hearing loss 45 dB) with normal discrimination score. Cochlear otosclerosis. Repeated controls show no progression. Corneometry: 440 μm.

The results of corneometry in the children and grandchildren are shown in Table 5.9. Cornea-positive individuals are found in three generations.

A typical example of a moderate non-progressive bilateral hearing disorder in a 79-year-old woman. A multiple-symptomatic risk mother, one of whose seven pregnancies resulted in a mongoloid child.

HCS 37·104, woman born in 1925 into a family with a severe tendency to hearing defects, some members being deaf-mute. The first examination at 42 years showed bilateral sensorineural hearing loss of 55 dB with a rather good discrimination score. Diagnosed as cochlear otosclerosis. Treated with bilateral ear hanger hearing aids under continued control. At 52 years, the deterioration of the hearing showed the threshold for pure tones to be 90 dB in both ears; these required treatment with the most powerful body aids. Corneometry: 550 μm. In Table 5.10

Table 5.9 Outcome of a couple father normal, mother cochlear otosclerosis). Where some of the hitherto examined children and grandchildren were cornea-positive, these results are italicised.

Diagnosis	Mother cornea	Father cornea	Children cornea		Grandchildren cornea
Cochlear					
otosclerosis	*440* μm	490 μm	?	Girl	
			475	Girl	B:*460* μm
(Bilateral)					G:475
			?	Girl	
			450	Girl	B:*450*
					B:*450*
					G:490
			500	Boy	G:*540*
					B:500
			440	Girl*	
23·335			?	Boy	
		*mongoloid			

Table 5.10 Outcome of a couple (father normal, mother progressive cochlear otosclerosis). All six children are cornea-positive (these results are italicised). Their birth weight and hearing disorders are indicated.

Diagnosis	Mother cornea	Father cornea	Children cornea		Birth weights	Diagnosis
Cochlear						
otosclerosis	*550* μm	520 μm	*565* μm	Girl	3·2 kg	High-tone loss
			605	Boy	4·0 kg	— — —
(Bilateral)			*550*	Girl	3·2 kg	— — —
			555	Girl	2·3 kg	— — —
			550	Girl	3·0 kg	— — —
37·104			*560*	Girl	4·2 kg	Normal

the birth weight, hearing disorders and corneometry of her six children are shown.

The contact with her children was established when the boy was examined for military service. The examination at the hearing centre, including family history and results of corneometry concluded that he was to be rejected. Apart from the severe, rapidly progressive hereditary hearing disorder, the mother had not had any illnesses, an example of a monosymptomatic risk-mother. The last example of an elderly person at risk was examined during her stay at the Geriatric Hospital, Århus.

HCA 65·564: 81-year old woman examined at the Geriatric Hospital. The hospital record showed:

myxoedema, 12 years
cancer colli uteri, 60 years
polypi recti, 72 years
sialolithiasis, 76 years
amputatio pedis dxt., 77 years
presbyacusis diagnosed, 79 years
Corneometry: 455 μm.

polypi uteri, 54 years
arthrosis varia, 70 years
osteitis hallucis dxt., 74 years
gangrena pedis dxt., 77 years
amputatio cruris dxt., 77 years
died, 81 years old

The patient and her two sisters unmarried, never pregnant.

The mother of the three women was operated for cancer pulmonis and possibly cancer coli (anus praeternaturalis).

One sister operated with extirpatio pulmonis dxt (cancer?)

The birth weight of all three between 4·0 and 4·5 kg.

Example of typical, cornea-positive, elderly person at risk; mother and sister had cancer.

Corneometry in patients over the age of 65 years

In an attempt to find the frequency of cornea-positive individuals among the patients at the hearing clinic, corneometry has for some time been performed routinely in this age group. In the past year the slit lamp used for this test has been part of the equipment at the hearing clinic, with nearly all measurements done by one observer. This objective measurement of the connective tissue organ is especially important at both ends of the life spectrum. Clinical judgement of the somatic constitution based on observation of hair, nails, skin, teeth and joints cannot be used in children under the age of 15 years because of lack of maturity. In individuals over 65 years of age this clinical observation is worthless as a consequence of degenerative changes in the ecto-mesodermally derived organ mentioned above. The thickness of the cornea seems, according to the experience gained at the Ophthalmological Department here, to be stable from four years of age until death, apart from cases in which diseases of the eye involve the corneal organ.

In total, a group of 175 individuals were cornea-positive in 31 per cent (among women 37 per cent and men 31 per cent). The distribution of cornea-positive individuals in the general population and the distribution among elderly persons in geriatric hospitals, old people's homes, etc., is still unknown. Ongoing examinations of the last categories of elderly individuals are in progress.

Table 5.11 The distribution of the thickness of the cornea in 175 individuals over 65 years of age visiting the hearing clinic.

| | Thinner | | Normal | Thicker | |
	440 μm	440–475	475–535	540–560	560 μm
Women		10	63	18	4
Men	1	13	55	11	
Total	1	23 (13%)	118 (69%)	29 (17%)	4 (1%)

Welfare programme for elderly persons at risk

An attempt to diagnose at risk or high-risk persons in this age group is made in order to try to establish a welfare programme for the elderly which can enable them to stay at home as long as possible under safe conditions. When, for example, two elderly persons of the same age need to be removed from their own home into a five-storey house without a lift, one to be placed on the ground floor and the other at the top storey, it is practical to know who would be most suitable for the flat or the top of the house. Other things being equal, the risk person among the two persons in question should be given the flat on the ground floor.

CONCLUSIONS

The high incidence of hearing disorders in the elderly (of whom 20 to 30 per cent feel their powers of communication and thereby their spiritual life threatened by disturbances in auditory contact) constitutes a great challenge to every facet of audiology. It is a challenge also to the medical, the educational, the social, the industrial, and last but not least, the administrative and economic services ready to secure the quality of life for the elderly.

Through services covering broad aspects of the whole problem it can be demonstrated that modern equipment, particularly hearing aids, is able to compensate very effectively for the age-related hearing loss. The mobilization of skilled and unskilled persons having enough foresight to realise that the quality of their own life after the age of 65 to 70 years will be determined by the efforts they now show to support the present representatives of this group. The integration of all handicapped into normal society also holds good for this part of the population in which minor or major defects are more the rule than the exception. Integration simply means keeping the elderly in their usual situation at all costs. Even when widowed or alone, these people must be maintained without losing daily contact with their children and close members of their family.

Changes in the mode of life, with a tendency to early retirement, increases the need to maximise hearing ability. This results in more motivated elderly patients consulting audiological centres. The remarkable development in electro-acoustic devices guarantees a service level never seen before. The elderly will call on this service for the many ways by which we can now improve their quality of life.

REFERENCES

Andersen H C, Warrer H 1966 Otosclerosis surgery on patients above the age of 64 years. In: G Lidén (ed) Geriatric audiology. Almqvist and Wiksell, Stockholm

Beasley W C 1940 General problem of deafness in the population. Laryngoscope 50 : 856–905

Bentzen O, Jelnes K 1955 Incidence of impaired hearing in Denmark. Acta Otolaryngolica, Stockholm 3 : 189–197

Bentzen O 1961 Skin abnormalities in otosclerosis. Excerpta (Amst.) Int. Congr. Ser. 35 : 40–41

Bentzen O 1961 Progressive affection of first and second acoustic neuron followed audiometrically for four years. Lyon, Audin

Bentzen O, Stadil P 1961 Akutte støjtraumer hos patienter med hudforandringer. Ugeskrift for Laeger 123 : 663–665 (English summary)

Bentzen O, Hastrup E 1966 Binaural hearing aids for the improvement of the discrimination-ability of hard of hearing patients over 65 years of age. In: Liden g (ed) Geriatric audiology. Almqvist and Wiksell, Stockh, pp 87–93

Bentzen O 1976 Audiological service in Denmark. In: 1976 O Bentzen, H Ewertsen and G Salomon (eds) Danish audiology, 1951–1976 Nyt Nordisk Forlag, Arnold Busck, Copenhagen, pp 35–48

Bentzen O 1980 Binaural hearing aid application-Denmark. In: Libby E R (ed) Binaural Hearing and Amplification. Zenetron, Inc, Chicago, Illinois vol. 2 pp 131–157

Bentzen O 1980 Unpublished data

Bentzen O, Jensen J H 1980 Early detection and treatment of deaf children. 3rd International Elks' Conference, Winnipeg.

Bentzen O, Ewertsen H, Salomon G (eds) Danish Audiology, 1951–1976 Nyt Nordisk Forlag. Arnold

Brandsborg K, Frost E 1976 The social paedo-audiological requirements of the patient, now in the future In: 1976 O Bentzen, H Ewertsen and G Salomon (eds) Danish audiology, 1951–1976 Nyt Nordisk Forlag, Arnold Busck, Copenhagen, pp 35–48

Hansen C C, Reske-Nielsen E 1963 Cortical hearing loss in patient with glioblastoma. Archives of Otolaryngology 77 : 461–464

Hansen C C, Reske-Nielsen E 1965 Pathological studies in presbyacusis. Archives of Otolaryngology
    82:115–132
Henriksen F, Ehlers N, Bentzen O 1976 Unpublished data
Jordan O, Greisen O, Bentzen O 1967 Treatment with binaural hearing aids. Archives of
    Otolaryngology 85:319–326
Jørgensen M B 1961 Changes of aging in the inner ear. Archives of Otolaryngology 74:164–170
Kristensen K, Kristensen K 1967 En auditiv skelnetest. Nordisk Tidsskrift, Tale og Stemme 1:30–35
    (English summary)
Kronholm A 1966 Auditory problems in a home for the aged. In: Liden G (ed) audiology. Almqvist and
    Witell, pp 58–62
Kruse F, Ehlers N, Bentzen O, Søgaard H 1971 Central corneal thickness in retinal detachment. Acta
    ophthalmologica 49:467–472
Olsen T, Busted N, Schmitz O 1980 Corneal thickness in diabetes mellitus. Lancet 19:883
Quaranta A, Cassano P, Amorso C 1980 Presbyacousie et reflexometrie stapedienne. Audiology
    19:310–315
Røjskjaer C 1952 Monaural speech audiometry. Thesis, University of Copenhagen. Poul Søndergaards
    bogtrykkeri, Odense
Schuknecht H F 1974 Pathology of the ear. Harvard University Press, Cambridge, Massachusetts,
    USA
Sindrason E, Eriksen P O, Halaburt H 1979 Rontgengeislagring a sjukdomum innra eyrans
    (otosclerosis cochlearis). Laknabladid, Reykjavik 65:91–97 (English summary)
Stadil P 1961 Histopathology of the corium in osteogenesis imperfecta. Danish Medical Bulletin
    8:131–134
Tonning F-M 1973 Directional audiometry. Thesis, University of Bergen

Central disorders of hearing in the elderly

In the chapter on Peripheral Disorders, Bentzen discusses the problems of age-related hearing loss. There is now increasing evidence that even in the absence of a significant loss of hearing sensitivity by the peripheral mechanism, age-associated changes take place in higher levels of the auditory perceptual system which markedly reduce the ability of ageing listeners to understand speech under less-than-optimal listening conditions. Such central changes, of course, additionally complicate the effects of impaired hearing due to peripheral changes.

It is the purpose of this chapter to present the findings of recent research studies on central auditory function in man to explore their implications in our understanding of ageing whether accompanied or unaccompanied by audiometric indications of significant hearing impairment.

The gerontologist views ageing as a life-long process. The implied continuous changes, which can be thought of as maturational, maximal and degenerative, may be monitored to provide reference guidelines for the clinician in his understanding of dysfunction in each individual who seeks his help. It is readily apparent that such changes, particularly those involving important inter-personal behaviour, as in the reception and expression of speech, often involve the function of more than a single system. Thus the perception of speech, at different stages of life, is related to the function of both peripheral and central mechanisms. While the auditory system is often viewed, in descriptive treatises, as beginning with the ear and ending in the primary auditory cortical centers, this topographic limitation is inadequate for clarifying age-related changes in the understanding of spoken messages under representative conditions of daily living. Each failure of speech perception is based upon the interaction of the linguistic content and physical attributes (i.e. of the phonological, transmission and environmental acoustics) of the message with the auditory, linguistic and psychological abilities and behaviour of the listener. Such failures can be understood by viewing the mechanism of audition as more than a simple reception and transmission system for individual auditory and neural events, and rather as a multistage complex in which the speech message is affected in a variety of ways as it ascends from the periphery and in which the brain is the final integrating system. This integrating system, when functioning efficiently, often overcomes widely varying combinations of the neurally coded messages pouring into it, resulting in an acceptable understanding of even highly unfavourable signal-to-noise conditions and of distortions and peripheral ear errors of audition. This is apparently due to a fortuitous confluence of external (the message itself) and internal (factors within the listener) redundancies. As the favourable aspects of message redundancy are reduced, either externally before being received, or internally by the failure of function of the peripheral auditory mechanism, the integrating brain comes under increasing stress to use its complex resources even more efficiently. This occurs repeatedly in everyday life, for example when we listen monaurally through the low-fidelity telephone system, or in situations with competing noise or other speech. Under such conditions the level of efficiency of brain function is usually the critical factor in speech perception, and it is there that we must look for the key to the socially disturbing changes in speech understanding which accompany ageing.

CHANGES IN THE CENTRAL AUDITORY NERVOUS SYSTEM

In a comprehensive review of the then state of knowledge about presbyacusis in 1962, Hinchcliffe forcefully emphasised the involvement of much of the entire auditory mechanism, particularly the central processes. This is supported by the findings of research studies reported here and elsewhere, that problems in hearing for speech are often disproportionately more disruptive than can be accounted for by the pure tone audiogram. Elsewhere in this book evidence is presented of specific degenerative changes in the peripheral ear mechanism. Coupled with the relatively advanced knowledge of the physiology of that mechanism, histopathologic findings can be related to pre-morbid hearing test results with considerable confidence. As we extend our interest to increasingly higher central levels of auditory function, however, we are confronted with the discouragingly (though highly valued) redundant and generalised linguistic and cognitive activity of speech perception. We have to content ourselves, at this stage of our knowledge, with emerging information about changes in parts of the central auditory nervous system (CANS), remaining aware of the undoubted importance of other parts of the brain in the observed degeneration of this complex function.

There have been conflicting reports of changes in the brain stem in older persons. Konigsmark (1969) and Konigsmark and Murphy (1972) in a study of the ventral cochlear nuclei found no evidence of age-related degeneration. Kirikae and his colleagues (1964), however, described age-associated degenerative changes in the cochlear nucleus, the superior olive, the inferior colliculus and the medial geniculate body, in addition to the changes in the internal ear tissues. Hansen and Reske-Nielsen (1965) found atrophic changes in parts of the central auditory pathways and their nuclei, as well as in cortical areas, in pathological studies of 12 aged patients.

Others have described generalised changes in the central nervous system in which areas thought to be essential to auditory perception are involved. Dublin (1976) points out that the central auditory pathway may be affected by the arterial insufficiency attendant upon degenerative arterial disease associated with ageing. He reported 'a correlation' between hearing loss and the degree of arteriosclerosis. In an often quoted study by Brody (1955) the greatest loss of brain neurons is reported to be in the superior temporal gyrus, followed by those of the inferior temporal gyrus, regions that apparently figure prominently in the understanding of speech. Samerajski (1976) reports that the older brain shows changes in the relative sizes of the gyri and sulci in the superior frontal and temporal lobes. While Roberts (1966) does not relate his report to ageing he links disturbances in immediate memory (so prominent in older listeners) to lesions in the inferior medial temporal region. Roberts also reports that 'the more anterior the lesion the more auditory aspects of speech are involved'. This takes on special meaning when coupled to Smith and Sethi's (1975) report that in many elderly persons there is a slowing in electrical brain waves, particularly over the anterior areas. In some older persons they found this to be more marked on the left side, which is usually the dominant side for speech processing.

Briefly, there is still a paucity of knowledge about age-associated changes in the central areas which are thought to be important to the understanding of speech. The documented shrinking of the ageing brain, however, suggests that its various areas which participate in the perception of speech lose some of their effectiveness for the critical integrative functions so necessary when speech undergoes degradation which reduces its redundancy.

Research approaches

Recent research efforts relating the understanding of speech to ageing have begun to explore various parts of the communication whole to determine their contributions, either singly or in interactions with other parts, to functional breakdown. The speech perception complex can be divided into two main divisions, that of the signal and that of the listener.

A. Aspects of the signal/message
  1. The talker
    a. His voice quality, patterns of articulation and prosody
    b. The linguistics of his message.
  2. The setting, topic of the communication, etc.
  3. The characteristics of the transmitting medium.
  4. The acoustic environment of the talker and of the listener.
B. Characteristics of the listener
  1. Peripheral reception
    a. His threshold sensitivity for various stimuli
    b. Distortions in the cochlea (i.e. the fidelity with which it encodes by frequency/intensity/time patterns)
  2. Brain stem alterations of the neural patterns
    a. Facilitation and inhibition, affecting such functions as binaural fusion and inhibition
    b. Changes in transmission time (aberrations may be noted through evoked electrical responses)
  3. Interactions between the cerebral cortex and other parts of the brain (Penfield and Roberts, 1959, suggest that connections between the main cortical areas for speech understanding may be through the upper brain stem rather than cortical).
  4. Processing skills
    a. Vigilance: for new stimuli; for continuing stimuli, as a function of time (e.g. visual perception is not as prompt, in older persons, and its maintenance span is shorter than in young persons.)

   b. Recognition of phonemic and prosodic patterns (i.e. intonation, stress, timbre, pause, pitch, etc.)
   c. Short-term memory
   d. Figure-ground selectivity (e.g. hearing in noisy surroundings)
   e. Linguistic processing: lexical (vocabulary), syntactic (rules of structure, grammar), and semantic (reasonableness of meaning)
   f. Hemispheric dominance for speech (This dominance by one hemisphere, usually the left, may be more pronounced, with ageing, in some persons)
   g. Inter-sensory integration (e.g. audio-visual, affecting the synthesis of facial clues and gestures with the auditory information)

A number of these factors and variables have been incorporated in published findings of research efforts. Some of these findings are summarised in the following, which is organised primarily according to the test materials employed.

Hearing for clinical word lists
It has long been observed by clinical audiologists that older patients often perform more poorly on tests of word discrimination than their audiometric hearing losses would suggest. Gaeth (1948) was one of the first to study this and apparently coined the term 'phonemic regression' to describe the abnormal mishearing of the consonants of speech by older persons. Since then his observations have been supported by, amongst others, Pestalozza and Shore (1955), primarily through the use of clinically available PB ('phonetically balanced') word lists (Harbert et al, 1966; Luterman et al, 1966; Toyoda and Yoshisuke, 1969; Punch and McConnell, 1969; Sticht and Gray, 1969).

   There have been conflicting reports about whether this decrement in word discrimination is gradual with ageing or occurs significantly only in older persons. Thus, Jerger (1973) drew a curve of the average maximum PB scores obtained by over 2000 clinic patients of different ages (6–89 years) (Fig. 6.1), showing a

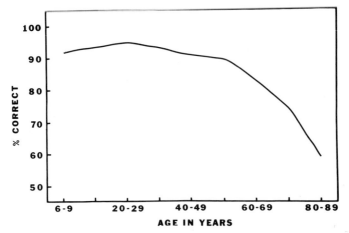

Fig. 6.1 Adaption of curve by Jerger (1973) showing average maximum speech discrimination scores for PB words, as a function of age. Jerger states that the curve follows 'the expected exponential form', for the equation $\log (y - 100) = a + 0.015x$, where y is the PB max score and x is the age in years.

continuous fall off in adults, particularly after the middle years. Blumenfeld and her colleagues (1969), on the other hand, used the Fairbanks Rhyme Test on an experimental population drawn from entirely outside the clinics and found that while there was a tendency for performance to decrease with age, the correlation was clearly more significant for subjects over the age of 60 years. The latter finding agrees with that of Feldman and Reger (1967) that the phonemic regression findings of Gaeth (1948) and Pestalozza and Shore (1955) and others is more pronounced in ageing adults seen in the audiology clinics than in non-clinic populations.

Hearing for degraded speech
The effects of ageing on the understanding of speech in everyday life are most clearly shown through the use of speech materials presented under conditions of distortion or in competition with other stimuli.

Bocca and Calearo (1956) were among the first to show reduced performance by aged subjects on tests using 'low redundancy' speech material, while Goetzinger and Rousey (1959) and Goetzinger and his colleagues (1961) reported that a poor quality recording of the standard clinical PB test more effectively revealed ageing decrement than the better recordings generally used in clinics. They therefore added the step of noting the difference in performance on a 'difficult' versus an 'easy' version of the same test to expose decline in central processing of speech as a function of age.

More recently investigators of ageing speech perception have degraded their test materials in a variety of ways. The following are some of the techniques used:

1. Filtering out the high or low frequencies (Teatini, 1970), or retaining only two narrow frequency bands, one low (surrounding 500 Hz) the other higher (centering around 2000 Hz) (Bergman, 1976).
2. Removing portions of the signal by electronic switching. For example, the sentence 'Please close the window' would be heard as 'P ea cl se e in ow' (Bocca and Calearo, 1963; Teatini, 1970; Bergman, 1971).
3. Compressing the material, in which portions are removed, as in the above, then closing up the resultant time gap so that the total time of the message is reduced, or compressed, by a given percentage. Thus, the above example would be heard as 'Pea clse e inow'. This technique has been applied to young versus older adults (Sticht and Gray, 1969; Konkle et al, 1977).
4. Altering the message's speed, e.g. by increasing the speaking rate from the normal average of 120 words per minute to 360 wpm (Calearo and Lazzaroni, 1957).
5. Submerging the message in noise (e.g. cafeteria noise) or in competing speech. Such speech may be either an unintelligible babble (Blumenfeld et al, 1969; Bergman, 1980) or competing intelligible speech by one or more talkers. The latter has been called 'perceptual masking' (Carhart and Nicholls, 1971), to distinguish its attentional interference from that posed by a meaningless but high intensity noise or speech competition, which is referred to simply as masking.
6. Overlapping messages, in which the listener is required to repeat *both* of the competing messages (Katz, 1962).

Other methods for measuring the understanding of speech under life-like conditions include studies under various listening environments (e.g. with reverberation, as in large halls and houses of worship) and with various transmitting media, such as the telephone (Bergman, 1968, 1980). Similarly, by employing talkers of different voice and speech characteristics in the preparation of recorded test materials it is possible to expose the relative difficulties in speech perception experienced by older listeners for different speakers (Bergman, 1980).

Finally, by manipulating the linguistics (vocabulary, syntax and semantics) of test materials as well as the length of messages it is possible to expose the role of such aspects as short-term memory failure and weakening of the automatic application of learned rules of grammar in the age-associated decline of speech understanding under difficult listening conditions (Bergman, 1980).

Findings

Time Processing

The most compelling evidence of ageing, in the understanding of degraded speech, involves time processing abilities. For example, older listeners are dramatically inferior to younger adults in their understanding of speech which is interrupted a number of times each second (Bocca and Calearo, 1956, 1963; Bergman, 1971) (see Fig. 6.2). Bergman (1980) explored his finding further by varying the amount of time the speech signal was on, in proportion to the silent intervals, in each interruption, on the assumption that for a given brief exposure to the signal older listeners may perceive less of it than younger ones. It was found that this premise was apparently supported and in addition it appears that as the proportion of signal is increased, in relation to the silent intervals, in each interruption, the ability to reap the advantages of the increased information is markedly reduced with increasing age. In short, older listeners are shown to be poor in central processing of brief speech exposures. This agrees with the general observations on ageing and brain damage by Hicks and Birren (1970) that perception and response are affected by slowing psychomotor performance in older persons.

Another example of apparently slower processing of speech is a report by Calearo and Lazzaroni (1957), who compared the performance of persons over age 70 with that of younger adults on the perception of speech produced at various speaking rates in Italian. Figure 6.3 shows the clear difference in performance between the young adults and the elderly group.

It appears that in addition to the probable breakdown of central auditory processing for fast speech, older persons experience anxiety, which then affects their performance. Eisdorfer (1968) measured the heart rate and blood fat concentrations. He noted the galvanic skin responses of older vs. younger Ss on rapidly paced tasks. The results indicated greater signs of stress as revealed by such measures.

Electronically compressed speech studies yield results similar to those of speeded speech. Sticht and Gray (1969) compared young vs. older persons who had similar types and amounts of sensorineural hearing loss. They interpreted the poorer performance of the older group as evidence of the role of central factors in the

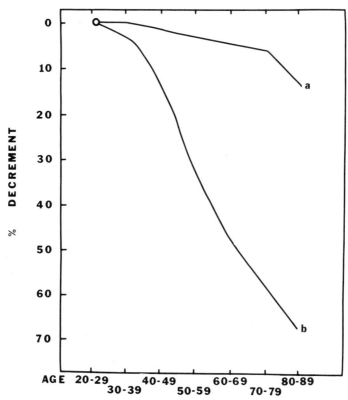

Fig. 6.2 Age decrement in the understanding of everyday sentences electronically interrupted 8 times per second. Curve 'b' represents the average scores for the interrupted sentences while curve 'a' depicts the scores for the sentences presented normally, to show the severely disturbing effect of the interruptions. N = 282.

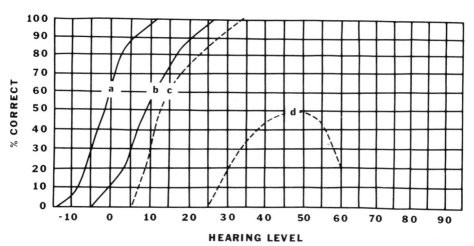

Fig. 6.3 The effect of age on the discrimination of Italian speech material produced at a normal rate and at a rapid rate. Curve a–Young adult scores for normal speech rate; b–Young adult scores for high speed speech; c–Older adult (over age 70) scores for normal speech; d–older for speeded speech (Adapted from Calearo and Lazzaroni, 1957).

differences. Others have supported these findings on tests with compressed speech (Konkle et al, 1977; Bergman, 1980).

Hearing speech in noise
Except for time-sharing transmission paradigms in long-distance telephone conversations we do not often experience speech mechanically interrupted by brief periods of silence, although that design does seem to have implications related to the time/intensity characteristics of speech at *all* times (McCroskey, 1979). A more readily familiar type of interrupted speech is that which is randomly masked by intrusion of noises around us. Experimental study of the disruptive effects of bursts of masking noise on speech perception shows this to be an even more age-revealing disturbance than the quiet-separated interruptions (Bergman, 1980). This is probably a major aspect of the breakdown of speech understanding in competing noise or babble by older listeners. Such difficulties have been repeatedly documented (Lindeman and Van Leeuwen, 1967/1969; Blumenfeld et al, 1969; Carhart and Nicholls, 1971; Smith and Prather, 1971; Jerger, 1973: Tillman et al, 1973; Mayer, 1978), and the increasing difficulty of hearing speech in noise is the most common complaint of older patients in audiology clinics.

Examples of 'typical' noises employed in studies of this difficulty include traffic noises and subway noises (Mayer, 1978), cafeteria noises (Corliss, et al, 1960; Cooper and Cutts, 1971), and cocktail party sounds (Groen, 1969), while artificial noise in such studies has included 'white noise' (a broad band hissing sound) (Dirks and Wilson, 1969). In such studies, and others in which speech is the interfering competition, the age-related drop in performance is most marked after age 65 years (Blumenfeld et al, 1969), but the correlation with age is poorer than for speech heard in quiet, indicating that there is considerable variation among older listeners in the difficulties encountered in hearing in noise.

Another approach is to determine how much above the competing noise levels a listener feels that the speech signal must be to be considered just comfortable for continued listening. Bergman (1980), reports that older listeners (aged 60–70) with essentially good hearing desired a significantly higher level (averaging 9 dB) of the prime message above the interfering noises than young adults (aged 20–30), but once again, there was greater variation of results among the older than among the younger adults.

It is probable that the dynamics of such time processing problems operate in the demonstrated disability older persons experience in understanding speech in large auditoria and in structures such as large churches, when the acoustics (reverberation characteristics) are unfavourable (Bergman, 1980). It may be that older persons do not benefit as well as younger from the precedence effect, in which a sound arriving at the ears immediately after a preceding sound is suppressed, apparently by the brain, so that it does not interfere with the perception of the first sound.

Effects of the voice of the talker
Middle-aged and older persons apparently experience increasing problems in understanding talkers who have poor voices, and with presbyacusic-type hearing loss the understanding of whispered speech becomes all but impossible (Bergman, 1980; see Fig. 6.4).

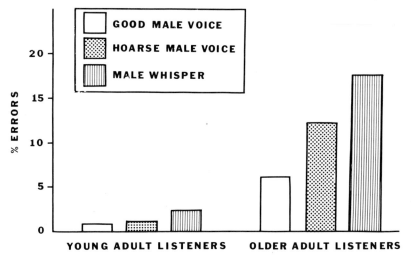

Fig. 6.4 Comparison of percentage of errors made by older vs young adult subjects listening to three different male speakers reading lists of words.

Telephone listening

It is a common observation that older persons have more difficulty hearing over the telephone than younger persons, and that this difficulty is exacerbated in the presence of noise in the listening room. One of the reasons for the inferior hearing over the telephone is its restricted frequency characteristics (300–3300 Hz) which is altered additionally by the characteristics of the particular handset in use and how the listener holds it to his ear (leakage dissipates low frequency response), and by how the talker inclines his mouth toward the telephone microphone and at what distance. Studies of the effect of such frequency distortions on the understanding of speech by older persons find significantly poorer performance than in young persons (Antonelli, 1970).

These are additional technical factors which introduce distortions in telephone communication, the sum total of which apparently account for the fact that even the best listeners frequently miss parts of the transmitted message. This is then a somewhat stressful listening situation, the kind which affects older persons disproportionately. It is not surprising, therefore, to find the common observation of this documented in quantitative studies (Fig. 6.5).

The role of the CANS in hearing through a hearing aid

A particularly unfortunate expression of the effect of an inferior transmission system on older persons is in the hearing for speech through a hearing aid. As with the telephone, the hearing aid also has a limited frequency range in which most of the energy must be devoted to the amplification of the consonants thought to be essential to the understanding of speech. The requirement that this be accomplished through severely miniaturised electronic components and their associated transducers (microphone and earphone) results in considerable reduction of the fidelity of representation of the speech signal. This alteration renders the understanding through a hearing aid somewhat difficult at best. Even in the absence of a

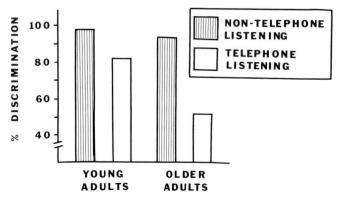

Fig. 6.5 Young adult vs older listeners' scores for everyday sentences spoken over a high fidelity system (non-telephone listening) and over a telephone system by a variety of talkers, including men, women and children. N = 16 for each of the 2 listener groups.

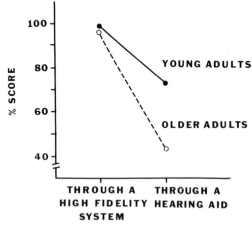

Fig. 6.6 Effect of listening with a hearing aid, young vs older listeners. Everyday sentences spoken by a variety of talkers was the test signal. N = 20 in each subject group.

clinically significant hearing loss older listeners experience demonstrably poorer speech perception through it than younger listeners (see Fig. 6.6). Since most users of hearing aids are hard of hearing adults of advanced age it is not difficult to perceive why for so many of them the benefits from their use are disappointingly limited.

Cerebral dominance

It is now clearly established that for most persons the left cerebral hemisphere is dominant for the processing of verbal material while the right hemisphere is more involved in nonlinguistic processing in addition to such activities as spatialisation and certain cognitive functions. The verbal processing dominance apparently obtains for visual as well as auditory material. In fact, Butters and his colleagues (1970), after studying patients with parietal or anterior damage of either hemisphere concluded that 'the left hemisphere is concerned with verbal material irrespective of sensory modality'. The differential activity of the cerebral hemispheres is supported further by reports such as that by Molfese and his colleagues (1975) which showed that auditory evoked responses (AERs) in infants, children and adults are larger in amplitude in the left hemisphere for speech stimuli while non-speech material evoked larger AERs in the right hemisphere.

Evidence is emerging to suggest that the relative weakness of the right hemisphere in the processing of verbal material becomes progressively more pronounced in ageing persons. For example, Johnson and his colleagues (1979) tested dichotic memory for spoken digits in Ss from age 50 to 79 years of age, divided into three groups of youngest, middle and oldest thirds. They found a substantial age-related decline in the performance of the left ear (right hemisphere) whereas the right-ear-left-hemisphere system showed no discernible decrement. They concluded from this and other of their experimental findings that abilities which depend more on the right hemisphere may show a real age-associated decline. This may mean that the contribution of the right cerebral hemisphere in the complex processing of speech becomes progressively weaker with ageing.

Memory

A generally accepted tenet of ageing is that short-term memory declines markedly. Early attempts to assess this in the retention of spoken numbers failed to support the supposition that older listeners have shorter 'auditory memory spans' when tested in this way for immediate repetition (Gilbert, 1941; Bromley, 1958). If, however, part of a message has to be held in storage while continuing to listen to incoming material it can be demonstrated that older listeners tend to forget the stored materials. This was shown for dichotic listening for groups of digits (Inglis and Tansley, 1967) and for understanding long sentences or sentences containing more than one noun phrase (Bergman, 1980). For example, when a sentence is split by a centrally intruding phrase, such as 'The man, who walks a mile every day, has two children in our school', the middle phrase will not be recalled as well by older as by younger listeners.

Effects of language and dialect background

In the mid–1960s, during the gathering of field data on ageing and the perception of speech we noted that among our 60–70 year old subjects there was a clear inferiority of performance by those for whom the test language, English, was their second-learned tongue, even though they had been speaking it regularly and fluently for an average of over 50 years. These findings were supported by additional studies in Israel in the test language of that country (Hebrew) with all results published in 1980 (Bergman, 1980). A brief study by Davis and his colleagues (1976) on hearing for frequency filtered speech compared the performance of 12 native English speakers with 12 for whom English was the second language. They found a significantly lower average score for the non-British Ss for the test material in which only the higher (intelligibility-bearing) frequencies were included.

Apparently even a difference in dialect between the speaker and listener introduces disproportionate difficulties for older listeners. An unpublished study by Kaen (reported by Bergman, 1980), of young and old White and Black Ss in the

USA found significantly poorer understanding of Negro non-standard dialect by the older White Ss than by younger White Ss, and of the standard American English by the older Black Ss than by the younger Black Ss. Such findings indicate that the understanding of speech heard under less-than-optimal conditions is even more difficult, for older persons, if communicated in a language or dialect other than that learned first in early childhood.

Judgmental rigidity, vigilance, etc

Psychological and behavioural patterns of listeners influence their anticipation of a message as well as their flexibility in correcting perceptual errors. There are some preliminary experimental indications that certain age-related tendencies contribute to declining speech perception. For example, older Ss often withold responses rather than risk the possibility of error (Craik, 1962; Silverman, 1963). Our own studies repeatedly exposed such caution as well as a rigidity in defending a first perception by our older Ss.

Although there is still a paucity of documented studies of alertness and continued vigilance to auditory stimulation by older persons, the effect of age on vigilance tasks has beem reported by Surwillo and Quilter (1964). These workers found that older Ss dropped significantly in their level of alertness on a vigilance task after a 45 minute period.

SUMMARY

The great success in human communication through speech is due in large part to the generous redundancies of language and its application to specific situations. Thus, efficient listeners are able to 'normalise' messages varying widely from speaker to speaker and under all but the most disadvantageous listening conditions (Miller, 1951). It is increasingly evident, however, that as these redundancies are reduced in the message itself and by unfavourable transmission and listening conditions, success in spoken communication is linked to the age of the listener, in whom central changes are operative. Particularly after 60 years of age, the average ageing adult experiences increasing failure of auditory processing under unfavourable listening conditions, whether or not he has a significant loss of hearing; the existence of a hearing loss complicates the problem even more. Since much of our daily listening involves the use of transmitting systems, such as the radio, television and telephone, as well as hearing in the presence of competing noises or other speech, the documentation of significant breakdown with age strongly suggests the urgency of greater attention to the physical (acoustical and environmental) and physiological (CNS and psychological) factors whose interactions are responsible, with a view to developing corrective measures to improve the quality of life for older persons.

REFERENCES

Antonelli A R 1970 Sensitized speech tests in aged people. In: Røjskaer C (ed) Speech audiometry Danavox, Borgergrade, Copenhagen, pp 66–79
Bergman M 1968 Unpublished study of 'Hearing and aging', Hunter College, New York
Bergman M 1971 Hearing and aging. Audiology 10:164–171

Bergman M 1980 Ageing and the perception of speech. Baltimore: University Park Press

Bergman M, Blumenfeld V G, Cascardo D, Dash B, Levitt H, Margulies M K 1976 Age-related decrement in heariing for speech. Journal of Gerontology 31: 533–538

Blumenfeld V G, Bergman M, Millner E 1969 Speech discrimination in an ageing population. Journal of Speech and Hearing Research 12: 210–217

Bocca E, Calearo C 1956 Aspects of auditory pathology of central origin in aged subjects. Annals of Laryngology 55: 365–369

Bocca E, Calearo C 1963 Central hearing processes. In: Jerger J (ed) Modern developments in audiology. New York, Academic Press

Brody H 1955 Organisation of the cerebral cortex. Journal Of Comparative Neurology 102: 511–556

Bromley D B 1958 Some effects of age on short-term learning and remembering. Journal of Gerontology 13: 398–406

Butters N, Samuels I, Goodglass H, Brody B 1970 Short-term visual and auditory memory disorders after parietal and frontal lobe damage. Cortex 6: 440–459

Calearo C, Lazzaroni A 1957 Speech intelligence in relation to the speed of the message. Laryngoscope 67: 410–419

Carhart R, Nicholls S 1971 Perceptual masking in elderly persons. Paper presented at the 1971 Annual Meeting of the American Speech and Hearing Association, Chicago

Cooper J G, Cutts B P 1971 Speech discrimination in noise. Journal of Speech and Hearing Research 14: 332–337

Corliss E, Kobal M, Burghorn S 1960 Reduction of signal-to-noise ratio induced by distortion in speech transmission systems. Journal of the Acoustic Society of America 32: 1502a

Craik F I M 1962 The effects of age and the experimental situation on confidence behaviour. Bulletin of the British Psychology Society 47: 21 (abstract)

Davis R J, Kastelanski W, Stephens S D G 1976 Some factors influencing the results of speech tests of central auditory function. Scandinavian Audiology 5: 179–186

Dirks D D, Wilson R 1969 The effect of spatially separated sound sources on speech intelligibility. Journal of Speech and Hearing Research, 12, 5–38

Dublin W B 1976 Fundamentals of sensorineural auditory pathology Thomas, Springfield, Illinois

Eisdorfer C 1968 Arousal and performance: Experiments in verbal learning and a tentative theory. In: Talland G A (ed) Human aging and behaviour. New York, Academic Press

Feldman R, Reger S 1967 Relations among hearing, reaction time and age. Journal of Speech and Hearing Research 10: 479–495

Gaeth J 1948 A study of phonemic regression in relation to hearing loss. Unpublished doctoral dissertation, Northwestern University Chicago, USA

Gilbert J G 1941 Memory loss in senescence. Journal of Abnormal Social Psychology 36: 73–86

Goetzinger C P, Rousey C 1959 Hearing problems in later life. Medical Times 87: 771–780

Goetzinger C P, Proud G O, Dirks D, Embry J 1961 A study of hearing in advanced age. AMA Archives of Otolaryngology 73: 662–674

Groen J 1969 Social hearing handicap: its measurement by speech audiometry in noise. International Audiology 8: 182–183

Hansen C C, Reske-Nielsen E 1965 Pathological studies in presbyacusis: cochlear and central findings in 12 aged patients. Archives of Otolaryngology 82: 115–132

Harbert R, Young I, Menduke H 1966 Audiological findings in presbycusis. Journal of Auditory Research 6: 297–312

Hicks L H, Birren J E 1970 Aging, brain damage and psychomotor slowing. Psychological Bulletin, 74: 377–396

Hinchcliffe R 1962 The anatomical locus of presbycusis. Journal of Speech and Hearing Disorders 27: 301–310

Inglis J, Tansey C L 1967 Age difference in dichotic listening performance. Journal of Psychology 66: 325–332

Jerger J 1973 Audiological findings in aging. Advances in Oto-rhino-laryngology 20: 115–124 (Basel)

Johnson R C, Coles R E, Bowers J K, Foiles S V, Nikaido A M, Patrick J W, Woliver R E 1979 Hemisphere efficiency in middle and later adulthood. Cortex 15: 109–119

Katz J 1962 The use of staggered spondaic words for assessing the integrity of the central nervous system. Journal of Auditory Research 2: 327–337

Konigsmark B W 1969 Aging cells and structures. International Audiology VIII Nos 2–3, 191–198

Konigsmark B W, Murphy E A 1972 Volume of the ventral cochlear nucleus in man: its relationship to neuronal population and age. Journal of Neuropathology and Experimental Neurology 31: 304–316

Konkle D F, Beasley D S, Bess F H 1977 Intelligibility of time-altered speech in relation to chronological aging. Journal of Speech and Hearing Research 20: 108–115

Kirikae I, Sato T, Shitara T 1964 Study of hearing in advanced age. Laryngoscope 74: 205–220

Lindeman H, Van Leeuwen P, 1967 Bepaling van de valideteir van het gehoor met behulp van een bedrijfsspraakandimeter. T. Soc. Geneesk, 45, 814–837 1967. English summary in International Audiology 8:626–632

Luterman D, Welsh O, Melrose J 1966 Responses of aged males to time-altered speech stimuli. Journal of Speech and Hearing Research 9:226–230

Mayer C 1978 The perception of speech in noise as a function of age. Unpublished doctoral dissertation, Doctoral Program in Speech and Hearing Sciences, City University of New York

McCroskey R L 1979 Some characteristics of temporal auditory behaviour among elderly persons., In Aural rehabilitation for the elderly (M A Henoch ed) New York, Grune and Stratton

Miller G A 1951 Language and communication, New York, McGraw-Hill

Molfese D L, Freeman R B, Palermo D S 1975 The ontogeny of brain lateralization for speech and nonspeech stimuli. Brain and Language 2, 356–368

Penfield W, Roberts L 1959 Speech and Brain Mechanism, Princeton N J, Princeton University Press

Pestalozza G, Shore I 1955 Clinical evaluation of presbyacusis on the basis of different tests of auditory function. Laryngoscope 65, 1136–1163

Punch J L, McConnell F 1969 The speech discrimination function of elderly adults. J Audit Res 9, 159–166

Roberts L 1966 Central brain mechanisms in speech. In: Brain Function, Vol. III Speech, language and communication (E. C. Carterette ed) Los Angeles, University of California

Samarajski T 1976 How the human brain responds to aging. J Amer Geriatrics Soc, 24, 4–11

Silverman I 1963 Age and the tendency to withold response. Journal of Gerontology 17:372–378

Smith R, Prather W 1971 Phoneme discrimination in older persons under varying signal-to-noise conditions. Journal of Speech and Hearing Research 14:630–638

Smith B H, Sethi P K 1975 Aging and the nervous system. Geriatrics 30:109–115

Sticht R, Gray B 1969 The intelligibility of time compressed words as a function of age and hearing loss. Journal of Speech and Hearing Research 12:443–448

Surwillo W, Quilter R 1964 Vigilance, age and response-time. American Journal of Psychology 77:614–620

Teatini G 1970 Sensitized speech tests (SST): Results in normal subjects. In: Røjskaer C (ed) Speech audiometry Danavox, Borgergade, Copenhagen, pp 37–43

Tillman T W, Carhart R, Nicholls S 1973 Release from multiple maskers in elderly persons. Journal of Speech and Hearing Research 16:152–160

Toyoda K, Yoshisuke G 1969 Speech discrimination in presbyacusis. International Audiology 12:135–139

Tinnitus in the elderly

The word tinnitus is derived from the Latin 'tinnire' which means to ring or to tinkle. The term is used to describe the sensation of any sound which appears to be arising in the head or ears of the sufferer. Occasionally, at its onset, the patient may have the impression that there is an external source for this sound, but he quickly realises that this is not so.

This last feature distinguishes the genuine tinnitus sufferer from the so-called 'hummers'. This name has been given by Walford (1980) to people, generally elderly widows or persons over 80 years of age, who complain of a low pitched hum. This humming is attributed by the sufferer to, for example, machinery, electric wires or secret defence installations. Paranoid features are often present. The noise troubles the patient mostly at night time and he often complains vociferously. Even after careful measurement of ambient sound such people are not easily convinced that there is no evidence for the sound they hear.

Auditory hallucinations, in which the noise takes the form of words, music or meaningful sounds are generally considered to be a manifestation of a neurological or psychiatric disorder and are not included in this definition of tinnitus. However, Goodwin (1980) reports five of her own cases and reviews the literature of eleven other cases in which these auditory perceptions changed, generally over a period of a few weeks, to the more recognisable form of tinnitus in the absence of identifiable psychiatric abnormality or organic neurological disease.

Hitherto 'tinnitus' has been subdivided into (a) subjective tinnitus, and (b) objective tinnitus, in which the sound is not only heard by the patient, but is also heard—or potentially can be heard—by another observer. Since, by definition, tinnitus is what is experienced by the patient, it might be argued that the term 'objective tinnitus' is inconsistent and there is no certainty that an observer is hearing the same sound. Nevertheless, the term is a useful one for clinicians in their management of patients.

PREVALENCE

It is probably normal to experience transitory episodes of tinnitus occurring perhaps once a month or thereabouts. These come on suddenly and die away over a few seconds. There is a concomitant, or immediately preceding, sense of dullness of hearing. Moreover, a proportion of normal people become aware of a continuous quiet sound when in a silent sound-proofed booth (Heller and Bergmann, 1953).

Hinchcliffe (1961) found in two samples of rural populations in the United Kingdom variously 17 to 30 per cent had experienced episodes of tinnitus and that the proportion increased with age. An epidemiological investigation is currently being carried out by the Medical Research Council's Institute of Hearing Research. Results so far available indicate that the prevalence of tinnitus lasting more than five minutes was 14·7 to 17·7 per cent in four cities in Great Britain (Cardiff, Glasgow, Nottingham and Southampton) (Haggard, 1980). Of those over 40 years old, 14·5 per cent reported tinnitus, whereas of those over 60 years old 22·2 per cent reported tinnitus. Severe annoyance was reported by 0·4 to 1·5 per cent, severe loss of ability to lead a normal life by 0·5 per cent and interference with getting to sleep by 4·0 to 6·8 per cent.

Recently Hazell (1979) produced an analysis of the ages of tinnitus patients attending his clinic for the first time. This analysis shows (Fig. 7.1) an increase in the late middle age group: men subject to acoustic trauma during the war years would fall in this age group. It can be expected that the ageing of this population will result in a further increase in the incidence of tinnitus in the elderly.

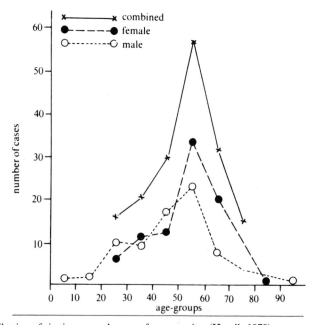

Fig. 7.1 Distribution of tinnitus cases by age of presentation (Hazell, 1979).

CHARACTERISTICS OF TINNITUS

Tinnitus has different attributes from a sound originating in the outside environment. Many patients, for example, will prefer to hear a background noise sufficiently loud to obliterate the sound of their own tinnitus, even though this background noise is louder and 'monotonous'. Feldmann (1971) makes the point that 'the pattern of hair cells or nerve fibres, whose spontaneous activity is responsible for the tinnitus, is not identical with the pattern which is activated by an external stimulus evoking the same subjective sensation'. However, at present tinnitus is probably best described in terms applicable to objective sound.

Number of sounds
Many patients are aware of more than one element of the tinnitus. In such cases drugs may abolish one or more sounds, yet leave other components of the tinnitus unchanged.

Constancy of tinnitus
In the majority of patients attending the author's tinnitus clinic, the noise is continuous throughout the waking hours—though it may become less intrusive at times of relaxation, of work, or in noisy backgrounds. The tinnitus may however be intermittent, either with a regular rhythmic quality or present for a few hours each day, particularly on waking or on retiring.

Loudness and pitch
The apparent loudness of tinnitus may well vary—unlike the pitch of the sound (or sounds) making up the tinnitus.

Localisation
The patient may state that the noise appears to come from one ear, both ears or elsewhere in the head. Fowler (1944) considered that the subject's sensation of localisation may be relevant to the aetiology and site of the lesion or disorder causing the tinnitus. However, if there is a relationship, it is not a simple one.

Annoyance
The patient may be asked about the annoyance of the tinnitus, the extent to which it interferes with daily activities and the enjoyment of life, and also, specifically, whether a background noise makes the tinnitus better or worse.

These features are probably best elucidated using a questionnaire. It may also be helpful in management if the patient keep a diary in which he can note the level of tinnitus, say three times a day (Fig. 7.2).

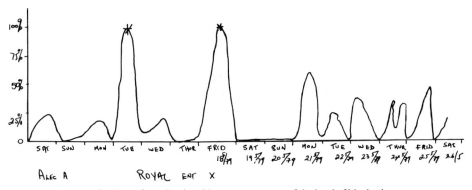

Fig. 7.2 Abstract of a diary of a patient's subjective assessment of the level of his tinnitus over a two week period. (Note this particular patient suffers most at periods of activity and concentration, and least when 'relaxed', including at weekends, and at night).

The recognition and recording of these features are of help in the management of the patient. With further study it may be possible to correlate these features with other factors e.g. causes of associated hearing loss, ease of masking.

MEASUREMENT

A thorough assessment of tinnitus uses psycho-acoustic methods employing matching and masking techniques.

Matching

If the patient can localise the tinnitus to one ear, or mainly one ear, and if, at the same time, the hearing in the contralateral ear is adequate, then the most commonly used procedure would be to present the matching sound to the contralateral ear (contralateral matching). Ipsilateral matching may be possible if a pulsed sound is used (Reed, 1960; Fowler, 1940). Even though the patient's tinnitus may take on a bizarre form, quite dissimilar from the noise output from the audiometer, the patient may nevertheless be willing to attempt to match the tinnitus with the output (be it pure tone, narrow band or wide band noise). A match in terms of frequency and intensity can thus be obtained. How meaningful these measurements are is uncertain.

Masking

Careful work on masking has been carried out by Feldmann (1971). He recorded the patient's pure tone audiogram, and then presented the patient with test tones at several frequencies increasing the intensity of these tones until the patient indicated his own tinnitus had been obliterated (Fig. 7.3).

Feldmann described five characteristic patterns. He considered whether or not there was a specific pattern related to the kind of tinnitus and whether or not the pattern revealed anything of the underlying pathological process. He also found that contralateral masking noise could sometimes abolish the tinnitus. If so, the requisite intensity could be greater or less than the ipsilateral tinnitus intensity.

In general, the technique of white noise masking is widely used (Morrison, 1975) and this is a more straight forward procedure. The level of such masking may be recorded as the sensation level. This is the difference between the threshold for the white noise and the level of the noise necessary to obliterate the tinnitus.

If the whole procedure of matching and masking is repeated the results obtained are rarely the same; indeed the author finds that they are often very different. This lack of reproducibility questions the value of one test only. It is possible that simply presenting the patient with various sounds, including those loud enough to mask and even overmask his tinnitus, may actually change the character of his tinnitus, albeit temporarily. This particularly applies to the elderly patient who may find it too demanding on his powers of concentration; and he may feel under pressure to respond too quickly. He is anxious to please and may too readily accept a match which is incorrect. With the method of adjustment (Voroba, 1979) the patient can vary the output of the instrument himself. This motivates the patient better and holds his attention. He can then produce a number of matches in a few minutes. However, this method has other drawbacks. Where the patient has a

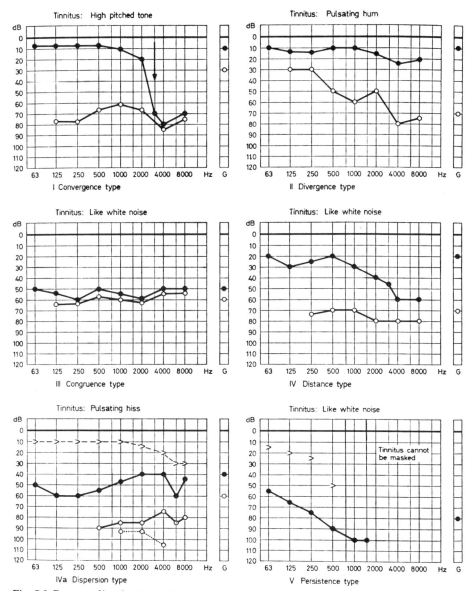

Fig. 7.3 Patterns of hearing loss and pure tone masking (Feldman, 1971).

hearing loss in the contralateral ear which affects some frequencies of sound more than others, then simply moving the frequency control will also influence the subjective magnitude of sound intensity (i.e. the loudness) more than would otherwise be the case, whether the intensity output is at constant sound pressure or at constant hearing level (decibels reaudiometric zero). Even in normally hearing subjects, equal loudness contours correspond neither to equal sound pressure contours nor to equal hearing level contours. He may thus accept as a 'best match' a sound which may not be so close to his tinnitus. There are other modifications

(Tyler, 1981) that can be used which may help but because of the time involved some of these facilities can only be of application in research and not in the day-to-day clinical situation.

The degree of disability produced by tinnitus is manifest in the behaviour of the patient. Two different individuals who are afflicted with tinnitus which is identical in respect of all features may nevertheless exhibit very different psychological reactions. Should the criterion for successful management be the reduction in the tinnitus loudness or an improvement in the patient's acceptance of it? It is possible for the loudness to be reduced but the psychological reactions to increase.

OBJECTIVE TINNITUS

In a small proportion of individuals the noise heard by the patient may also be heard by another person, typically, for example, by the spouse when both are lying in bed. The causes of such objective tinnitus can usefully be divided into muscular and vascular. Involuntary arrhythmic contractions (myoclonus) of the palatal, tensor tympani or stapedial muscles may give rise to an irregular 'clicking' type of tinnitus. Although the onset of this symptom is generally in the young and middle aged (Bjork, 1954), it may well persist to affect the elderly.

Haemodynamic disorders may give rise to a pulsatile tinnitus in rhythm with the heartbeat. The cause may be vascular malformation (Arenberg and McGeary, 1971), an arteriovenous aneurysm or a glomus tumour. In a series of 15 patients with pulse-synchronous tinnitus, three patients had no audible murmur and no abnormal findings on angiography whereas the remaining twelve had both a murmur and a demonstrable vascular abnormality (Harris et al, 1979). A haemodynamic cause for objective tinnitus is found in Paget's disease (Gibson, 1973); this has been helped by carotid ligation.

Turbulent blood flow over atherosclerotic plaques might also be expected to produce a pulsatile tinnitus. Cervical arterial bruits increase with age and a prospective study (Heyman et al, 1980) has shown that such bruits are associated with a significantly higher risk of stroke and death from ischaemic heart disease in men (but not in women). The inference is that this finding is an indication of the general state of the arterial system. The prevalence of these cervical bruits was 8 per cent in the age group 75 years and over. Many of these patients do not complain of tinnitus. Nevertheless the symptom of a pulsatile tinnitus affected, and often relieved temporarily, by firm pressure on the neck over the carotid artery below the angle of the jaw, or by posture, is common in this group of late-middle-aged or elderly patients; it is presumably due to similar changes. In some patients one can hear a pulsatile sound from a sensitive microphone introduced into the patient's external acoustic meatus. It is possible to confirm that this objective sound is obliterated at the same time the subject says he has obliterated the sound by gentle pressure on the neck. House (1981) says that in such cases ipsilateral ligature of the internal jugular vein abolishes the noise and may be well worth carrying out.

Thus in the examination of patients with tinnitus the mastoid, neck, skull and eye should be auscultated. The electronic stethoscope, though not widely used, has been shown to have a place in the examination of young people with pulsatile tinnitus (Goldie, 1960) and may prove worthwhile in the elderly. Tewfik (1974) used electronic recording equipment and found that, where objective tinnitus was associated with hypertension, adequate treatment of the hypertension abolished both the sound as recorded in his instrument and the patient's tinnitus. In this connection, however, a case of tinnitus apparently caused by propranolol (an antihypertensive drug) has been reported (Mostyn, 1969). It is probably advisable to avoid reserpine also as this may exacerbate the depression suffered by so many elderly tinnitus patients.

Although the contrary view is sometimes stated, in general the cause of objective tinnitus, particularly of vascular origin, is often not easy to find or to treat. In the absence of alarming symptoms, angiography can seldom be recommended because of the risks, particularly to the elderly. Moreover, surgery for localised atheromatous plaques in the carotid arteries has not been shown to have a worthwhile result in terms of survival (Heyman, 1980). Angiography itself has apparently caused tinnitus. Embolism by gelatine sponge after selective angiography has been reported to give a temporary cure for pulsatile tinnitus (Harris, 1979). A glomus jugulare or a glomus tympanicum may present with pulsatile tinnitus, a conductive hearing loss and a red mass seen in the external canal or seen through an intact tympanic membrane. Myoclonus of the middle ear muscles may be demonstrated by impedance audiometry even though movement of the tympanic membrane may not be visible on otoscopy (Coles, 1975). The tinnitus of stapedial myclonus may be helped, but not always permanently, by stapedius tendon section. Carbamazepine is also said to have been helpful in the treatment of palatal myoclonus (Rahko and Häkkinen, 1979). A case of synkinesis between facial nerve and the stapes tendon presenting with tinnitus which was abolished by surgical division of the fibrous attachment has been described.

Kemp (1979) has found that the healthy ear can generate a sound, the evoked cochlear mechanical response (ECMR), or echo[*]. This can be detected by a microphone in the external acoustic meatus a few milliseconds after the input of sound into the ipsilateral ear. Subsequently, Wilson (1980), using the same recording equipment, found some normal subjects not complaining of tinnitus emit noise continuously from the ear. This spontaneous acoustic emission from the cochlea has also been found in some subjects who complain of tinnitus. The tinnitus in these subjects does not necessarily have the same frequency characteristics as that of the acoustic emission. Only certain defined areas of the basilar membrane are apparently responsible for the re-emissions which have been studied. Of the tinnitus sufferers with a sensory hearing loss the regions of the basilar membrane corresponding to the hearing loss are not the same regions as are the source of the 'objective component'. In this connection, Wilson has observed that the emission appears at times to come from a location on the basilar membrane adjacent to an area which corresponds to a hearing loss on the pure tone audiogram. This may be relevant to the clinical observation that tinnitus is not always matched to the portion of the pure tone audiogram showing the greatest hearing loss. It is usually considered that such a disordered physiology, whether from dying hair cells or from affected nerve fibres, results in abnormal afferent impulses in the auditory nerve; this may be interpreted as tinnitus (Tonndorf, 1979). Clearly this spontaneous emission of sound from the cochlea is not what

[*]an oto-acoustic emission

clinicians would call tinnitus unless it corresponds to the patient's complaint; it may possibly be relevant to the tinnitus found immediately after noise exposure. The relevance of the ECMR to the subject of tinnitus needs much further study.

AETIOLOGY

Theoretically, tinnitus could arise from anywhere along the auditory pathway. There is, in the absence of any external sound, a steady resting discharge in the cochlear nerve. Several workers are now postulating that, with time, a circular pathway is established at a higher level in the brain so that even though the original cause might have been within the ear, the tinnitus is no longer 'peripheral' but 'central' (Emmett and Shea, 1980; Melding et al, 1978). A lesion of the temporal cortex can produce, interestingly, bilateral tinnitus. At the level of the colliculus, tinnitus has occurred after cingulectomy. Tinnitus may be a feature of multiple sclerosis affecting the midbrain. Pulec (1979) has discussed 'cervical' tinnitus. He postulates that, as a consequence of degenerative changes in the cervical spine, afferent impulses reach the vestibular nuclei (presumably producing the so-called 'cervical vertigo') and spill over into the cochlear nuclei. He proposes a diagnostic test. Local tender areas in the neck are injected with local anaesthetic. If the test is positive the tinnitus is abolished.

The majority of patients with tinnitus have some degree of hearing impairment. An analysis of two groups of tinnitus patients showing the cause of the hearing loss (if present) is given in Figure 7.4. In addition to the causes listed, tinnitus may be a presenting feature of a vestibulocochlear schwannoma. It also occurs with syphilitic hearing loss. Dyslipoproteinaemia and diabetes are associated with partial occlusion of vascular channels in the cochlea and resultant hearing loss; tinnitus may well be a feature also. Conductive hearing loss with tinnitus occurs in chronic suppurative otitis media (CSOM) and particularly after mastoidectomy,

	JACKSON	HAZELL
		%
UNKNOWN	24	58
ACOUSTIC TRAUMA	17	10
CSOM	10	7
POST STAPEDECTOMY	7	6
VIRAL/VASCULAR	0	6
MENIERES	10	4
MENINGITIS	0	4
CONGENITAL	3	3
H.INJURY	7	2
? DRUG INDUCED	10	
BAROTRAUMA	3	
OTOSCLEROSIS	3	
POST MIDDLE EAR SURGERY	3	

Fig. 7.4 Aetiology of hearing loss (where this is present) in patients with tinnitus.

after middle ear surgery and myringoplasty. It is also a feature of otosclerosis, but usually not a distressing one.

Many clinicians expect that patients with tinnitus will also have impaired hearing. There is, however, a substantial proportion of patients attending tinnitus clinics who have apparently normal hearing. The Medical Research Council epidemiological survey found (by questionnaire) that about half the people who have tinnitus do not report a hearing impairment (Coles, 1981). However, it remains to be seen how many would have a normal audiogram.

INVESTIGATION

Probably any type of hearing loss may be associated with tinnitus. With regard to the history, examination and investigation, these will be along the general lines of those for the investigation of hearing loss. Of particular relevance are enquiries about previous and current drug administration. Brown (1981) made two lists of drugs which produce tinnitus: one in which the drugs also cause a hearing loss, either temporary or permanent (this includes aminoglycosides), and a second in which there is no associated hearing loss. He found experimental evidence (using both electric response audiometry and scanning electron microscopy) that some drugs, e.g. aminoglycosides and chloramphenicol, potentiated the damage caused by noise: some, e.g. salicylates, did not. Could it be that this potentiation occurs when either effect separately produces an area of temporary or subliminal damage and this is only revealed when there is a further insult?

In analysing the cases of vestibulocochlear nerve tumours House (1981) found that 11 per cent had tinnitus as the only, or principal, feature.

Auscultation, with electronic amplification where possible, is particularly important in those with a rhythmic element to the tinnitus. Electrophysiological methods in which the electrical activity in the auditory pathway can be detected is so far without promise in measuring or assessing tinnitus as it depends on the use of computer to 'average out' the background activity; in doing this, any activity due to, or associated with, continuous tinnitus would be lost. However, electrocochleography may be of value in the examination of the totally deaf ear (Graham, 1979) in that the site of the deafness, whether cochlear or retro-cochlear and hence the presumed site of tinnitus, can be revealed.

MANAGEMENT

Perhaps 80 per cent or so of patients referred to a tinnitus clinic can be helped simply by interview together with the relevant examination and investigation, followed by reassurance where this can be given. Patients often describe their tinnitus in words with emotional overtones such as screeching, hissing and shrieking. This is particularly a feature of the elderly patient with tinnitus when activity and other interests are waning and time seems to hang heavily. In general, once tinnitus is troublesome it can be expected to persist so that its prevalence in the population increases with age. Most elderly patients with tinnitus will have had this symptom for many years and although the loudness may not have changed, it has become for them a 'fact of life'. The patient involved in community work for her peers will generally make light of her symptoms.

People in this age group are prone to depression and the depressed patient with tinnitus is a not infrequent attender both at psychiatric and tinnitus clinics. It seems the state of mind makes the tinnitus worse. The patient with endogenous depression may tend to rationalise his feelings, and if tinnitus is present 'as it often is in the early evolutional period the patient becomes preoccupied with it to the exclusion of all else . . . telling himself (or more generally herself) that 'these noises are spoiling my life and driving me mad' (Kennedy, 1953). Although it is demanding to see such patients, particularly where the physician may feel himself unable to help, nevertheless it is probably beneficial to the patient to have follow up appointments at suitably long intervals. Some of these patients may already be on tranquillisers. Instances occur where, after taking the patient off whatever psychotropic drug she (or he) is on, one is rewarded by seeing, at the next visit a much brighter happy patient, even though the tinnitus is still present. Others may be on an inappropriate anti-hypertensive—reserpine for example—which may cause or exacerbate the depressive mood.

For those who have a hearing loss, a hearing aid may not only give improved communication, but also amplification of the ambient sound such as to effectively mask the tinnitus. Unfortunately some patients will find that the amplification distorts speech sounds and makes communication more difficult. However, before hearing aids are abandoned consideration should be given not only to the use of bilateral hearing aids (if the hearing loss affects both ears) but also to the response characteristics of whatever aids are employed.

Provided he is not profoundly deaf, a sound of sufficient intensity can often make the patient oblivious to his tinnitus and many prefer hearing this exter-nal noise to their own noises. It is now possible to provide a *masking device* (structurally similar to a hearing aid). As its name implies, this device produces a masking noise. With simpler devices which produce 'white noise', the volume control can be adjusted by the patient. Other devices have, additionally, a frequency adjustment and some have a hearing aid as well (a masking instrument) (Fig. 7.5). Vernon who has considerable experience in this field stresses the importance of matching the masker (or masking instrument) to the patient's own tinnitus, and of carefully assessing the patient's tinnitus. In addition to the procedures already given he looks for *residual inhibition*. This is a phenomenon, inconstantly found, in which tinnitus is suppressed for a varying period of time following the removal of a masking sound.

A patient may find maskers in both ears a significant improvement on the unilateral masker and yet find that conversation is still possible. The percentage of patients who can be helped in this way varies in different series (Schleuring et al, 1980; Rosen and Price, 1980; Rose, 1980). If, as commonly occurs, a patient finds the tinnitus most obtrusive when trying to get to sleep, it may be possible to try a masker which fits under the pillow. However, no more expensive and at least as effective is a bedside radio which will switch itself off after the patient has gone to sleep. A masker is of no help to the profoundly deaf as the masking tone will not be heard loudly enough to obliterate the tinnitus. Moreover, there is also a sizeable group of patients in whom the tinnitus is more troublesome when there is back-ground noise, or when trying to concentrate or engage in activity; these too are not helped by maskers.

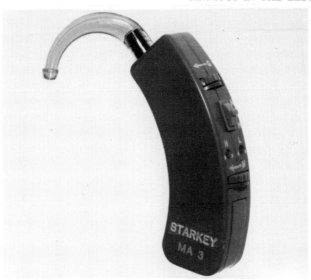

Fig. 7.5 A masking instrument with independent controls for the hearing aid attenuation and for the masking sound.

Surgery

For those with a conductive hearing loss associated with the tinnitus it is tempting to consider reconstructive surgery in the hope that by improving the hearing there would be an increased awareness of ambient sound which would have a masking effect. All too frequently, however, this type of surgery, be it myringoplasty or ossicular reconstruction, while it may improve the hearing, does not improve the tinnitus and may make it worse. Tinnitus with otosclerosis is not necessarily improved by stapedectomy and in the group of otosclerotics whose main presenting complaint is tinnitus (rather than hearing impairment) perhaps 50 per cent or more are made worse by stapedectomy: those who have suffered a 'failed stapedectomy' are among the sufferers from the worst tinnitus. If the patient has a profoundly deaf ear which is the source of tinnitus, then destruction of the ipsilateral vestibulocochlear nerve may be considered. Ideally the patient should be shown to have poor speech discrimination even with amplification, and good hearing on the opposite side. However, here again the results are disappointing, the tinnitus being improved in only 25 to 50 per cent of patients in various series (Morrison, 1975). Failure to respond must be because the tinnitus is arising 'centrally'. Even if the cause of the associated hearing loss is peripheral, e.g. from perilymph fistula or after stapedectomy, there is no certainty that the tinnitus, by the time the patient is seen, is arising peripherally. It may be possible in the future to determine what is the site of origin of the tinnitus and so lead to a better pre-operative selection.

It has recently been shown to be possible to abolish tinnitus by *electrical stimulation*. Aran has applied an electrode variously to the round window and to the promontory of patients with tinnitus and delivered positive and negative currents at various frequencies. With the positive electrode in position, he found the patient would report suppression of the tinnitus using current strength generally between 50 to 300 μA at frequencies between 200 to 3200 Hz. One could envisage the development of a simple device which may be of benefit particularly to those with a dead ear or perhaps with a mastoid cavity. This may pose another good reason for not embarking too readily on nerve section since treatment by an electrical suppression technique could then no longer be offered.

Drugs

Gejrot (1976) reported that, when using intravenous lidocaine (lignocaine) for the treatment of acute attacks of Ménière's Disease, there was suppression of both the vertigo and the tinnitus. Melding and her colleagues (1978) confirmed this observation and also found that the tinnitus which accompanied middle ear disease was not affected by lidocaine. They felt at that time that the value of lidocaine may be in determining the source of the noise. They and others (Emmett and Shea, 1980) considered that those patients in whom lidocaine abolishes the tinnitus, the tinnitus is arising centrally. However, in those patients selected for cochlear nerve section to treat the tinnitus, there has been some correlation between the abolition of the tinnitus by lidocaine and its abolition by the section. Conversely those who fail preoperatively to respond to lidocaine do not have tinnitus abolished by subsequent nerve section (though there has been one exception to this observation in a small series). The tinnitus of the failures after nerve section has not been abolished by lidocaine (Jackson, 1981). The early approach that response or non-response to lidocaine might be useful in classifying tinnitus (Melding, 1978) has now been succeeded by hopes that a similar orally effective drug could be produced which would have a prolonged bioavailability and be suitable to treat tinnitus. A number of such drugs which are allied to lidocaine and have a similar cardiac antidysrhythmia action is at present undergoing evaluation and preliminary reports are encouraging (Emmett and Shea, 1980) (Fig. 7.6).

Naftidrofuryl is also a powerful local anaesthetic and apparently inhibits the destruction of ATP. Gibson (1977) found that this drug altered the electrococh-leogram in Ménière's Disease. Patients have occasionally reported that their tinnitus seems to be helped by this drug. Also one sees patients from time to time who claim that their tinnitus has been relieved by betahistine or by prochlorper-azine. Donaldson (1979) found that amylobarbitone relieved tinnitus. Martin and Coleman (1980) reported that their patients with tinnitus did not respond to a placebo given in the form of either saline injection or inactive oral preparations.

Because lidocaine proved effective in abolishing epileptic attacks in the ex-perimental animal (Bernhard and Bohm, 1954), anti-epileptic drugs have been used in tinnitus. In this connection perhaps most work has been done with carbamazepine. In spite of some encouraging initial reports, Shea (1979) has now abandoned it in the treatment of subjective tinnitus because of its side effects. A psychotherapeutic drug to improve the mood of the depressed patient with tinnitus is often helpful (Williams, 1980) but such long term drug therapy may be criticised as threatening the wholeness of the personality. Consequently, a drug which would specifically abolish the tinnitus would be preferable. In this connection it is remarkable how the mood of the depressed patient with tinnitus immediately improves if the tinnitus is abolished, even temporarily by a bolus injection of lidocaine. Infrequently, the patient may find other complaints if the tinnitus is abolished.

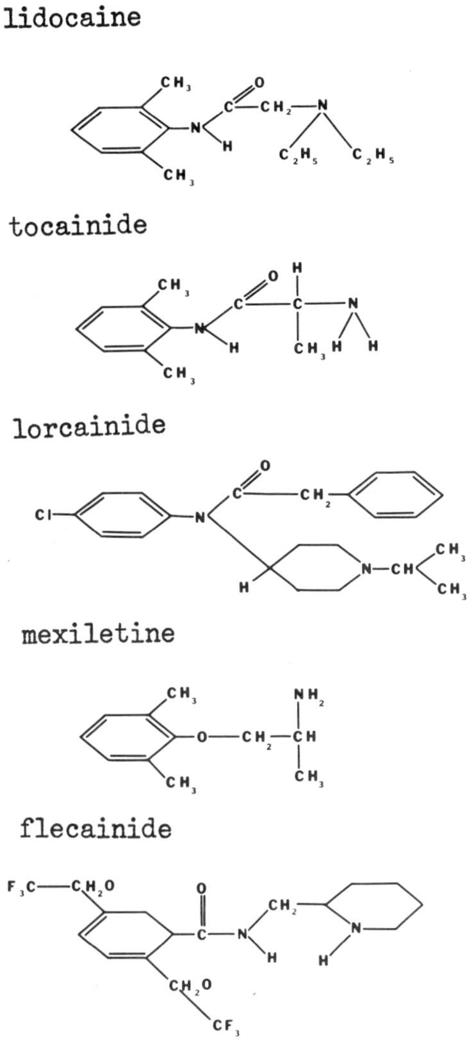

lidocaine

tocainide

lorcainide

mexiletine

flecainide

Fig. 7.6 Structural formulae of lidocaine and allied drugs currently undergoing trials in tinnitus suppression.

Diabetes and dyslipoproteinaemia, if discovered in the course of investigations of tinnitus, may themselves require medical treatment. The hearing impairment associated with dyslipoproteinaemia may at times be reversed by dieting. There may also be an improvement in the serum lipoprotein levels; it is reasonable to hope that the tinnitus too would be improved.

On the basis that, in the elderly, cochlear damage and hence the tinnitus might be due to impaired circulation, drugs aimed at improving the circulation have been used. As well as naftidrofuryl, as mentioned earlier, cyclandelate and nicotinic acid have been prescribed. Again in a small series, naftidrofuryl given intravenously or by mouth has abolished the tinnitus of patients with treated syphilis.

Biofeedback

Some success has been claimed in the USA for biofeedback (House, 1978; Grossman, 1977). The principle is to induce the patients to relax by registering action potentials in, for example, the frontalis muscle, and making this electrical activity visible or audible to the patient. House (1978) reported that 47 per cent of his patients undergoing this form of therapy were improved. However, it was accepted that it could well be the patient's attitude to his tinnitus that improved rather than that there was any change in the loudness of the tinnitus.

CONCLUSION

Many patients experiencing tinnitus for the first time are particularly anxious lest they have a cerebral tumour or that it may be a feature of impending deafness. If after appropriate investigations it is possible to reassure the patient, then this in itself is therapeutic and the patient may well find the symptom more acceptable. Likewise, for the severely depressed patient, psychotherapy and encouragement to become involved in active pursuits can improve the quality of life, so reducing the effect of the tinnitus.

The recently formed British Tinnitus Association provides the opportunity for tinnitus patients to meet fellow sufferers (who are likely to be sympathetic) for keeping them informed of progress in the field and of facilities available. The American Tinnitus Association performs a similar service. These Associations have given hope to many patients who had endured their symptoms for years.

There is thus no simple panacea for tinnitus. At the present time when the doctor is expected to 'cure' the patient he himself may feel inadequate and helpless. It is therefore not surprising that some doctors dread seeing the tinnitus patient and are glad when she is gone. However, current research work is giving grounds for hoping that ere long much more help will be available.

REFERENCES

Arenberg I K, McGeary H S 1971 Objective tinnitus aurium and dural arteriovenous malformation of the posterior fossa. Annals of Otology Rhinology and Laryngology 80:112–120

Bernhard C G, Bohm E 1954 Epilepsy abolished by lignocaine. Acta Physiologica Scandinavia, Supplement 114:5

Bjork H 1954 Objective tinnitus due to clonus of the soft palate. Acta Otolaryngologica, Supplement 16:39–45

Brown D 1981 Tinnitus. CIBA Foundation Symposium 85

Coles R R A 1981 Tinnitus CIBA Foundation Symposium 85

Coles R R A, Snashall S E, Stephens S D G 1975 Some varieties of objective tinnitus. British Journal of Audiology 9:1–6

Donaldson I 1978 Tinnitus: a theoretical view and a therapeutic study using amylobarbitone. Journal of Laryngology and Otology 92:123–130

Emett J R, Shea J J 1980 Treatment of tinnitus with tocainide hydrochloride. Otolaryngology, Head and Neck Surgery 88:442–446

Feldman H 1971 Homolateral and contralateral masking of tinnitus by noise bands and pure tones. Audiology 10:138–144

Fowler E P 1940 Head noises significance, measurement and importance—diagnosis and treatment. Archives of Otolaryngology 32:904–914

Fowler E P 1944 Head noises in normal and disordered ears: significance, measurement differentiation and treatment. Archives of Otolaryngology 39:498–503

Gejrot T 1976 Ménière's, tinnitus and lignocaine. Acta Otolaryngologica 82:301
Gibson R 1973 Tinnitus in Paget's Disease with external carotid ligation. Journal of Laryngology and
    Otology 87:299–301
Gibson W P R, Moffat D, Ramsden M 1977 The immediate effects of naftidrofuryl on the human
    electrocochleogram in Ménière's Disorder. Journal of Laryngology and Otology 91:679–696
Goldie L 1960 Phonocraniography, the recording of cephalic bruits. Third International Conference
    on Medical Electronics. Motor and Nervous Systems II
Goodwin P E 1980 Tinnitus and auditory imagery. American Journal of Otology 2:5–9
Graham J 1979 The role of evoked response and audiometry in evaluation of the tinnitus patient. Paper
    read at 1st International Tinnitus Seminar, New York City, June 1979
Grossman M 1977 Biofeedback treatment of tinnitus. Hearing Instruments 28:46–47
Haggard M 1980 Epidemiology of Tinnitus. Paper read at meeting of British Society of Audiology,
    Nottingham, July 1980
Harris S, Brishar J, Cronqvist S 1979 Pulsatile tinnitus and therapeutic Embolism. Acta
    Otolaryngology 88:220–226
Hazell J W P 1975 Determination of tinnitus quality. Presented to British Society of Audiology, 12th
    December, 1975
Hazell J W P 1979 Tinnitus. British Journal of Hospital Medicine 22:468–471
Hazell J W P 1981 Tinnitus. CIBA Foundation Symposium 85
Heller M F, Bergman M 1953 Tinnitus aurium in normally hearing persons. Annals of Otology,
    Rhinology and Laryngology 62:73–82
Heyman A, Wilkinson W E, Heyden S 1980 Risk of stroke in asymptomatic persons with cervical
    arterial bruits. New England Journal of Medicine 302:838–841
Hinchcliffe R 1961 Prevalence of the commoner ear nose and throat conditions in the adult rural
    populations of Great Britain. British Journal of Presentive and Social Medicine 15:128–134
House J 1981 Tinnitus CIBA Foundation Symposium, 85
Jackson P D 1980 Tinnitus: an enigma with variations. Paper read at the Royal College of Surgeons of
    England (Feb. 1979)
Kemp D T, Chum R 1980 Properties of the generator of stimulated acoustic emissions. Hearing
    Research 2:213–332
Kennedy A 1953 Cochlear, neural and subjective factors in tinnitus. Proceedings of the Royal Society of
    Medicine 825:829–832
Melding P S, Goodey R J, Thorne P R 1978 The Treatment of tinnitus with oral anticonvulsants.
    Journal of Laryngology and Otology 93:111–122
Morrison A 1975 Management of sensorineural deafness. Butterworth, London, ch 5
Mostyn R H L 1969 Tinnitus and propranolol. British Medical Journal 1:766–768
Portmann M, Cazais Y, Negrevergne M, Aran J M 1979 Temporary tinnnitus suppression in man
    through electrical stimulation of the cochlea. Acta Otolaryngologica 87:294–299
Pulec J L, Hodell S F, Anthony P F 1978 Tinnitus–diagnosis and treatment. Annals of Otology,
    Rhinology and Laryngology 87:821–833
Rahko T, Häkkinen V 1979 Carbamazepine in the treatment of objective mycoclonus tinnitus, Journal
    of Laryngology and Otology 93:123–127
Reed G F 1960 An audiometric study of 200 cases of subjective tinnitus. Archives of Otolaryngology
    71:84–94
Rose E D 1980 Tinnitus maskers: A follow-up. Ear and Hearing 1:69–70
Rosen R J, Price D R 1980 Clinical experience with tinnitus maskers. Ear and Hearing 1:63–68
Schleuring A J, Johnson R A, Vernon J 1980 Evaluation of a tinnitus masking program. Ear and
    Hearing 1:71–74
Shea J J, Harrell M 1978 Management of tinnitus with lignocaine and carbamazapine. Laryngoscope
    88:1477–1484
Tewfik S 1974 Phonocephalography—an objective diagnosis of tinnitus. Journal of Laryngology and
    Otology 88:869–875
Tonndorf J 1979 Tinnitus and Physiological correlates of the cochleo vestibular system. Paper read at
    1st International Tinnitus Seminar New York City, June 1979
Tyler R S 1981 Tinnitus CIBA Foundation Symposium, 85
Voroba B 1979 Tinnitus Research Frontiers Hearing Instruments 30:9, 31–33
Walford R 1980 Acoustical techniques for diagnosing low frequency tinnitus in noise complainants
    known as hummers. Proceedings of the Institute of Acoustics Spring Meeting, 1980
Williamson J 1980 Aspects of depression. Geriatric Medicine 9:15–19
Wilson J F 1980 Evidence for cochlear origin for acoustic re-emission threshold, fine structure and tonal
    tinnitus. Hearing Research 2:233–252

Psycho-social consequences of disorders of hearing in the elderly

INTRODUCTION

Prevalence of the disorder

Hearing loss has been documented as one of the disabilities concomitant with the ageing process since the time of the early British studies of the state of the health and welfare of the elderly in this country (Sheldon, 1948). It has traditionally been noted by clinicians and social researchers alongside many other conditions such as failing sight, poor teeth and bad feet, either as an incidental part of their research, or with the intention of disclosing to health care administrators and policy makers areas of unmet need amongst the elderly population. It was, and is, generally accepted by these researchers that 'deafness' implies a level of impairment at which it is generally considered necessary for individuals to obtain amplification from a hearing aid. Indeed, it is the unmet need for hearing aids that has been the dominant interest of studies when enquiring about hearing loss in the elderly.

It is now generally believed that between 30 and 40 per cent of all people beyond retirement age have some defect of hearing constituting a significant disability. These figures have been arrived at by various methods—some studies have emphasised functional hearing impairment by using questions about actual ability to hear, while others have been orientated more towards hearing impairment as a physiological entity, using questions such as 'Do you suffer from deafness?'; yet others have observed whether elderly respondents could hear the whispered questions of the interviewer.

Table 8.1 shows estimates of prevalence of hearing loss in community studies on elderly populations when assessed by self-report and Table 8.2 shows estimates based on clinician or interviewer assessment. Whilst each of these studies has its own particular way of ascertaining the information, an examination of the two tables shows that the prevalence of the disorder is fairly consistently estimated by whichever method is used. Similarly, the proportion of hearing impaired is consistently found to increase with age.

The prevalence of hearing loss amongst elderly persons in residential accommodation has been estimated at 42 per cent using self-report methods (Townsend and Wedderburn, 1965) and is thought to be higher than in the community because of the advanced age and greater infirmity of residents. These estimates, whilst accepted as being of questionable validity (Rawson, 1973), are nonetheless being used by the DHSS when considering rehabilitation services for the hearing

Table 8.1 Estimates of prevalence of hearing impairment in the elderly population based on self-assessment by respondents.

author	date	age in years 60+	65+	70+	75+	80+	85+
		F	M				M F
Sheldon	1948	29%	38%	—	—	—	60% 68%
Wilkins	1948	—	—	—	M F 28% 25%	—	—
Harris	1962	M F 35% 30%			—	—	—
Kay et al Pt. I	1964		37%		—	—	—
Richardson	1964	—	—	—	—	50%	—
Townsend & Wedderburn	1965	—	30%	—	—	—	—
Brockington & Lempert	1966	—	—	—	—	54%	—
Goldberg	1970	—	—	31%	—	—	—
Notts. Social Services	1973	—	—	—	32%	—	—
Milne	1976	39%	—	44%	—	53%	—
Abrams	1978	—	—	—	36%	—	—
Gilhome Herbst & Humphrey	1980a	—	—	38%	39%	54%	69%

Table 8.2 Estimates of prevalence of hearing impairment based upon clinician or interviewer assessment.

author	date	65+	age in years 70+	75+	80+
Stockport C C	1958	—	—	—	54·6%
Williamson	1964	36%	—	—	—
Sheard	1971	—	30%	—	—
Cumbria C C.	1973	—	—	31%	—

impaired (DHSS, 1977). It is important to note that none of the studies mentioned above provides estimates of the prevalence of hearing loss based upon the assessment of auditory deficit using audiometric techniques. In contrast to the considerable number of community studies listed on Tables 8.1 and 8.2 (a list which is probably not exhaustive), there is, at present, probably only one British study providing audiometrically-based estimates of the prevalence of hearing loss amongst the elderly living in the community—that carried out by Gilhome Herbst and Humphrey (1980a) (See Table 8.3). Audiometry was employed by Milne (1976) in a longitudinal study of ageing begun in Edinburgh in 1968, but results have not been published in terms of audiometrically-assessed prevalence. Milne's figures reported in Table 8.3 are based upon personal communication.

Figures based on audiometric assessment are also provided by two recent studies carried out in local authority homes for the elderly (Burton, 1977; Martin and Peckford, 1978). These studies suggest that between 60 and 90 per cent of residents have impaired hearing.

Table 8.3 Estimates of prevalence of hearing impairment in elderly populations based upon audiometric measurement.[1]

author	date	sample size	age in years			
			70+	75+	80+	85+
Gilhome Herbst & Humphrey	1980a	253	60%	69%	82%	84%
Milne	1980	221	68%	—	94%	—

[1] Gilhome Herbst and Humphrey define hearing impairment as an average hearing loss of 35 dB or more over the speech frequencies at 1 kHz, 2 kHz and 4 kHz in the better ear. Milne has provided his results in such a way as to be compatible with this criterion.

The audiometrically-based studies provide results which, whilst consistent with each other, are alarmingly at odds with all the other studies where no audiometry was used. They suggest that significant bilateral hearing impairment is almost twice as prevalent as has hitherto been assumed. On this basis, indeed, hearing impairment must now be seen as almost synonymous with ageing and, as such, as a contributing factor to the social and psychological experience of nearly all old people.

The discrepancy between the estimates of prevalence based upon audiometry and those based on self-report or observation has been presented as the introduction to this chapter on the social and psychological impact of hearing loss in the elderly because it is hardly likely to be purely an artefact or accident. It is likely that the high prevalence of hearing impairment which is only now coming to light has been a considerable, if unnoticed, influence on attitudes to hearing loss and to ageing itself at both personal and professional levels and for social theorists.

Some origins of prevailing social attitudes to impaired hearing
Intuitively we all 'know' the prevalence findings presented in the previous section. This knowledge has been used by playwrights and novelists throughout the centuries when depicting old age. Hearing impairment, used in an allegorical sense as synonymous with old age, usually represents a breakdown in meaningful communication with the world, or it is depicted as a characteristic of unimportant or mildy ludicrous characters. It is used to emphasise frailty and proximity to untimely death, and it is sometimes regarded as a condition that can be turned on or off at will to break communication with another person in a premeditated sense. Hence the saying 'None so deaf as those who will not hear'. 'To hear is to conform; not to hear may mean to rebel. . . . Perhaps here is reason for the resentment which society feels for deaf ears of whatever cause' (Knapp, 1948, p. 221). As Knapp has recognised, to deliberately withhold communication can also be an act of aggression. This is highlighted in the subtle distinction between the sayings 'turning a blind eye' which is conventionally associated with the obliging ignoring of harmless peccadilloes, and 'casting a deaf ear' which has connotations of selfish and unsympathetic dismissal. Most similes related to hearing impairment (reviewed by Stephens, 1979) reinforce the rebuff of hearing impairment by depicting it in relationship to hard, solid, immovable objects, 'as deaf as a post', 'stone deaf', 'deaf as a door nail' (though Stephens interprets these in terms of sound-reflecting

objects). The 'none-so-deaf-as-those-who-will-not-hear' connotations of hearing impairment also imply that it is a 'hoax' disorder which can be overcome if there is a will to do so. No parallel proverb exists which accuses blind men of peeping when they want to see. From these few examples it seems fair to say that there is built into our cultural heritage some mistrust and dislike of hearing impairment, which, unlike its sister handicap, blindness, holds no romance, no poignant beauty, no heroic mysticism.

Whereas most physical handicap, including blindness, cuts people off from things (usually doing things, which thus begs a helping hand), hearing impairment cuts people away from other people and defies help. In this sense it may be seen as a form of dreadful isolation with only God as company, much as are many forms of mental disorder. This latter parallel is reinforced by the apparent similarity between the symptoms of hearing impairment and those of some types of mental disorders (particularly defects of reason) namely, indistinct speech, not answering when spoken to, or answering inappropriately or out of context, pitching the voice incorrectly and so on. These symptoms often encourage people to talk to and treat the hearing impaired as if their cognitive abilities were also impaired.

The dislike of hearing impairment and the blurring in the popular mind between mental disorder and hearing impairment are not peculiar to contemporary society. The ancients also failed to differentiate between hearing impairment and mental disorder or retardation. Probably the most detrimental influence on attitudes towards the deaf came from Aristotle, whose philosophies affected the Western world for over a thousand years. According to Greek philosophy, language (or speech) was a human instinct, closely linked to man's ability to reason. Aristotle noted (in History of Animals, Bk. IV. No. 9) that 'men that are deaf are in all cases also dumb; that is they can make vocal sounds, but they cannot speak'. Throughout the ages until the Renaissance, Aristotle's analysis of the link between deafness and the inability to use speech was written and re-written until it was interpreted as meaning that all those who are deaf (and therefore dumb) are without speech and therefore without reason. Gradually the Greek words for 'deaf' and 'speechless' took on the meaning 'dumb' and 'stupid' (Hodgson, 1953; Bender, 1970). The latter meanings are also inextricably linked in modern English—particularly in America—where the term 'dumb' is currently used to mean 'silly' or 'stupid'. We now know that the interpretations given to Aristotle's writing are quite incorrect and that people who have little speech because they are deaf are just as likely to be as intelligent as anyone else; but traditional associations die hard.

Of course Aristotle was really writing about the pre-lingually deaf, that is those who were born deaf or who lose their hearing before the normal acquisition of language, and not about the adventitiously deaf who constitute the bulk of elderly hearing impaired. But, nevertheless, the stigma suffered by the one group seems to have rubbed off onto the other.

Deafness was viewed with compassion by the early Hebrews who protected the deaf with laws similar to those governing their children. Hence the code of conduct, expressed in Leviticus IX, v. 14, 'Thou shalt not curse the deaf'. Subsequently, however, the deaf suffered at the time of the early Christians from the fact that they were deprived from hearing the word of God. Paul, in his letter to the Romans X,

v. 17, had said 'So then faith cometh by hearing and hearing by the word of God'. By implication therefore, deafness hindered faith itself. It is no wonder that for centuries, until, indeed, reading and writing became universal alternatives, deafness was regarded as the most horrendous of misfortunes.

Thus we have a disability which is stigmatised in its own right and associated very closely with two other 'conditions' which we might well say are equally as sitgmatised, mental disorder and old age. Indeed, in our ageist society, it could be argued that much of the dislike of hearing impairment is derived from its very synonymity with old age and its attendant frailties. To admit to hearing impairment is tantamount to admitting being old and to the role of one with impaired reason. It is this stereotypical fusion between hearing impairment and old age that is probably the root cause of the neglect of reporting and treating the disorder.

Impaired hearing and social theories of ageing

An awareness of the synonymity of impaired hearing and ageing can provide some useful insights into social theories of ageing, particularly Cumming and Henry's disengagement theory (Cumming and Henry, 1961). This theory, which was first propounded in America during the early 1960's and subsequently reappraised by others (eg. Havighurst et al, 1968), strove to explain the observed phenomenon of social withdrawal which may often accompany advancing years. It suggests that ageing people naturally and voluntarily withdraw from too great an involvement with others, thus also diminishing their emotional investment in personal relationships. It further suggests that the elderly are generally satisfied with comparatively casual, surface social contacts and proposes that this diminution in social involvement is also convenient for the young–society being content to release its elderly from the normal demands of responsibility and accountability. The emphasis is on this being a 'natural' and 'mutual' process and, as such, one to be condoned and promulgated. Such a theory, which naturally has its followers and its dissenters, seems to draw directly, if unwittingly, on the effects of impaired hearing as a communication interrupter. Impaired hearing supports, or at least explains, the observed phenomenon of mutual release, or should one say breakdown, in communication between young and old in a very literal sense. Consequently, from a disengagement perspective, impaired hearing can be seen as a normal and natural part of ageing which may not therefore demand attention.

The opposing view, sometimes known as the activity or continuity approach to explaining the observed social changes that accompany old age, is that the diminishing world of the older person is largely societally constructed and reinforced. It suggests that in fact people continue throughout their life-spans with very much the same social and emotional requirements (Cavan et al, 1949; Maddox, 1963 and 1968; Abrams, 1979) and that it is therefore a fallacy that older people are content with less because they are old and physically less robust.

Thus the very recent interest in the social implications of impaired hearing in ageing goes hand in hand with the wide-spread rejection of disengagement. Indeed there is a general antagonism to the acceptance of any of the disorders of ageing as unalterable and inexorable. Impaired hearing must now be seen as another physical disorder requiring treatment and care for which an understanding of the social and psychological implications of the disorder is a necessary pre-requisite.

THE SOCIAL IMPLICATIONS OF HEARING IMPAIRMENT

Definitions of impairment, disability and handicap

Before discussing the personal implications of impaired hearing, some thought must be given to a discussion of concepts surrounding the terminology of disability. This is not to be viewed purely as a semantic exercise, but rather as an attempt to expand beyond the dangerously narrow view that the social restrictions caused by a physiological impairment may in some way be determined merely from a clinical assessment of the extent of malfunction and may be equally simply dispelled by the issue of a prosthetic instrument—in this case a hearing aid.

A more specific terminology to describe the life experience of disabled people evolved from the interest of social psychologists—particularly in America (Barker et al, 1953; Wright, 1960; Goffman, 1963; Safilios-Rothschild, 1970)—who wrote extensively on the broad psycho-social implications of physical disability. Their writings contributed considerably to the creation of a climate of opinion in this country in which legislation concerning welfare services, cash benefits and recompense for injury for disabled persons could slowly expand. The development of a common parlance to define specific, yet shared, physical, social and emotional problems attendant on physiological impairments reflects the need of health care administrators and policy makers to identify disabled persons coming within the boundaries of their jurisdiction*. Evidently the motivating force behind such interests is economic as well as humanitarian, involving as it does complicated issues concerning the allocation of resources according to some defined priority.

During the 1960s the Office of Population Censuses and Surveys was commissioned to undertake a national survey of handicapped people in Great Britain (Harris et al, 1971), which was published just after the passing of the Chronically Sick and Disabled Persons Act and gave it much of its force. Although other definitions are used by other writers, the terminology used by Harris and her colleagues in that study has slipped into fairly general use.[†] Harris and her colleagues distinguish between three major types of loss caused by a physiological deficiency and use the following terms:

impairment: "lacking part or all of a limb, or having a defective limb, organ or mechanism of the body"

disability: "the loss or reduction of functional ability"

[‡]handicap: "the disadvantage or restriction of activity caused by the disability"

Impairment and even disability can be fairly objectively assessed. Handicap is a relative concept and is therefore less amenable to being measured, although serious

---

* A requirement now placed upon all local authorities under Section I of the Chronically Sick and Disabled Persons Act of 1970.

† The Open University uses it in its course on the Handicapped Person in the Community (P853). Local authorities recognise it, and so do training bodies such as the Central Council for Education and Training in Social Work whose task it is to provide some of the suitably trained personnel for the care of the disabled (CCETSW, 1974).

‡ It is acknowledged that 'In general usage, disablement and handicap are often used interchangeably. The Department of Employment (now the Manpower Services Commission) has a register for disabled persons, while local authorities keep a register for the substantially and permanently handicapped. . . . . . and so on, (Harris et al, 1971).

attempts are being made to do so by the World Health Organisation for inclusion in the International Classification of Diseases (Wood, 1975).

The hearing impaired were excluded from the terms of reference of the Harris study probably because of criterial difficulties and probably also because the major preoccupation of service providers has always been with disorders which demand literal physical help. It remains open to debate whether such a terminology can usefully be applied to hearing impairment. The following discussion suggests that it can and, further, that the terminology in itself focuses attention on the different problems faced by hearing impaired people and the difficulties in assessing or measuring them.

The impairment resulting from a hearing disorder is the actual degree of auditory loss, which is clinically assessed using pure-tone audiometry. The impairment will inevitably have a great influence on the disability, that is, the practical or functional restriction caused by an individual person's inability to hear sounds—in particular speech.

Speech discrimination testing (Fry, 1961; Boothroyd, 1968) is recommended by Wood (1975) as a measure of the disability. But there is much debate as to the validity of this practice on the grounds that, used under clinical conditions, speech discrimination tests may not reflect the real world experience (Hood and Poole, 1977; Noble, 1978).

Other scales also claim to measure the disability by using questionnnaire techniques to assess the practical problems faced by the hearing impaired individual. At the outset, these tests were primarily concerned with assessing functional problems and activity restrictions before and after the issue of a hearing aid as part of a rehabilitation programme (High, Fairbanks and Glorig, 1964; Ewertsen and Birk-Nielsen, 1973). However, the Hearing Measurement Scale devised by Noble and Atherley (1970) does include some assessment of the handicap attendant on the disability as well as measuring the disability itself.

The extent to which the disability caused by an impairment will become a handicap is very contentious. A lot will depend upon the needs and requirements of the individual's life-style, his personal responsibilities, his personality, his age and so on. Thus Shakespeare (1975) suggests: 'to assess the degree of a person's handicap, we need to assess how many of the demands of his surroundings he fails to meet and how far removed from the normal level is his response.' Added to this, is another important factor determining the somatopsychological relationship (a term coined by Barker et al, 1954) between physical impairment and handicap, and that is the societally determined attitude of the sufferer, and of those people around him, towards his particular disability. In the final instance, whether or not a disability is assessed as handicapping may, in an extreme sense, be seen to depend on the extent to which restrictions cause psychological disturbance.

If we now turn to the social implications of hearing impairment in old age, we see that we must discuss both the disability and the handicap and their effect on mental state if we are to fully understand the implications for elderly people.

Factors differentiating the hearing impaired from normally hearing subjects
The major pre-occupation of research on hearing loss in the elderly has been its measurement and definition and suggestions for initiatives in aural rehabilitation.

Few writers can therefore do more than comment, in passing, on the social and psychological effects upon the sufferers of the disability which improved methods of assessment and improved rehabilitation are designed to alleviate.

In the UK there has been one relevant piece of systematic research which has examined the social and psychological implications of deafness in old age. Funded by the Nuffield Foundation, this study has been conducted by the Department of Applied Social Studies at the Polytechnic of North London (Gilhome Herbst and Humphrey, 1980ab). Its overall aim is to see whether there is any association between hearing loss and mental disorder in the elderly living at home. It is a direct development of previous work by the same team (Thomas and Gilhome Herbst, 1980) in which a systematic investigation was made of the social and psychological implications of acquired hearing impairment in adults of employment age passing through NHS hearing aid centres. The results of that study showed that, when comparing hearing-impaired to hearing people, the overriding effect of acquired hearing loss in that age group, even after 'rehabilitation', was loneliness and a tendency to anxiety and depression. The use of some similar questions in the two studies has made possible a comparison of the responses of the hearing impaired of employment age and those in retirement. Although the sample sources of the two studies are different, the overall research design of the present study is similar to that of the previous one in that the elderly with a hearing loss are compared against a hearing control group in order to have some yardstick by which it is possible to see the influence of hearing loss upon the lives of elderly people living in the community.

The sample consisted of all 365 persons aged 70 years and over who were registered with a group practice in an Inner London borough. 48 refused to take part and 46 were in hospital, on holiday, or untraceable. 18 people were subsequently excluded from analysis because of inadequate audiometry, poor English or inebriation. 253 subjects, representing 69 per cent of the sample, were studied. The age and sex distribution is shown in Table 8.4. There were no significant differences between respondents and non-respondents on these measures.

Table 8.4 Age and sex distribution of the sample.

sex	70–74	75–79	age in years 80–84	85+	total
male	46 (41%)	34 (46%)	7 (20%)	5 (16%)	92 (36%)
female	66 (59%)	40 (54%)	28 (80%)	27 (84%)	161 (64%)
total	112 (100%)	74 (100%)	35 (100%)	32 (100%)	253 (100%)

Audiometric measurements were made and scales to screen for organic brain syndrome and depression were extracted from the Comprehensive Assessment and Referral Evaluation (CARE) Schedule (Gurland et al, 1977), and were administered to each respondent. The interview schedule also comprised detailed questions about three other life domains: general health and use of primary and secondary health and welfare services; the experience of loneliness and contacts with friends and relations; the experience of hearing impairment (where it was found to be in evidence from the audiogram).

Hearing impairment was defined as an average loss of 35 dB HL (Hearing Level) or more averaged over the speech frequencies at 1 kHz, 2 kHz and 4 kHz.

A more detailed breakdown of the prevalence of hearing loss using this criterion is to be found in Table 8.3. By this criterion, 60 per cent (153) of the sample were assessed as being 'deaf' with a mean dB loss of 54·75 dB (sd. 16.96).

Only 19 respondents were wearing a hearing aid at time of interview. They have not been singled out for special consideration in the overall debate on the effects of hearing impairment. If anything, the presence of this small group of people within the larger hearing-impaired group would be reflected in an underestimation of the impact of hearing loss.

However, 19 persons assessed as probably suffering from marked dementia according to their scores on the organic brain syndrome scale are not included in the present analysis as their responses to the interview schedule were not deemed to be valid. Thus the sample for the subsequent discussion comprises 136 hearing impaired and 98 normally-hearing subjects.

Those factors which were found to significantly differentiate the hearing-impaired group from the normally hearing will be discussed first. The experience of hearing loss itself as reported by those afflicted will then be considered. The completed schedules of the sample were divided into hearing impaired and normally hearing groups. ANOVA, a sub-programme of the Statistical Package for the Social Sciences (Nie et al, 1975) designed to produce a chi-square test of significance whilst allowing for multi-control of nuisance variables, was used. In the case of the present study such 'nuisance' variables are age and socio-economic status. Both these variables are themselves significantly associated with hearing impairment.

The following eight factors on Table 8.5 were found to significantly differentiate the hearing impaired from the normally hearing elderly.

Table 8.5 Factors differentiating the hearing impaired from the normally hearing elderly.

Differentiating factors		Level of significance
1. Self-assessment of health:	the hearing impaired rate their health worse	$p < 0·05$
2. Extent of mobility:	the hearing impaired are less likely to be able to get out without help	$p < 0·01$
3. Range of excursions in the past week:	the hearing impaired have ventured out less far	$p < 0·05$
4. Satisfaction with amount of going out:	the hearing impaired are more likely to say they do not get out enough	$p < 0·05$
5. Number of friends relative to the past:	the hearing impaired are more likely to say they have fewer friends than in the past	$p < 0·05$
6. Having a relationship to which they make an active contribution:	the hearing impaired are less likely to be assessed as having such a relationship	$p < 0·05$
7. Enjoyment of things relative to the past:	the hearing impaired are more likely to say they enjoy less than previously	$p < 0·01$
8. Depression rating:	the hearing impaired are more likely to be rated as depressed	$p < 0·05$

None of these associations are exceptionally strong, but together they seem to constitute a clearly interpretable picture of the aspects of life affected by defective hearing in old age. Taken together, they show that hearing impairment in old age may be said to contribute to a significantly impoverished quality of life. They also show that, in general terms, hearing loss is both disabling in its influence on activity and handicapping in its effect on personal happiness.

First, as regards the first four variables in Table 8.5, hearing loss is apparently associated with poor general health (see also Thomas and Gilhome Herbst, 1980a) and, as such, can be seen to be linked with reduced mobility and a reduction in both range of activities and numbers of excursions outside the home. Alternatively, hearing loss may be a direct cause of reduced mobility outside the home due to, let us say, fears of managing with poor hearing. In fact, when further controlling for general health status and limiting and non-limiting physical disabilities, hearing loss was still found to be significantly associated with a restricted range of outdoor activities and thus this latter hypothesis is supported. In either case, the association remains: the hearing impaired are more likely to be physically restricted and thus disabled.

Insofar as this restricted mobility associated with hearing impairment is irksome (not getting out as much as wanted; variable 4), it can be seen to be handicapping.

However, it should be remembered that defective hearing is only disruptive to the maintenance of an 'active' life insofar as an active life is desired. Hence the trap (recognised by Alpiner, 1979) of generalising about the effects of hearing impairment upon the lives of elderly people, who probably differ in their life-style patterns more than any other age group (Heron and Chown, 1967).

The second main area of influence of hearing loss (variables 5 and 6) is its association with a significant reduction in personal contacts. No doubt in part this is due to reduced mobility, but a major cause of this diminution must also be because of problems with communication. This mirrors the findings of the study on the hearing impaired of employment age. It is indeed the most obvious and the most frequently noted effect of hearing loss in all age groups (von Leden, 1977; Jackson, 1979).

All eight factors in Table 8.5 present a picture which one might easily associate with ageing per se. One can now see more readily why hearing impairment is popularly synonymous with ageing and may thus be overlooked. Variables 1, 2, 3, 5 and 6 in particular may be viewed from a disengagement perspective as 'normal' ageing. However, the cumulative handicapping effect of the restrictions discussed above can be seen in the association of hearing impairment with reduced enjoyment of life as a whole (variable 7) and with depression (variable 8). Indeed, the first seven variables are each themselves significantly associated with depression. This association of hearing impairment with depression confirms how, in the extreme case, the handicapping effect may engender psychiatric disturbance. It also underlines the previous suggestion that hearing impairment must be seen as a disorder requiring treatment and care.

Insofar as the reduction in mobility and reduction in personal contacts associated with hearing impairment may be said (objectively) to constitute conditions of living which together create an isolated life-style, hearing loss in the elderly can be said to be working primarily as a determinant of isolation. This finding systematically supports the observations of other writers (Myklebust, 1964; Gilad and Glorig, 1979; Garland, 1978; Alpiner, 1979). However, whilst both hearing impaired and normally hearing elderly people were asked in considerable detail about feelings of loneliness, no significant difference between the two groups could be found on any of those measures (see also Powers and Powers 1978). This was despite the fact that four variables in Table 8.5 were found to correlate significantly with loneliness: rating one's health as 'poor', feeling one has fewer friends than in the past, feeling that one enjoys less than previously and being screened as depressed. Therefore the assumption made by some writers (Burton, 1977; McCall, 1979) that defective hearing is associated with loneliness in old age is not supported.

Deafness in old age appears by itself not to be a strong determinant of loneliness (which we may call the lack of companionship of the desired kind). In old age, loneliness is probably more a consequence of lack or loss of kindred spirits, or possibly follows a lifelong predisposition (Shanas et al, 1964; Tunstall, 1966). The very 'normality' of hearing loss in old age probably renders it less influential in disrupting such relationships as remain.

The personal experience of hearing impairment

In that a handicapped person may be defined as one who deviates, against his own wishes, from the norms and social values of the group of which he is a member, one key question is whether having trouble with his hearing makes an elderly person feel differently about himself and, if so, in what way.

There were 136 people who had impaired hearing (as defined in the text) and it was to these people that it was intended that a detailed series of questions concerning their experience of the disability would be directed. However, 27 per cent of this group (36 people) refused to admit that they had any trouble with their hearing even after audiometry was performed.* The mean hearing loss of these respondents was 43·8 db HL (sd 10.1). It is possible that elderly people are unaware of their defective hearing because their life-styles do not demand better hearing, but conscious denial of the disorder even in the face of obvious difficulties (arguably because of the stigma associated with defective hearing) is equally as likely and has been noted since early times by psychologists and social researchers (Menninger, 1924; Berry, 1933; Wilkins, 1948; Gregory, 1961; Townsend and Wedderburn, 1965). The above finding seems most likely to be direct evidence of denial of hearing impairment.

This denial reduces the sample under consideration to 100, which means that the numbers on which the following discussion is based may not really be large enough for firm conclusions to be drawn. The interpretations made should rather be seen as providing possible guidelines to thinking. One third of the respondents (30) who admitted their hearing defect suggested that being 'deaf' did make them feel differently about themselves. When asked what their feelings were, these respondents fell into four categories. Defective hearing made people 'feel closed in', 'feel

---

* Alpiner (1963) also found fairly extensive denial of hearing defect amongst a sample in 'homes for the aged' and in a 'self sustaining retirement centre'. At that stage in his research he was led to generalise that this was the general reaction of elderly people to their hearing loss. In a more recent article (Alpiner, 1979), he corrects this assumption and concludes that a sizeable number of elderly hearing impaired people do not only admit they have a hearing defect, but also actually take steps to see a doctor about it, possibly with a view to rehabilitation. The present study confirms Alpiner's realigned position.

inferior', 'get frustrated or depressed', 'tend to evade other people'. All these are sentiments which have a familiar ring to them: they are feelings that one would expect to be associated with having defective hearing and thus 'feeling different' compared to what one had been, and what one would expect for oneself at the moment. They also express the feeling of personal degradation associated with having a hearing defect.

The question remains as to why only some hearing impaired people have such feelings. To this end the following Table was drawn up (Table 8.6) to show those factors which were found to be significantly associated with 'feeling different'. A chi-square test was used. The variables have been ranked according to the strength of the association. Taken together they express a fusion of perceptions of the practical interference, the external pressure of the attitudes of others and the affective disturbance caused by difficulties in hearing the spoken word—indeed all those factors which contribute to the definition of handicap. 'Feeling different' can arguably be redefined as 'feeling handicapped'.

Table 8.6 Factors significantly associated with 'feeling different' (handicapped) because of hearing defect.

Factors	Level of significance
Onset of defective hearing before retirement age	$p < 0.0001$
A feeling that hearing defect 'matters'	$p < 0.0001$
Depression	$p < 0.004$
Describing oneself as a lonely person	$p < 0.005$
A feeling that having a hearing defect is 'bothersome'	$p < 0.008$
Severity of hearing loss (pure tone audiometry)	$p < 0.01$
A feeling that people get irritable with one because of defective hearing	$p < 0.02$
A feeling that people mistake the hearing impairment for absentmindedness	$p < 0.02$

Some of the above factors will now be discussed. 22 of the 30 people who may be said to feel handicapped said they had had impaired hearing before reaching retirement age. When present age and the present degree of hearing loss were controlled for, early onset of hearing impairment remained a crucial indicator of handicap. This implies that people who experience hearing impairment as younger adults retain negative feelings specifically related to having defective hearing when younger and carry these through into their retirement years.

In the whole sample (100) of those who would admit to having defective hearing, 45 per cent thought that they had been impaired before reaching retirement age. As a group they were significantly more likely than those whose hearing impairment was of onset after the age of 65 years to have acknowledged the disabling effect of their impairment and to have taken some steps to improve their lot. That is, they were more likely to have gone to see their doctor ($p < 0.005$), had their ears examined ($p < 0.03$), had their hearing tested ($p < 0.0001$) and to be wearing a hearing aid ($p < 0.002$)*. They were also significantly more likely to feel that those

* At the time of interview, 19 of the sample of 136 hearing impaired elderly people were evidently using and wearing an aid. Only 4 of these people said their hearing loss had developed since their retirement.

nearest to them (relatives and friends) understood that they were hearing impaired and had some appreciation of their problems ($p < 0.03$).

The mean hearing loss (as previously defined) of those who felt handicapped by their loss was 63·6 dB (sd 14.89). For those who did not, it was 50·7 dB (sd 15.71). Using a two-tail t-test for calculating significant differences between means, it is possible to say that, as a group, those who feel handicapped by their hearing defect are significantly more impaired than those who do not ($p < 0.005$). In this way, too, we can see that both groups are significantly more impaired than those who deny their hearing impairment outright ($p < 0.005$). Nonetheless, the degree of hearing loss objectively assessed (the impairment) is one of the least significant of all the determinants of the handicap. The perception of how much loss actually matters and is bothersome is more closely associated with handicap. This confirms the notion that the severity of deafness, clinically assessed, is less crucial to the individual than his personal perceptions of the amount that it interferes with his life. This is exactly what one could have predicted, in that personal feelings must relate to handicap by definition. This mirrors the findings of the study on the younger hearing impaired sample (Gilhome Herbst, 1980).

It was suggested that handicap is a relative concept—relative also to others. Thus another important determinant is the perception of other people's attitudes to the disability twenty one of the thirty who felt handicapped said that other people got irritable with them because of their hearing loss. Eleven felt that people sometimes mistook their hearing loss for 'absent mindedness'. The negative attitudes of other people were, in fact, important to the whole sample who admitted they had defective hearing: 54 per cent experienced the irritation of others and 24 per cent felt their hearing defect was mistaken for 'absent mindedness'. Goffman (1963) and other writers on disability suggest that, given the opportunity of hiding a stigmatised disorder, most disabled people will try to do so in order to protect themselves from such negative attitudes as those just mentioned. The corollary of this argument is that, if people can be seen to be hiding their disorder from others, it may be deduced that the disorder is socially stigmatising.

To test this notion in both the present study and the one previously undertaken by Thomas and Gilhome Herbst, respondents were asked whether they tended to tell other people of their hearing loss soon after meeting them or not: 60 per cent (125) of the sample of persons of employment age said they certainly did not, compared to 75 per cent (75) of the elderly. This shows a fair degree of conscious withholding of information about hearing impairment.

The overall mean hearing loss of the two sets of respondents was 55·8 dB (sd.14.5) for the elderly and 55·3 dB (sd.14.4) for the younger sample. This gives some clue to the level of disability and the subsequent practical problems for the normally hearing with whom the hearing impaired may be in conversation. With losses of this degree it seems unlikely that normally hearing people would not have detected some abnormalities in their communication which would have remained unexplained—possibly fuelling the commonly held stereotype, mentioned by the elderly themselves, of the hearing impaired being mentally impaired.

On the face of it it would appear that more elderly people are hiding their defective hearing than are the younger sample. This may be true, but life-style requirements and the expectation of hearing impairment as normal in old age must be taken into account and, when they are, the results take on a different complexion. Both samples were asked to explain why it was that they consciously withheld knowledge of their disability. The results are shown in Table 8.7.

Table 8.7 Reasons given for withholding knowledge of impaired hearing from others.

Reasons for withholding knowledge of impaired hearing	Hearing impaired elderly	Hearing impaired of employment age
I don't need to tell (I manage)	26 (35%)	53 (42%)
I don't know why	25 (33%)	5 (4%)
It's obvious to others	8 (10%)	—
I don't meet anyone	7 (9%)	—
I am ashamed	5 (7%)	40 (32%)
People treat me badly when I do	4 (5%)	27 (22%)
Total	75 (100%)	125 (100%)

The elderly are generally more vague in their understanding of why they suppress information about their hearing loss—one third saying they 'did not know'. It is most likely that they had not thought about the matter before being asked because hearing impairment at that time of life is so normal. Very few of the younger people were as undecided. Indeed, over half the hearing impaired of employment age who concealed their hearing loss did so as a conscious response to the shame and stigma associated with having defective hearing at their age. Only 12 per cent of the elderly with impaired hearing expressed any recognition of stigma associated with their loss, confirming that hearing loss in old age is by and large part of the social identity of the old and to that extent is also generally less handicapping.

People who report that having a hearing defect makes them feel handicapped are significantly more likely to feel lonely and significantly more likely to feel depressed—exactly as were the hearing impaired of employment age in the previous study. It seems likely that the association of loneliness and depression with feeling handicapped is associated either with the frustrations of the active elderly who wish to maintain an outward-going life-style more conventionally associated with the young or with those who for other reasons (living alone) need to remain in command of their senses. For it was such people who found themselves handicapped by their hearing impairment and for whom a hearing loss was truly bothersome and mattered a lot.

From these findings there would seem to be a danger of concluding that, in order to reduce the handicapping effect of impaired hearing, situations in which an individual is made to feel inadequate and rebuffed should be reduced. Withdrawing from situations which will expose the disability in order to reduce negative experiences is a strategy frequently employed by handicapped persons. Goffman (1963) elaborates very fully on this issue, as does Wright (1960). Indeed, with specific regard to hearing impairment, such strategies were seriously recommended by the first hearing impaired authors writing advice-giving texts on how to cope with the impairment (Jackson, 1902; Murphy, 1913; Collingwood, 1923). 'One of my rules, which I will dare to commend is to make myself as little obtrusive as possible. . . . . . Thus by holding curiosity under constraint, I save myself embarrassment and others annoyance' (Jackson, 1902). By withdrawing, the elderly may find that at least one of the many problems they have to face is minimised: they become less impaired and thus less handicapped if they need to hear less. But, in that social isolation and withdrawal in the elderly is associated with psychiatric disturbance and the need for admission to hospital (Grad d'Alarcon, 1971), the implications of such behaviour are quite serious.

PSYCHOLOGICAL EFFECTS OF HEARING IMPAIRMENT IN OLD AGE

The previous discussion has indicated that the social implications of hearing impairment, though diverse, are in the main two-pronged, stemming both from the disability and from the handicap. Thus we saw that the major social effects of hearing defect in old age are an increased tendency to social isolation and an increased tendency to feelings of personal malaise and discomfort. There is also a third issue which must now be discussed, namely the extent to which the socio-somatic imbalances associated with hearing impairment may produce or contribute to more serious psychological disorders.

Hearing defect and organic mental states

Research reports reviewed by Gilmore (1974) consistently suggest that between 5 and 10 per cent of the elderly population suffer from some form of organic brain disorder. Because the care of persons suffering from dementia soaks up some 50 per cent of all finances allocated to the health care of the elderly (Age Concern, 1977), and because these disorders create deep personal misery to supporters and sufferers alike (Grad d'Alarcon op cit; Jolley and Arie, 1980), a lot of research has been directed towards studying the social and medical aetiology of this condition (Cosin et al, 1957; Post, 1958; Kay et al, 1964 Pt. II; Hodkinson, 1973; Bergmann, 1977). Two of these studies suggest that impaired hearing may play some part in the development of organic mental disorders. The first major study in which such a suggestion was made was carried out by a team of psycho-geriatricians investigating the possible social and medical causes of mental disorders in the elderly in Newcastle-upon-Tyne (Kay et al, 1964 Pt. II). This team estimated that 62 per cent of the elderly with organic brain syndromes in their sample had impaired hearing while only 31 per cent of the mentally normal had impaired hearing. They therefore concluded that: 'It is possible that those defects of sight and hearing may have sometimes played a part in the production of the mental symptoms by reducing the subjects' contact with the outside world; for the association of sensory defects with organic mental states seemed to be too strong to be wholly explicable by the advanced age of the subjects' (Kay et al, 1964 Pt. II, p. 676). This opinion was tentatively supported by Hodkinson in a London-based study on mental impairment in the elderly (Hodkinson op cit), where he estimated that, in a sample of 588 geriatric inpatients, 52 per cent of the confused, 47·5 per cent of the demented and 29 per cent of the mentally normal had an impairment of hearing. Audiometry was not used in the assessment of hearing defect by either team of geriatricians.

In their study of the relationship between mental disorder and defective hearing in the elderly living at home, Gilhome Herbst and Humphrey (1980b) found an apparently closer association between impaired hearing and dementia, such that 79 per cent of the dements also had a hearing defect. They further report a significant association between the severity of the dementia and the severity of the hearing loss, such that as people lose their hearing they are significantly more likely to be demented and the severely demented are significantly more likely to have a hearing defect. However, their results do not support the suggestion made by Kay and his colleagues that the connection between impaired hearing and dementia is 'too strong to be wholly explicable by the advanced age of the subjects'. Gilhome Herbst and Humphrey report that, once age is controlled for, the apparent relationship between hearing impairment and dementia is lost. They suggest that hearing defect and dementia are merely contiguous conditions, both being a function of age.

A simple explanation for the discrepancy between this finding and those of other researchers is to be found in the fact that no audiometry was performed in any previous studies looking at the possible aetiology of dementia (see Tables 8.1 to 8.3). Albeit Gilhome Herbst and Humphrey found an apparently closer relationship between hearing loss and dementia than other studies, in that 79 per cent of the demented also had a hearing defect, and they also showed that impaired hearing is the norm, and not the exception, in all those over the age of eighty. If 60 per cent of the population aged 70 years and over are found to be significantly hearing-impaired, common sense suggests that the prevalence of the disorder amongst the middle-aged must be far higher than is now assumed (DHSS, 1977). Gilhome Herbst and Humphrey's work suggests that at least a third of the hearing impairment found in the elderly is probably of onset in middle age (see also D' Souza et al, 1975). It is still possible that there is some causal link between impaired hearing and dementia derived from a complicated interweave of cause and effect of time of onset, type of hearing defect and type of dementia. Since a strong component of organic brain syndrome is poor memory recall, it is not possible to determine in any accurate way the duration of hearing impairment amongst the demented without recourse to longitudinal studies.

Impaired hearing and depression
An association between impaired hearing and depression has been constantly reported by psychologists and psychiatrists over the years (Menninger, 1924; Ingalls, 1946; Knapp, 1948; Ramsdell, 1966; Mahapatra, 1974; Denmark, 1976). However, reviewers (Rosen, 1979; Cooper, 1976) have pointed out that this association was an assumption based primarily on clinical observation and not upon systematic research on unbiased samples. Thomas and Gilhome Herbst (1980b) saw their study as filling this gap, since it investigated the social and psychological implications of acquired hearing loss on a unbiased hearing impaired sample possessing NHS hearing aids and used psychological measuring techniques which were not likely to mis-classify the hearing impaired. Moreover, as has been stated, their results were stringently controlled on a normally hearing population. In that study they confirmed the association between hearing loss and depression. They estimated that the hearing impaired were four to five times as likely as the normally

hearing to suffer from anxiety and depression (Thomas and Gilhome Herbst, 1980b). Their sample, like those of most other writers, was restricted to adults of employment age.

A review of the literature on the prevalence of depression in community-based populations of persons of retirement age suggests that between 20 and 30 per cent of the elderly suffer from depression (Kay et al, 1964, Pt. I; Blessed, 1979; Milne et al, 1971). Indeed, Williamson (1978) suggests that depression is probably the most common mental illness in this age group, except for the very old where organic brain syndromes may become more prevalent.

Community studies which have observed a specific relationship between defective hearing and depression in old age (Goldberg 1970; Charatan, 1975; Garland, 1978) have not used audiometric techniques to establish the presence of a hearing loss, nor has this association been established on the basis of systematic enquiry. In particular, these studies have not distinguished endogenous depression from exogenous or reactive depression. It is proposed here to follow the lead of these studies by not differentiating between types of depression.

Gilhome Herbst and Humphrey's study will once again be referred to in detail.

Using the depression scale taken from the CARE schedule (Garland et al, 1978), they found that 35 per cent (82 people) of their sample of 253 elderly people could be assessed as suffering from some degree of depression (Gilhome Herbst and Humphrey, 1980b). These figures are higher than those of other community studies (Kay et al, 1964, Pt. I; Blessed, 1979), but this may be partly explained by the greater age of respondents in the study and the consequently higher proportion of women, among whom the incidence of depression is apparently greater (Kay et al, 1964, Pt. II). It will be remembered that the schedules of the 19 respondents assessed as suffering from dementia were excluded from analysis on the grounds that their responses to the interview were judged not to be valid. A significant relationship was found between the occurrence of hearing impairment and the occurrence of depression ($p < 0.01$; see Table 8.8).

Table 8.8 The relationship between depression and hearing loss.

Hearing threshold level	depression		
	not depressed	depressed	total
0—34 dB HL	73 (50%)	50 (69%)	123 (57%)
≥35 dB HL	72 (50%)	22 (31%)	94 (43%)
total	145 (100%)	72 (100%)	217 (100%)
	$X^2 = 6.39$ with ldf $p < 0.01$		

The relationship remained even when other contributing factors to depression, such as age and lower socio-economic status, were allowed for. However, no relationship could be be found between the severity of depression and the severity of the hearing loss as measured by pure-tone audiometry. In other words, there was no direct linear association between the severity of the impairment and its effect on mental health (wearing an aid made no difference, nor did the time of onset of the hearing impairment before retirement age).

The association between a hearing loss and personal wellbeing has already been discussed in the previous section on the social implications of hearing impairment. From this we have some indication as to why a hearing loss is associated with depression in old age. One can also understand why the association is not as strong as previous research on younger hearing impaired people might have suggested.

In persons of employment age, the overriding effect of a hearing defect was found to be loneliness (an unwelcome feeling of being alone, even in the midst of others—at work and at home). However, this is not the case among the elderly, where the main consequences of impaired hearing seem rather to be in the direction of isolation.

The link between loneliness and depression is accepted as being strong (Post, 1958; Shanas et al 1964; Weiss, 1973). The link between isolation and depression is probably less strong, in that isolation is not necessarily a personally perceived lack or loss and thus may lead less directly to depression by definition (Lowenthal, 1968).* Nonetheless, the relationship between impaired hearing and depression is of great interest for, as has been said, it is effectively an expression of unhappiness specifically related to having a hearing defect and therefore embodies the major handicapping effect of hearing defect and the major challenge to rehabilitation.

If we return now to our previous definition of handicap, it will be remembered that it was suggested that a disability is handicapping to the extent that it restricts a persons' activities to a level below what is felt to be a normal requirement for a particular life-style, or to the extent that it undermines the self-image.

We must therefore consider the impact of hearing impairment on elderly persons with different life-styles and, as Grad d'Alarcon (1971) suggests, use the sociological theories of ageing discussed earlier in the text for the sake of 'the hypothesis they can provide'. Thus, for the sake of discussion, Gilhome Herbst and Humphrey propose that elderly people living 'active' lives (much as they would have normally done during their middle years) were those who reported good health, did not describe themselves as lonely people, had no mobility problems and maintained an active relationship with friends as well as their families. Indeed, these are the active elderly whom Isaacs would have considered in their 'silver age' (Isaacs, 1974).

Against these 'active' elderly, can be balanced the elderly living 'disengaged' lives. That is those who reported living alone, had little or no supportive family network, no relationships with persons other than their family, no contacts outside the home and had not left their homes during the last week.

Hearing impairment interfered most with people at each of these extremes. For those with a way of life that might be more traditionally associated with the middle-aged, hearing impairment was found to be as irksome as it is to people of younger years and a stronger association between depression and hearing impairment was found. At the other end of the spectrum, hearing impairment was particularly bothersome for elderly people leading 'disengaged' lives. For such people, hearing impairment increased their fears of personal insecurity and

* Long-term social isolation seems to have a stronger role to play in producing predispositions to psychoses of non-affective type in old age—e.g. late schizophrenia and late paraphrenia—and it may be for this reason that hearing impairment has traditionally been associated with those disorders rather than with depression.

underlined the losses in their lives which had 'reduced them to this'. These people were also far more likely to feel lonely than any other group of elderly people and, most important, were most likely to be depressed.

Extrapolations by the author from the work of Abrams (1978) gives support to the latter finding. Abrams found the incidence of loneliness amongst those living alone to be at least double that expressed by elderly persons living with others and suggested that living alone is the most significant contributory factor to loneliness in old age, ageing itself making comparatively little difference. 27 per cent of Abrams' whole sample of 1646 persons aged 65 or more, admitted to the interviewer that they were hard-of-hearing. On all the measures of loneliness, those living alone who volunteered that they were also hard-of-hearing rated themselves more unhappy and lonely than the normally hearing living alone.

For the bulk of the elderly people who live neither particularly active lives nor particularly withdrawn lives, hearing impairment seems to matter far less. This again explains the weak association with depression overall and underlines the important role of life-style and life expectations in determining whether hearing impairment is handicapping.

Hearing impairment and paranoid psychosis, late paraphrenia or late schizophrenia

The relationship between paranoid, paraphrenic and schizophrenic illness is not yet agreed upon, but Kay and Roth (1961), Post (1966) and Bromley (1966) support the suggestion that paranoid psychosis is a part of the schizophrenic syndromes found in later life which they call 'late paraphrenia'.

Psychiatrists are also not yet in agreement as to whether there is an association between hearing impairment and paranoia in younger adults. The evidence (reviewed exhaustively by Cooper, 1976) suggests that, on balance, it is unlikely. Nonetheless, the debate remains open. The relationship between hearing impairment and late paranoid psychosis or late paraphrenia appears to have been well accepted for some time (Post, 1966; Roth, 1971) and indeed, Bromley (1966) suggests quite firmly in his section on late paraphrenia that: 'partial or total deafness occurs more frequently than in other psychiatric groups of the same age, but physical health is not usually impaired'. Nonetheless, there has been a recent upsurge of interest in the relationship of impaired hearing to paranoid psychosis in the elderly, as can be seen by the quantity of research on this matter stemming from the Medical School at Newcastle-upon-Tyne (Cooper et al, 1974; Kay et al, 1976; Cooper, Garside and Kay, 1976; Cooper and Curry, 1976; Cooper, 1978). In their examination of evidence regarding a 'psychosis of the deaf' Cooper, Garside and Kay (1976) remind the reader that: 'an association between deafness and paranoid psychosis in later life has often been reported, but few comparisons have been made of the clinical and other characteristics of deaf and non-deaf patients'.

The 'other' characteristics of hearing impaired and normally hearing patients that were investigated by the team are singled out here from the vast body of research on the matter because they contribute to the existing body of knowledge concerning the influence exerted by hearing impairment on social life and show how it, in turn, affects mental state.

Cooper, Garside and Kay (1976) confirm the earlier finding of Houston and Royse (1954) that paranoid patients who also have a hearing defect exhibit less constitutional pre-disposition and have fewer hereditary factors which might predispose them to psychosis than the normally-hearing. They further identify an important sub-group for whom this is particularly true, namely patients with impaired hearing of onset in middle or early age. From this finding they conclude that impaired hearing, working in its role as an isolating agent over a long period of time, may be capable of exerting pathogenic effects of its own (Cooper, Garside and Kay, 1976). At the same time, the team could find little evidence to suggest that hearing impairment, even of long duration, produced any consistent personality changes which might have resulted in an increased liability to psychotic illness. They recommend that the presence of impaired hearing is a useful diagnostic tool to discriminate between patients with paranoid and affective psychoses.

The relationship which has just been discussed between impaired hearing of onset in early life and paranoid psychoses in later life seems to be similar to the mechanism by which impaired hearing of onset in early life has been found to play some part in the development of late schizophrenia (late paraphrenia) (Kay and Roth, 1961). In their exploration of the role of social isolation as a factor in the causation of late schizophrenia, Kay and Roth suggest that the isolated circumstances of a high proportion of such cases (in their study) 'must be attributed to some extent to accidental factors such as deafness'. Indeed, they found that 40 per cent of their paraphrenic cases had a hearing defect—a proportion far in excess of those with affective disorders, though they note that 'assessments (of impaired hearing) were made by rough methods only'. They also recommend, as do others (McClelland et al, 1966), that the presence of impaired hearing should be a useful diagnostic tool to discriminate affective from late paraphrenic disorders.

CONCLUSIONS

Throughout this text, considerable issue has been made of the high prevalence of disorders of hearing in persons of retirement age. It was suggested that defective hearing is almost synonymous with old age and, as such, part of the social and psychological experience of most elderly people. It was proposed that impaired hearing is to be generally expected with advancing years and generally *is* anticipated—to the extent that any of us wait for the maladies of mortal life.* However, this prevalence and the subsequent expectation of being hearing impaired in one's old age has had the general effect of forestalling any true appreciation of the specific social and psychological implication of the disorder. In the text, a distinction was made between the overriding impact of impaired hearing on the elderly as a whole—whether perceived or not—and the specific experience of impaired hearing by affected individuals.

The first analysis showed that there is a significant overall association between impaired hearing and low socio-economic status, advanced age, poor health,

---

* In his report of his study on self-perceptions of ageing, Vischer (1966) was able to rank disorders of ears and eyes third on the list of those defects of mind and body which his test subjects gave as the first indication of the onset of old age.

reduced out-of-door activity due to fears of managing with poor hearing, loss of friends, loss of enjoyment of life and depression. Indeed, there was sufficient evidence to support the notion that impaired hearing in old age is strongly associated with isolation and an artificially imposed loss of personal autonomy and physical independence. These associations were not necessarily perceived by the elderly themselves.

The second analysis drew attention to the fact that, although the majority admit to withholding information about their disorder and experience negative attitudes towards it from others impaired hearing is only perceived as distressing to a substantial minority of the elderly with this defect. For this minority, whom it was estimated may constitute nearly a third of those who admit to hearing loss, their distress at their loss was attributable primarily to their experience of having had a hearing defect before reaching retirement age, to a significantly greater degree of impairment, and to an acute perception of the interference of their hearing defect with their particular life-styles. This distress was evidenced by an increased incidence of loneliness and depression among this group. Using the terminology of Harris (1971) in order to express these life losses associated with impaired hearing, one can see that such impairment is disabling to most elderly people in that it can be seen to generally restrict function, both in terms of literally reduced physical mobility and in terms of maintaining relationships with others. Impaired hearing is handicapping only when it causes personal unhappiness. More elderly people who have a hearing defect experience the disabling effects than feel handicapped. The reason for this is to be found in the 'normality of hearing impairment' in ageing and the reduced demands for social activity that tend to accompany the retirement years. Thus, whilst impaired hearing in old age may be as disabling for the elderly as it is for people of employment age, it is found to be less handicapping and is consequently less strongly associated with depression than in the young.

Nonetheless, the association of hearing impairment and depression remains, and whilst it may not therefore be possible to say that such impairment is a *major* cause of depression in old age, it is certainly a contributing factor, and one which may be more readily ameliorated than many others.

Some consensus has also been reached as to the role that hearing impairment has to play with regard to the schizophrenias and paranoias of later life. It is a premorbid characteristic of these psychoses, in particular those of a paranoid type, and it is probably a pathogenic factor capable of producing breakdown in cases where there is otherwise insufficient predisposition. The manner in which it affects or contributes to psychosis is by causing a breakdown in communication early on in life, which in turn produces a life-style of withdrawal and social isolation. Furthermore, impaired hearing has been found to be useful as a discriminating tool in the differentation of affective psychoses from paranoid psychoses, late paraphrenia or schizophrenia.

Contrary to popular belief, however, impaired hearing is not found to be associated with dementia. It is still possible that there is some link between impaired hearing and dementia associated with early onset. However, since a strong component of organic brain syndrome is poor memory recall, without recourse to longitudinal studies using audiometric techniques no causal associations can be made.

The frequent co-existence of impaired hearing and advanced age has considerable implications for the diagnosis of mental states in the elderly, particularly organic brain syndrome. It is increasingly common practice for both research and clinical purposes to use screening devices, in the form of standardised tests, as an aid to establishing the presence of mental disorders, in particular, dementia (Blessed, Tomlinson and Roth, 1968; Isaacs and Kennie, 1973; Bergmann, Gaber and Foster, 1975). Many compilers of these measures caution would-be users that the tests, being essentially verbal, may be unsuitable for use with hearing impaired subjects (Irving, Robinson and McAdam, 1970; Isaacs and Kennie, 1973). In that some 82 per cent of those aged 80 years or over are likely to be substantially hearing impaired, the validity of all such screening devices would therefore seem to be questionable. However, by tackling the assessment and diagnosis procedure with the firm expectation that the majority of elderly people also have defective hearing, it should be possible to overcome this problem.

The danger of regarding, and therefore treating, elderly people as demented or confused when they actually have a severe hearing loss is not hard to imagine, particularly as the manifestations of both these disorders are in many ways so similar. Such fears have already been voiced by researchers, particularly with regard to residents in local authority homes for the elderly (Townsend, 1964; Martin and Peckford, 1977). Similarly, the apathetic or negative answers which may be the easy way out for the severely hearing-impaired should not be mistaken for depressive responses.

The scope for early intervention is evidently wide, particularly amongst those of employment age or those in their 'silver years'—the young old. Unfortunately, however, early diagnosis and treatment is substantially hampered by prevailing social attitudes to hearing impairment, particularly amongst the old.

Indeed, Beaver (1973) suggests that doctors, as well as their patients, may overlook hearing impairment as a disorder to be treated[*] and consider it a mere irritant of advancing age, to be expected and borne with fortitude and a stiff upper lip. Arguably this is because of its insidious nature.

Disinterest by physicians is reflected in the disinterest of other para-medical staff in, for example, residential homes for the elderly where impaired hearing is found to be most prevalent. The few authors who have made specific enquiries into the care of hearing loss in these homes, express, without exception, their dismay at the lack of staff training in the care and use of available hearing aids and the general lack of knowledge of the implications of unattended hearing loss. (Symington, 1975; Jones, 1977; Burton 1977; Martin and Peckford 1977, 1978; Ward, 1980). Whilst the NHS provides rehabilitation services on demand, lack of interest in hearing impairment and the expectation of poor hearing must of course mean a suppression in taking-up services specific for hearing impairment, particularly the hearing aid. Clearly there is a big gap between admitting to having a hearing loss and making a demand for a 'deafness-labelling' device such as the hearing aid;

---

[*] Thus Harris (1962) found only 55 per cent of those who admitted to being hard-of-hearing said that their doctor knew about it. Sheikh and Verney (1972) report similar results, though more recently Gilhome Herbst and Humphrey found that 64 per cent of those who admitted, or suspected, a hearing loss had mentioned it to their doctor.

hence demand can be seen to fall far behind potential need*. This has considerable implications not only for the elderly but also for service providers.

Because they receive little encouragement to do otherwise, the elderly either defer a demand for hearing aids indefinitely, or postpone it as long as possible. Thus one sees that the hearing aid clinics are by and large servicing a very elderly population, who are already substantially hearing impaired (Brooks, 1979), likely to be physically and mentally quite frail (Alberti, 1977; Ward, Gowers and Morgan, 1979) and often in need of a domiciliary service (Gilhome Herbst and Humphrey, 1980a).

There is a danger, highlighted by Alberti (1977), that attempting to initiate auditory rehabilitation with the very old is a wasteful use of staff time: 'for those who had learnt to wear an aid when they were younger . . . continued to wear them well beyond the stage at which we were unable to make any impression on their equally hard-of-hearing contemporaries'.

Moreover, rumours of the failure of rehabilitative measures when undertaken at this very late stage may well reinforce the belief of the unrehabilitated elderly, their doctors, and their supporters that there is little *point* in getting an aid. So the original causes of withholding recognition of impaired hearing and therefore demand for an aid, namely the stigma of defective hearing, the expectation of poor hearing and life-styles which apparently demand little communication, come full circle to disrupt attempts to overcome the disability by making appropriate or sensible use of existing services.

Not only does the disinterest of medical men and others act to suppress report of the disorder and concern amongst other health workers, but ignorance of the extent of hearing impairment and therefore ignorance of the unmet need at grass roots level, also suppresses interest at policy level. It is true that, in comparison with other pressing needs of the elderly, impaired hearing hardly appears to present itself as an important issue. It is not a matter of life of death, it has little emotional appeal, it rarely produces a crisis, nor is it a disability which in itself produces financial or physical dependancy on others. Yet, nonetheless, sufficient evidence has been provided in this text to recommend that impaired hearing may no longer be disregarded and overlooked with impunity.

ACKNOWLEDGEMENT

The author wishes to express her thanks to her colleague Charlotte Humphrey for her careful commentary on earlier drafts of this text.

REFERENCES

Abrams M 1978 Beyond Three-Score and Ten. A First Report on a Survey of the Elderly. Age Concern Research Publication: Mitcham
Abrams M 1979 Transitions in Middle and Later Life. Paper presented to the British Society of Social and Behavioural Gerontology. Keble College, Oxford. September 1979

* Community studies such as Townsend and Wedderburn's have estimated that in 1965 6·3 per cent of their sample of elderly people possessed hearing aids. By 1978, Abrams estimated that 9·2 per cent of those aged 65+ had aids, and more recently Gilhome Herbst and Humphrey suggest that of those aged 70+, 11·8 per cent have aids. Of those who do admit to a hearing loss, there is some indication that about one third will possess an aid (Harris, 1962; Sheikh and Verney 1972; Gilhome Herbst and Humphrey 1972, 1980a).

Age Concern 1977 Profiles of the Elderly, Vol. 2, 4. Their Health and the Health Services. Age Concern: Mitcham

Alberti P W 1977 Hearing aids and aural rehabilitation. Journal of Otolaryngology; 6: Supplement 4

Alpiner J G 1963 Audiological problems of the aged. Geriatrics 18:19–26

Alpiner J G 1979 Psychological and Social Aspects of Aging as Related to Hearing Rehabilitation of Elderly Clients. In: Henoch MA (ed) Aural rehabilitation for the elderly. Grune and Stratton, New York

Barker R G, Wright B A 1954 Disablement: the somatopsychological problem. In: Wittkower E D, Cleghorn R A (ed) Recent developments in psychosomatic medicine. Lippincott, Philadelphia pp 419–435

Barker R G, Wright B A, Myerson L, Gonick M R 1953 Adjustment to Physical Handicap and Illness: A Survey of the Social Psychology of Physique and Disability. 2nd edn. New York: Social Science Research Council, Bulletin 55

Beaver R 1973 Hearing loss in the elderly—a community health perspective. Public Health London 88:19–25

Bender R 1970 The Conquest of Deafness. The Press of Case Western Reserve University

Bergmann K 1977 Chronic brain failure—epidemiological aspects. Age and Ageing 6, Supplement: 4–8

Bergmann K, Gaber L B, Foster E 1975 The Development of an Instrument for Early Ascertainment of Psychiatric Disorder in Elderly Community Residents: A Pilot Study. Gerontopsychiatr. Arbeitsgem. Janssen Symp. Freiburg.

Berry G 1933 The psychology of progressive deafness. Journal of the American Medical Association: 101:1599–1603

Blessed G 1979 Depression: Assessing the patient behind the mask. Geriatric Medicine, May 1979:29–32

Blessed G, Tomlinson B E, Roth M 1968 The association between quantitative measures of dementia and of senile change in the cerebral grey matter of elderly subjects. British Journal of Psychiatry 114:797–811

Boothroyd A 1968 Developments in speech audiometry. Sound 2:3–10

Brockington F and Lempert S M 1966 The Social Needs of the Overs-80's. Manchester University Press

Bromley D B 1966 The Psychology of Human Ageing. Penguin Books, Harmondsworth

Brooks D N 1979 Hearing aid candidates—some relevant features. British Journal of Audiology; 13:81–84

Burton D K 1977 Hearing Impaired Residents in Local Authority Homes for the Elderly. Unpublished M Sc dissertation, Salford University

Cavan R S, Burgess E W, Havighurst R J, Goldhamer H 1949 Personality Adjustment in Old Age. Science Research Associates

Central Council for Education and Training in Social Work 1974 People with Handicaps Need Better Trained Workers. CCESTW paper 5

Charatan F B 1975 Depression in old age. New York State Journal of Medicine 75:2505–2507

Collingwood H W 1923 Adventures in Silence. Distributed by the Rural New Yorker

Cooper A F 1976 Deafness and psychiatric illness. British Journal of Psychiatry 129:216–226

Cooper A F 1978 Paranoid Psychosis and Late Hearing Impairment. In: Montgomery G (ed) Deafness, Personality and Mental Health. Scottish Workshop with the Deaf

Cooper A F, Curry A R 1976 The pathology of deafness in the paranoid and affective psychoses of later life. Journal of Psychosomatic Research 20:97–105

Cooper A F, Curry A R, Kay D W K, Garside R F, Roth M 1974 Hearing loss in paranoid and affective psychoses of the elderly. Lancet ii: 851–854

Cooper A F, Garside R F, Kay D W K 1976 A comparison of deaf and non-deaf patients with paranoid and affective psychoses. British Journal of Psychiatry 129:532–538

Cosin L Z, Mort M, Post F, Westropp C, Williams M 1957 Persistent senile confusion: A study of 50 consecutive cases. International Journal of Social Psychiatry 3:195–202

Cumbria County Council 1973 Survey of the Handicapped and Impaired and Elderly Over Seventy-five in Cumberland. Cumbria County Council

Cumming E, Henry W E 1961 Growing Old: The Process of Disengagement. Basic Books, Southport

Denmark J C 1976 The psycho-social implications of deafness. Modern Perspectives in Psychiatry 7:188–205

Department of Health and Social Security 1977 Report of a Sub-Committee Appointed to Consider the Role of Social Services in the Care of the Deaf of All Ages. Advisory Committee on Services for Hearing Impaired People, London

D'Souza M F, Irwig L M, Trevelyan H T, Swan A V, Shannon D, Tuckman E, Woodall J D 1975 Deafness in middle age—how big is the problem? Journal of the Royal College of General Practitioners 25:472–478

Ewertsen H W, Birk-Nielsen H 1973 Social hearing handicap index. Audiology 12:180–187

Fry D B 1961 Word and sentence tests for use in speech audiometry. Lancet ii:197–199

Garland M H 1978 Depression and dementia. Hospital Update June 1978:313–319

Gilad O, Glorig A 1979 Presbycusis: The ageing ear. Part I. Journal of the American Auditory Society 4 (5):195–206

Gilhome Herbst K R 1980 The social consequences of acquired hearing loss. Hearing 35 (2):54–57

Gilhome Herbst K R, Humphrey C M 1980a The prevalence of hearing impairment in the elderly living at home. Journal of the Royal College of General Practitioners 31:155–160

Gilhome Herbst K R, Humphrey C M 1980b Hearing impairment and mental state in the elderly living at home. British Medical Journal 281:903–905

Gilmore A J J 1974 Community Surveys and Mental Health. In: Anderson W F, Judge T G (eds) Geriatric Medicine. Academic Press, London

Goffman E 1963 Stigma: Notes on the Management of a Spoilt Identity. Penguin Books, Harmondsworth

Goldberg F M 1970 Helping the Aged. National Institute of Social Work. Training Series 19; Allen and Unwin, London

Grad d'Alarcon J 1971 Social Causes and Social Consequences of Mental Illness in Old Age. In: Kay DWK, Walk A (eds) Recent Developments in Psychogeriatrics. A Symposium. Headly Bros. for Royal Medico-Psychological Association, London

Gregory P 1961 Deafness and Public Responsibility. Occasional Papers on Social Administration. No. 7. Welyn: Codicote Press

Gurland B J, Kuriansky J B, Sharpe L, Simon R, Stiller P, Birkett P 1977 The Comprehensive Assessment and Referral Evaluation (CARE)-rationale, development and reliability. International Journal of Aging and Human Development 8 (1):9–42

Harris A I 1962 The Social Survey. Health and Welfare of Older People in Lewisham. Central Office of Information, London

Harris A I, Cox E, Smith C R W 1971 Handicapped and Impaired in Great Britain. Pt I HMSO London

Havighurst R J, Neugarten B L, Tobin S S 1968 Disengagement and Patterns of Aging. In: Neugarten B L (ed) Middle Age and Aging. Pt. III. University of Chicago Press, pp 161–177

Heron A, Crown S 1967 Age and Function. Churchill, London

High W S, Fairbanks G, Glorig A 1964 Scale for self assessment of hearing handicap. Journal of Speech and Hearing Disorders 29:215–230

Hodgson K 1953 The Deaf and Their Problems: A study in Special Education. Watts, London

Hodkinson H M 1973 Mental impairment in the elderly. Journal of the Royal College of Physicians, London 7 (4):305–317

Hood J D, Poole J P 1977 Improving the reliability of speech audiometry. British Journal of Audiology 11:93–101

Houston F, Royse A B 1954 Relationship between deafness and psychotic illness. Journal of Mental Science 100:990–993

Ingalls G C 1946 Some psychiatric observations on patients with hearing defects. Occupational Therapy and Rehabilitation 25:62–66

Irving G, Robinson R A, McAdam W 1970 The validity of some cognitive tests in the diagnosis of dementia. British Journal of Psychiatry 117:149–156

Isaacs B 1974 The silver age. New Society 30:417–418

Isaacs B, Kennie A 1973 The Set Test as an aid to the detection of dementia in old people. British Journal of Psychiatry 123:467–470

Jackson A W 1902 Deafness and Cheerfulness. Little, Brown & Co., Boston.

Jackson P H 1979 Special problems of the hard of hearing. Journal of Rehabilitation of the Deaf 12 (4):13–26

Jolley D, Arie T 1980 Dementia in old age: An outline of current issues. Health Trends 12:1–4

Jones S 1977 Many old people are unnecessarily deaf. Residential Social Work 17 (2):36–38

Kay D W K, Beamish P, Roth M 1964 Old age mental disorders in Newcastle upon Tyne. Pt. I: A study of prevalence. British Journal of Psychiatry 110:146–158

Kay D W K, Beamish P, Roth M 1964 Old age mental disorders in Newcastle upon Tyne. Pt. II: A study of possible social and medical causes. British Journal of Psychiatry 110:668–682

Kay D W K, Cooper A F, Garside R F, Roth M 1976 The differentiation of paranoid from affective psychoses by patient's premorbid characteristics. British Journal of Psychiatry 129:207–15

Kay D W K, Roth M 1961 Environmental and hereditary factors in schizophrenias of old age. Journal of Mental Science 107:649–686

Knapp P H 1948 Emotional aspects of hearing loss. Psychosomatic Medicine 10:203–222

Lowenthal M F 1968 Socio-Psychological Theories of Aging. Introduction to Part III of Middle Age and Aging. Ed Neugarten B L. The University of Chicago Press, pp 159–160

Maddox G L 1963 Activity and morale: A longitudinal study of selected elderly subjects. Social Forces 42:195–204
Maddox G L 1968 Persistence of Life Style Among the Elderly: A Longitudinal Study of Patterns of Social Activity in Relation of Life Satisfaction. In: Middle Age and Aging, Pt. III Ed. Neugarten B L University of Chicago Press, pp 181–1833
Mahapatra S B 1974 Deafness and mental health: Psychiatric and psychosomatic illness in the deaf. Acta Psychiatrica Scandinavia 50:596–611
Martin D N, Peckford R W 1977 Hearing Impairment in Homes for the Elderly. North Yorkshire County Council Social Services Department
Martin D N, Peckford R W 1978 Hearing impairment in homes for the elderly. Social Work Service 17:52–62
McCall R 1979 Understanding the sounds of silence. New Age 6 Spring:28–29
McClelland H A, Roth M, Neuhauer H, Garside R 1966 Some observations on case-material based on patients with certain common schizophrenic symptoms. Proceedings of 4th World Congress on Psychiatry, pp 2955–2957
Menninger K A 1924 The mental effects of deafness. Psychoanalytic Review 11:144–155
Milne J S 1976 Hearing loss related to some signs and symptoms in older people. British Journal of Audiology 10:65–73
Milne J S, Maule M M, Williamson J 1971 Method of sampling in a study of older people with a comparison of respondents and non-respondents. British Journal of Preventive and Social Medicine 25:37–41
Murphy G E B 1913 Your Deafness is Not You. The World's Work Ltd: Survey
Myklebust H R 1964 The Psychology of Deafness. Grune and Stratton, New York
Nie N H, Hadlai Hull C, Jenkins J G, Steinbrenner K, Bent D H 1975 The statistical package for the social sciences. 2nd edn. McGraw Hill, New York
Nobble W G 1978 Assessment of impaired hearing: a critique and a new method. Academic Press, New York
Noble W G, Atherley G R C 1970 The Hearing Measurement Scale: A questionnaire for the assessment of auditory disability. Journal of Auditory Research 10:229–250
Nottingham Social Services 1973 The Elderly in Nottingham. Report on Phase I of a Survey of Persons aged 75+. Nottingham Social Services Committee
Post F 1958 Social factors in old age psychiatry. Geriatrics 13:567–580
Post F 1966 Persistent Persecutory States of the Elderly. Pergamon Press, Oxford
Powers J K, Powers E A 1978 Hearing problems of elderly persons: Social consequences and prevalence. Asha 20 (2):79–83
Ramsdell D A 1966 The Psychology of the Hard of Hearing and the Deafened Adult. In: Davis H, Silverman S R (eds): Hearing and Deafness, Holt, Rinehart & Winston, New York
Rawson A 1973 Deafness: Report of a Departmental Enquiry into the Promotion of Research. HMSO, London
Richardson I M 1964 Age and Need. A Study of Older People in the North-East of Scotland. Livingstone, Edinburgh
Rosen J K 1979 Psychological and social aspects of the evaluation of acquired hearing impairment. Audiology 18:238–252
Roth M 1971 Classification and Aetiology in Mental Disorders of Old Age: Some Recent Developments. In: Kay D W K, Walk A (eds): Recent Developments in Psychogeriatrics. Royal Medico-Psychological Association. Headley Brothers, Ashford
Safilios-Rothschild C 1970 Sociology and Social Psychology of Disability and Rehabilitation. Random House, New York
Shakespeare R 1975 The Psychology of Handicap. Methuen, London
Shanas E, Townsend P, Wedderburn D, Friis H, Milhoj P, Stehouwer J 1964 Old People in Three Industrial Societies. Routledge & Kegan Paul, London
Sheard A V 1971 Survey of the elderly in Scunthorpe. Public Health London 85:208–218
Sheikh J. Verney A R 1972 Report on the Survey of Hearing Impaired Persons in Blaby Rd. Leicestershire County Council, Social Services Dept
Sheldon J H 1948 The Social Medicine of Old Age. Report of an Enquiry in Wolverhampton. Oxford University Press, London
Stephens S D G 1979 Deaf as a post. Hearing 34:197–198
Stockport County Council 1958 Report on the Survey of the Aged in Stockport. Stockport County Council
Symington B 1975 A Service for Elderly Hearing Impaired People in Residential Care. Paper presented to the National Council of Social Workers for the Deaf. Birmingham: April 1975

Thomas A J. Gilhome Herbst K R 1980a Social and psychological implications of acquired hearing loss for adults of employment age. British Journal of Audiology 14:76–85

Thomas A J. Gilhome Herbst K R 1980b Acquired Deafness and Psychological Disorder From: Disorders of Auditory Function. Vol III proceedings of Third Conference of British Society of Audiology July 1979

Townsend P 1964 The Last Refuge. Routledge & Kegan Paul, London

Townsend P, Wedderburn D 1965 The Aged in the Welfare State. Occasional Papers on Social Administration No. 14. Bell, London

Tunstall J 1965 Old and Alone: A Sociological Study of Old People. Routledge & Kegan Paul, London

Vischer A L 1978 On Growing Old. In: Carver V, Liddiard P (eds) An Ageing Population. University Press, London

Von Leden H 1977 Speech and hearing problems in the geriatric patient. Journal of the American Geriatrics Society 25 (9):422–426

Ward P R 1980 Treatment of elderly adults with impaired hearing: Resources, outcome and efficiency. Journal of Epidemiology and Community Health 34:65–68

Ward P R, Gowers, J I. Morgan D C 1979 Problems with handling the BEIO series hearing aids among elderly people. British Journal of Audiology 13 (1):31–36

Weiss R S 1973 Loneliness: The Experience of Emotional and Social Isolation. M. I. T

Wilkins L T 1948 The Social Survey. Survey of the Prevalence of Deafness in the population of England, Scotland and Wales. Central Office of Information, London

Williamson J 1978 Depression in the elderly. Age and Aging 7: Supplement

Williamson J, Stokoe I H, Gray S, Fisher M, Smith A, McGhee A, Stephenson E. 1964 Old people at home: Their unreported needs. Lancet i:1117–1120

Wood P H N 1975 Classification of Impairments and Handicaps. Paper presented to the International Conference for the Ninth Revision of the International Classification of Diseases. WHO. Geneva 30 Sept—6 Oct 1975. WHO/ICDG/REV.CONF/75·15

Wright B A 1960 Physical Disability: A Psychological Approach. Harper & Row, New York

Auditory rehabilitation for the elderly

INTRODUCTION

The elderly population constitute the vast majority of the hearing impaired. There have been a number of studies (e.g. Henoch, 1979; Bentzen et al, 1969; Gilhome-Herbst and Humphrey, 1980) which have considered many different aspects of their audiological rehabilitation. The aim of this account is to present an integrated approach in the context of the comprehensive overall model proposed by Goldstein and Stephens (1981).

This model, which places considerable emphasis on non-auditory factors in the evaluation of the patients and on non-instrumental factors in the remediation process, appears particularly pertinent in any consideration of the problems of the elderly population. This presentation will consist first of an outline description of the model followed by a discussion of the application of its individual components to the elderly population.

MODEL

The two columns of Figure 9.1 summarise the overall outline of the processes involved in audiological rehabilitation in increasing complexity. Column 1 shows that the actual process of audiological rehabilitation may be divided into two main components of evaluation and remediation. Column 2 shows that each of these may be further subdivided into major sections, three in the case of evaluation and five in remediation. These further sections may then be subdivided and this process of elaboration may be continued over many further stages. However, as the model is meant to be global and not setting-specific, a detailed elaboration has been avoided at this stage.

There is considerable evidence (e.g. Markides, 1977; Davis, 1980; Humphrey et al, 1981) that less than one quarter of patients in Western Countries, who have a hearing loss and who might reasonably benefit from amplification, actually possess hearing aids. This varies considerably from country to country when the rest of the world is considered (e.g. Bentzen and Courtois, 1973) and is related in part, at least, to the wealth of the countries concerned (Stephens, 1977). Other factors such as the nature of the social provisions of the particular country, whether aids are provided free or have to be purchased by the hearing impaired individual, account for further, if smaller, components of the difference between countries.

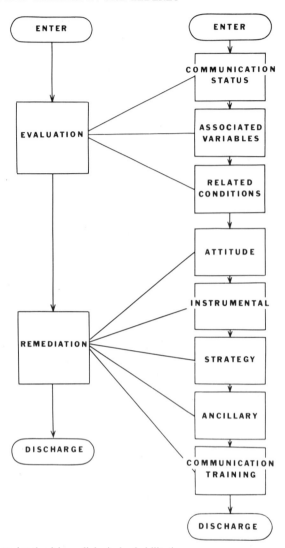

Fig. 9.1 The process involved in audiological rehabilitation

Even within countries it may be argued that such factors as the distance which the patient lives from the hearing aid providors, the attitude of the patient, his family, and his professional advisors towards rehabilitation, earlier experiences with aids, together with his social situation, may further influence whether he seeks help. In addition those patients with more severe hearing losses are more likely to seek help than those with relatively mild losses. Furthermore, those who develop a hearing loss before retirement age are more likely to have a hearing aid than those impaired after retirement (Humphrey et al, 1981). Such factors were deliberately excluded by Goldstein and Stephens (1981) from their model which concentrates solely on what happens or should happen to the patient once he has sought appropriate help.

Whether or not a patient enters into a system may be influenced by publicity and propaganda, education of personnel likely to come into contact with the elderly, and the provision of mobile or domiciliary services. Some of these approaches have been adopted in various places (e.g. Bentzen et al, 1976; Stephens, et al, 1980; Brooks and Johnson, 1981) but there are still few data as to their effectiveness.

Returning to the outline of the process of Audiological Rehabilitation shown in Figure 9.1, it may be seen that each stage is portrayed as being sequential. However, certain aspects of the remediation process may highlight a need for further evaluative stages or even a repeat of earlier stages of the remediation process. This is allowed for in detailed flow charts developed with the model described.

In addition, it must be emphasised that certain stages may take place very rapidly with a 'no action' decision being made. Others, and in particular communication training, may last for months or even longer.

EVALUATION

Communication status

This entails an evaluation of the existing communication abilities of the patient. It involves a consideration of both receptive and productive capabilities, together with an assessment of overall integrative capacity. These are summarised in Figure 9.2, which shows the communication status section of Figure 9.1 splitting into these six components.

1. Auditory

In the auditory component, one is concerned both with what the patient considers to be his problems resulting from the hearing loss and also with an assessment of his auditory capacity. In the elderly in particular it is important to focus on the specific needs and problems faced by the patient within his individual lifestyle and social situation. Often a patient may be somewhat overawed when questioned about this in the context of a hospital clinic or hearing aid department, and much useful information may be obtained by the use of a 'hearing problem questionnaire' (Barcham and Stephens, 1980). This is an open ended form which may be sent to the patient before his appointment and which may be completed in the relaxed atmosphere of his own home, where he will be more aware of his real needs. It consists of a simple form worded as follows: 'Please make a list of the difficulties which you have as a result of your hearing loss. List these in order of importance starting with the biggest difficulties. Write down as many as you can think of'.

It is important to emphasise at this stage that audiological rehabilitation is concerned with helping an individual with a specific set of problems arising from an auditory disorder. It is most definitely not the fitting of one (or two) hearing aids to match an audiometric configuration. This emphasis is particularly true of the elderly in some of whom a hearing aid may be only a very minor component of the rehabilitation process. In fact, in some circumstances, in spite of a hearing loss, mitigating factors may rule out the use of a hearing aid.

Specific difficulties encountered by the patient may further be elicited by direct questioning and also by the use of structured questionnaires, some of which have

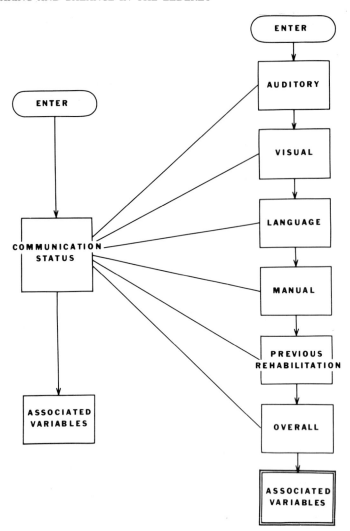

Fig. 9.2 Evaluation of the communication abilities of a patient

been discussed elsewhere (Stephens, 1980). These may be pencil and paper based and completed by the patient before he is seen, or may be administered in interview form. In many ways they are less pertinent to the problems of the elderly patients, although modified forms have been developed for use with such a population (e.g. McCartney et al, 1976).

Assessment of auditory capacity in the elderly may vary from an intensive audiometric workup of an alert mobile individual to a careful clinical assessment which may be all that is possible in the case of certain bedbound individuals. However, such an assessment, using only the spoken and whispered voice, and certain tuning fork tests, may provide considerable information as to the auditory status of the patient (e.g. Hinchcliffe, 1981). In certain senile patients even this may not be possible, and in those cases emphasis will be put on helping the nursing/care staff to communicate with the patient.

Ideally, however, it is important, where possible, to obtain three measures of auditory function when considering the patient from a rehabilitative point of view. These are measures of auditory sensitivity, tolerance levels and speech discrimination.

Measurement of sensitivity is based normally on pure tone audiometric thresholds which also provide a guide as to the frequency characteristics of the hearing aid which might ultimately be the most appropriate. Speech reception thresholds are often obtained, although it is arguable that these may be predicted relatively easily from the patient's pure tone thresholds.

Measurement of the patient's tolerance levels, or uncomfortable loudness levels, is important in order to ensure that the patient is not fitted with amplification in which the maximum output is at a level causing discomfort. This would lead to rejection of any amplification and could ultimately set back the rehabilitative procedure.

Speech discrimination measures may be obtained in different ways. The aim of all techniques is to derive a measure of the best discrimination of speech which may be possible for the particular individual for the ear under test. The measures may be obtained by plotting a discrimination curve, measuring a fixed point above the threshold level or measuring at the comfortable listening level. Each approach has both advantages and disadvantages but, in general, similar results may be obtained with the three techniques. Speech discrimination measures provide an idea of the optimal level of performance for that individual by the auditory modality alone, and also give information as to which ear should be aided if monaural amplification is to be used.

Visual
Visual performance measures cover two aspects of vision, basic visual acuity and speechreading (lipreading) ability. In addition note is taken as to whether the patient normally uses spectacles to correct a visual defect and, if so, whether he uses one or more pairs. This is important in any consideration as to whether one or two hearing aids are to be incorporated in a spectacle frame.

Knowledge of the patient's corrected level of visual acuity is important. One must bear in mind that, even when fitted with a hearing aid the patient will be more dependent than a normally hearing person on visual cues in order to achieve maximum communication in a one to one conversation. It is thus important that he should be made aware of any defect and advised to take steps to remedy this, if possible.

If the patient has a severe uncorrectable visual deficit, and such a problem occurs more commonly among the elderly, it is essential that more than normal emphasis should be put on a binaural fitting of hearing aids. This is particularly important if the patient is to be able to adequately directionalise warning or danger signals.

Speech-reading (lip-reading) performance may be assessed simply in an interview situation in a gross manner using unvoiced speech material. In most patients this serves a therapeutic role, indicating to them that they are in fact able to speech read, and indeed some of the best speech-readers encountered in practice are found among elderly patients with lifelong chronic middle ear disease but who have not received any formal training in speechreading.

Patients with with severe hearing loss who are shown in such tests to be poor speech-readers will require more sophisticated measures of speechreading performance based on standardised video-recorded material. By such means it is possible to define the specific difficulty which the patient encounters, the recognition of particular visemes*, their integration into words, or the discrimination of running speech, and hence indicate appropriate remediation.

Language
In inner city populations in particular a number of the elderly hearing impaired patients who are seen will not be native speakers of the language of the clinic nor particularly fluent in that language. The problems associated with such reduced fluency will be enhanced by the acquisition of a hearing loss. It is important therefore, that in such patients evaluation and remediation be performed as far as possible within their maternal language, through intermediaries such as members of their family where necessary. If such approaches are not possible, the professional concerned with rehabilitation of this individual must be aware of this linguistic problem and allow for it in all stages of rehabilitation.

It is important to assess the general vocabulary of all patients so that the approach adopted be appropriate to their vocabulary and explanations be understandable to them. This is also pertinent in any communication training which should be concentrated on speech material related to the patient's specific vocabulary needs.

Consideration of the syntactic approach used by the patient will generally be pertinent only in the case of the prelingually deaf, who constitute a very small minority of the hearing impaired elderly. In this group, however, it is important to be aware of the syntactic differences between the manual communication (sign language) system of the country and the normal spoken language. Daily use of manual communication within a deaf community will bias the patient's use of syntax in the spoken language and may lead to confusion on the part of the unprepared professional. Syntactic changes are, however, most unlikely to occur in those individuals with acquired hearing loss even if the loss is severe.

Phonological changes, on the other hand, occur quite frequently in this latter group due to impaired monitoring and feedback to the patient of the sound of his own speech. This is most marked in those patients with a profound or complete hearing loss, but characteristic changes also occur in those with a high frequency impairment. Even those with a moderate loss may have some difficulty in monitoring the intensity of their speech, patients with sensorineural losses tending to speak too loud and those with conductive losses speaking too softly. This can, however, be remedied reasonably easily by appropriate counselling.

The more severe disorders of rhythm, intonation and sound substitutions found in those with severe acquired losses and in those with prelingual hearing losses may require more intensive speech therapy if this is indicated by their lifestyle and communicative circumstances. It is thus important to evaluate the patient's needs in a global context and also to carefully define the specific speech problems from which the patient suffers.

---

* A viseme is visual equivalent of a phoneme. It is a unit of speech which depends on visual contrasts.

Manual communication

This is of minor importance in the evaluation of the vast majority of elderly hearing impaired individuals. It is important, however, to consider and enquire as to whether the patient has any knowledge of manual communication.

For those with some knowledge of manual communication it may be important to determine the system used and the patient's fluency in this although such factors are less relevant in the elderly. The only exception to this is in the case of an individual with a sudden profound or complete hearing loss. In such a person, the introduction of a system such as the mouth-hand system or finger spelling to supplement speech reading within the family circle may be of some relevance.

Previous rehabilitation

It is essential to be aware of any previous rehabilitative treatment which the patient may have received, as this may well have biased his attitude and approach to any management which may be proposed subsequently. If the previous management has been poor it behoves the professional to take great care to restore the patient's faith in such a process in order that positive steps may be taken to help him. On the other hand, if the patient has previously had a positive experience and has returned for help only to seek improved amplification or other specific assistance, the task of rehabilitation may be considerably easier.

In this context it is important to enquire about amplification systems previously used, approaches to audiovisual communication and other aids and to evaluate the patient's experience with these.

Overall communication

In the previous sections consideration has been given to specific aspects of factors influencing the patient's communication. In a consideration of the parts it is important not to neglect the entirety and to consider the patient's total communication status. This entails a determination of how well he functions in this respect within his own environment using all the means which he has at his disposal. This will give guidance as to the degree of emphasis and effort which may be needed, and indeed justified in order to help him to perform optimally. Thus an individual assessed as performing almost as well as might be expected, given his sensory deficit, will require considerably less help than an individual who, because of minor discrimination problems, withdraws completely from any communication situation, including those well within his auditory capabilities.

Associated variables

This section deals with psychosocial factors which will considerably influence the patient's needs and handicap. Figure 9.3 illustrates the components of this within a general rehabilitative context. It is important, however, to realise that, in an elderly population, the first two components of psychological and sociological factors predominate, whereas the educational and vocational factors play a relatively minor role. It is, however, pertinent to consider these last two sections as many elderly individuals still work at least on a part-time basis and the nature of their former work may colour their attitude towards auditory rehabilitation. Their

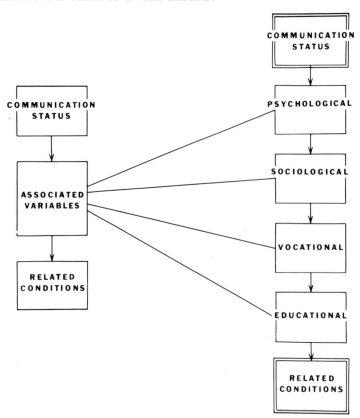

Fig. 9.3 Psychosocial factors influencing patients' needs and handicaps

educational experiences, albeit some 50 years previously, may also bias their attitude and approach to any procedures which may be proposed.

Psychological factors
The patient's psychological makeup and status comprise a variety of components which must influence the rehabilitative approach to be adopted. These components may be grouped into three sections under the general headings of attitude, personality and intelligence.

The patient's attitude towards his handicap and towards proposed rehabilitative procedures will have a critical effect upon the outcome of such procedures. This is so central to the entire rehabilitative process that different detailed approaches must be adopted according to the patient's overall attitude and this is discussed further in the sections concerned with remediation.

The attitudinal factors may be further subdivided into components of acceptance of the impairment and the proposed procedures, the individual's expectation of the ultimate outcome, and his motivation to obtain a satisfactory result.

The patient's personality will undoubtedly interact with his attitude, and indeed there is a strong relationship between certain aspects of emotional stability and failure avoidance motivation (e.g. Broadbent, 1972). However, on the whole the patient's emotional stability is more likely to influence the professional's attitude towards him, which should be to ensure that the overall procedure takes place in as relaxed an atmosphere as possible. In this respect more attention to detail will be required by the anxious apprehensive patient than by the stoic, although the latter may need some additional positive stimulation in order to attract his interest.

Aspects of the patient's personality with regard to his assertiveness and sociability will govern the approach to the rehabilitative strategy to be encouraged. While much of the Danish Hearing Tactics (Vognsen, 1976) is based on encouraging the patient to adopt a positive and assertive attitude towards his hearing loss, this will not be appropriate to a patient who all his life has been a shy reticent individual.

Further, in structuring an appropriate rehabilitative programme it is important to know how obsessional the patient may be in his behaviour and hence how conscientiously he may follow his guidelines. It is also useful to be aware of his adaptability.

The final consideration within the context of psychological factors will cover the intelligence of the patient. This will have important bearings on the way in which the rehabilitative programme is structured and presented.

Sociological factors
These will have a vital bearing on the approach and outcome of any rehabilitative programme. They cover the life situation of the patient, cultural factors, his communication lifestyle and aspects of stigma related to the society as a whole.

Relevant factors in this context cover such matters as whether the patient lives alone, with his spouse, in a wider family circle or in an institution. Studies both in Manchester (Brooks, 1972) and in London (Stephens, et al, 1980) indicate that approximately a quarter to a third of patients fitted with hearing aids live alone. The vast majority of these are elderly. The auditory communication needs of such individuals will be very different from those living with their children and grandchildren or again from those, albeit only about 5 per cent of the population, living in an institution. The communication needs of those living alone, and who have only a moderate hearing loss may, arguably, be better met by concentrating on a judicious use of environmental aids rather than on a personal hearing aid. Close liaison with social services to avoid further isolation will also be necessary.

Sociological factors will also have an important bearing within the larger community in which the patient lives. For example, within a relatively small community, a large proportion of whom have worked within a particularly noisy industry for much of their working lives, the understanding, cameraderie and sympathy for the hearing impaired individual will be strong. In such circumstances the individual with normal hearing may be the exception. On the other hand, a hearing impaired individual living in a predominantly normally hearing community will be faced with a completely different set of circumstances.

This also has a bearing on the stigma associated with hearing loss. In the former circumstances there will be no emotional pressure on the individual to conceal his impairment, indeed it will be regarded as something quite normal. In the latter society the hearing impaired individual may feel a need to hide his impairment little realising that although he is in an essentially 'normally hearing' society, that society still contains a significant proportion of hearing impaired individuals. These factors will have a considerable influence on the strategy to be adopted in the process of rehabilitation, the involvement of outside professional workers and even the instrumental approach itself.

Vocational and educational
Although these factors are important in younger subjects, they are of secondary importance in the elderly.

Related conditions
This section, the last component of evaluation, is concerned with factors which will influence a number of the practical, and particularly instrumental, components of the rehabilitative process. They are summarised in Figure 9.4 which shows a breakdown of these into mobility, upper limb function and related aural pathology.

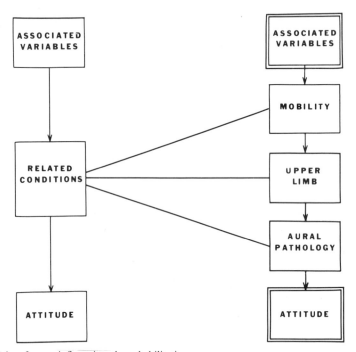

Fig. 9.4 Other factors influencing the rehabilitative process

Mobility
The patient's mobility, whether or not he is able to leave his residence, or for that matter his bed, unassisted to seek audiological help, will influence the organisation of the rehabilitative help. It will also influence the nature of instrumental support. Hence, if a patient is housebound there is a compelling requirement that the rehabilitation should be performed on a domiciliary basis. This of necessity means a foregoing of some of the more sophisticated aspects of auditory and visual evaluation, but can be compensated for by the more realistic picture which may be obtained of the patient's needs. Rehabilitation on a domiciliary basis should not be

regarded as an exceptional process, particularly among the elderly. In a re
of the rehabilitation offered within an inner London Borough, it was judg
17 per cent needed all, or most, of their rehabilitation on a domiciliary
(Stephens et al, 1980). This proportion will increase with the increasing age of t
population being served.

Despite the limited equipment and test facilities which the audiologist can
take to the patient's home, with the aid of basic clinical tests (Hinchcliffe, 1981)
and a portable audiometer with sound attenuating cushions, a good assessment of
the patient's communication status may generally be obtained. Being on site then
gives the audiologist more insight as to the patient's communication needs and the
means of overcoming these may be related more to the use of a variety of
environmental aids rather than wearable hearing aids.

The wheelchair-bound patient must be taken into consideration in the design of
any rehabilitation centre to ensure easy access for such individuals. This entails
replacing steps with ramps, providing doors of adequate width, and also appropriate toilet facilities.

Upper limb function

The patient's upper limb function will limit his ability to control or insert any form
of wearable amplification. The factors which may have a bearing here will range
from moderately impaired hand and finger dexterity and sensitivity through tremor
of varying degree to paralysis; there may even be lack of upper limbs following
amputation.

The milder disorders will lead to more emphasis and time put on aspects of
fitting the earmould and handling the hearing aid together with the choice of
devices with more easily manageable controls. These controls may be made larger
in bodyworn hearing aids. Thus for patients with moderate to severe manipulative
problems, there is a strong indication for switching to such devices despite the
initial objection, on cosmetic grounds, by the patient. Such an approach may have
to be taken in gradual stages so that the patient comes to accept the need for it.

One of the greatest handling problems for the individual with defective upper
limb function is that of fitting the earmould properly into the ear. Various
approaches have been adopted to overcome this problem including headsets,
earmoulds with handles, and stetoclips (Stephens, 1981). In the authors' experience, the last have been found to be extremely effective provided that the patient
can be persuaded to accept the idea.

In cases of patients with bilateral upper limb deficits, who have only a mild to
moderate hearing loss, it is often best to meet the patient's needs by means of
environmental aids rather than by wearable hearing aids.

Aural pathology

This section is concerned with the problems arising from the presence of aural
discharge (otorrhoea), sensation of pressure in the ear(s), tinnitus and vertigo.
Each is important in that it may have a significant bearing on the instrumental
approach to be followed.

Otorrhoea due to otitis media or otitis externa may be exacerbated by the use of a
closed meatal earmould on the infected ear. It is thus important to avoid, where

to an ear in which there is any evidence of active infection,
rforation. In certain cases with severe bilateral otitis media,
in order to prevent exacerbation of the infection, it may be
conduction receivers. Another approach is to use open or
h may be fitted alternately to each ear but, in those patients
ss, such an approach can lead to feedback problems. A
way out is by the use of a mould with a sintered filter* (French St. George
and Barr Hamilton, 1978) which allows slow pressure equilibration while reducing
audiofrequency feedback problems. Such approaches may also be important for
patients complaining of pressure in their ears, whether, related to auditory tubal
dysfunction or to endolymphatic hydrops. Such pressure sensations may be
enhanced by the occlusion of the meatus with a tight fitting earmould so that an
open or vented mould fitting will be necessary if the patient is not to reject the
hearing aid system altogether.

The presence of disturbing tinnitus in one ear may influence the choice of that
ear for a hearing aid if a monaural fitting is being used. This is related to the finding
that, in many patients with both tinnitus and hearing loss, such a hearing aid fitting
may help suppress the tinnitus (e.g. Vernon, 1977). However, in a minority of
patients the tinnitus may be aggravated by a hearing aid fitting, so that in such a
case the presence of tinnitus will have the opposite effect on the choice of ear for a
monaural fitting.

Vertigo is of relevance in that some 25 per cent of patients with episodic vertigo
suffer from the Tullio phenomenon (Stephens and Ballam, 1974). That is to say
that loud sounds may precipitate episodes of vertigo. In such cases it will be
important to apply amplification either to the ear not affected in this way, or to
limit the output of the hearing aid so that it does not exceed the threshold level of
this Tullio effect.

REMEDIATION

Attitude
This important first step in the remedial process consists of three major
components and is summarised in Figure 9.5. These comprise the integration of
the information obtained in the evaluative sections, particularly in the 'Associated
Variables' sections, the modification of such attitude, where possible, and the
classification of the patient into one of four attitude types. This classification will
then determine the approach to be followed in the subsequent management of the
patient.

Integration
The integration entails the bringing together of all the information, collected in the
evaluative section, which may have some bearing on the patient's attitude towards
his disability and what may have to be done to help him overcome this. Such
information will largely be derived from the psychological and sociological sections

* A small cylinder of sintered metal, i.e. metal particles coalesced under heat treatment; the porous
nature provides an acoustical resistance

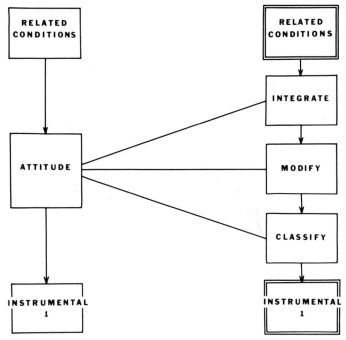

Fig. 9.5 Attitude and patient categorization

of the evaluation, but other factors, such as his physical handicaps, visual acuity and severity of hearing loss will also influence this attitude.

The attitude may be subdivided into three components, which we referred to, for convenience, as acceptance, understanding and expectation. The first, acceptance, entails the patient's approach to his disorder, and whether he is prepared to accept the concept that he has a hearing loss, with consequent communication problems. Some patients may persist in maintaining that the problem lies in the unclear way in which the 'younger' generation speak, rather than in the distortions encountered as a result of their auditory deficit. Others, while accepting that they do have a hearing problem may refuse to accept that it is permanent. Yet others may have the approach that it is 'something to be expected at their age' and not accept any need or potential of it being helped.

Understanding, or lack of it, will bias this approach of the patient and reinforce his limited acceptance. He may insist, despite repeated explanations, that an operation could restore his hearing. Alternatively he may not appreciate the effects of his auditory deficit on those around him. On a more subtle level he may not appreciate why he appears to hear 'normally' under certain circumstances, and be completely lost under others.

The expectations deal with the patient's attitude to the ultimate outcome of the rehabilitative process. Here it is extremely important to strike a fine balance between an over optimistic high expectancy and a pessimistic 'no help' approach. No rehabilitative process can restore the patient's auditory performance to normality, but an appropriate approach can be of considerable benefit. Should the patient have too high an expectancy, he may rapidly become disenchanted as the help he receives from his hearing aid(s) and the other aspects of the rehabilitative process does not reach his expectations. There is a serious danger then that he may then reject the entire process. On the other hand, the patient who initially expects too little from the rehabilitative process and who has come for a consultation only as a result from pressure from the family or friends, is likely not to return even for a fitting session.

Modification

The purpose of this stage of the rehabilitative process then is, having made a preliminary evaluation of the patient's attitude, to attempt some initial modification so that it is more appropriate to the degree and nature of his disorder and to the potential outcome. In this the aspects of acceptance, understanding and expectations will be taken in parallel either together or with emphasis on whichever appears to need most attention. Such an attitude modification session will not be a long drawn out approach at this stage. The purpose here will be to overcome outstanding misconceptions and attitudinal prejudices as far as possible to facilitate the subsequent rehabilitative approach. More extensive and in-depth aspects of attitude modification are more appropriately dealt with in the communication training stage of the remedial process.

Classification

The initial stage of attitudinal modification will lead to a further assessment of the patient's consequent attitude and its classification into one of four categories which will determine the subsequent remedial approach.

Category I comprises the majority of patients and represents the 'straight forward' case from a rehabilitative point of view. The patient is positively motivated to obtain help, may have had previously successful rehabilitative processes, and has a relatively uncomplicated audiometric configuration. He will pass very rapidly through the subsequent rehabilitative stages and require little follow-up.

Category II describes the patient who is still basically positively motivated, but in whom there are actual or potential complicating factors. These may be directly apparent and include such points as a poor previous experience with rehabilitation, a relatively mild hearing loss, handling problems, otorrhoea and other related factors. On the other hand they may not be particularly apparent to the patient but more obvious to the audiologist. Especially in this last group will be patients with audiometric configurations which are difficult to fit. This type of case requires additional time to go through hearing aid modifications and communication training processes.

The vast majority of patients seen in audiological clinics come within these two categories. A minority of those who reach the clinics come in categories III and IV.

Category III describes the patient who basically has a negative attitude towards the rehabilitative process and in particular towards the idea of a hearing aid. He does, however, have an element of motivation and should be considered for a different approach, concentrating initially on a discussion of stategy and environmental aids and then moving on to the communication training component. There, particularly in a group context with others who wear hearing aids, he can have the opportunity to try such devices in an informal setting and may be gradually encouraged to adopt a more positive attitude towards such sources of help.

Category IV describes a patient with a strong negative attitude towards rehabilitation who has come along solely as a result of intense pressure from his family or associates. Many of such patients will not return for further sessions, but it is important to endeavour to encourage such an individual by routing him directly to the communication training component, if only to illustrate to him what can be done. By means of such a 'gently-gently' approach a certain proportion of this group can come to develop a more positive attitude to seeking help. If such a patient is merely fitted with a hearing aid when first seen it is certain that the device will never be worn once the patient has left the rehabilitation centre.

Instrumental I

This section deals with the initial approach to instrumental help for the patient. In many places it is the sole aspect of the rehabilitation process which is given any consideration whatsoever. The present authors would argue that in any process of auditory rehabilitation, and particularly in one concerned with the elderly, the hearing aid is only one component and even only part of one component of the total rehabilitative process. It must be admitted however, that even in well structured schemes of auditory rehabilitation, the wearable aid(s) may be identified by the patient as the most important of these components, partly because of its unique role, and partly because of the patient's expectancy.

Figure 9.6 shows a breakdown of what for convenience may be referred to as Instrumental I (Instrumental II is a component of the Communication Training section of the remedial process). Instrumental I may be seen to consist of amplification, alerting and warning systems, other sensory aids, and training. One of the aims of this classification is to emphasise that, particularly with the elderly, the hearing aids comprise only one aspect of the approach to instrumental help for the patient.

Amplification

In the process of selection of appropriate amplification it is important to consider the approach most relevant to the particular individual. The first question to be answered is whether the patient can cope with and be helped by a headworn aid. If so, then further decisions need to be made as to whether it should be postaural, intra-aural, or spectacle type, and whether one or two aids should be used. Parallel decisions consider the power and frequency characteristics of the aid(s), the nature of its controls and, most important, the type of earmoulds/coupling to be used to link the aid to the ear.

There is not sufficient space here for a detailed consideration of these different points but some general principles must be recalled. First, it is essential to consider the benefit of any fitting to be recommended in terms of the additional burdens which it will impose on the patient. A binaural fitting, for example, may be acoustically ideal for a particular individual but his handling difficulties may mean that even a single aid presents a severe challenge to him. A CROS or BICROS fitting may be of value to the patient active in committees and other difficult

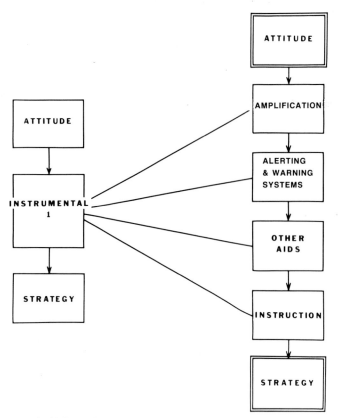

Fig. 9.6 Instrumental aid for patients

listening situations but not for his counterpart living a sedentary life in semi-isolation. Handling problems are particularly important in consideration of a specific aid, and spectacle aids may be limited by the fact that the patient uses two different pairs of spectacles.

If it is decided that for acoustical or ergonomic reasons, a headworn aid may not be appropriate, the next stage must be to consider a bodyworn hearing aid. Such devices will have the advantage of higher gain without problems of feedback, and also of larger controls. They may thus be more appropriate for patients with handling difficulties and for those with a severe or profound hearing loss requiring high levels of amplification. Before considering fitting a particular aid for an ergonomic point of view, it is however, worth remembering that a number of existing bodyworn aids present considerable handling difficulties, particularly with respect to access to the battery compartment.

Bodyworn aids with bone conduction receivers may also be considered for those patients with recurrent otorrhoea. Those patients who have difficulty in fitting the earmoulds for the use of the receivers for bodyworn aids into their ears may be helped by the use of stetoclips as used by audio-typists (Stephens, 1981).

Some elderly patients may not be able to cope with the controls of a bodyworn aid with ergonomic modifications, and in such cases, particularly when the hearing loss is not severe, the possibility of an eartrumpet or speaking tube must be considered. Many elderly patients may happily accept such an approach. Berger (1974) and Grover (1977) have shown that such devices have a gain of some 20–30 dB. Indeed within the UK National Health Service some 300 non-electric aids are fitted every year (Stephens, 1979).

Patients who have difficulty in handling wearable electronic aids may also derive considerable benefit from other types of electronic amplification designed for specific purposes. Such devices may include an amplifier handset for the telephone or an additional amplifier linked to a stetoclip headset or headphones for picking up the output of the television or radio. Indeed, for the elderly person living alone, such an approach may be more relevant than the use of a personal hearing aid. Such devices should also be considered for those patients with hearing aids, who may require particular help in those circumstances. In a recent survey of patients seeking help for their hearing at the Royal National Throat, Nose and Ear Hospital, almost 50 per cent complained that one of their main problems was with hearing the radio and television (Barcham and Stephens, 1980).

Alerting or warning systems
Related to these aids offering amplification are those instruments providing alerting and warning signals for the hearing impaired. Such devices can include extra loud, or flashing lights, doorbells and telephone bells. Barcham and Stephens suggested that these would meet the need of some 25 per cent of the patients whom they investigated. Other devices include alarm clocks, which activate lights, fans or vibrators, although these are of less relevance to those who have retired. Even baby alarms, with a microphone placed over the baby's cot which leads to an amplifier activating a light circuit when the intensity of sound reaches a threshold level, may be useful for those elderly individuals who babysit for their children.

Other aids to communication
Other communication aids are relevant only to those individuals with a profound or complete hearing loss, and are often orientated towards those with a prelingual loss. They include teletype telephones, the pallantype device (Newall, 1978), and various sensory substitution aids. These last may be used to help with a complete acquired bilateral hearing loss and include vibrotactile devices, modified visual clues incorporated into special spectacles, and direct electrical stimulation of the cochlear nerve (e.g. Fourcin et al, 1979). Such patients are extremely few and probably constitute less than 0·1 per cent of the hearing impaired population.

Instruction
The final section here, instruction, applies to all of the devices fitted in this section and should cover the basic aspects of the devices used and include advice to the patient as to how to use them optimally in different circumstances. In the case of many patients this will require reinforcement in the 'communication training' section.

Strategy
This section deals with the development of an initial plan by which the patient and the audiologist together will develop an overall approach most likely to minimise

the patient's handicap. In organising this the audiologist must take into account and integrate all he knows about the patient, his impairment, attitude, lifestyle, personality and the like. It is particularly important to develop a stategy appropriate to the patient's individual needs.

The components of 'strategy' are shown in Figure 9.7 which considers the goals, philosophy and tactics. In the past some consideration has been given to 'hearing tactics' (e.g. Vognsen, 1976) but it is considered important here to deal with these in this wider context.

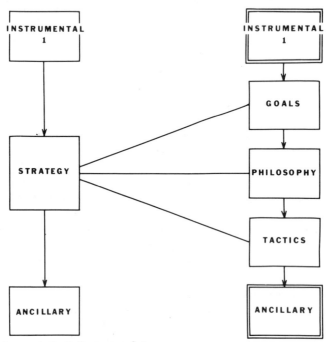

Fig. 9.7 Development of individual rehabilitative strategy

Goals

Only a limited number of goals can be achieved at any particular time, so initially it is important to determine with the patient what he regards as important goals which he is prevented from achieving because of his hearing loss. It is important to consider which of these might be achievable given appropriate rehabilitation and to discuss with and explain to the patient those which will never be possible. Thus, for example, the aim of the elderly musician may be to continue teaching music on a part-time basis, but if he suffers from a severe distortion in both ears, this will never be possible. On the other hand the elderly naturalist interested in bats may continue his interest and study of these animals by the modification of the output frequency transposition of a bat detector to the frequencies and level which he is able to hear.

Most elderly people, however, have more modest goals and generally the most difficult auditory situation aimed at may well be continued participation in committees and meetings within the individual's general field of interest and activity. Once such reasonable goals are selected a discussion must take place between the audiologist and patient as to how they might most effectively be achieved.

Philosophy

The approach to be followed will depend on the philosophy, personality and established lifestyle of the individual patient, which must be considered before any detailed consideration of tactics can be made. Thus although the importance of the hearing impaired person adopting an assertive approach towards his handicap has been emphasised elsewhere (Vognsen, 1976) this will be most inappropriate to an individual who throughout his life has been a shy person. In such an individual a very different approach will be necessary.

Tactics

Once this overall approach has been determined it is then important to discuss the basic tactics which must be followed by the individual in order to achieve his particular goals. At a committee meeting, for example, this will entail him sitting so that his better hearing ear is on the side of the most important participants, he should also able to clearly see the faces of such speakers who should be well illuminated, more over, he should encourage the speakers to face him and speak without their hands infront of their faces. Depending on the personality of the individual concerned and his assertiveness, some of these aims may be achieved by him stating his difficulties at the beginning of the meeting and explaining to the others how they can best help him. Alternatively, a shyer individual may speak to each other participant individually or even ask the Chairman of the meeting to do so for him.

Such approaches in all cases must specifically be geared to the goals selected and to the basic philosophy of the particular individual.

Ancillary

This section, summarised in Figure 9.8, is concerned with an assessment as to whether the audiologist requires the help of other professional workers in the global management of the patient. In the younger patient this will include educational and vocational assistance but these components are not generally pertinent to the elderly population. This leaves the two elements of social worker referral or medical referral. The exact form which these will take depends very much on the sociomedical system extant in the country concerned. Thus in certain countries (e.g. UK, Denmark) there may be specialist Social Workers for the Deaf and the Hearing Impaired, although even between these countries there are differences in their roles. For example, in the UK under the terms of the Chronically Sick and Disabled Persons Act (1970) it is the social worker who has the responsibility and facility for the provision of environmental aids.

Likewise, the role of the medical practitioner in the rehabilitative team varies from country to country and even within countries. In certain places there may be no medical involvement whatsoever within the rehabilitative process, or it may be restricted to perfunctory otoscopy. In others an Audiological Physician may play a major role and perform much or all of the rehabilitation himself.

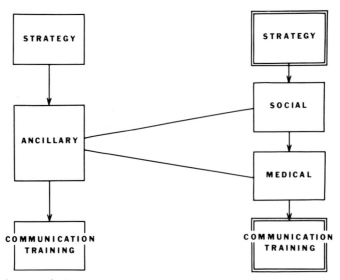

Fig. 9.8 Involvement of other agencies

The important point in all these different situations is that the Audiologist, whatever his background, who has assumed responsibility for the particular patient, should retain a central co-ordinating role, and it is vital that one person should have such an overview of the total rehabilitative process involved. He can organise certain aspects of the social service management himself by direct liaison with clubs for the elderly, but more concrete provisions, such as the organisation of home helps, environmental aids, and other support requires close links between the audiologist and the social worker. This is relatively easy in small discrete communities, but in larger cities may present more problems. Within the present authors' experience (e.g. Stephens et al, 1980) it is possible to establish a very close working relationship, which is essential to the wellbeing of the patient, between the audiology centre and social services departments, even within an inner city area.

The question of medical referral depends very much upon the structure of the audiological rehabilitation team. If an audiological physician or otologist forms an integral part of the team, he will generally be able to cope with such problems as otorrhoea or vertigo as they arise without further referral. Often, however, in the long term management of the elderly hearing impaired individual, evidence of more generalised systemic disease may present itself and will necessitate referral to the primary physician or to other specialists for its further investigation and treatment.

In other circumstances where there is no medical member of the rehabilitative team, referral of the patient back to his primary physician or otologist may additionally be necessary when otorrhoea, allergy, vertigo or other difficulties interfere with the audiological management of the patient. It is, however, important in both sets of circumstances that the audiologist responsible for the patient retains overall co-ordinative responsibility for the patient's audiological management and does not merely use the action of referral as a means of ridding himself of a troublesome patient.

Communication training

This stage, summarised in Figure 9.9, is far more complicated than the previous components of the rehabilitative process. It is the basis of the ongoing remediation and will often entail repeated sessions devoted to one or more of its components. A possible flow diagram to illustrate this repeated looping has been presented elsewhere (Goldstein and Stephens, 1981). It illustrates the fact that, at this stage, detailed, in depth attention can be given to whatever parts of the rehabilitative process are considered necessary to achieve optimal remediation. As a result of information obtained by the audiologist in this session, it can also lead to further evaluation.

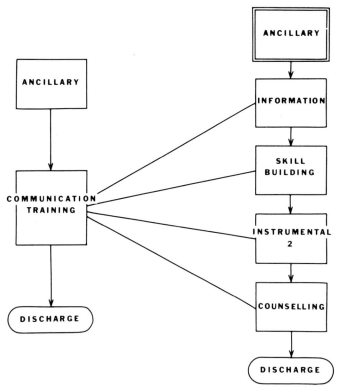

Fig. 9.9 Communication training in patients

Many, if not most, patients will require relatively little attention in this section, but even in those cases it is important that the audiologist asks himself whether he has achieved as much as he can reasonably hope to achieve in the way of helping his patients with all aspects of the remedial process. Communication training may take many different forms, on an individual or group basis, in regular weekly sessions, or an intensive residential basis, in the patient's home, or elsewhere. Generally speaking the degree of communication training needed will be related to the severity of the patient's handicap, and here it must again be emphasised that handicap is not synonymous with hearing loss.

From Figure 9.9 it will be seen that the communication training has been broken down into four components, Information, Skill building, Instrumental II and Counselling. The degree of need for each of these components will depend on the individual concerned and the programme must be tailored to meet these needs.

Information
The information component aims at giving the patient as much understanding as possible about the cause, nature and effects of his hearing loss as a means of helping him to come to terms with his sensory deficit. This can cover such diverse aspects as the mechanism of audition, some detailed discussion of the nature and site of hearing loss in the individual concerned, an explanation of the audiometric measures and a discussion of the remedial processes. Usually the choice of topic will be the result of questions posed by, or misconceptions held by, the patient. It is, however, important in every case that the patient be as aware as possible of the causes and severity of his loss, and of steps which he may take to avoid unnecessary further risk to his hearing. Again if a structured set of group sessions are planned different information topics may be considered in each session, along the lines of 'the mechanism of hearing', 'causes of hearing loss', 'audiometric procedures', 'aids to hearing' and so on.

Skill building
The skill building component covers all different aspects of skill development for difficult situations by the hearing impaired. It can cover the further development and discussion of hearing tactics necessary to achieve particular goals, listening skills with their new amplification and in particular the improvement of the patient's audiovisual communication skill.

For many readers this last may be the essential component of auditory rehabilitation and this view is reflected in the plethora of 'lipreading' classes organised in so many centres throughout the world. This concept of lipreading (speechreading) classes has been discussed elsewhere (e.g. Anon, 1980; McCormick, 1979). Essentially the evidence currently available would appear to suggest that speechreading tuition closely tied to the specific needs and abilities of an individual patient may be of value, but merely presenting repeated non-specific training to a group varying in ability, visual acuity, and vocabulary needs can be expected to achieve little in this respect. This is not to deny that such an approach can be of great benefit to the patient because of the group dynamics involved. Many of the better teachers of lipreading are aware of this and structure their classes accordingly. It is arguable that a more open and public acceptance of such an approach would be of great benefit to the hearing impaired population.

The question then arises as to what aspects should be taught within this skill building component. Certainly general aspects of speechreading tactics, a discussion of the ways by which lipreading can be facilitated, together with a discussion of the general processes involved will be of benefit to all patients. This will include aspects of lighting, articulation, speed of speech, the importance of contextual cues and the tactics for obtaining information from running speech. In patients with particularly severe handicaps and specific vocabulary needs, training to meet those needs may be given on an individual small group or video basis (e.g. Jacobs, 1979) although there will be little real call for this amongst the elderly. Consequently in the elderly population, the individual with a profound acquired hearing loss will merit individual training, the need for this being accentuated by the likely different learning speeds, visual acuity and vocabulary skills amongst the individuals concerned.

Overall, however, most of the elderly hearing impaired population will have a mild to moderate hearing loss and their needs will be largely for some basic information and encouragement together with guidance as to how they can meaningfully work to improve their own communication skills. The call for, and value of, sensory substitution aids in this population is likely to be minimal.

Instrumental II

Instrumental II is concerned more with the adjustment, modification and supplementation of instrumental aids rather than their basic selection and fitting. This will include further instruction to the patient as to their optimal use, the modification of frequency responses, as the patient adapts to the aid (Barfod, 1979), the introduction of binaural aids as the patient comes to better accept their potential benefit, and the consideration of further environmental aids.

Within this section it behoves the audiologist to ensure that the patient is capable of adequately handling his aid and of fitting the earmould into his ear. In practice this is one of the greatest problems for many elderly patients (e.g. Ward et al, 1979), but one which may be overcome by sufficient patience, practice and encouragement from the audiologist. He must, however, be prepared at some stage to consider alternative forms of amplification if it appears that the patient is not going to be able to cope with the approach initially selected. Here there may need to be a strong counselling component so that the patient will come to accept a modified bodyworn or hand-held approach, but this will have been facilitated by the experience of the patient becoming convinced that he cannot cope with the postaural approach first selected. At this stage, when the decision has been made in principle, there would be a looping back to the Instrumental I section for detailed aid selection.

Modifications to the aid which may be performed at this stage include further reduction of the low frequencies as the patient adjusts more to such an approach, the introduction of filters and modifications of the earmoulds. The question of a binaural fitting can be raised again at this stage if the reason for rejecting it earlier was patient opposition. Once the patient has experienced the asymmetrical listening situation of a monaural aid fitting to a binaurally symmetrical hearing loss he is more likely to accept the concept of a binaural approach. His attitude is also likely to be helped by his increasing acceptance of the idea of hearing aids in general, to which he might well have been opposed earlier for cosmetic reasons.

The other instrumental modifications which may be considered at this stage are in the field of environmental aids in the home. Once the patient has adjusted to his wearable aid or aids, it is easier to determine the further help he may need in the context of specific amplification, or alerting/warning devices. Thus for example, he may still have considerable difficulty in hearing the telephone bell and doorbell while he is in his living room watching television so that under these circumstances the fitting of extension bells can be reconsidered.

Counselling

The final component of communication training is that of counselling. Some reference has been made to aspects of this earlier and indeed this can be a wide field dealing with whatever the audiologist and/or patient may consider necessary. Much counselling can come from other patients in a group situation in which problems are discussed, and many individuals respond better to criticism and advice with regard to the hearing tactics which they adopt when such criticism comes from other hearing impaired individuals. Counselling forms an important part of all the sections of communication training and even the information providing section can have a valuable counselling role. Furthermore, this is a section in which any outstanding problems can be picked up and discussed either on an individual or group basis.

It must be emphasised that the structure of the communication training sessions should be regarded as flexible and potentially repetitive with all or some of the components being repeated as often as necessary on further occasions. Although each component may not be used on every occasion it is important that the audiologist should ask himself as to whether it is necessary. The breakdown into the four overlapping components is also valuable in the structuring of group sessions in order to maintain the patient's interest and ensure that there is sufficient of relevance for all the patients concerned. It is also important to consider at each session whether information derived there leads to a need for further repetition of earlier stages of the rehabilitative process on an individual basis.

Finally the audiologist must assess whether the patient is coping as well as he ever is likely to, given his sensory deficit. This entails the criterion for discharge from the active remedial process. There is considerable controversy as to how the completeness of rehabilitation may be assessed. However it is done, it must be emphasised to the patient that he should return for further advice and/or assessment should he encounter new problems with his hearing or his aids and his approaches to his hearing difficulties. It is arguable that patients should be further assessed at appropriate intervals (e.g. six months) after the initial rehabilitative process is deemed to be complete.

The final assessment may be performed by simply asking the patient how he is coping, how effectively he has resolved his difficulties, and how much he is using his hearing aid(s). Unfortunately there is an element of wanting to please the professional which occurs at this stage and the patient may give unrealitically optimistic reports (e.g. Stephens et al, 1980).

More quantitative approaches may be to present handicap scale measures such as the Hearing Handicap Scale (High et al, 1964) the Social Hearing Handicap Index (Ewertsen and Birk Nielsen, 1973) or the Hearing Measurement Scale (Noble and Atherley, 1970) at this stage. What is important to note here is the change in scores of such scales as compared with the values at the beginning of the rehabilitative process, rather than the absolute values obtained. Likewise, the 'Problems Questionnaire' (Barcham and Stephens, 1980) may be readministered.

Further approaches could be a repeat evaluation of the patient's audiovisual discrimination (McCormick, 1980) or his speech in noise discrimination, but there is little evidence as to the value of these measures in assessing the effectiveness of the rehabilitation. On a completely different front is the assessment as to whether the rehabilitative process has made the patient less dependent on the medical and social services provisions in general. One of the problems here, as Gilhome Herbst and Humphrey (1980) have shown, is that, for the elderly individual, hearing problems may be only one of several difficulties or handicaps which he may have. Even within this hierarchy of handicaps it may come fairly low down in the list as far as the patient is concerned. Hence, any changes which the audiologist may bring about in the individual's wellbeing and in the way of alleviating his dependence may be marginal as compared with what might be achieved in a younger individual whose sole complaint stems from his hearing difficulties.

The final assessment then in practise at the present time must be a joint clinical assessment by the audiologist in discussion with the patient as to whether he has achieved as much as he can reasonably have hope to achieve for the individual concerned.

ACKNOWLEDGEMENTS

The authors are grateful to Mr. D. Connolly and the staff of the Department of Clinical Photography of the Institute of Laryngology and Otology for the preparation of the figures.

REFERENCES

Anon 1980 Can lipreading be taught? Clinical Otolaryngology 4:3–4

Barcham L J, Stephens S D G 1980 The use of an open-ended problems questionnaire in auditory rehabilitation. British Journal of Audiology 14:49–54

Barfod J 1979 Speech perception processes and the fitting of hearing aids. Audiology 18:430–441

Bentzen O, Courtois J 1973 Statistical analysis of the problem for the deaf and hard of hearing in the world of 1970. Scandinavian Audiology 2:17–26

Bentzen O, Ewertson H W, Salomon G (eds.) 1976 Danish Audiology 1951–1976. Copenhagen, Nyt Norisk Forlag Arnold Busck

Bentzen O, Frost E, Skafrason S 1969 Treatment with binaural hearing aids in presbyacusis. International Audiology 8:529–533

Berger K W 1974 The hearing aid, 2nd edn. National Hearing Aid Society, Livonia

Broadbent D E 1972 Individual differences in annoyance by noise. Sound 6:56–61

Brooks D N 1972 The use and disuse of medresco hearing aids. Sound, 6:80–85

Brooks D N, Johnson D I 1981 Pre-issue assessment and counselling as a component of hearing-aid provision. British Journal of Audiology 15:13–19

Davis A 1980 Personal communication

Ewertsen H W, Birk Nielsen H 1973 Social hearing handicap index. Audiology 12:180–187

Fourcin A J, Rosen S M, Moore B C J, Douek E E, Clarke G P, Dodson M, Bannister L H 1979 External electrical stimulation of the cochlea. British Journal of Audiology 13:85–107

French St George M, Barr-Hamilton R 1978 Relief of the occluded ear sensation to improve earmould comfort. Journal of the American Auditory Society 4:30–35

Gilhome-Herbst K R, Humphrey C M 1980 Hearing impairment and mental state in the elderly living at home. British Medical Journal 2:903–905

Goldstein D P, Stephens S D G 1981 Audiological Rehabilitation: Management Model I. Audiology 20:432–452

Grover B C 1977 A note on acoustic hearing aids. British Journal of Audiology 11:75–76

Henoch M A (ed) 1979 Aural rehabilitation for the elderly. Grune and Stratton, New York

High W S, Fairbanks G, Glorig A 1964 Scale for self-assessment of hearing handicap. Journal of Speech and Hearing Disorders 19:215–230

Hinchcliffe R 1981 Clinical tests of auditory function in the adult and the school child. In: Beagley, H A (ed) Audiology and audiological medicine. Oxford University Press, Oxford pp 319–364

Humphrey C, Gilhome-Herbst K, Faruqi S 1981 Some characteristics of the hearing impaired who do not present themselves for rehabilitation. British Journal of Audiology 15:25–30

Jacobs M 1979 Speechreading instruction for the Ntid student. Report. National Technical Institute for the Deaf, Rochester, New York.

McCartney J H, Maurer J F, Sorensen F D 1976 A comparison of the hearing handicap scale and the hearing measurement scale with standard audiometric measures on a geriatric population. Journal of Auditory Research 16:51–58

McCormick B 1979 The skill of lipreading: a review. Hearing 34:126–130

McCormick B 1980 The assessment of audio-visual and visual speech discrimination skills in aural rehabilitation programmes. In: Taylor, I G, Markides A (eds) Disorders of Auditory Function III. Academic Press, London pp 307–320

Markides A 1977 Rehabilitation of people with acquired deafness in adulthood. British Journal of Audiology Suppplement 1

Newall A 1978 Palantype transcription units. Hearing 33:99–104

Noble W G, Atherley G R C 1970 The hearing measurement scale: A questionnaire for the assessment of auditory disability. Journal of Auditory Research 10:229–250

Stephens S D G 1977 Hearing aid use by adults: a survey of surveys. Clinical Otolaryngology 2:385–402

Stephens S D G 1979 La prothèse auditive dans le système socio-medical Britannique. Audition et Parole 1:116–121

Stephens S D G 1980 Evaluating the problems of the hearing impaired. Audiology 19:205–220

Stephens S D G 1981 Auditory rehabilitation. In: Beagley H A (ed) Audiology and audiological medicine, Oxford University Press, Oxford pp 516–540

Stephens S D G, Ballam H M 1974 The sono-ocular test. Journal of Laryngology and Otology 88:1049–1059

Stephens S D G, Barcham L J, Corcoran A L, Parsons N 1980 Evaluation of an auditory rehabilitation scheme. In: Taylor I G, Markides A (eds) Disorders of Auditory Function III. Academic Press. London pp 265–273

Vernon J 1977 Attempts to relieve tinnitus. Journal of the American Audiology Society 2:124–131

Vognsen S (ed) 1976 Hearing tactics. Oticon, Copenhagen

Ward P R, Gowers J I, Morgan D C 1979 Problems with handling the BE10 series hearing aids among elderly people. British Journal of Audiology 12:31–36

Balance

Epidemiology of balance disorders in the elderly

INTRODUCTION

Compared to the epidemiology of hearing and its disorders, the epidemiology of balance and its disorders is relatively unexplored. However, there are a number of scattered reports in the literature which are relevant to the epidemiology of balance disorders in the elderly. It will be the purpose of this chapter to refer to, and discuss, these reports. First it will be appropriate to mention the mechanisms and measurement of balancing function and changes in these measures with age. This will be followed by a discussion of the epidemiology of falls and ataxias. These can be equated with acute and chronic imbalance conditions respectively.

Although dizziness is, as Luxon points out in Chapter 16, a symptom spectrum encompassing a number of different symptoms, it is generally included in the ambit of imbalance disorders. This is justified on the basis that some of the disorders underlying the symptom of dizziness are disorders of the body systems providing postural stability. This applies particularly to the symptom of vertigo (a halluciation of movement, whether rotary or non-rotary, subjective or objective), which is indicative of a disorder of the vestibular labyrinth or its neurological connections. However, vertigo itself, together with some other specific dizzy symptoms, is a symptom of spatial disorientation. Thus, unlike falls, unsteadiness and staggering, vertigo is not a prime imbalance symptom, but it may be associated with these symptoms.

The discussion of the epidemiology of dizziness will be followed first by mention of the prevalence of nystagmus and the epidemiology of what might be termed the quasi-imbalances. These are symptoms which relate to restrictions of gait or movement that are not quite indicative of primary disorders of body balancing systems. For example, epidemiological data has been collected on limitations on movement outside the house in older people, as well as difficulties experienced in moving in the dark and difficulties experienced in negotiating stairs. It is appropriate to bear these deficiencies in mind when considering the overall pattern of balance disorders in the elderly.

MECHANISMS AND MEASUREMENT OF BALANCE

As Roberts (1978) points out, the neurophysiology of postural mechanisms is complex. Under the conditions of everyday living, vision, the vestibular labyrinth and joint mechanoreceptors all have a part to play, and in varying degrees of importance, in controlling posture and gait.

The support of the body in the standing position requires that each of the limbs should act as a fairly rigid pillar. When the foot is placed on the ground the distribution of forces in the interphalangeal joints is changed and the interosseus muscles are stretched by the splaying out of the foot. The appropriate stretch reflexes are facilitated so that the limb is converted into a stiff pillar ready to support whatever load is imposed on it (positive supporting reaction; Sherrington's antigravity mechanism).

In conjunction with information derived from other receptors, information from the vestibular labyrinth is used by the vertebrate nervous system in the formulation of the reflexes of balance. These include accelerating reflexes from the semicircular canals and positional reflexes from the otolith (saccule and utricle) organs. The reflexes of balance serve to stabilise the attitudes of the head and trunk, to stabilise the direction of gaze of the eyeballs when the head moves, and to adjust the attitudes of the limbs and neck to compensate for asymmetries in the disposition of support.

Joint mechanoreceptors, especially those in the cervical spinal apophyseal joints (De Jong, De Jong, Choen and Jongkees, 1977; Wyke, 1975) are particularly important in determining the stability of posture and of gait. Indeed Wyke (1979) has emphasised the importance of apophyseal joint disorders in the genesis of ataxia and disequilibrium in older people.

If the combination of stabilising and compensation fails to preserve balance, the rescue reactions are introduced at the point of overbalancing. These rescue operations themselves consist of a sequence of events; sway reactions, staggering (a series of small hops whereby the area of support is extended in the direction of impending fall) and the reaction of sweeping (use of a limb in a rapid movement to act as an inertia paddle). If these reactions fail, then fall-breaking reactions are invoked. For example, the arms may be flung out to protect the head.

Magnus (1924) first pointed out, and both Purdon Martin (1967) and Wyke (1979) have emphasised, that the importance of the vestibular mechanism in the control of posture and movement decreases with ascent of the evolutionary scale. Based upon clinical observations, Purdon Martin concluded that the vestibular mechanism plays no essential part in the maintenance of static posture in man. In animals, as Wilson and Melville Jones (1979) point out, even after bilateral section of the vestibulocochlear nerves, or complete bilateral extirpation of the vestibular labyrinths, an acceptable degree of behavioural recovery usually occurs provided that taxing movement environments are avoided. However, in a taxing environment, serious permanent behavioural defects become apparent. This is illustrated by the experiments of Igarashi, Watanabe and Maxian (1970) on the squirrel monkey. Trained monkeys readily scamper from one end to the other of a horizontal bar which is rotating about its longitudinal axis. After unilateral labyrinthectomy, there is a severe but temporary inability to do so; compensatory processes progressively restore skill to normal. However, after bilateral labyrinthectomy the ability is permanently lost.

Melvill Jones (1973) has suggested that the timing of pre-contact extensor activity during a downward step, hopping or running, might be partially dependent on vestibular cues, resulting from the vertical head movements occurring during these manoeuvres. Experiments on cats by Watt (1976) have indicated that a sacculospinal effect produced early activity in antigravity muscles to cushion the effects of landing from a fall. In man, Greenwood and Hopkins (1976a) demonstrated that electromyographic activity in response to an unexpected fall may show two peaks. The initial peak of activity, which is found in muscles throughout the body, occurs during the period 80 ms to 200 ms after release; it is considered to be a startle response. The peak could not be recorded in two subjects with absent vestibular function. The amplitude of the peak was later (Greenwood and Hopkins, 1976b) found to be proportional to the acceleration during falls; the authors consider that the effective stimulus was the rate of change of acceleration. A second peak, which is found only in lower limb muscles occurs before landing provided that the fall is from a sufficient height; its timing depends primarily upon knowledge of the height of a fall and not on ongoing visual information. The two subjects with absent vestibular function were unable to time this second peak of activity normally and landed heavily. This suggested that the otolith organs were involved in the timing of the co-ordinated pattern of electromyographic activity during downward motion that reached a peak before the moment of landing. However, during downward stepping, this effect occurred only with higher steps.

Purdon Martin has pointed out that man also becomes more dependent on his vestibular mechanism when the supporting base is unstable (including underwater). This function of the vestibular mechanism also encompasses walking over an uneven surface. Thus patients without vestibular function are particularly vulnerable to tilting; there are no other mechanisms during tilting that can compensate for loss of vestibular reflexes (Purdon Martin, 1965).

It is thus apparent that different disease processes can conceivably produce impairment of posture and movement control in a variety of ways, depending upon which receptors or reflexes are impaired. Thus there are considerably a number of ways in which postural stability could be measured. However, the quantitative measurement of postural stability has, in general, concentrated primarily on the measurement of either body sway (Vierordt, 1862; Tomlinson and Stevens, 1971) or the movement of the centre of foot pressure (Kelso and Hellebrandt, 1937; Terekhov, 1976). Although postural stability must always be essentially dynamic, some workers have endeavoured to distinguish between static and dynamic postural stability by using unstable platforms (Travis, 1945; Begbie, 1967; Shipley and Harley, 1971). Notwithstanding previous claims, the recent studies by Koles and Castelein (1980) showed that the relationship between body sway and the movement of the centre of foot pressure during upright stance, even in normal man, is not a simple one. These workers made simultaneous measurement of body sway and foot pressure variation. Optical detection units (planar sources of collimated light on one side of the subject and photo-detectors on the other side) were placed at the three levels: hips, shoulders, head, and the centre foot pressure was measured with a force platform. The single force considered (the centre of foot pressure) could not stabilise the three segments (ankle-hip; hip-shoulder; shoulder-head) stick model used for the human body. A second force, i.e. a horizontal force of reaction, is also required. The authors also suggested that a distinction should be made between steadiness and stance and stability and stance.

Measurement of the centre of foot pressure requires a moderate degree of sophisticated technology and the validity of the measure yet requires to be clarified. Consequently, measurement of body balance for epidemiological purposes has been essentially restricted to the measurement of body sway, where simple procedures are available.

Body sway

Sheldon (1963) has studied body sway as a function of age on a group with ages ranging from six years to 96 years. Sway was measured under two conditions. One was with the eyes closed and the other with the eyes open. In both conditions the subjects stood with the feet comfortably apart. Such a stance should minimise vestibular influences. The test with the eyes closed enables one to assess the influence of neurophysiological mechanisms other than vision and vestibular function.

The results of Sheldon's study are shown in Figures 10.1a and b. Vision clearly brings about a marked improvement in postural stability. With or without vision, postural stability shows an initial period of maturation before a progressive decline

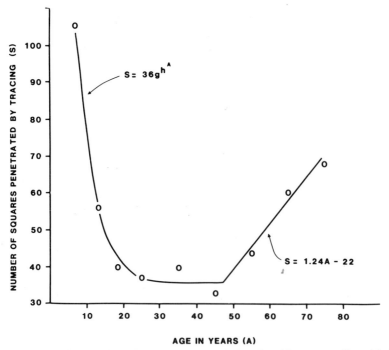

Fig. 10.1a Sway as a function of age. Body sway was tested when the subject was standing with the eyes closed and the feet comfortably apart. A triangular light aluminium frame fitted to the shoulders of the subject recorded sway by means of a vertical spring-loaded pencil recording on a horizontal sheet of graph paper. The graph paper was ruled at ten lines to the inch. Sway was measured as the number of squares penetrated by the tracing over a period of one minute. Data from a total of 268 subjects (116 males; 152 females) with ages ranging from 6 years to 97 years. The first part of the graph, where there is maturation of balance has been fitted to a Gompertz function; the second part has been fitted to a linear function. The values for the constants in the Gompertz function are 140 and 0·8253 for g and h respectively (after Sheldon, 1963).

sets in about the age of 45 years. The period of maturation may be complete before the age of 20 years and be followed by an intermediate stationary period before the deterioration develops (Fig. 10.1b).

The data plotted in Figure 10.1a has been fitted to two functions, i.e. an initial growth (Gompertz function) followed by a decline (linear function). The Gompertz function takes the form:

$$S = 36\ g^{h^A} \tag{1}$$

where   S = body sway measured by the number of
squares penetrated by the tracing
that registers shoulder sway

   g = a constant (140)

   h = a constant (0·8253)

and   A = age of subject in years

and the linear degeneration after the age of 45 years the form

$$S = 1·24A–22 \tag{2}$$

where   S = body sway measured as above

and   A = age of subject in years.

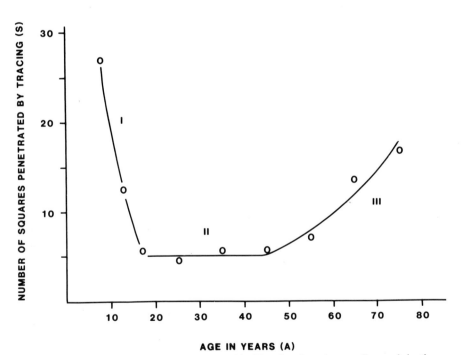

Fig. 10.1b As for Fig. 10.1a but with eyes open and looking directly at the recording made by the pencil. The curve is considered to have three parts, i.e. an initial (phase I) period of maturation, an intermediate (phase II) period during which sway is stable, and then a final (phase III) period of deterioration. The first and third parts of the curve have been fitted with exponential functions (after Sheldon, 1963).

In Figure 10.1b, the initial phase (I) of maturation has been fitted with an exponential function of the type

$$S = 100e^{-0.166A} \tag{3}$$

and the phase III of deterioration with an exponential function of the type

$$S = 0.847e^{0.0403A} \tag{4}$$

where S and A have the same meaning as in Eq. 1.

As Sheldon pointed out, the performance of the children was surprisingly bad. However, the tests were concerned with what is termed static posture. The children would have undoubtedly done better in tests involving movement.

The results shown in Figures 10.1a and b are not strictly comparable since, in presenting the data for the eyes open conditions, Sheldon deliberately excluded 36 subjects who were 'quite unable to control their stance in obedience to a visual signal'. Yet with the eyes closed, some of these subjects were able to achieve an essentially normal postural stability for their age. 29 of these 36 subjects were over the age of 60 years and 28 of the 36 were women. Sheldon considered that this accentuation of postural instability with the eyes open, and with visual feedback of the sway being provided, was not primarily due to defective vision. As Sheldon hypothesised, the phenomenon may be relevant to the genesis of falls in older people, especially in view of the sex incidence.

In a more recent study, Overstall, Exton-Smith, Imms and Johnson (1977) studied the body sway of 306 subjects, including 243 who were in the age range 60 years to 96 years. The latter group were also questioned about falls. Sway was measured with Wright's (1971) ataxiameter. This instrument expresses body sway as total angular movement, summed regardless of sign, but in the anteroposterior plane only. The justification for measurement in the anteroposterior plane only is not only because it is simpler but also because lateral sway is appreciably influenced by the position of the feet. The measuring instrument consists of a mast extending up from a box on the floor. A thread connects the mast with the subject's waist. The instrument can detect movements down to 300 μrad (about 1 minute of arc) and can communicate movements of up to 90 mrad (about 5 degrees of arc) to a double ratchet mechanism in the box which causes a pointer to rotate continuously over a dial graduated from 0 to 100. Full scale deflection corresponds to 580 mrad. Since the subjects stood with their feet comfortably apart and looked at a distant object, the results are broadly comparable to those shown in Figure 10.1b. Both sets of data show an exponential deterioration with age. However, Overstall separately analysed the results for the men and the women. The performance of the women is significantly poorer than that of the men.

The exponential functions fitted to Overstall's data are, for the men

$$S = 0.87e^{0.0166A} \tag{5}$$

for the women

$$S = 1.2e^{0.0153A} \tag{6}$$

where   S = body sway in nominal units

and   A = subject's age in years.

In both sexes, sway was significantly increased in subjects who fell because of loss of balance and in women whose falls were due to giddiness, drop attacks, turning their head and rising from bed or a chair.

There is considerable inter-individual variability in measured body sway. A number of factors other than vision, vestibular function and the integrity of the nervous system have been shown to influence sway. With the feet together, the hands hanging down by the sides and the eyes closed, 81 per cent of normals show a maximum sway (forwards or backwards) of less than 2·5 cm; the corresponding value for neurotics is 32 per cent. No normal swayed more than 5 cm, but 31 per cent of neurotics did (Eysenck, 1952). Ingham (1954) has sinced confirmed that neurotics tend to sway more than normals. There is some uncertainty as to whether or not, with suggestion, neurotics sway more than normals.

In considering various positions of the feet, Miles (1922) found that the most favourable position reduced sway by nearly two-thirds. Listening to music increases sway about as much as does closing the eyes (Husband, 1943; Edwards, 1947).

FALLS

Sheldon (1948) reported the results of questioning a random sample of elderly people living at home in Wolverhampton. Subjects were visited in their homes and an extensive questionnaire completed. One of the questions concerned a liability to falls (Table 10.1; Fig. 10.2). The data show that the liability to falls increases linearly with age but is much more marked in women than in men. The data for men have been fitted with an equation of the type

$$P = 1\cdot74\,(A-62) \tag{7}$$

and for women

$$P = 3\cdot24\,(A-59) \tag{8}$$

where   P = per cent prevalence of liability to falls

and   A = age in years.

The data thus infer that (a) liability to falls starts about the age of 60 years in both sexes, (b) the rate of growth for women is nearly twice that for men and (c) by the age of 90 years all women will give a history of liability to falls.

Table 10.1 Prevalence of 'liability to falls' as a function of age and sex in a sample of older people living at home in Wolverhampton, England (Sheldon, 1948).

Age group (yrs)	Prevalence of 'Liability to falls'	
	Men	Women
65–69	11%	27%
70–74	19	48
75–79	25	60
80–84	38	77
≥85	33	69

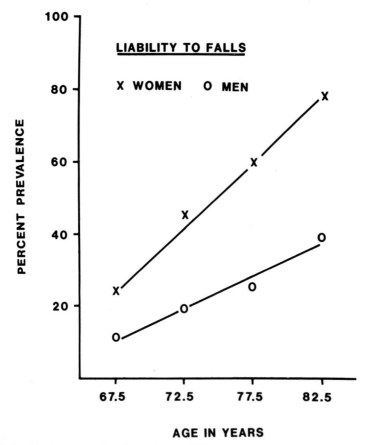

Fig. 10.2 Graphical representation of data given in Table 10.1.

The apparent drop in prevalence after 85 years of age may be partly due to the small numbers involved as well as to the fact that one is dealing with a survivor population. However, this drop in prevalence for men after 85 years of age is also seen in the data reported by Exton-Smith (1977). These data were obtained from a group of 963 people over the age of 65 years who participated in a nutrition survey. These London data confirmed the Wolverhampton finding that women show a greater liability to falls than men. However, the rates of growth of the liability to falls were different for the two populations. Liability to falls increased by about 1 per cent per annum for both sexes in Exton-Smith's population, compared with 1·74 per cent for men and 3·24 per cent for women in Sheldon's population. Moreover, extrapolation (admittedly always a dangerous procedure) would indicate that the liability to fall starts an appreciably earlier age in Exton-Smith's population. It is unlikely that the different criteria for determining 'liability to fall' account for these differences. Whether the differences point to geographic differences in the prevalence of falls is yet to be determined. However, the cause of falls is almost certainly multifactorial and there are indications that these causes differ in different populations. For example, Sheldon (1960) considered that tripping was responsible for only 11 per cent of the falls of his population

Table 10.2 Causes of 500 falls which happened to 202 individuals aged between 50 years and more than 85 years (Sheldon, 1960).

Accidental falls		34%
On stairs		13%
Missing last step	3%	
Poor illumination	3%	
Vertigo	2%	
Various	5%	
Slipping		10%
Falling over unexpected objects		3%
Dark		2%
Various		6%
Drop attacks		25%
Trips		11%
Vertigo		7%
CNS lesion		5%
Head back		4%
Postural hypotension		4%
Weakness in leg		3%
Falling out of bed or chair		2%
Uncertain		5%

(Table 10.2), but tripping was the single most important cause of falls in Exton-Smith's (1977) population. Exton-Smith also pointed out that the relative importance of causes of falls depended upon the age. For example, in women between the age of 65 years and 74 years, tripping accounted for 37 per cent of falls; in women of 75 years and over, it accounted for 22 per cent of falls. Giddiness was put as the cause in 6 per cent of women fallers in the age range 65 to 74 years; for women 75 years and over, the prevalence rose to 16 per cent (Table 10.3).

In 1960, Sheldon reported a study of 500 falls (involving 202 subjects). He said that 'it proved surprisingly easy to classify' the falls (Table 10.2). One-third of falls sustained by old people living at home were accidental. Stairs, in turn, accounted for one-third of accidental falls. Thus the small amount of time actually spent at risk is a measure of the great hazard that stairs afford to older people. Vertigo on the stairs accounted for 12 of the 63 falls. Some older people are apt to be giddy when looking down from the top of stairs, but vertigo seemed to be most dangerous when an individual was ascending. Sheldon attributed this to the danger of falling backwards with obvious risk of severe injury. However, only 9 per cent of all the falls were attributed to vertigo. As Sheldon pointed out, this is a surprisingly small proportion in view of popular belief ascribing all unexplained falls in old people to

Table 10.3 Major causes of falls in 190 women over the age of 65 years who were drawn from a random sample population (Exton-Smith, 1977).

	Age group	
	65–74 yrs	⩾75 yrs
Cause	(N = 77)	(N = 113)
Giddiness	6%	16%
Loss of balance	10%	9%
Drop attacks	14%	12%
Tripping	37%	22%

an attack of giddiness. The low proportion is attributed to the development of an attack of vertigo usually being slow enough to allow the subject to sit down or hold on to something.

In a quarter of individuals to whom Sheldon administered the Romberg test, there was a severe degree of Rombergism, 'the subjects being quite unable to remain erect with the eyes closed, even when standing on a wide base'. A fifth of the subjects showed a severe deterioration of gait. 'With an attitude of general flexion they walk with everted feet on a wide base while holding on at the same time to the furniture or walls for support. It is a truly senile gait for, of the 24 subjects concerned, 23 were over the age of 70 and 18 were over 80.'

Abnormal plantar responses without other evidence of corticospinal tract damage were four times as common in the fallers as in the general old age population.

Sheldon concluded from his study that the general insecurity of postural control and the liability to fall which are characteristic of old age are based ultimately on a decline in the number of nerve cells in the brain stem, cerebellum and other centres. The adverse effects of this cellular poverty will inevitably be accentuated by interference with the blood supply to the region which, in two ways, is particularly apt to happen in old age. First, there is the liability of the vertebral arteries to temporary obstruction; secondly there is a general proneness to episodes of hypotension which are attributable to postural and other causes. It is to be noted that postural hypotension occurs in from 11 per cent (Rodstein and Zeman, 1957) to 24 per cent (Caird, Andrews and Kennedy, 1973) of elderly populations. However, following a study of 125 people aged 65 and over (from a survey of six general practices) who had fallen in their homes, Deidre Wild and her colleagues (1981) concluded that there was little evidence to support statements that falls in old age are often caused by vertebrobasilar ischaemia and cervical spondylosis. They consider it much more common for falls to result from errors in environmental perception, slowing of responses and weakness of support. The appreciably greater mortality of the fallers is depicted in Figure 14.2 on page 384. One quarter of these patients died within one year of the fall; this was five times as much as in an age- and sex-matched control group. Of those who lay on the floor after the fall for more than an hour (20 patients) half died within six months of the fall.

ATAXIAS

An oto-neuro-ophthalmological syndrome (or syndromes) exists in varying degrees of prevalence and severity in many parts of the tropics (Cruickshank, 1956; Money, 1959; Haddock, Ebrahim and Kapur, 1962). In its fullest expression this syndrome comprises a neuromyelopathy in association with a retrobulbar neuropathy and a sensorineural hearing loss.

An epidemiological study, encompassing the direct examination of a random sample of a suburban Jamaican community aged between 35 years and 74 years, indicated that Jamaican neuropathy (or neuropathies) was the most prevalent neurological disorder in that population (Ashcroft et al, 1967). The syndrome occurred in about 5 per cent of women and 4 per cent of men in the age group studied, with a trend towards higher prevalences in older subjects. The syndrome is three and a half times as common as cerebrovascular accident, which was the second most common neurological disorder found in that population.

A variety of audiometric patterns are found to be associated with the syndrome (Hinchcliffe, Osontokun and Adeuja 1972) but frequently an audiogram is characterised with peaks or islands of better hearing superimposed upon the overall hearing loss (Osuntokun, 1968; Hinchcliffe, 1972).

There is evidence that this syndrome comprises at least two disorders. In Jamaica, for example, it is possible to distinguish an ataxic neuropathy and a spastic neuropathy. The ataxic type is more particularly associated with auditory and vestibular defects; sensorineural hearing loss occurs in about 80 per cent of ataxic cases and in about 7 per cent of spastic cases; retrobulbar neuropathy in 72 per cent of ataxic cases and 15 per cent of spastic cases (Montgomery, Cruickshank, Robertson and McMenemy, 1964). Moreover, the spastic type has clinical features indicating a syphilitic aetiology (Rodgers, 1965). Furthermore, histopathologically this type exhibits the picture of a chronic meningomyelitis (Montgomery et al, 1964). Epidemiological and other studies in Jamaica have failed to elucidate the aetiology of the ataxic type of neuropathy.

Osuntokun (1968) has extensively investigated the ataxic neuropathy, colloquially termed *raserase* or *lagero*, which is endemic in southwest Nigeria, particularly Ijebu Province. The age of onset of the condition may range from eight years to 60 years. This Nigerian ataxic neuropathy is characterised by bilateral optic atrophy, bilateral sensorineural hearing loss and a predominantly posterior column myelopathy and polyneuropathy. Osuntokun describes the gait as follows: the typical gait is ataxic and wide based. If foot drop is present, it becomes high steppage with the patient's eyes fixed to the ground, as in tabetic gait. More than two thirds of the patient with ataxic gait volunteered that the gait was worse at night; half said that they fell frequently in the dark. The gait varies in severity; in severe cases patients may resort to walking sticks. Osuntokun reported that all his patients gave a history of poor diet in which the staple food, cassava (*Manioc utilissima*) was eaten in one form or another (*gari, eba, puru puru*) at least twice a day. Cassava contains a cyanogenetic glycoside, linamarin. Osuntokun, Monekosso and Wilson (1969) studied two Nigerian villages, Akinmorin and Ososa, in which there were different consumptions of cassava. Akinmorin has a relatively low consumption of cassava; Ososa has a relatively high consumption. Differences in the prevalences of certain balance descriptors are shown in Table 10.4. Plasma thiocyanate concentration were greater in the Ososa villagers and even

Table 10.4 Frequency of balancing dysfunctions in two villages (Akinmorin and Ososa) in Southwestern Nigeria. Cassava consumption is higher in Ososa. The mean plasma thiocyanate concentrations are also greater in the Ososa villagers who also show a higher prevalence of a degenerative neuropathy (Nigerian ataxic neuropathy). Cassava contains a cyanogenetic glycoside, linamarin (Osuntokun, Monekosso and Wilson, 1969).

Balance descriptor	Frequency	
	Ososa	Akinmorin
Ataxic gait	3·8%	0·7%
Inability to walk heel-to-toe	10·3%	0·7
Romberg	0·9	0·7

greater in those with the neurological disorder. Subsequently, Osuntokun, Ala-detoyinbo and Adeuja (1970) showed that increased blood free cyanide concentrations were characteristic of this ataxic neuropathy.

It is to be concluded that the inhabitants, particularly Africans, and including older people, in many parts of the tropics may be afflicted with a nutritional ataxic neuropathy which is due to chronic cyanide poisoning.

DIZZINESS

Epidemiological studies of dizziness in the elderly have been made principally by Sheldon (1948) and by Droller and Pemberton (1953) in England, by Orma and Koskenoja (1957ab) in Finland, and by Tanja, Hofman and Valkenburg (1979) in the Netherlands.

As mentioned previously, Sheldon studied a random sample of older people living at home in Wolverhampton, England. A questionnaire was administered to people in their homes. Sheldon's team was able to interview 477 people (143 men; 334 women) out of a random sample of 585, i.e. an 82 per cent yield. This was done during the period May 1945 to January 1947. Droller and Pemberton were able to interview and medically examine 476 (71 per cent) out of a random sample of 672 older people living at home in Sheffield, England. There were 192 men aged 67 years or over and 284 women aged 62 years or over. Examination included measurement of the blood pressure and a chest X-ray.

The sampling procedures used by Orma and Koskenoja in Finland were somewhat complex. One group of older dizzy subjects were solicited through a newspaper advertisement in Helsinki. One hundred and twelve people (36 men; 76 women) responded to this advertisement. All these subjects underwent a general medical examination, as well as special examinations in neurology, ophthamology and otolaryngology. Chest X-rays and a number of laboratory tests were also done. Orma and Koskenoja also sent out a questionnaire about dizziness and related matters to a random sample of 1085 individuals who had attended their out-patient department for older people in the previous two years. Of the questionnaires which were returned, 811 were considered to be suitable for analysis. In this group there were only 121 patients who reported no dizziness. Of these, it was possible to examine what they termed their 'control group', i.e. a group of older people (18 men; 44 women) with no history of dizziness.

Tanja and his colleagues studied 750 subjects who were obtained from the population of people over the age 65 years (1285) who were living in one of three communities (Dorp, Palenstein, Zoetermeer) not far from the Hague. The study was conducted during the period April 1975 to June 1978. Each subject was interviewed and given a general medical examination. The cervical spine was X-rayed and the serum creatinine concentration (used as an indicant of renal function) determined.

An indication of the sensations that are subsumed under the term dizziness is provided by Orma and Koskenoja (1957a) (Table 10.5). These data are based upon the group who responded to the advertisement. It will be noted that the sum of more specific symptoms exceeds 100 per cent. This is because many individuals had more than one symptom which they included under the term 'dizziness'.

Table 10.5 Sensations subsumed under the term 'dizziness' amongst elderly people living in Helsinki (Orma and Koskenoja, 1957a).

Descriptor	Frequency
Sensation subsumed under the term 'dizziness'	
Momentary equilibrium disturbance	46%
Blackout or spots before the eyes	41
Turning sensation	35
Staggering or loss of balance	19
Feeling of falling	14
Heaviness or confusion in the head	7
Fainting	7
Buzzing in the ears	1

Table 10.6 Prevalence of dizziness (currently present) as a function of age and sex. Based upon a random sample of an elderly population in the Netherlands (Tanja, Hofman and Valkenburg, 1979).

	Prevalence of dizziness as a current complaint	
Age group (yrs)	Men	Women
65–69	8·9%	20·7%
70–74	13·4	21·4
75–79	24·1	24·3
≥80	16·0	23·9

Table 10.7 Prevalence of vertigo as a function of age and sex. Based upon a sample of older people living at home in Wolverhampton, England. The apparent decline in prevalence for older men is not significant since the two oldest groups comprise 13 men only (Sheldon, 1948).

	Prevalence of vertigo	
Age group (yrs)	Men	Women
65–69	28%	49%
70–74	33	65
75–79	62	62
80–84	33	63
≥85	25	70

The prevalence of dizziness in the elderly is indicated by Tanja's study. Table 10.6 shows that the prevalence is higher in women than in men, the relative prevalence being dependent on the age; the prevalence ratio is least marked for the 75 to 79 years age group. The absence of a sex difference for this age group is associated with the peak prevalence for this age group in men. One might wonder whether the peak really exists. However, the data on the prevalence of 'vertigo' which were presented by Sheldon and by Droller and Pemberton also shows this pattern (Tables 10.7 and 10.8) (see also Fig. 10.3). Surprisingly, the demonstrated prevalence of vertigo, which is only one component in the broad symptom-spectrum of dizziness, is greater than that for dizziness. A possible explanation is

Table 10.8 Prevalence of vertigo ('rarely', 'often' or 'continuous') as a function of age and sex. Based upon a sample of older people living at home in Sheffield, England (Droller and Pemberton, 1953).

	Prevalence of vertigo	
Age group (yrs)	Men	Women
65–69	34%	58%
70–74	47	67
75–79	63	64
≥80	43	62

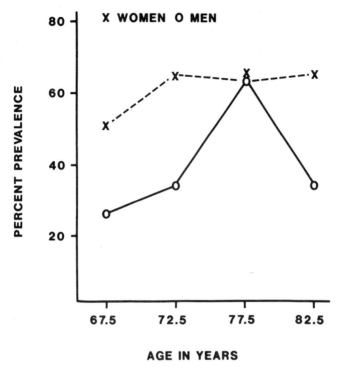

Fig. 10.3 Graphical representation of data shown in Table 10.7.

Table 10.9 Prevalence of a history of vertigo as a function of age; based upon a random sample of a rural population in Southwest Scotland (Hinchcliffe, 1961).

Age group (yrs)	Prevalence of a history of vertigo
18–24	17%
25–34	20
35–44	19
44–54	23
55–64	35
65–74	29

Table 10.10 Prevalence of people who 'often' have vertigo; as a function of age and sex. Based upon a sample of older people living at home in Sheffield, England (Droller and Pemberton, 1953).

Age group (yrs)	Prevalence of people who 'often' have vertigo	
	Men	Women
65–69	3%	23%
70–74	11	30
75–79	15	30
≥80	19	37

that the prevalence of vertigo is subject to geographic variation. Nevertheless, Tables 10.6 to 10.8 inclusive indicate the relatively high prevalence of dizziness and vertigo in the elderly.

The prevalence of vertigo determined on a random sample of a rural population in Scotland (Hinchcliffe, 1961) showed values for older subjects (Table 10.9) that were compatible with those obtained by Sheldon and by Droller and Pemberton. It is therefore probable that the values obtained from these three studies apply to Britain as a whole. The principal criticism which can be applied to these measures of vertigo is that they encompass vertigo of all degrees of severity; they could also include subjects who were no longer troubled with the symptom. However, Droller and Pemberton provided data on the prevalence of older people who 'often

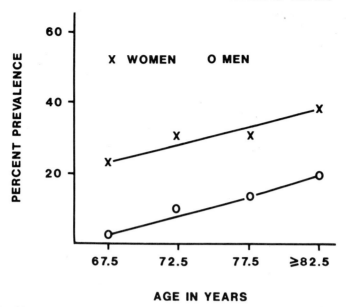

Fig. 10.4 Graphical representation of data shown in Table 10.10.

have vertigo' (Table 10.10; Fig. 10.4). The data indicate, for both sexes, a linear increase with age according to the expressions.

$$\text{for men} \quad P = (A - 63) \tag{9}$$

$$\text{and for women} \quad P = 0.84\,(A - 39) \tag{10}$$

where P = per cent prevalence of people who 'often have vertigo'
and A = age in years.

It will be noted that there is no peak for the 75 to 79 years old males in this data. The sex ratio is even more pronounced, falling from 7·7 for the 65 to 69 years group to about 2·0 for people greater than 75 years of age.

Perhaps greater interest has been shown in the correlative studies and the attempts to assign causes for the dizziness and vertigo in these various groups.

Table 10.11 shows the attributed cause of the symptom in Orma and Koskenoja's group of elderly subjects with episodic, non-postural dizziness. It will be noted that aural causes are in the minority. The pattern of 'postural dizziness' is indicated in Table 10.12 and the results of a correlation study for this symptom are shown in Table 10.13. It will be noted that postural dizziness in the elderly is particularly associated with, first, neurological disorders, especially cerebro-vascular disease, and, secondly, cardiac failure, but not with hypertension. Droller and Pemberton concluded from their studies that arteriosclerosis was the principal cause of vertigo in the elderly. The absence of any association between vertigo and hypertension was demonstrated by Droller, Pemberton, Rosen and Grout (1952) (Table 10.14). One might suppose that Orma and Koskenoja's failure to demonstrate any association between retinal arteriosclerosis and postural dizziness was due to this ophthalmoscopic sign being a poor index of arteriosclerosis involving the labyrinth and the vestibular pathways.

le 10.11 Classification of episodic, non-postural
ness in a group of 45 people over 64 years of age who
recruited by newspaper advertising in Helsinki.
ᴐatient with Ménière's disease also had a 'neurologic
ᴈ' (Orma and Koskenoja, 1957b).

Probable cause	Frequency
Neurological	49%
Ménière's disease	11
Post-infectious	11
Associated with angina pectoris	7
Chronic otitis media complicated by labyrinthitis	4
Cardiac arrhythmia	4
Toxic	4
Labyrinthine vascular accident	2
Post-traumatic	2
Tussive syncope	2
Agoraphobia	1

Table 10.12 Symptomatology of postural dizziness in 103 people over 64 years of age who were recruited by newspaper advertising in Helsinki (Orma and Koskenoja, 1957a).

Descriptor	Frequency
Movements producing 'postural dizziness'	
All sudden movements of head or body	63%
Walking	56
Rising from bed or sitting position	50
Lying down	20
Looking up	13
Bending forward	12
Definite position in bed	11
Looking down	9
Turning onto one side in bed	9
Other precipitating factors	
Physical exertion	26%
Associated with angina pectoris	8
Duration of episodes	
'A moment or a few seconds'	56%
'a few seconds to one minute'	23
'one to five minutes'	9
'more than five minutes'	12

Failure of Koskenoja and Orma to demonstrate a significant correlation of postural dizziness with aural disease might be partially attributed to the term 'dizziness' in their subjects encompassing symptoms other than vertigo.

Tanja and his colleagues were the first to introduce a psychosomatic measure into epidemiological surveys of dizziness. As Table 10.15 shows, a complaint of dizziness was highly correlated with the presence of psychosomatic symptoms. In addition, neck pain was the anamnestic variable showing the highest correlation with a complaint of dizziness. The occurrence of dizziness, however, showed no correlation with objective clinical evidence for cervical spine disorders. Radiological studies of the cervical spine showed that the occurrence of dizziness was significantly correlated ($p < 0.05$) with cervical osteoarthritis but not with simple

Table 10.13 Vertigo and blood pressure in the elderly. Data obtained from 457 men and women who were drawn from a random sample of elderly people living at home in Sheffield, England (after Droller, Pemberton, Roseman and Grout, 1952).

Blood pressure	Vertigo		
	none	occasional	frequent or continuous
MEN			
Number	87	74	25
Mean systolic BP	22·2	22·5	22·1 kPa
Mean diastolic BP	12·1	12·3	12·3 kPa
WOMEN			
Number	103	87	81
Mean systolic BP	23·7	23·7	24·3 kPa
Mean diastolic BP	13·2	13·2	13·2 kPa

Table 10.14 Correlation of a present complaint of dizziness with a history of psychosomatic symptoms and various disorders. Based upon a random sample of an elderly population in the Netherlands. n.s. = not significant (after Tanja, Hofman and Valkenburg, 1979).

Anamnestic variable	Significance of correlation with present complaint of dizziness
Neck pain	$p < 0.0001$
Psychosomatic symptoms	< 0.001
'weak heart'	< 0.001
Heart infarct	< 0.01
Epilepsy	< 0.01
Diabetes	< 0.05
'bleeding from the brain'	n.s.

intervertebral disc degeneration. Kuilman (1959) had previously demonstrated a correlation between the occurrence of vertigo and radiological changes in the cervical spine.

Beek and van Zonneveld (1977) appears to have conducted the only longitudinal study of dizziness in the elderly. In a study in the Netherlands, these authors found that a complaint of dizziness was correlated with a lower life expectancy. Moreover, these authors were of the opinion that the symptom was primarily due to cerebro-vascular processes and not to aural disease.

NYSTAGMUS

Koskenoja and Orma (1956) have reported the results of testing for spontaneous and positional nystagmus in their 103 postural dizziness patients and 62 non-dizzy patients who were the subject of the epidemiological study discussed in the preceding section. All the subjects were more than 64 years of age. Nystagmus was examined on the ordinary examining table in the following positions: sitting upright, leaning to the left and to the right, bending forwards, in the supine position, in the lateral position, lying on the left side and on the right side, lying on the back with the head hanging and after quickly rising from the supine position.

Table 10.15 Correlation of 'postural dizziness' with other symptoms and signs. The *relative frequency ratio* refers to the ratio of the frequency of a particular symptom or sign in the postural dizziness group to that in a similar group of elderly patients who did not have any dizziness. A 'neurologic attack' means an attack with neurological symptoms; unconsciousness was also considered as a neurological symptom if no other cause for it could be determined. An asterisk denotes that the required information to determine the ratio was not reported. The relative frequency ratios are expressed to the nearest integer. The third column gives the level of significance where a particular symptom or sign is correlated with postural dizziness; n.s. indicates that there was no significant association (after Orma and Koskenoja, 1957a).

Other symptoms or signs	Relative frequency ratio	Significance of correlation with postural dizziness
Neuro		
'Neurologic attack'	∞	$p < 0.001$
Focal cerebral signs	8	$p < 0.001$
Mental symptoms	5	$p < 0.001$
Diffuse cerebral signs	4	$p < 0.001$
Headache	3	$p < 0.001$
CVS		
'Pulmonary stasis'	2	$p < 0.005$
Cardiac enlargement	1	n.s.
Elevated blood pressure	1	n.s.
Retinal arteriosclerosis	1	n.s.
ENT		
Cerumen	1	n.s.
Chronic middle ear disease	1	n.s.
Hearing loss	⋆	n.s.
Tinnitus	2	$p < 0.001$
Caloric test response	⋆	n.s.
Maxillary sinusitis	1	n.s.
Other		
Elevated blood sugar	7	$p < 0.02$

The change from one position to another happened 'fairly rapidly'. The patient's eyes were viewed with the naked eye. Neck torsion was avoided as far as possible.

In the postural dizziness group, a first degree spontaneous nystagmus was observed in five patients. In 26 other patients, nystagmus was observed in one or more position other than the upright sitting position. Five of these patients had a direction-changing nystagmus. In all positional nystagmus cases, the nystagmus appeared as soon as the head reached the critical position. Only in three patients was the appearance of nystagmus associated with a concomitant sensation of dizziness. However, in 13 patients, the position and movements which provoked positional nystagmus corresponded to the position and movements in which the postural dizziness usually appeared.

In the control group, neither a spontaneous nystagmus nor a direction-changing positional nystagmus were observed. However, eight subjects exhibited a positional nystagmus other than a direction-changing type. As with the postural dizziness group, the nystagmus appeared as soon as the head reached the critical position. None of this group experienced a sensation of dizziness concomitant with the appearance of the nystagmus.

Koskenoja and Orma compared the group of patients with nystagmus to the group without nystagmus. Focal cerebral signs compatible with cerebral arteriosclerosis were found in 10 of the 39 subjects with nystagmus, and in 14 of the 126 subjects without nystagmus. Focal or diffuse cerebral signs were found in 22 subjects in the nystagmus group and in 41 subjects in the non-nystagmus group (significant at $p < 0.01$).

There was no difference between the nystagmus and the non-nystagmus groups in respect of ear disease, hearing acuity or caloric test responses.

QUASI-IMBALANCES

Limitation for movement out of doors

Part of Sheldon's questionnaire related to capacity for movement. It was noted whether the subject was bedfast, limited to the house, limited in outside movements or with unlimited capacity for movement. The data indicated that about 3 per cent of elderly men and 2 per cent of elderly women are bedfast, and that 7 per cent of elderly men and 9 per cent of elderly women are restricted to their homes. As Table 10.16 indicates, the prevalence of limited capacity for movement appears to increase exponentially with age. The data have been fitted to a curve of the type

$$\text{for men} \quad P = 0.16e^{0.0678A} \tag{11}$$

$$\text{and for women} \quad P = 0.24e^{0.0678A} \tag{12}$$

where P = per cent prevalence of people who have limited capacity for movement

and A = age in years.

The conditions which Sheldon considered to be responsible for limitation of outside movement are listed in Table 10.17. Vertigo was sixth down in the list as a cause for limiting movement and neurological disease (presumably including ataxia) was near the bottom of the list. However, since this list was constructed from the questionnaire, it is highly likely that a medical examination would have shown that balance disorders are more important than the list indicates. There is no doubt that the symptom 'weakness' would cover a whole spectrum of neurological and medical disorders.

Table 10.16 Prevalence of individuals with a limited capacity for movement, as a function of age and sex, in a random sample of older people living at home in Wolverhampton, England (Sheldon, 1948).

Age group (year)	Prevalence of limited capacity for movement	
	Men	Women
65–69	26%	24%
70–74	23	31
75–79	31	57
80–84	33	50
≥85	67	91

Table 10.17 Conditions responsible for limited capacity of movement in elderly people living at home in a random sample of the population in Wolverhampton, England (Sheldon, 1948).

Condition		Cases
Weakness	..	32
Dyspnoea	..	30
Arthritis	..	20
Fear of traffic	..	17
Pain in feet	..	13
Vertigo	..	8
Effects of accident or operation	..	7
Lack of desire	..	6
Defective vision	..	6
Angina of effort	..	5
Spinal deformity	..	5
Oedema of legs	..	3
Previous stroke	..	3
Varicose veins	..	3
Sensitivity to cold	..	2
Neurological disease	..	2
Effects of fall	..	2

Difficulty in the dark

It would appear that about half of older people find difficulty when in the dark. The prevalence of the condition increases with age (Table 10.18) and women are more affected than men. The prevalence of this difficulty can be expressed in men as

$$P = 2 \cdot 36 \, (A - 59) \tag{13}$$

and for women $\quad P = 2 \cdot 82 \, (A - 55)$ (14)

where $\quad P =$ per cent prevalence of people who have difficulty in the dark

and $\quad A =$ age in years.

There are a number of reasons for this difficulty. A degenerative night blindness may have been responsible for about 8 per cent of cases; 4 per cent were afraid of the dark for psychological reasons; in 6 per cent of cases it was because the subject had lost all sense of direction. However, Sheldon considered that the primary cause

Table 10.18 Prevalence of 'difficulty in the dark' as a function of age and sex in a sample of older people living at home in Wolverhampton, England (Sheldon, 1948).

Age group (years)	Prevalence of difficulty in the dark	
	Men	Women
65–69	20%	36%
70–74	31	50
75–79	52	63
80–84	43	83
≥85	67	90

Table 10.19 Prevalence of individuals finding 'difficulty with the stairs' as a function of age and sex in a random sample of older people living at home in Wolverhampton, England (Sheldon, 1948).

Age group (years)	Prevalence of 'difficulty with stairs'	
	Men	Women
65–69	19%	40%
70–74	25	48
75–79	29	54
80–84	58	40
≥85	40	67

Table 10.20 Conditions causing difficulty in ascent of stairs in elderly people living at home in Wolverhampton, England (Sheldon, 1948).

Condition	Cases
Dyspnoea	15
Intermittent claudication	3
Weakness	3
Angina of effort	2
Arthritis	2
Painful feet	2
Effects of stroke	1
Obesity	1
Sciatica	1

was failure of the mechanisms subserving posture and orientation, as a result of 'ageing' processes.

Difficulty with stairs

Table 10.19 shows the prevalence of 'difficulty with stairs'. Again women are more affected than men and a linear increase in prevalence is suggested. The expression describing this trend for men could be

$$P = 1 \cdot 03 \, (A - 49) \tag{15}$$

and for women $\quad P = 1 \cdot 33 \, (A - 37)$ $\hfill$ (16)

where $\quad$ P = per cent prevalence of people who have difficulty with stairs

and $\quad$ A = age in years.

As Tables 10.20 to 10.22 show, a different pattern of causes is responsible for difficulty ascending stairs, descending stairs, or both ways. Vertigo is the commonest cause of difficulty descending stairs, the fourth commonest cause in cases where there is difficulty both ascending and descending, but of no importance where the difficulty concerns ascent only.

Table 10.21 Conditions causing difficulty in descent of stairs in elderly people living at home in Wolverhampton, England (Sheldon, 1948).

Condition	Cases
Arthritis or spondylitis	12
Lack of confidence	5
Vertigo	4
Stiff leg	3
Difficulty in feet	2
Old stroke	1

Table 10.22 Conditions causing difficulty with stairs both coming up and down in elderly people living at home in Wolverhampton, England (Sheldon, 1948).

Condition	Cases
Arthritis or spondylitis	25
Weakness	8
Dyspnoea	8
Vertigo	7
Rheumatism	7
Feet	6
Stroke	4
Obesity	2
Oedema (varicose veins)	2
Nervousness	2
Fear of heights	1
Defective sight	1
Amputation (leg)	1

Sheldon found that 6 per cent of old people have to have their bedroom downstairs because it was impossible for them to manage stairs at all. Vertigo appeared to be the cause of about 10 per cent of this group of cases.

CONCLUSIONS

Epidemiological data available to date, although still somewhat patchy, indicate that balance disorders, including dizziness, are important causes of impaired well being in older people. These conditions show an increase in prevalence with increasing age. This increase in prevalence applies particularly to the liability to falls. Indeed, extrapolation of available data would indicate that 100 per cent of women will be liable to falls by the age of 90 years.

People subject to falls or dizziness would appear to have a shorter life expectancy.

It would seem that degenerative arterial disease and degenerative changes in the central nervous system are the principal pathological processes underlying balance disorders in the elderly.

The experience accrued from previous epidemiological studies will be useful in planning further epidemiological studies which are clearly required. Future studies should include not only the use of appropriate questionnaires but also the direct examination of random samples of appropriate populations. General medical, including cardio-vascular (particularly measures of degenerative arterial disease) and neurological examination will be required, as well as psychological and sociological measures to determine the pattern of interaction of these factors and their magnitude. It will also be necessary to solve some of the semantic problems which clearly arise in the use of this and similar terms in even a single, let alone several, linguistic groups.

REFERENCES

Ashcroft M T, Cruickshank E K, Hinchcliffe R, Jones W I, Miall W E, Wallace J 1967 A neurological, ophthalmological and audiological survey of a suburban Jamaican community. West Indian Medical Journal 16:222–245

Beek A, Zonneveld, R J van 1977 De gezondheid in de voortschrijdende ouderdom. Gezondheidsorganisatie TNO

Begbie, G H 1967 Some problems of postural sway. In: de Reuck AVS, Knight J (eds) Myotatic, Kinesthetic and Vestibular Mechanisms. Ciba Foundation Symposium. Churchill, London, p 80

Caird F I, Andrews G R, Kennedy R D 1973 Effect of posture on blood pressure in the elderly. British Heart Journal 35:527–530

Cruickshank E K 1956 A neuropathic syndrome of uncertain origin. Review of 100 cases. West Indian Medical Journal 5:147–158

De Jong P T V M, De Jong J M B V, Cohen B, Jongkees L B W 1977 Ataxia and nystagmus induced by injection of local anaesthetics in the neck. Annals of Neurology 1:240–246

Droller H, Pemberton J 1953 Vertigo in a random sample of elderly people living in their homes. Journal of Laryngology and Otology 67:689–694

Droller H, Pemberton J, Roseman C, Grout J L A 1952 High blood-pressure in the elderly. British Medical Journal 2:968–970

Edwards A S 1947 Body sway and non-visual factors. Journal of Psychology 23:241–254

Exton-Smith A N 1977 In: Exton-Smith A N, Grimley Evans J (eds) Care of the elderly: Meeting the Challenge of dependency. Academic Press, London

Eysenck H J 1952 The scientific study of personality. Routledge and Kegan Paul, London

Greenwood R, Hopkins A 1976a Muscle responses during sudden falls in man. Journal of Physiology 254:507–518

Greenwood R, Hopkins A 1976b Landing from an unexpected fall and a voluntary step. Brain 99:375–386

Haddock D R W, Ebrahim G J, Kapur B B 1962 Ataxic Neurological syndrome found in Tanganyika. British Medical Journal 2:1442–1443

Hinchcliffe R 1961 Prevalence of the Commoner Ear, Nose and Throat Conditions in the Adult Rural Population of Great Britain. British Journal of Preventive and Social Medicine 15:128–140

Hinchcliffe R 1972 Some geographical aspects of neuro-otology with particular reference to the African. African Journal of Medical Sciences 3:137–148

Hinchcliffe R, Osuntokun B O, Adeuja A O G 1972 Hearing Levels in Nigerian Ataxic Neuropathy. Audiology 11:218–230

Husband R W 1943 The effect of musical rhythms and pure rhythms on body sway. Journal of Genetic Psychology 10:328–335

Igarashi M, Watanabe T, Maxian P M 1970 Dynamic equilibrium in squirrel monkeys after unilateral and bilateral labyrinthectomy. Acta otolaryngologica 69:247–253

Ingham J G 1954 Body-sway suggestibility and neurosis. Journal of Mental Science 100:432–441

Kelso L E A, Hellebrandt F A 1937 Devices for the study of two plane shifts in the centre of gravity of a swaying body. Science 86:451–452

Koles Z J, Castelein R D 1980 The relationship between body sway and foot pressure in normal man. Journal of Medical Engineering and Technology 4:279–285

Koskenoja M, Orma E J 1956 Positional nystagmus in elderly patients with postural dizziness. Annals of Otology, Rhinology and Laryngology 65:707–713

Kuilman J 1959 The importance of the cervical syndrome in otorhinolaryngology. Practica oto-rhino-laryngologica 21:174–185

Magnus R 1924 Körperstellung. Springer, Berlin

Melvill Jones G 1973 Is there a vestibulo-spinal reflex contribution to running? Advances in Oto-rhino-laryngology 19:128–133

Miles W R 1922 Static equilibrium as a useful test of motor control. Journal of Industrial Hygiene 3:316–331

Money G L 1959 Endemic neuropathies in the Epe district of southern Nigeria. West African Medical Journal 7:58–62

Montgomery R D, Cruickshank E K, Robertson W B, McMenemy W H 1964 Clinical and pathological observations on Jamaican Neuropathy—A report on 206 cases. Brain 87:425–462

Orma E J, Koskenoja M 1957a Postural dizziness in the aged. Geriatrics 12:49–59

Orma E J, Koskenoja M 1957b Dizziness attacks and continuous dizziness in the aged. Geriatrics 12:92–100

Osuntokun B O 1968 An ataxic neuropathy in Nigeria. A clinical, biochemical and electrophysiological study. Brain 91:215–248

Osuntokun B O, Aladetoyinbo A, Adeuja A O G 1970 Free-cyanide levels in tropical ataxic neuropathy. Lancet 2:372–373

Osuntokun B O, Monekosso G L, Wilson J 1969 Relationship of a degenerative tropical neuropathy to diet. Report of a field survey. British Medical Journal 1:547–550

Overstall P W, Exton-Smith A N, Imms F J, Johnson A L 1977 Falls in the elderly related to postural imbalance. British Medical Journal 1:261–264

Purdon Martin J 1965 Tilting reactions and disorders of the basal ganglia. Brain 88:855–874

Purdon Martin J 1967 The basal ganglia and posture. Pitman, London

Roberts T D M 1978 Neurophysiology of postural mechanisms. Butterworths, London

Rodstein M, Zeman F D 1957 Postural blood pressure changes in the elderly. Journal of Chronic Diseases 6:581–588

Rodgers P E B 1965 The clinical features and aetiology of the neuropathic syndrome in Jamaica. West Indian Medical Journal 14:36–37

Sheldon J H 1948 The Social Medicine of Old Age. Oxford University Press, London

Sheldon J H 1960 On the natural history of falls in old age. British Medical Journal 2:1685–1690

Sheldon J H 1963 The effect of age on the control of sway. Gerontologia Clinica 5:129–138

Shipley R, Harley R J 1971 A device for estimating stability of stance in human subjects. Psychophysiology 7:287–292

Tanja T A, Hofman A, Valkenburg H A C 1979 Een epidemiologisch onderzoek onder bejaarden (EPOZ) II: Duizeligheid bij bejaarden; mogelijko oorzaken en gevolgen. Nederlandsch Tijdschrift voor Gerontologie 10:195–201

Terekhov Y 1976 Stabilometry and some aspects of its applications—a review. Biomedical Engineering 11:12–15

Tomlinson G E, Stevens D L 1971 Measurement of postural sway. Biomedical Engineering 6 : 162–163
Travis R C 1945 An experimental analysis of dynamic and static equilibrium. Journal of Experimental Psychology 35 : 216–234
Vierordt K 1862 Grundriss der Physiologie des Menschen. Tübingen
Watt D G D 1976 Responses of cats to sudden falls: An otolith-originating reflex assisting landing. Journal of Neurophysiology 39 : 257–265
Wild, Nayak U S L, Isaacs B 1981 How dangerous are falls in old people at home? British Medical Journal 282 : 266–268
Wilson V J, Melvill Jones G 1979 Mammalian vestibular physiology. Plenum Press, New York
Wright B M 1971 A simple mechanical ataxia-meter. Journal of Physiology 218 : 27P–28P
Wyke B D 1975 The neurological basis of movement: a developmental review. In: Holt K S (ed.). Movement and child development. Heinemann, London pp 19–37
Wyke B D 1979 Cervical articular contributions to Posture and Gait: Their relation to Senile Disequilibrium. Age and Ageing 8 : 251–258

G. R. Barnes

Vestibular mechanisms

INTRODUCTION

The vestibular system of the internal ear forms a very small part of the body of man, the main components being no larger than 10 mm across, and yet it has attracted increasing interest over the last 10–20 years. There appear to be three principal reasons for this. First, the vestibular system offers to the neurophysiologist several examples of reflex mechanisms which can be studied at a sub-cortical level with considerable success using modern micro-electrode techniques. Secondly, a number of practical problems have arisen in the use of high speed vehicles and in particular in space flight through stimulation of the vestibular organs. Thirdly, the relative lack of complexity in the vestibular response has led to this being one of the most fertile areas for the use of mathematical modelling techniques akin to those used extensively in the inanimate world. The object of this review is to chart current progress in these areas of vestibular physiology.

In normal human subjects, as in other vertebrates, the vestibular apparatus is an important transducer governing the reflex control of eye, head and body movements. In addition it provides sensory information concerning our orientation in space. There are two types of endorgan, the semicircular canals and the maculae, the receptors of which are responsive to angular and linear accelerations respectively. In general the reflex mechanisms of which they form a part are concerned with providing responses within the effector systems, the head, eyes and limbs, which are compensatory for imposed accelerations and thus tend to stabilise the body in space.

Functionally the mechanisms may be divided into two parts: the vestibulo-ocular reflex which controls the movement of the eyes in all rotational planes through a system of neural networks contained within the brain-stem, and the vestibulospinal reflexes which control the activity of postural muscles through neural pathways which descend in the spinal cord. These mechanisms will be considered separately, preceded by a discussion of the behaviour of the vestibular endorgans that are common on both reflex mechanisms.

ANATOMY AND FUNCTIONAL CHARACTERISTICS OF THE VESTIBULAR APPARATUS

System components

The components involved in the many reflex and sensory mechanisms of the vestibular system have been extensively investigated since the time of Breuer

(1889). The principal components are the vestibular endorgans and the vestibular nuclei which relay sensory information via motoneurones to control head, body and eye movements. Secondary, but equally important, centres within the cerebellum and the reticular formation of the brainstem serve principally as response modifying and coordinating centres, receiving convergent sensory information from the visual cortex and from proprioceptors which monitor the positions of body components with respect to each other.

The vestibular system

The bony labyrinth of the internal ear contains two sets of endorgans with distinct, and apparently separate sensory functions; that of hearing, mediated by the cochlea, and that of balance subserved by the vestibular apparatus. The three components of the labyrinth, the vestibule, the semicircular canals and the cochlea are cavities within the petrous part of the temporal bone and as such are firmly located within the skull. The receptor mechanisms are contained within the membranous labyrinth (Fig. 11.1) which is filled with endolymph, a fluid similar to intracellular fluid, and is separated from the bony labyrinth by a slightly less dense fluid, the perilymph. In the human, the non-auditory membraneous labyrinth is divided functionally into two parts: the semicircular ducts and the maculae or otoliths.

The semicircular canals

On each side of the skull there are three semicircular ducts* lying in planes which are approximately mutually orthogonal as indicated in Figure 11.1. The two lateral ducts lie in a plane which is horizontal when the head is tilted approximately 30° forward from the upright position (Fig. 11.2). The diameter of the semicircular duct is only 150 μm and the toroidal outer diameter is of the order of 6 mm (Igarashi, 1966). All three semicircular ducts have their origin in the utricle, a sac-like structure which resides in the vestibule. Near the junction with the utricle lies an enlarged area, the ampulla, within which is a raised section of the inner wall called the crista ampullaris (Fig. 11.3a). The crista contains specialised hair cells of neurological origin which are connected via the vestibulocochlear (VIIIth cranial) nerve to the vestibular nuclei of the brain stem. The cilia associated with these hair cells are invested by a gelatinous structure, the cupula, which forms a seal with the walls of the ampulla. There are two types of cilia within each hair cell, the stereocilia, of which there are 60–100 per cell and a single kinocilium which is longer and thicker in cross-section (Fig. 11.3b) (Wersall and Lundquist, 1966). The cilia are arranged with a morphological polarisation which results in a specificity of directional sensitivity, the maximal response being found when the stereocilia are bent towards the kinocilium (Lowenstein and Wersall, 1959). In the cristae, the hair cells are arranged with a common direction of maximum sensitivity in the plane of the canal (Fig. 11.3b).

---

* Although the term 'duct' refers strictly to the membranous part which contains the sensory cells, the term 'canal' is frequently used to denote the system as a whole.

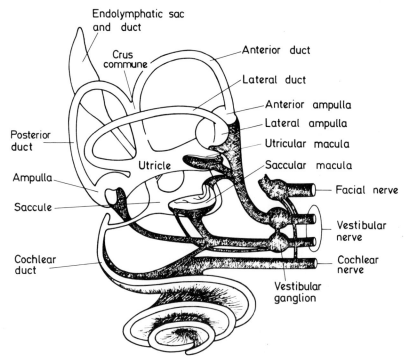

Fig. 11.1 A simplified, expanded diagram of the membranous labyrinth of the right side as viewed from the right. Hatched areas indicate the neural pathways by which the ampullae and maculae are in communication with the vestibular nuclei of the brainstem.

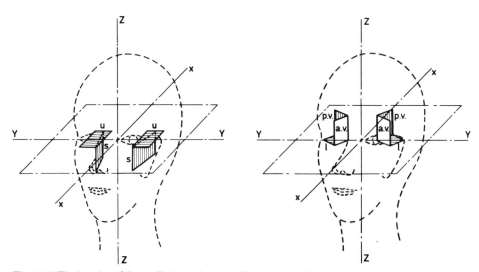

Fig. 11.2 The location of the vestibular endorgans within the head. The lateral semicircular canals (l) and the utricular maculae (u) lie in the horizontal plane when the head is tilted forward approximately 30° from the normal upright position.

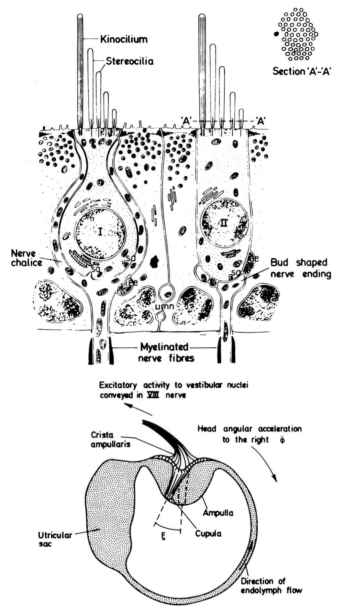

Fig. 11.3 (a) A simplified plan diagram of the right lateral semicircular duct indicating the manner in which the cupula and endolymph respond to head rotation to the right. (b) The arrangement of hair cells within the sensory epithelium of the crista ampullaris, showing the relationship between the kinocilium and the stereocilia which project into the body of the cupula.

Dynamics of the semicircular canals

The semicircular canal system is sensitive to angular motion of the head. As the head is rotated the endolymph within the duct tends to remain stationary in space because of its inherent inertia. The resultant flow of endolymph with respect to the duct is resisted by the elasticity of the gelatinous cupula which thus becomes deflected (Fig. 11.3a). The motion is also resisted by viscous forces proportional to flow velocity.

Deflection of the cupula induces bending of the cilia and consequent changes in firing level of the sensory cells. The exact mechanism of transduction has not been established although various hypotheses have been put forward (e.g. Malcolm, 1974; Goldberg and Fernandez, 1975).

The dynamics of the cupula-endolymph system have been compared to that of a damped torsion pendulum (Steinhausen, 1931) in which the angular displacement of the cupula (ξ) is related to the angular acceleration of the head ($\ddot{\phi}$) by the differential equation:

$$\Theta \cdot \ddot{\xi} + \Pi \cdot \dot{\xi} + \triangle \cdot \xi = \Theta \cdot \ddot{\phi}(t) \tag{1}$$

θ is the effective moment of inertia of the endolymphatic toroid, Π is the viscous damping couple provided by the interaction of the endolymph with the walls of the duct and $\triangle$ is the restraining couple provided by the elasticity of the cupula. The system is heavily damped so that the governing equation may be conveniently rewritten in Laplace notation

$$(1 + T_1 s)(1 + T_2 s)\xi = \Theta/\triangle \cdot \ddot{\phi}(s) \tag{2}$$

where $T_1 \approx \Pi/\triangle$ & $T_2 \approx \Theta/\Pi$

Early attempts were made (van Egmond et al, 1949; Groen et al, 1952) to estimate the parameters of equation (2) from subjective assessments associated with the sensation of turning engendered by rotational stimuli. Values thus obtained were 10 s for the long time constant (T_1) and 100 ms for the short time constant (T_2). It is doubtful if such an assessment is valid since higher central processing is involved and may modify the endorgan response. In particular the value of T_2 is not in accord with theoretical calculations for the damping to inertia ratio made by van Egmond and his colleagues (1949) based on the assumption of laminar flow within the duct which led to a value for T_1 of 5 ms. A similar value was obtained in a subsequent and more detailed theoretical investigation by Steer (1967), who also attempted to estimate cupular elasticity ($\triangle$). Oman and Young (1972) were able to indicate the extreme sensitivity of the hair cells by showing that cupula deflection would lie in the range 0·01 to 5 μm in the normal physiological range of head movements.

A more direct method of measuring cupula-endolymph dynamics is by the recording of neural activity within the primary afferent fibres innervating the cupula. A number of such studies have now been performed for the responses of all three canals (Lowenstein and Sand, 1940; Groen et al, 1952; Fernandez and Goldberg, 1971; Precht et al, 1971; Correia and Landolt, 1973; Estes et al, 1975).

The intensity of cupula deflection is registered as changes in the rate of discharge of neural impulses in the afferent fibres. There is a high resting discharge rate ($\approx$90 spikes/sec in the squirrel monkey) and the afferents exhibit a bidirectional response with a slightly higher gain in the excitatory response (Ewald's 2nd law). Fernandez and Goldberg (1971) were able to show that the response of first order afferents of the squirrel monkey which is shown in Figure 11.4 could not adequately be represented by the simple model expressed by equation (2), but

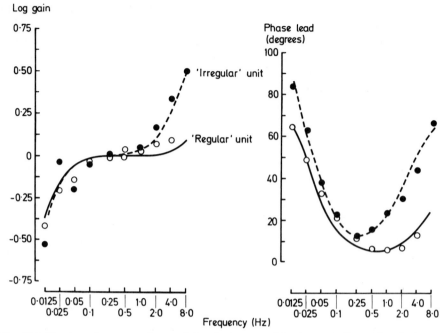

Fig. 11.4 The dynamic response characteristics of primary semicircular canal afferent fibres in the squirrel monkey indicating two different types of unit response to sinusoidal oscillation. Gain and phase are with respect to the angular velocity of the stimulus, the gain being represented by the firing rate above resting discharge level (From Fernandez and Goldberg, 1971).

rather by an equation of the form:

$$\frac{f_C}{\dot{\phi}(s)} = \frac{\kappa_C \tau_A s}{(1 + \tau_A s)} \frac{(1 + \tau_L s)s}{(1 + \tau_1 s)(1 + \tau_2 s)} \tag{3}$$

where f_C is the frequency of firing in a single canal unit and typical values for the time constants were: $\tau_A = 80$ s; $\tau_L = \cdot05$ s; $\tau_1 = 5\cdot7$ s; $\tau_2 = \cdot003$ s

The time constants τ_1 and τ_2 appear to conform with those of the simple model of equation (2). However there are two additional components. First, there is a rate sensitive component $(1 + \tau_L s)$ which introduces gain enhancement and phase lead at high frequencies $(\omega > 1/\tau_L)$. Second, there is an adaptation component $(\tau_A s/(1 + \tau_A s))$ which is necessary to explain the phase lead observed at low frequencies and the departure from the expected response of the torsion pendulum model to transient stimuli. Later it will be shown that these features are also observed in the vestibulo-ocular response.

The utricular and saccular maculae

The utricle and saccule of the membranous labyrinth (Fig. 1) contain within their walls the endorgans (frequently referred to as the otoliths) responsible for transducing linear accelerations. The positions of the two sensors on either side of the head are illustrated in Figure 11.2b. As a general approximation it is often assumed that the utricular maculae lie in the horizontal plane when the head is tilted some 30° forward from its normal position and the saccules in the normal vertical plane when the head is upright, although both have considerable representations in other planes.

The structure of the maculae is illustrated in Figure 11.5. The base is a thickening of the membranous labyrinth which contains supporting cells and hair cells similar to those in the ampullae. The macula is overlayed by a gelatinous substrate containing an aggregation of minute crystals of calcium carbonate (the statoconia*) which collectively form a plaque with an area of approximately 1·5 to 2 mm² and a density approximately twice that of the surrounding endolymph.

In the utricular maculae the directional sensitivities of sensory cells in each half of the macula have an approximately radial distribution (as shown in Fig. 11.5a) and are of opposite polarity on either side of the dividing crest which is known as the striola (Spoendlin, 1965). The arrangement for the saccular macula is similar but geometrically more complex (Fig. 11.5b).

It is not certain how the neural signals from these multitudinous receptors are organised but it has been postulated (Benson and Barnes, 1973) that the radially distributed sensitivities are integrated spatially over each half macula so that the utricle can provide independent signals in response to both fore-aft (X-axis) and lateral (Y-axis) acceleration of the head. This is partially supported by the eye movements resulting from electrical stimulation of the otoliths observed by Fluur and Mellstrom (1971). The sensory cells synapse on afferent fibres which project to the vestibular nuclei in the vestibulocochlear nerve:

Dynamics of otolith behaviour

The mechanism by which linear acceleration is transduced is thought to be as follows. The component of acceleration in the plane of the macula ($\ddot{y}$) induces an inertial force on the statoconial plaque which is denser than the surrounding endolymph. The resultant shear force applied across the gelatinous substrate causes the hair cells to be deflected (Fig. 11.6) with a consequent change in firing rate of the sensory cells. The deflection (r) may be represented (Barnes, 1972; Benson & Barnes, 1973) by a differential equation of the form:

$$m \cdot \ddot{r} + \lambda \cdot \dot{r} + \left(k - \frac{m \cdot \ddot{z}}{1}\right) \cdot r = m \cdot \ddot{y} \tag{4}$$

where m = effective mass of statoconial plaque, λ = damping coefficient, k = elasticity provided by supporting structures, and $\ddot{z}$ = acceleration normal to the macula. Since the system appears over-damped this equation may be rewritten as:

$$(1 + T_3 s)(1 + T_4 s) \, r = \ddot{y}/(k - m \cdot \ddot{z}/1) \tag{5}$$

where
$$T_3 = \lambda/(k - m \cdot \ddot{z}/1);$$
$$T_4 = m/\lambda$$

The effect of acceleration ($\ddot{z}$) normal to the plane of the macula is to increase the deflection of the statoconial plaque when some deflection has already taken place, although this factor is often ignored. The parameters of equation (5) have been estimated from threshold detection studies (Young and Meiry, 1967; Young, 1969) to be of the order of 5 s for T_3 and 0·7 s for T_4. In conflict with these values, theoretical calculations based on the observed deflections of the otolith (de Vries,

---

* now referred to as otoliths or otoconia

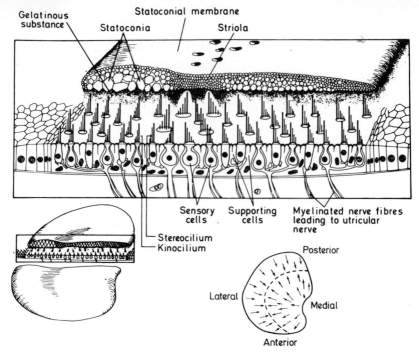

(a) UTRICULAR MACULA

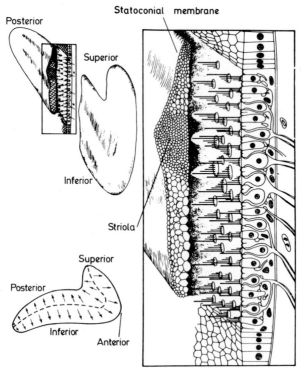

(b) SACCULAR MACULA

Fig. 11.5 The microstructure of the utricular and saccular maculae, showing the disposition of the statoconia with respect to the sensory epithelium. The directional specificities of the sensory cells are radially distributed on either side of the central striola.

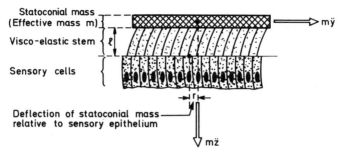

Fig. 11.6 A simplified representation of the utricular otolith organ to illustrate the manner in which the statoconial mass is deflected by accelerations acting in shear ($\ddot{y}$) and normal to ($\ddot{z}$) the macula.

1950) have provided estimates for the product of T_3 and T_4 of approximately 4×10^{-6} s². Goldberg and Fernandez (1975) estimated the sensitivity of mammalian otolith organs to be 0·5 μ/g, again emphasising the exquisite mechanical sensitivity of the vestibular organs.

As with semicircular canal responses, the response of first order afferents has been extensively investigated for both static stimuli (Lowenstein and Roberts, 1950; Vidal et al, 1971; Fernandez et al, 1972; Loe et al, 1973) and dynamic stimuli (Lowenstein and Saunders, 1975; Fernandez and Goldberg, 1976). The primary afferents exhibit a resting discharge level with some units having a tonic response ('regular' units) and some a more phasic response ('irregular' units). In general the firing rate is related to applied acceleration with a greater sensitivity to excitatory stimuli. Fernandez and Goldberg (1976) derived a rather complex transfer function to fit their data (Fig. 11.7): a simplified and possibly adequate

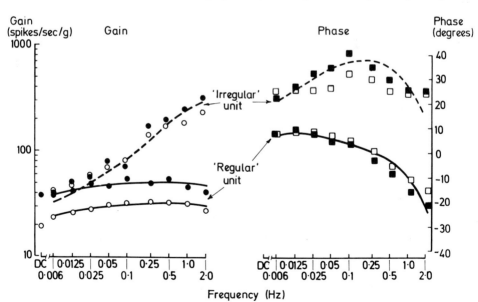

Fig. 11.7 The dynamic response characteristics of primary afferent fibres of the utricular macula of the squirrel monkey, indicating the two different types of unit response ('regular' and 'irregular') to sinusoidal oscillation. Gain and phase are with respect to linear acceleration. ■ and ● excitatory stimuli; □ and ○—inhibitory stimuli. (After Fermandez and Goldberg 1976).

description is afforded by the equation:

$$\frac{f_M}{\ddot{x}(s)} = \frac{k_M \cdot (1 + k \cdot \tau_{AM}s)}{(1 + \tau_{AM}s)} \frac{(1 + \tau_Ms)}{(1 + \tau_3s)(1 + \tau_4s)} \tag{6}$$

Typical values for the parameters of this equation are: $\tau_3 = 0\cdot6$ s; $\tau_4 = 0\cdot01$ s; $\tau_{AM} = 80$ s; $k = 2\cdot5$; $\tau_M = 2\cdot4$ s for 'irregular' units, $= 0\cdot65$ s for 'regular' units.

Thus, as for the canals, there is an adaptation term $(1 + k \cdot \tau_{AM}s)/(1 + \tau_{AM}s)$ and a gain augmenting phase lead component $(1 + \tau_Ms)$ at high frequency in addition to the expected response, a feature predicted from sensory threshold experiments (Young and Meiry, 1967; Young, 1969).

The vestibular nuclei

The majority of the afferent fibres from the receptor areas of the vestibular apparatus terminate in the vestibular nuclei. Before the neuronal impulses relayed to the nuclei can be transmitted further they must pass at least one synapse and thus may be modified by impulses entering the nuclei from other sources. The vestibular nuclei thus occupy a stragetic position in relation to vestibular function.

The location of the vestibular nuclei is the dorsal area of the medulla oblongata caudal to the pons and just ventral to the floor of the fourth ventricle. The complex consists of four major cell groups; the superior, medial, lateral and descending nuclei, together with some smaller groups of less significance. There are many uncertainties concerning the exact afferent connections and projections of these cell groups, but the consensus of available information (Brodal, 1974; McMasters et al, 1966; Goldberg and Fernandez, 1975; Wilson and Peterson, 1978), points to the following general arrangement. Afferents from the semicircular canals project mainly to the superior and lateral nuclei and to rostral parts of the medial nuclei. Fibres from the maculae project principally to the descending and medial nuclei and to caudal parts of the lateral nuclei.

The activity of neurones within the vestibular nuclei during vestibular stimulation has been investigated for canal dependent units (Gernandt, 1949; Shimazu and Precht, 1965; Benson et al, 1970; Melvill Jones and Milsum, 1971; Shinoda and Yoshida, 1974; Fuchs and Kimm, 1975; Schneider and Anderson, 1976) and for otolith dependent units (Milsum and Melvill Jones, 1967; Fujita et al, 1968; Melvill Jones and Milsum, 1970; Peterson, 1970). These indicate that the nuclei apparently function primarily as a relay station for primary vestibular afferents since, in general, the same frequency-modulated characteristics are exhibited. However, this is not the only role of the vestibular nuclei, which are important integrating centres for spinal, cerebellar and reticular formation afferents as will be discussed later.

THE VESTIBULO-OCULAR REFLEX MECHANISMS

Function of the vestibulo-ocular mechanisms

In general, the function of the vestibular apparatus is to enable an organism to induce activity in the effector system which is compensatory for disturbances of the reference platform, that is, the head. But, in particular, it was recognised by Breuer (1889) and by Dodge (1903) that the ocular movements with respect to the head induced by stimulation of the semicircular canals are in the opposite direction to the movement of the head itself. The eye movement is thus of a compensatory nature, so that the eye is stabilised in space whilst the head is in motion. Consequently, objects which are fixed in space may be viewed without smearing of the retinal image during body motion, a feature which has recently been substantiated by Benson (1972) (see also Benson and Barnes, 1978).

The need for a system to stabilise the retinal image becomes apparent when one considers the limitations of the reflex mechanisms by which man is able to maintain fixation on a moving object. Pursuit tracking movements of the head and eyes can result from visual stimulation alone. However, it has been well established (Dodge and Cline, 1901; Westheimer, 1954; Rashbass, 1961; Young and Stark, 1963), that the visually driven response breaks down when either the velocity of target movement is too great (>approximately 60°/s) or when the frequency of a direction changing movement is too high (>1–2 Hz).

During an imposed movement of the head the effect on the retinal image of attempts to fixate an earth-fixed object is similar to that which obtains during pursuit tracking, since in both instances the object is moving in relation to the retina. However, the ability of the vestibular system to induce movements of the eyes which compensate for head movement enables the retinal image to be stabilised at levels of velocity and frequency of head movement at which the visual pursuit system alone is not capable of controlling eye movement (Fig. 11.8). This feature is of importance during natural high frequency body movements, such as

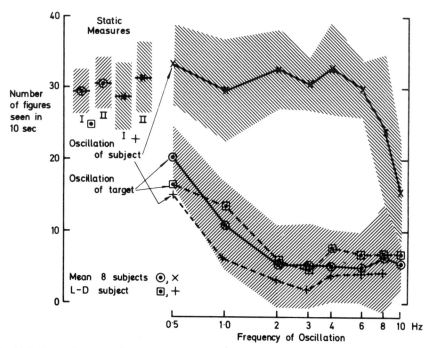

Fig. 11.8 Comparison of reading performance during sinusoidal angular oscillation in yaw of the observer (x) or of the target (○). Hatched areas represent ±1 S.D. The performance of a subject without functioning labyrinths is denoted by (L—D subjects). The results indicate the importance of the vestibulo-ocular reflex during oscillation of the subject.

occur during walking and running. Subjects without functioning labyrinths experience difficulty in preserving visual acuity during such manoeuvres. Fortuitously, modern man also finds this feature of great assistance during vehicular travel where frequencies of stimulation are often well above the range at which the visual pursuit system will function.

The compensatory nature of the vestibulo-ocular reflex response is most apparent in the presence of visual stimulation. However, when the vestibular system is stimulated in the absence of vision the evoked eye movement is most frequently of an oscillatory nature and is referred to as nystagmus. There are two components of the nystagmus as indicated in Figure 11.9. One is the compensatory

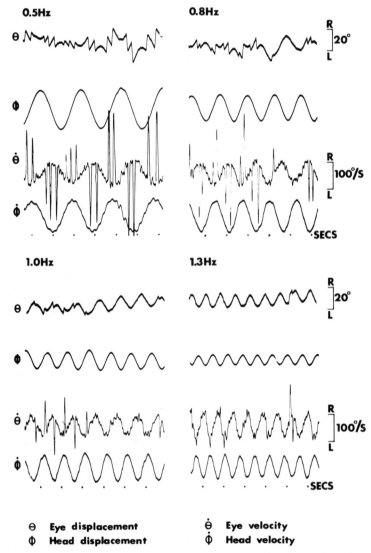

Fig. 11.9 Examples of vestibular nystagmus evoked during sinusoidal oscillation about the yaw axis at different frequencies, indicating the manner in which slow-phase eye velocity compensates for head velocity. Note the relative paucity of saccadic activity at high frequencies.

(or slow-phase) component, the nature of which has already been described. The other is referred to as the fast-phase or saccadic component, the velocity of which is of opposite polarity to the compensatory component, thus giving rise to the oscillatory appearance of the nystagmus. Whilst the velocity of the compensatory components reflects the varying velocity of head movement, the saccadic components are of approximately constant velocity (up to 400°/s) and constitute a fast resetting mechanism.

Neurophysiology of the vestibulo-ocular reflex

Despite the fact that many of the anatomical relations within the vestibulo-ocular reflex pathways are not known, many of the inter-connections have been revealed by electrophysiological experiments (Fig. 11.10).

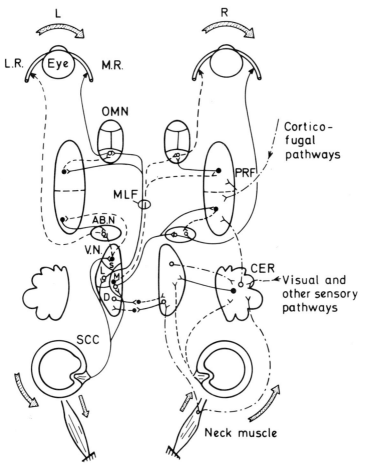

Fig. 11.10 The activity within vestibulo-ocular pathways involved in the control of lateral eye movements, during a counterclockwise rotation of the head. ○—excitatory, ●—inhibitory synapses. SCC—Lateral semicircular canal; CER—Cerebellum; MLF—Medial longitudinal fasciculus; PRF—Pontine reticular formation; VN—Vestibular nuclei; S,L,M,D.;—Superior, lateral, medial, descending vestibular nuclei; ABN—Abducens nucleus; OMN—Oculomotor nuclei; LR & MR—Lateral and medial rectus muscles.

The most basic component of the system is a 3-neurone arc consisting of (1) the primary (or 1st order) vestibular afferent fibres connecting the sensory cells of the crista ampullaris with neurones in the vestibular nuclei, (2) the secondary (or 2nd order) vestibular neurones sending axons to the nuclei of the oculomotor complex via the ascending medial longitudinal fasciculus, and (3) motoneurones which innervate the various extra-ocular muscles. Stimulation and ablation of individual semicircular canals (Lorente de No, 1933; Szentagothai, 1950; Cohen et al, 1964) has indicated that there is a high degree of specifity between individual canals and extra-ocular muscles, so that, for example, the horizontal semi-circular canal, which is stimulated by rotation about the longitudinal (Z) body axis, projects directly and principally to the ipsilateral medial and contralateral lateral rectus muscles of the eye. A similar basic disynaptic arc has also been established for utricular stimulation (Baker et al, 1973; Schwindt et al, 1973).

The most direct pathway from the vestibular nuclei to the nuclei of the oculomotor neurones is via the ascending medial longitudinal fasciculus. Lesions in this pathway abolish the short latency crista reflexes normally observed (Szentogothai, 1950, 1952) but do not completely remove the control of eye movement. A powerful synaptic connection is made by second order vestibular neurones directly onto oculomotor neurones as demonstrated anatomically by Szentogothai (1964).

Stimulation of the vestibulocochlear nerve or the medial vestibular nucleus induces, respectively, disynaptic or monosynaptic responses in the abducens and trochlear motoneurones (Richter & Precht, 1968; Baker et al, 1969; Precht & Baker, 1972). Thus, as shown in Figure 11.10, excitatory activity in the left lateral semicircular canal induced by a counterclockwise angular acceleration is conveyed to the contralateral lateral rectus muscle via the ipsilateral medial vestibular nucleus and the contralateral abducens nucleus, initiating eye movement to the right. In the left eye, deviation to the right is induced by excitatory activity in the medial rectus muscle conveyed by the ipsilateral lateral vestibular and oculomotor nuclei (Yules and Gault, 1966; Highstein, 1971). Conversely, the concommitant inhibitory activity in the right lateral canal stimulates inhibition of the left lateral rectus and right medial rectus muscles which thus act as a coordinated agonist/antagonist pair.

However, a unilateral vestibular stimulus such as that induced by caloric irrigation (a clinical technique in which the density of the endolymph within the duct is modified by a thermal stimulus (Barnes and Benson, 1978)) is, of itself, able to bring about a conjugate pattern of eye deviation as a result of two further sets of pathways. First, in addition to the excitatory connections described above, the vestibular nuclei also exhibit inhibitory connections to the oculomotor neurones (Baker et al, 1969; Highstein et al, 1971; Precht and Baker, 1972). The organisation is such that the horizontal canal inhibits the ipsilateral lateral rectus via the superior vestibular nucleus and the contralateral medial rectus via the medial vestibular nucleus. Secondly, it has been demonstrated that there is a reciprocal inhibition between the vestibular nuclei of both sides (Shimazu and Precht, 1966).

In addition to the main disynaptic pathways there are polysynaptic pathways through the reticular formation of the brainstem and through the cerebellum. These will be discussed in more detail later.

The activity of single neurones in the oculomotor nuclei and nerve fibres has been studied during vestibular stimulation (Sasaki, 1963; Schaeffer, 1965; Precht et al, 1967, 1969; Yamanaka and Bach-y-Rita, 1968; Maeda et al, 1972). At this level the frequency of discharge is modulated in accord with the different phases of nystagmus. Both tonically active and inactive neurones apparently participate in both fast and slow phases of nystagmus.

Finally, for the basic disynaptic arc there have been various attempts to correlate activity in the oculomotor neurones with eye movements (Zuber, 1968; Robinson, 1970; Schiller, 1970; Barmack, et al, 1971; Skavenski and Robinson, 1973; Barmack, 1974). All of these authors agree on the high tetanus frequency observed in extra-ocular muscle (frequency 500 Hz) which is essential for the production of saccadic eye movements. Moreover, none were able to find any distinction between the response of fast and slow twitch muscle fibres during either fast- or slow-phase eye movements.

Dynamic response of the canal-ocular reflex

The action of a single canal has been compared to that of a damped torsion pendulum, an analogy which may be represented by a second order differential equation. The vestibulo-ocular reflex exhibits dynamic characteristics which are very similar to those observed in the endorgan itself and early attempts to estimate the parameters of equation (2) were made by consideration of the oculomotor response to head rotational stimuli with the underlying assumption that slow-phase eye velocity was proportional to cupula deflection. Two principal methods of stimulation have been used; transient and periodic acceleration. The response to yaw movements is lateral eye movement, that for pitch rotation is vertical eye movement and that for roll movements is counter-rolling of the eye (i.e rotation about the antero-posterior axis) (Melvill Jones et al, 1964).

Transient stimuli

The transient stimuli used most frequently are those of constant angular acceleration and impulsive deceleration (van Egmond et al, 1949; Hallpike and Hood, 1953; Stahle, 1958; Guedry and Lauver, 1961). The latter is a stimulus induced by an abrupt cessation of rotation after a prolonged period of constant angular velocity and is frequently used for diagnostic assessment of vestibular function (Jongkees, 1967).

The response of the simple model represented by equation (2) to such a stimulus is:

$$\dot{\theta} \propto \xi = \frac{\Theta}{\Delta} \frac{1}{(T_1 - T_2)} (e^{-t/T_1} - e^{-t/T_2}) \tag{7}$$

Since $T_1 \gg T_2$, the response is dominated, as with all transient responses, by the long time constant (T_1) of the cupula-endolymph system. As a first order approximation, the observed slow phase eye velocity does exhibit the response indicated by equation (7), that is an exponentially decaying response. The time constant for the lateral canals thus obtained is generally of the order of 15–20 s, which is considerably higher than the value of approximately 6 s observed in the first order afferent responses of primates (Fernandez and Goldberg, 1971) and the value of 10 s estimated in humans from sensory thresholds (Meiry, 1965). The oculomotor response elicited by stimulation of the vertical canals exhibits a faster decay with long time constants of approximately 7 and 4 s for the pitch and roll axes respectively (Melvill Jones et al, 1964).

Benson and Bodin (1966b) observed differences in the value of T_1 in the postrotational response of the lateral canals, dependent upon the position of the subject with respect to gravity. When rotated about the horizontal axis the long time constant was reduced to about 7 s, probably indicating some central interaction between the semicircular canals and the otolith organs (Benson, 1970, 1974).

Adaptation in the transient response

A further aspect of the vestibulo-ocular response to angular acceleration is a demonstrable adaptation which occurs with prolonged stimulation, a feature which, as noted previously, can also be observed in first order afferent units (Goldberg and Fernandez, 1971a). The response to an impulsive angular decelera-tion about the yaw axis decays exponentially towards zero in some 20–30 s (Fig. 11.11) but is followed by a period of reversed slow-phase velocity not predicted by equation (7).

Attempts were made by Young and Oman (1969) and Malcolm (1971) to simulate this effect using a transfer function for the adaptation of the form:

$$A(s) = \frac{T_{AD}s}{(1 + T_{AD}s)}$$

where $T_{AD} \approx 80 - 120$ s.

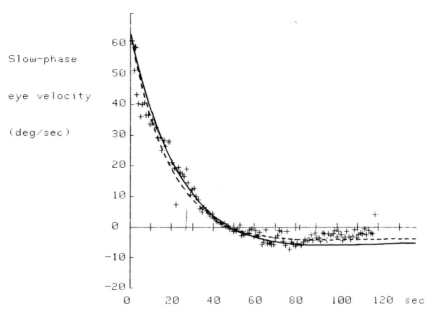

Fig. 11.11 The response of the canal-ocular reflex to a sudden cessation of rotation (100°/s) about the yaw axis. The reversal of slow phase eye velocity after a period of 40 s is referred to as secondary nystagmus. The curves drawn through the data are the predictions of the adaptation model.
(——— $T_B = 25$ s; $T_{AD} = 114$ s: ––– $T_B = 20$ s; $T_{AD} = 171$ s).

The validity of this model of adaptation in the canal-ocular response has recently been further substantiated by Barnes and Benson (1978) using the clinical test of caloric irrigation.

It is important that considerable caution be exercised in the interpretation of time constants obtained from transient stimuli. In Figure 11.11 the oculomotor response observed within the initial 40 s period may be approximated by a single exponential function with a time constant of 17 s, but modelling of the adaptation effect suggests that the value of the long time constant should be approximately 20–25 s.

Periodic stimuli

In more recent years the response of the vestibulo-ocular reflex has been extensively investigated through the use of sinusoidal angular oscillation. The response can be characterised in terms of the gain (or amplitude ratio between slow phase eye velocity and head velocity) and the phase relationship as a function of frequency. Phase is defined on the assumption that eye and head movements are of opposite sign as indicated by the crossed connections within the vestibulo-ocular pathways (Fig. 11.10). Studies have been made in lower animals (Skavenski and Robinson, 1973; Landers and Taylor, 1975; Keller, 1978) and in man (Niven and Hixson, 1961; Benson, 1970; Hixson, 1974; Barr et al, 1976; Wolfe et al, 1978; Barnes and Forbat, 1979). Wall et al (1978) have investigated the reflex using pseudo-random binary sequence stimuli. Some of the human responses and those obtained in the monkey (Keller, 1978) are illustrated in Figure 11.12, all being for rotation about the yaw axis. The response departs significantly from that expected from equation (2) particularly at frequencies above 1 Hz where there is gain enhancement of the kind observed for first order afferents by Fernandez and Goldberg (1971).

The response may be represented by an equation of the form:

$$\frac{\dot{\theta}}{\dot{\phi}} = \frac{-K_C T_B s(1 + T_A s)e^{-Ts}}{(1 + T_B s)(1 + T_C s)(1 + T_D s)} \cdot \frac{T_{AD} s}{(1 + T_{AD} s)} \tag{9}$$

where $T_A \approx 0.2$ s; $T_B \approx 15$ s; $T_C \approx 0.125$ s; $T_D \approx .002$ s; $T \approx .005$ s; $T_{AD} \approx 80$ s; $K_C \approx 0.7$.

Over the frequency range 0·02–0·5 Hz, eye velocity is approximately proportional to head velocity and almost exactly in phase, although the gain is less than unity, indicating that compensation is not complete and must be enhanced by visual feedback for maintenance of visual acuity. At higher frequencies the studies in both monkey and man indicate that gain increases beyond unity. But in the important frequency range, 0·5–2 Hz in which most voluntary head movements (Barnes, 1976b, 1977) and those induced by locomotor activities (Melvill Jones and Watt, 1971a) are made the gain is closest to unity. It is of interest to compare equation (9) with the transfer function for single canal afferent units in the monkey (equation 3). They are similar in form if allowance is made for the species difference and if it is assumed that eye velocity $(\dot{\theta})$ is proportional to firing rate (f_C) in first order afferents, with the exception that the time constant T_C is additional to the oculomotor response. In the human response it is the need to simulate the near zero phase angle at frequencies above 1 Hz which dictates the inclusion of this

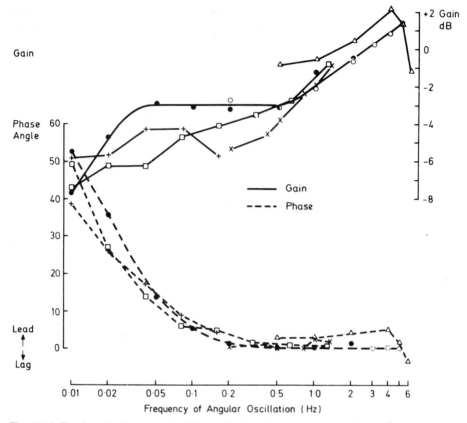

Fig. 11.12 The dynamic characteristics of the vestibulo-ocular response to angular oscillation in yaw. Gain is defined as the ratio of slow phase eye velocity to head angular velocity. Phase is defined on the assumption that eye velocity is compensatory for head velocity. Results obtained from the following sources with peak angular velocities ($\dot\theta p$) as indicated:

○ & ●—Benson (1970)	—man	$\dot\theta_p = 30°/s$	(N = 9)
☐ —Hixson (1974)	—man	$\dot\theta_p = 50°/s$	(N = 10)
+ —Wolfe et al (1978)	—man	$\dot\theta_p = 50°/s$	(N = 50)
× —Barnes & Forbat (1979)	—man	$\dot\theta_p = 50°/s$	(N = 12)
△ —Keller (1978)	—monkey	$\dot\theta_p = 100°/s$	(N = 4)

component, although circumstantial evidence from reading performance during angular oscillation (Fig. 11.8) also indicates that such a component is required to maintain the gain near unity at frequencies up to 10 Hz, as observed in the monkey (Keller, 1978). It seems most likely that T_D represents the short time constant of the canal response and that T_C arises from the dynamic response of the extra-ocular muscle system.

Response of the otolith-ocular reflex

The static reflex

Unlike the cupula-endolymph system the otolith-ocular reflex can provide static eye rotations as well as dynamic responses. In man and other species with frontal eyes the static reflexes are very weak, whereas in animals, such as the rabbit, with lateral eyes the eyes move in an appropriate manner to compensate for head deviations up to 70° in pitch (de Kleijn, 1921).

In man the only static reflex response normally observed is the counter-rolling of the eye resulting from a lateral tilt of the head (Merton, 1956; Miller, 1962; Belcher, 1964; Petrov and Zenkin, 1973). However, the eye movements appear vestigial and are certainly not effective in compensation, since maximum rotational displacements are only of the order of 5–7 degrees.

The dynamic response
The static responses are frequently referred to as the only otolith-ocular reflex responses, the semicircular canals being attributed with providing all phasic responses. However, in recent years a number of experiments have shown that a potent dynamic response can be elicited from different types of linear acceleration stimuli. The lateral eye movement responses resulting from utricular stimulation were collated by Benson and Barnes (1973) and the results are shown in Figure 11.12. The stimuli included sinusoidally modulated linear acceleration on a horizontal track (Niven et al, 1966) and various forms of constant rotation with respect to a linear acceleration acting in shear on the utricular maculae (Benson and Bodin, 1966a; Correia and Guedry, 1966; Niven et al, 1966; Steer, 1967; Benson, 1968; Stockwell et al, 1971). In the latter condition the effective stimulus in the latero-medial axis of the head is equivalent to a sinusoidally modulated linear acceleration and, as might be expected, both types of stimulus gave rise to a nystagmus with a sinusoidally modulated, slow-phase eye velocity. In general, eye velocity exhibited a steady increase with frequency in a manner similar to that observed for 'irregular' first order afferent units in the vestibular nerve as shown in Figure 11.7 (Fernandez and Goldberg, 1976). Thus, as with the canal-ocular reflex the otolith reflex response appears to exhibit some rate sensitivity over and above that which could be expected from the simple model (equation 4).

The otolith-ocular reflex response was originally modelled by Barnes (1972) and has subsequently been modified (unpublished observations) using a describing equation of the form:

$$\frac{\dot{\theta}}{\ddot{y}} = \frac{-K_M T_\beta (1 + T_\alpha s)}{(1 + T_\beta s)(1 + T_\gamma s)(1 + T_\delta s)} \tag{10}$$

where $\ddot{y}$ is the acceleration acting in shear along the latero-medial (Y) axis of the head. Typical values for the parameters when $\ddot{z} = \lg$ are: $T_\alpha = 2$ s; $T_\beta = 0 \cdot 2$ s; $T_\gamma = 0 \cdot 1$ s; $T_\delta = 0 \cdot 001$ s; $K_M = 7 \cdot 5°/s/g$. When $\ddot{z} = 0$ the approximate value of T_β is $0 \cdot 8$ s. As for the canal-ocular response, the value T_β reflects the long time constant (T_3) of the model and is consequently modified by acceleration normal to the plane of the maculae (see equation (4)), whereas T_δ appears similar to the expected value of T_4, the short time constant. There is a phase advance component $(1 + T_\alpha s)$ which corresponds with that observed in first order afferents but in addition there is a further lag with a time constant T_γ which may reflect the dynamic response of the eye globe.

In addition to the sinusoidal component, the responses of the utricles to a rotating acceleration acting in shear exhibited a constant velocity offset or 'bias' component. Benson and Barnes (1973) suggested that this might be attributable to twisting of the statoconial plaque with respect to the macula. It is unlikely that this response was of canalicular origin since blockage of all semicircular canals (Correia and Money, 1970) was unable to completely abolish the response, whereas after cutting the afferent fibres from the maculae (Janeke, 1968) no such response was observed.

Vertical eye movements induced by linear accelerations in the plane of the saccular maculae have been examined by Niven and his colleagues (1966) in humans and found to be of very low amplitude without significant saccadic activity. More recently Melvill Jones and his colleagues (1976) made similar observations and determined that the phase is similar to that depicted in Figure 11.13.

The usefulness of the otolith-ocular reflex response is not immediately apparent since the effectiveness of compensatory rotational eye movements in response to linear acceleration is dependent upon the distance of the viewed object from the observer. Whether there is some interaction with the accommodative mechanisms of the eye to increase the amplitude of the response for near fixation is a possibility which remains to be investigated.

Evidence for a neural integrator in the vestibulo-ocular reflex

As noted earlier the response of first and second order vestibular afferent neurones is essentially coded for head angular velocity over a large range of frequencies for which eye velocity is porportional to head velocity (Shimazu and Precht, 1965; Melvill Jones and Milsum, 1971; Shinoda and Yoshida 1974). However, studies made at the level of the oculomotor neurones (Yamanaka and Bach-y-Rita, 1968; Reinhart and Zuber, 1970; Maeda et al, 1972; Shinoda and Yoshida, 1974) show that at this point the signal is coded for eye position. It is therefore evident that some form of neural integration must take place between the vestibular nuclei and the oculomotor neurones. The presence of an integrating mechanism has been postulated by many authors (Cohen et al, 1965; Young, 1969; Schmid, 1970; Robinson, 1971). It is evident that the process cannot be one of pure integration since this would result in a constant eye velocity in response to a constant cupular deviation. However, the effect may be equally well produced by a partial integrator with a long time constant (e.g. 10 s) which would effectively integrate periodic waveforms even at very low frequencies (>0.02 Hz). The equation relating firing rate in the oculomotor neurones to firing rate in the vestibular nuclei is then:

$$\frac{f_{OMN}}{f_C} = \frac{T_I}{(1 + T_I s)} \tag{11}$$

where $T_I \approx 10$ s.

In fact the time constant of the neural integrator need not be as high as 10 s, because of the presence of fast phase activity in nystagmus, a point which will be explained later when discussing models of the saccadic mechanism.

The site of the neural integrating mechanism is not known at present, although the most probable site is within the reticular formation of the brainstem where the necessary multisynaptic pathways are known to exist. Skavenski and Robinson, (1973) have shown how such a secondary pathway acting in parallel with the

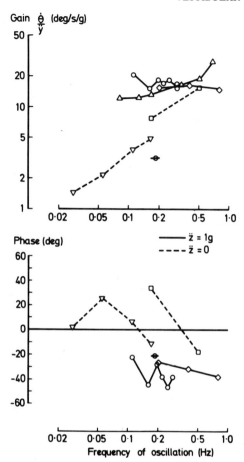

Fig. 11.13 The dynamic characteristics of the utriculo-ocular response to sinusoidal oscillation about the latero-medial (Y) axis of the head. Gain is defined as the ratio of slow-phase eye velocity to effective linear acceleration. Phase is defined on the assumption that eye velocity is compensatory for head movement. Results obtained from the following sources:

▽ —Benson & Bodin (1966) —horizontal Z-axis rotation
□ —Correia & Guedry (1966)—horizontal Z-axis rotation
⊖ —Stockwell et al (1971) —horizontal Z-axis rotation
△ —Steer (1967) —rotation about Z-axis at end of centrifuge arm: effective acceleration in shear ±0·3 g.
◇ —Niven et al (1966) —linear oscillation on horizontal track, peak acceleration = ±0·58 g.
⊙ —Benson & Barnes (1973) —counter-rotation at end of centrifuge arm: peak acceleration in shear = ±0·15ω^2g.

disynaptic pathway could provide not only partial integration but also a phase lead component which could compensate for the phase lag imposed by orbital dynamics, although as demonstrated earlier this may be provided at first order afferent level. It has been suggested by Carpenter (1972) that integration may take place within the cerebellum on the basis of phase changes observed in the vestibulo-ocular response of cerebellectomised cats, although it is possible that this may reflect the behaviour of adaptive centres within the cerebellum.

In addition to this integrative mechanism it is probable that a further integrator also exists (Robinson, 1976; Raphan et al, 1977), since the long time constant observed in vestibulocochlear nerve neurons ($\approx$4 s in the cat; Blanks et al, 1975) appears to be smaller than that observed in the oculomotor response ($\approx$12 s). However, this is not supported by the work of Landers and Taylor (1975) who found a value of 4·7 s for the long time constant in the oculomotor response. Sugie and Melvill Jones (1971) observed a decrease in the long time constant T_B of the vestibulo-ocular response of drowsy subjects to a value of less than 2 s. This effect was undoubtedly partially brought about by the lack of saccadic activity with such a low level of arousal (Melvill Jones and Sugie, 1972).

The dynamic response of the extra-ocular muscles
It has been suggested that integration is effectively carried out by the eye globe dynamics (Melvill Jones, 1971). However, this would seem to be unlikely for two reasons: first, as stated previously, the signal at the level of the oculomotor neurones is already coded for eye position, and, second, available experimental evidence (Robinson, 1964, 1971; Reinhart and Zuber, 1970) indicates that the principal time constant of the eye globe dynamics is not higher than 200 ms, a value too low for effective integration at low frequencies.

The relationship between eye velocity and oculomotor firing rate is complex but may be given approximately by the equation:

$$\frac{\dot{\theta}}{f_{OMN}} = \frac{s}{(1 + T_E s)} \tag{12}$$

where $T_E \approx 150 - 200$ ms.

There is no doubt that the dynamic response of the eye and its musculature ought to have a significant effect on the overall vestibular response. In fact, at the frequency ($\approx$1 Hz) at which the eye globe dynamics ought to introduce attenuation in the canal-ocular reflex there is gain enhancement (see Fig. 11.4) in the response of first order afferents (equation 3). As noted earlier the canal-ocular response can only be effectively simulated by the introduction of a further time constant T_C, the value (0·12 s) of which is very close to that expected for the eye-globe dynamics. However, if the compensation for eye-globe dynamics does take place peripherally, it is necessary to invoke a further central mechanism to expain the oculomotor response during saccadic eye movements as explained by Robinson (1971).

The contribution of eye muscle proprioceptors
The role played by eye muscle proprioceptors is not at all clear at present, although they certainly exist (Whitteridge, 1960) and have some afferent representation within the brain (Fuchs and Kornhuber, 1969). Early experimental results indicated that they are not used to give conscious sensation of eye position (Brindley and Merton, 1960) although more recent experimental results (Brindley et al, 1976) have cast doubt upon this conclusion. It is doubtful whether they play a major part in the control of vestibular nystagmus, since experiments involving either cutting of the oculomotor nerve fibres (Maeda et al, 1972) curarization of eye muscles (Taylor, 1965) or clamping of the eye (Carpenter, 1972) do not appear to bring about any significant change in the output of the oculomotor neurones,

although recent work by Maffei and Fiorentini (1977) suggests there may be a modification of saccadic activity. Bach-y-Rita (1975) has carried out a detailed survey on the role of extraocular proprioceptors.

The contribution of neck proprioception to oculomotor responses

The ascending spinal afferents from the muscles of the neck are known to influence the vestibular (Rubin et al, 1975, 1977) and the oculomotor (Hikosaka and Maeda, 1973) nuclei via vestibulo-ocular pathways. The influence of neck receptors on sensations normally associated with vestibular stimulation has aroused considerable interest (Cohen, 1961; Biemond and Dejong, 1975; de Jong et al, 1978).

The existence of a cervico-ocular reflex in man has been demonstrated by Meiry (1965), Takemori and Suzuki (1971) and Barnes and Forbat (1979), although it is of a very weak nature. At low frequencies (0·1 Hz) when the subject's trunk was oscillated about the yaw axis while maintaining the head fixed in space, the slow phase eye movement was compensatory, being driven in phase with the motion of the trunk.

Meiry (1965) claimed that the responses of the cervico-ocular and vestibulo-ocular systems could be added to obtain the response during voluntary head movement. However, this would appear to be of little functional significance since the amplitude of neck induced eye movements is so small at frequencies of voluntary head movement (0·5–2 Hz) that there is no detectable difference in the oculomotor response during voluntary and passive head movement (Barnes, 1979a).

Neural mechanisms underlying modifications of the vestibulo-ocular response

Although discussion so far has assumed the vestibular response to be firmly established, in recent years it has been shown that the vestibulo-ocular response may be considerably modified. First, Gonshor and Melvill Jones (1976) have shown that the direction of the nystagmic eye movements may actually be reversed if the subject is presented with a long-term reversal of the visual world through the wearing of suitable prism lenses. In a similar experiment Robinson (1976) showed that such an extreme modification of the vestibulo-ocular response is probably brought about by the action of the vestibulo-cerebellum, which is known to receive both visual and vestibular afferents (Maekawa and Simpson, 1973; Brodal and Hoivik, 1964) and to project inhibitory fibres onto the vestibular nuclei (Brodal et al, 1962; Fernandez and Fredrickson, 1963; Shimazu and Smith, 1971). It is probable that a similar mechanism is brought into play in the adaptation which follows a unilateral labyrinthectomy, when the spontaneous nystagmus observed in the immediate post-operative period, resulting from the unbalanced spontaneous activity of the intact labyrinth progressively disappears over a period of one to two weeks (Dow and Moruzzi, 1968). However, it is likely that reciprocal inhibitory connections between the vestibular nuclei (Shimazu and Precht, 1966) also play an important part in this adaptation.

Secondly, as a result of recent experiments it has been suggested that the vestibulo-ocular response may be modified by mental set or by imaginary visual stimulus conditions. Collins and his colleagues (1961) and Melvill Jones and Sugie

(1972) showed that the level of mental arousal of the subject could affect the response considerably, the saccadic activity in particular tending to become diminished when the subject was drowsy. Barr and his colleagues (1976) have shown that the instruction set to the subject is also very important since subjects were able to decrease vestibulo-ocular response when attempting to fixate an imaginary head-fixed target or augment the response when imagining an earth-fixed target during head movement. Yasui and Young (1975) have also shown that the gain of the canal-ocular reflex can be enhanced when fixating upon an after-image.

Saccadic eye movements and their role in head-eye coordination
Whereas the velocity of the slow-phase components of nystagmus reflects the varying velocity of head movement, the saccadic, or fast phase components are of approximately constant velocity and constitute a fast resetting mechanism. However, it has become apparent from recent experiments that the saccade serves a functionally more important role during voluntary head movements. Melvill Jones (1964) was the first to show that the fast phase component becomes the dominant feature of the nystagmic response during high-rate angular oscillatory head movement. On the basis of these observations it was suggested that the saccade might serve the important function of introducing a rapid offset of the eye in the direction of head rotation during voluntary head movement.

During coordinated movements of the head and eyes to acquire offset visual targets there is a characteristic pattern of eye movement which consists of an initial saccadic component in the direction of head movement followed by a slower return towards orbital centre (Bartz, 1966; Bizzi et al, 1972; Gresty, 1974). The slow return serves to compensate for remaining head movement so that the eye attains its final position at the end of the saccade (Fig. 11.14). The experiments of Barnes (1975, 1976a, 1979b) showed that a similar pattern of responses could be elicited even in the absence of any visual information during voluntary head movements and during passive head movements in which the response was presumably elicited by stimulation of the lateral semicircular canals. The relationship between the amplitude of the gaze saccade and both head displacement and velocity were indistinguishable in all conditions. However differences in the latency of saccadic initiation with respect to head acceleration indicate that the vestibular system probably plays a subsidiary role to the visual control system in the initiation and control of the saccadic eye movement.

The mechanism of saccadic generation
Several attempts have been made to produce a mathematical model of the mechanism by which the saccadic eye movements of nystagmus are generated. Sugie and Melvill Jones (1965, 1971) first put forward the concept of a model having a primary and secondary pathway for vestibulo-ocular control in the manner suggested by Lorente de Nó (1933). In this model the primary pathway was responsible for the slow phase of nystagmus and the secondary contained a sampling mechanism responsible for the generation of fast phases. The sampling mechanism was assumed to operate at regular intervals of time; a feature also used in a model by Schmid (1970). As a consequence these models were unable to

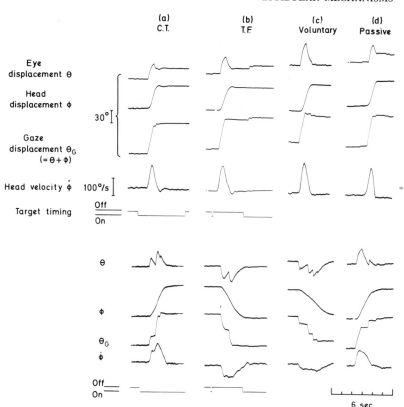

Fig. 11.14 Typical responses of the head and eyes during visual target acquisition (a and b) and during head movements in the dark (c and d) for approximately equivalent gaze displacements of 75° from centre. The head movements in the lower set of traces (ii) had peak velocities which were lower than normal as compared with those in the upper set (i).

account for the variation in the duration of slow-phase components that accompany changes in the amplitude and frequency of vestibular stimulation.

An attempt was made by Barnes (1973) (see also Barnes and Benson, 1973) to explain how the occurence of fast phases is controlled, using a model which was similar to that of Sugie and Melvill Jones (1965), but in which the secondary pathway contained a threshold detector. It was assumed that saccades would be generated whenever the vestibular afferent signal, which is coded for eye velocity, exceeded the threshold level. A feedback system operated around the threshold detector to inhibit its input following onset of a saccade; the resultant delay before the onset of another saccade was thus a function of the input level to the detector. This model was later modified (see Fig. 11.15) to simulate more effectively responses during voluntary head movements (Barnes, 1976b, 1977). It was able to explain the increase in saccadic beat frequency with increasing stimulus level, the paucity of saccadic activity at frequencies above 1 Hz and the preponderance of eye displacement in the direction of the fast phases (Mishkin and Melvill Jones, 1966). Models similar in concept but different in detail have been produced by Schmid and Lardini (1976) and by Chun (1977), the latter model incorporating an important component for the stochastic nature of the threshold detection.

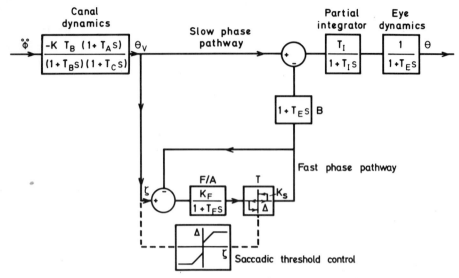

Fig. 11.15 A mathematical model of the vestibulo-ocular reflex for the control of lateral eye movements. The reflex consists of a basic slow-phase pathway and a secondary fast-phase pathway responsible for the generation of saccadic eye movements, both feeding into a partial integrator prior to eye muscle activation. Approximate values of the parameters not indicated in the text are: $T_F \approx 1$ s; $K_F \approx 1$.

An important feature of the models is that they indicate how the introduction of saccades enables the partial integrator to be continuously reset provided it lies downstream of the saccadic mechanism. The resultant transient response approximates a pure integration and thus increases the effectiveness of the neural integrating mechanism.

The neural basis of the saccadic mechanism

There is now a large body of experimental evidence which appears to link the reticular formation of the brainstem with saccadic eye movements of all kinds. Manni and Giretti (1970) were able to show that horizontal nystagmus could be evoked by stimulation of the superior colliculus when only the oculomotor nuclei and the associated reticular formation were intact. It has also been shown that units on both sides of the pons are active both before and during the fast phase of nystagmus (Duensing and Schaeffer, 1957; Sparks and Travis, 1971; Cohen and Henn, 1972; Luschei and Fuchs, 1972) and during saccades induced visually or by stimulation of the frontal cortex (Robinson and Fuchs, 1969; Robinson, 1970; Ron et al, 1972; Keller, 1974; Hikosaka et al, 1978). There appears to be little difference in the response of such units during saccades of all types (Cohen and Henn, 1972). The responses take the form of bursts of activity whose duration is related to the ensuing saccade. At any particular site there are some units which increase their rate of discharge during a horizontal saccade in one direction and decrease it for the other direction; other units show the opposite response.

Stimulation of reticular neurones induces predominantly constant velocity eye movements (Cohen and Komatsuzaki, 1972) and Bender and Shanzer (1964) found that there is a specificity in the direction of the induced eye movement which is dependent on the site of stimulation. Stimuli applied below the level of the trochlear nucleus induced ipsilateral deviations and those above the oculomotor nucleus, contra-lateral deviations, with mixed responses in the area around these two nuclei (see Fig. 11.10). The results of ablation studies in this area have been somewhat equivocal, but the body of evidence (Bender and Shanzer, 1964; McCabe, 1965; Cohen et al, 1968) appears to support the original findings of Lorente de Nó (1933) that ablation of the pontine reticular formation results in loss of saccadic eye movement of all types in the ipsilateral visual field. Finally, it must be mentioned that Duensing and Schaefer (1957) found neurones in the reticular formation closely associated with oculomotor activity which appeared to be influenced by the state of behavioural arousal of the experimental animal and it is reasonable to assume that these may represent the neurophysiological substrate of the arousal effects observed in vestibular nystagmus (Collins et al, 1961).

The interaction of visual and vestibular mechanisms

In recent years there has been considerable interest in the manner in which the visual and vestibular systems interact in the control of eye movement. This has stemmed from the realisation that visual stimuli can induce strong sensations of both linear motion (Berthoz et al, 1975) and rotation (Dichgans and Brandt, 1972, 1973) indicating a close relationship between the visual and vestibular systems. Considerable practical interest has also arisen from the need to maintain visual acuity in moving vehicles. The vestibulo-ocular reflex functions to stabilise the eye and enable fixation of objects fixed in space during vibration. Viewing of objects within a moving vehicle is thus made more difficult by the need to suppress inappropriate vestibular eye movements (Guedry, 1968; Gilson et al, 1970; Benson and Guedry, 1971). Barnes et al (1978) were able to show that during angular oscillation about the yaw and pitch axes visual acuity became impaired at frequencies above 1–2 Hz. Comparison of oculomotor responses during suppression of the vestibular reflex and during tracking of a moving display showed that the breakdown in performance occurred over a similar frequency range. Thus it was inferred that the pursuit reflex is responsible for visual suppression of inappropriate eye movements. Various models have been developed which describe the interaction of the visual and vestibular mechanisms (Barnes, 1976b; Raphan et al, 1977; Zacharias and Young, 1977; Benson and Barnes, 1978; Lau et al, 1978) which reflect the way in which visual information dominates at low frequencies (<0.5 Hz) and the vestibular system at higher frequencies.

There is now considerable neurophysiological evidence showing that the integration of visual and vestibular afferents takes place within the vestibular nuclei (Dichgans and Brandt, 1972; Henn et al, 1974; Fuchs and Kimm, 1975; Waespe and Henn, 1977) and it is probable that the modification of vestibular afferent activity is carried out by visual pathways through the cerebellum. Experiments by Takemori and Cohen (1974) have show that ablation of the flocculus, an area of the cerebellum known to be in receipt of visual afferents (Maekawa and Simpson, 1973) can result in defective optokinetic nystagmus and an inability to suppress vestibular nystagmus, a finding also supported by Lau et al, (1978).

THE VESTIBULO-SPINAL REFLEX MECHANISMS

The function of vestibulo-spinal reflexes

Whereas the effects of vestibular stimulation on the movements of the eyes are fairly circumscribed the influence upon the postural muscles is more difficult to define, principally because of the multiplicity of possible arrangements of the body as a whole and the interactions caused by body movement on the labyrinths themselves. In general, however, the reflex mechanisms serve, as for the eye, to compensate for imposed accelerations. Many of the reflex mechanisms are most easily demonstrated in lower animals; in man they are still functional but usually swamped by voluntary actions and learned responses. The vestibular reflex mechanisms from part of a total equilibratory system which includes basic spinal reflexes, neck reflexes, and visual control mechanisms.

Neurophysiology of vestibulo-spinal mechanisms

Vestibulo-spinal pathways
The manner in which the vestibular afferent fibres innervate the postural muscles is similar in many ways to that of the vestibulo-ocular reflex. There are two pathways by which direct disynaptic connections are made upon motoneurones, principally those of the axial musculature. The lateral vestibulo-spinal tract carries neurones originating in the lateral vestibular nucleus which descend ipsilaterally to all levels of the spinal cord (Brodal et al, 1962; Wilson and Yoshida, 1969; Wilson et al, 1970). Wilson and Maeda (1974) have shown that this pathway carries excitatory fibres from the ipsilateral anterior semicircular canal. Fibres in this tract also influence limb muscles, principally through polysynaptic connections upon spinal interneurones (Lund and Pompeiano, 1968; Grillner et al, 1970). The second major pathway, the medial vestibulo-spinal tract, carries fibres from the lateral, medial and descending vestibular nuclei to cervical and thoracic levels. Stimulation of individual semicircular canal afferents (Wilson and Maeda, 1974) has shown that the innervation of neck extensor muscles responsible for dorsiflexion of the head is as demonstrated Figure 11.16.

Pitching the head forward increases the discharge from the anterior canals and decreases that from the posterior which leads to compensatory neck extension. On the other hand, a rolling movement of the head would produce no activity in neck extensors if the excitatory and inhibitory effects exactly cancelled out. It is probable that a similar, but converse, reciprocal arrangement exists for the muscles responsible for lateral flexion of the head.

As with vestibular control of eye movement the disynaptic pathways are supplemented by projections from the vestibular nuclei onto reticular formation neurons which send fibres in the reticulo-spinal tract (Wilson and Yoshida, 1969; Wilson et al, 1970). These fibres make monosynaptic and disynaptic connections with both flexor and extensor motoneurones (Wilson and Peterson, 1978). The effects of stimulation of the maculae upon the spinal motoneurones was investigated by Szentagothai (1952), using mechanical stimulation of the utricle. More recently Wilson and his colleagues (1977) have shown that electrical stimulation of the saccular nerve normally inhibits contralateral but excites ipsilateral neck extensor motoneurones, whereas this pattern appears to be reversed for stimulation

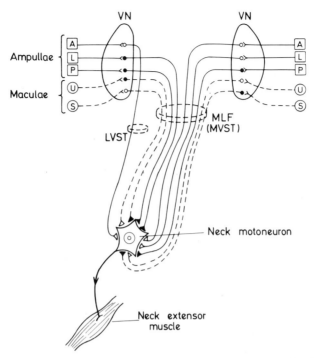

Fig. 11.16 A simplified diagram of the major pathways by which semicircular canal and macular afferents innervate the motoneurones of the neck extensors VN—vestibular nuclei. MLF— medial longitudinal fasciculus which becomes medial vestibulo-spinal tract (MVST). LVST—lateral vestibulo-spinal tract. A, L, and P—anterior, lateral and posterior semicircular canals. U. and S— utricular and saccular maculae (modified from Wilson and Maeda, 1974)

of the utricular nerve (Fig. 11.16). Many of the responses exhibited disynaptic connections.

Spino-vestibular pathways

The major difference between the vestibulo-spinal and the vestibulo-ocular reflexes is that in the latter the afferent fibres from the extra-ocular muscles appear to exert little or no direct effect upon the oculomotor response and have no direct representation within the vestibular nuclei; whereas the spinal afferent fibres, particularly from the cervical joint receptors (McCouch et al, 1951; Biemond and de Jong, 1969) are heavily represented within the vestibular nuclei (Rubin et al, 1975, 1977). Thus the oculomotor reflex is essentially open-loop, whereas the spinal mechanisms have the potential of operating as a closed-loop system.

The nature of vestibular myoneural control

The reflexes controlling posture have been divided into three categories: the positional, acceleratory and righting reflexes (Roberts, 1978). An example of the nature of vestibular reflex control is seen in the compensatory responses of extensor muscles when the body is titled in such a manner as to produce an acceleration of the vestibular system. Thus, for example in a quadruped, the sudden removal of support to the right forelimb induces an angular acceleration which stimulates excitatory activity in the right anterior vertical canal. This engenders an increase in the activity of the extensor muscle of the right forelimb and, by reciprocal action, a decrease in tone of the left hindlimb extensor muscle. The nett result is to stabilise the body so that the head remains in its normal position.

Positional reflexes

The vestibular system plays a key role in the positional reflexes, which are static postural adjustments adopted when the animals reference platform is displaced from its normal earth reference (Roberts, 1978). However, it has recently been shown (Lindsay et al, 1976; Roberts, 1978) that the labyrinthine reflex mechanisms act in a coordinated antagonistic manner with afferent responses arising from the proprioceptors in the neck, chiefly from the intervertebral joints. The evidence comes from an experiment in the cat in which, by deafferentation of the first two cervical nerves, the head and neck could be rotated independently. Right side-down stimulation of the vestibular system induced ipsilateral forelimb extension and contralateral flexion. In contrast, right side-down rotation of the neck induced contralateral extension and ipsilateral flexion. Thus when the support to the right forelimb induces an angular acceleration which stimulates excitatory activity in the right anterior vertical canal. This engenders an increase vestibulo-collic reflex attempts to bring the head back to its vertical position, thus twisting the neck to the left with respect to the body which serves to maintain the extension of the right-hand limbs. Linsday and his colleagues (1976) showed that the neck and labyrinthine influences in the limbs tended to be cancelled out when the neck and head were moved together, an obvious necessity to enable the animal to make voluntary head movements without postural adjustment.

These findings are in accord with the neurophysiological evidence for the projection of otolithic afferents (see Fig. 11.16). It is possible that the interaction of neck and vestibular afferents may take place within the vestibular nuclei where such effects have been demonstrated by Rubin and his associates (1975, 1977). This is supported by the apparent absence of any local spinal reflex mechanisms in the cervical muscles (Abrahams et al, 1975).

The reflex effects of angular acceleration on the limbs

Berthoz and Anderson (1971a) investigated the dynamic response of the vestibular reflex in forelimb extensors (triceps brachii) of the cat with sinusoidal angular oscillations about the roll axis. An essentially linear response was recorded in which the motor unit activity was modulated in accord with the stimulus waveform at frequencies between 0·1 and 1·5 Hz, with little response at higher frequencies. The response exhibited a phase lag of 20° to 30° on head angular velocity and a gain which decreased slightly over the frequency range tested (Fig. 11.17). Activity was similar in both forelimbs, leading to ipsilateral extension and contralateral flexion in the same manner as the responses to static tilt (Lindsay et al, 1976). No modulation could be observed after labyrinthectomy. Similar frequency response characteristics were recently obtained by Anderson and his colleagues (1977b) for oscillation in yaw.

It is difficult to assess the exact significance of these findings in relation to actual limb movement. Experiments by Rosentahl and his associates (1970) and Par-

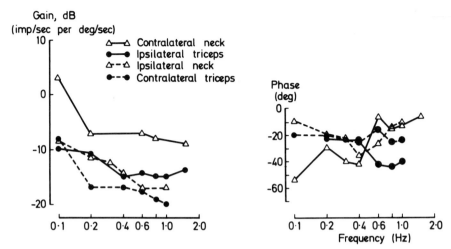

Fig. 11.17 The effect of sinusoidal oscillation about the roll axis on the motor unit discharge frequency in extensor muscles of the neck and forelimbs. Solid lines represent excitation, broken lines inhibition. (Redrawn from Berthoz and Anderson, 1971b.)

tridge and Kim (1969) indicate that muscle tension will lag behind motor unit activity in a manner which may be approximated as a first order response (time constant ≈ 0.2 s). However, the exact dynamic effect of this muscle tension will depend largely on the animals body mass distribution and the movement of the body, and of the head itself, will modify the vestibular outflow.

In humans, the contribution of the vestibular system to control of the standing posture is important, since in the absence of vision patients without functioning labyrinths are disorientated and find balance difficult. Nashner (1970) investigated the contribution of the various control mechanisms by selectively eliminating visual cues and ankle proprioception. He concluded that the acceleratory reflex from the vestibule could be principally attributed to the semicircular canals, as angular velocity transducers. Interestingly, the reflex response exhibited a mean reaction time of 220 ms which precludes its effectiveness as a high frequency control mechanism.

Nashner (1970) further showed that when the vestibular and proprioceptive reflex mechanisms were combined a much tighter control of postural equilibrium could be achieved with reduced thresholds of tilt detection and less overall sway displacement. Introduction of visual control both with and without the ankle reflex resulted in an improved damping of body movement and a better low frequency response. Thus, as for oculomotor control, the visual system appears to dominate postural control at low frequencies, vestibular and exteroceptive cues being preeminent at high frequency. Lee and Lishman (1975) have also shown that visual cues are very important in the reflex control of standing. Transient displacements of the peripheral visual field caused overbalancing in young children and adults deprived of an effective ankle reflex. It is clear that although the proprioceptive mechanisms appear to be the most effective component of the response, they alone are not sufficient in the absence of vision, as is demonstrated by the response of patients without functioning labyrinths. It is possible that the vestibular system influences the proprioceptive mechanisms via spinal interneurones (Wilson and

Peterson, 1978). Nashner, (1970) reported that labyrinthectomised patients compensate by increasing the stiffness of the ankle reflex and Benson (1959) observed a similar modification of the myotatic reflex during angular acceleration.

The reflex effects of angular acceleration on the neck

Clearly it is a gross oversimplification to consider that, in man, the body acts as a rigid structure, such that tilt from the vertical is compensated only by activity in the limbs. The process of stabilisation is a complex one in which the predominant corrective effects of vestibular influence are probably upon the muscles of the neck. In the cat, Berthoz and Anderson (1971b) have shown that during oscillation about the roll axis neck motoneurons responsible for head tilt exhibit a modulated response which is essentially similar to that of the contralateral forelimb extensor (Fig. 11.17). Thus a tilt to the right induces increased firing in neck motoneurones on the left-side which tends to bring the head upright. A similar finding has been published by Wilson and Peterson (1978). During oscillation about the yaw axis Berthoz and Anderson (1971b) found negligible response in forelimb extensors but a strong, modulated response in neck motoneurons with dynamic properties similar to those in roll.

The movement of the head induced by the EMG activity recorded in neck muscles is more predictable than that of the limbs since the mass distribution of the head is normally constant. Bizzi and his colleagues (1976) have shown that visually directed head movements in the monkey are of a ballistic nature, not affected by feedback of head position, whereas it might be expected that vestibular feedback would exert some effect upon the response. However, as discussed earlier, it is probable that neck proprioceptive information cancels out the vestibular response within the vestibular nuclei in the manner demonstrated by Rubin and his colleagues (1975, 1977), so that the head displacement depends solely upon the EMG activity initiated by voluntary command.

In animals such as the pigeon (Dunlap and Mowrer, 1930) it is possible to observe nystagmic head movements during vestibular stimulation similar to those of the eye which are brought about by the vestibulo-ocular reflex. Outerbridge and Melvill Jones (1971) have shown that it can even be observed in man when the subject is in a relaxed state.

It is of interest that the response observed in both forelimb and neck motoneurons is phase lagged with respect to head velocity and thus to the output of the vestibular system (cf. Fig. 11.4). Some form of integration of the vestibular afferent signal must take place, probably within the reticular formation of the brain-stem. In this respect there is a close similarity in the vestibular reflex control of neck and eye muscles.

The reflex effects of linear acceleration on the limbs

The effects of periodic linear acceleration on the forelimbs of the cat have been investigated by Anderson and his colleagues (1977b) for all three orthogonal body axes. The EMG activity in motor units of triceps brachii is illustrated in Figure 11.18 as a function of the frequency of oscillation. It is apparent that the response to acceleration in all three axes is very similar. Comparison of these responses with those of macular afferent units (regular) in the monkey (Fig. 11.7) indicates that a

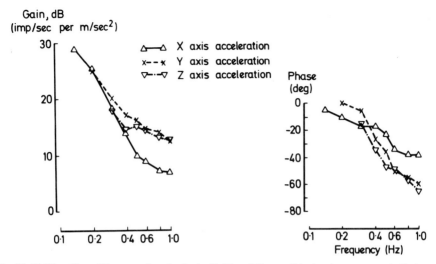

Fig. 11.18 The effect of linear acceleration in the X, Y, and Z axes of the head on motor unit discharge frequency in triceps brachii of the cat. During Y axis acceleration, activity is excitatory in the limb ipsilateral to the direction in which the animal is accelerated. (Redrawn from Anderson et al 1977a.)

considerable modification has taken place with a decrease in gain and increasing phase lag at high frequency, indicative of a process of central integration.

The functional significance of these findings is shown in Fig. 11.19a. Acceleration along the Y axis from left to right induces excitation in the right extensor and flexion in the left triceps, thus resisting body tilt to the right. Similarly, acceleration along the X axis of the body from tail to head induces an extensor propping reaction in the forelimbs and presumably flexion of the hindlimbs which serves to reduce the effective angular momentum. In these conditions the hopping reflex (see p. 285) is likely to be invoked in order to broaden the stance and improve the usefulness of the propping reactions. It is probable also that other limb muscles will be brought into play, for example those resisting rotation at the shoulder. Upward acceleration along the Z axis in the normal standing posture induces flexion in the forelimbs (and probably also in the hindlimbs) and thus tends to absorb much of the movement and stabilise the head, an effect which may be observed in skiers on rough terrain.

The role of the otoliths and canals in the reflex response

The relative roles of the semicircular canals and otoliths in the compensatory response of the neck is not certain. However, as Roberts (1978) points out it is logical to assume that the system operates as a conventional servo-system, in which positional feedback is provided by the otoliths, whereas the canals provide damping to the response with velocity feedback. This is supported by the evidence that damage to the semicircular canals can result in undamped oscillations of the head.

However, as Nashner (1970) has pointed out, the information arising from the otoliths is often equivocal. Thus, in the human subject, a backward tilt of the

whole body would result in an increased component of the gravitational acceleration upon the utricle. If the body is undergoing acceleration towards the earth the
tangential component of the acceleration will serve to counteract the effects of
gravity and may even reverse the direction of deviation of the statoconia. The
ability of the otoliths alone to sense deviation from the vertical has been called into
question by the experiments of Guedry and Harris (1963) on the parallel swing,
where a purely linear acceleration was unable to induce a sensation of tilt in normal
subjects.

The anomaly may be clearly demonstrated when comparing the response of the
reflex mechanisms to linear acceleration and body tilt. As we have seen in the
previous section, a linear acceleration (such as might be induced by pushing
the animal from the left side) induces increased tone in the limbs on the right side,
as is appropriate (Fig. 11.19a). However, this response would be inappropriate if
a similar linear acceleration in the plane of the utricular otoliths were introduced
by acceleration to the right, of a platform, upon which the animal is standing.
(Fig. 11.19b). Although in both examples the utricular otoliths experience an
acceleration to the right, there are important differences in the angular accelerations in the two conditions, which will be to the animal's right in the first example,
to its left in the second. As shown earlier (Berthoz and Anderson, 1971b), during
dynamic tilt about the roll axis the side-down limb is extended—the appropriate
response for the second condition (Fig. 11.19b). Thus it appears that the response
of the canal-forelimb reflex is able to modify the response of the utricular otoliths to
the extent of reversing the pattern of excitation and inhibition in the forelimbs.

Anderson and his colleagues (1977b) have shown that the responses of the
otoliths and canals are combined in an apparently linear manner during concomi-

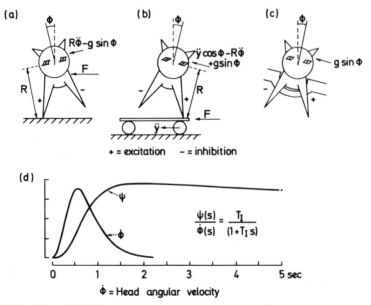

+ = excitation   − = inhibition

$$\frac{\psi(s)}{\phi(s)} = \frac{T_1}{(1+T_1 s)}$$

$\dot{\phi}$ = Head angular velocity

Fig. 11.19 The different forelimb responses to be expected during various stimuli all involving linear
acceleration to the animal's right side (and thus otolith deflection to the left). The expected response (Ψ)
in the limb extensors from stimulation of the vertical semicircular canals is shown in (d).

tant angular oscillation about the yaw axis and linear accelerations about the X or Y axes. One of the effects was that of changing the phase of the response. It is possible that a similar interaction takes place between the vertical canals and the otoliths.

It is more difficult, however, to explain the difference in the response when the body is pushed from the left side (Fig. 11.19a) and that observed when the whole body is tilted to the left (Fig. 11.19c) (Lindsay et al, 1976). In both examples the acceleration and resultant otolithic deflection is in the same sense and yet the pattern of excitation in the forelimbs is reversed. At first sight it would appear that in the tilt condition the only stimulus is to the maculae, since the canal response will decay after the cessation of rotation (Roberts, 1978).

However, as noted earlier, for all the vestibular-forelimb reflex responses there is some central process of integration. Thus during a rotational displacement, the canals fairly accurately signal head angular velocity, but after integration the output more closely represents head position as demonstrated in Fig. 11.19d. As this is only a partial integration it is to be expected that the response in the muscle would decay over a period related to the time constant of the integrator. Just such a response decay was observed by Berthoz and Anderson (1971a) to take place over a period of 10–20s. Lindsay and his colleagues (1976) do not report this effect, possibly because head tilt in their experiment was maintained for a period of only 5 s. An exactly similar response may be observed in the canal-ocular reflex as a result of rotational displacement (Barnes, 1979b). It seems probable that the canals and otoliths interact in a complex manner in normal circumstances to maintain the appropriate activity in the limbs.

Righting reflexes and other complex postural adjustments

The righting reflexes are essentially a particular example of the behaviour of the vestibular, neck and limb reflex mechanisms already discussed. When an animal is lying with head and body constrained on one side the labyrinthine reflexes are ineffective in attempting to bring the animal to the upright position. However, if the head is free, labyrinthine reflexes initiate activity which brings the head toward the upright position thus stimulating neck receptors which, in turn, excite the axial musculature to twist the trunk. At the same time, the action of the labyrinthine and/or neck reflexes is to draw the side-down limbs into the body and extend those of the opposite side so that the animal is in a position to lever itself into the upright position. In fact, these involuntary postural adjustments can be observed in animals without functional labyrinths and are then thought to be initiated by pressure receptors. In higher animals such reflex mechanisms tend to be overriden or dominated by higher cerebral functions such as vision.

Another example of the complex interaction of labyrinths and exteroceptive cues is seen in the hopping reaction in which the limbs are repositioned to achieve greater stabilisation in response to body tilt. This has been investigated by Roberts (1978) in man, who concludes that stimulation of any one of the sites involved in transducing body tilt (i.e. ankle, hip joint, otolith, canal) is of itself insufficient to establish the hopping reflex. What is required is the combination of a change in the force vector sensed by the labyrinths (i.e. whole body tilt) together with a change in the leg-ankle angle. Again, as was observed with the interaction of neck and labyrinth reflexes, an essential mechanism has been built in to allow voluntary independent movements of the head or the ankle to be made without the effect of a countermanding reflex mechanism. If this hopping reaction fails to reinstate body stability, further hopping or staggering movements may be initiated, but if this also fails then attempts are made to redistribute the body mass by sweeping actions of the limbs, the inertial effects of which may be sufficient to restore equilibrium. Failure of this manoeuvre results in more complex reactions being invoked to break the fall, and more particularly to protect the head against injury. The vestibular labyrinths probably play little direct part in this response since it can also be observed in labyrinthine-defective subjects (Purdon-Martin, 1967). In addition, Melvill Jones and Watt (1971b) have estimated that the reaction time involved in the muscle response to a sudden fall is considerable (≈ 100 ms) and may be too great to initiate a reaction before impact.

CONCLUSIONS

Many different techniques are currently being used to investigate the various components of the vestibulo-ocular and vestibulo-spinal reflex mechanisms. Electrophysiological experiments on animals have provided vital information about the neural mechanisms and response characteristics of the vestibular end-organs, the brain-stem relay centres and of the motoneurones which carry out the reflex actions. In humans such investigations are not usually possible except by inference from the responses of those with certain disease states. In most experimental studies in man the system has been investigated as a whole, particularly through the use of control system analysis techniques. Psycho-physical techniques such as threshold detection and visual acuity tests have also been used extensively to assess human system behaviour.

In general all these methods have combined to provide the following scheme for the vestibular reflex mechanisms. The semicircular canals provide information about head angular velocity, whereas the otolith organs give a response related to head linear acceleration. Both groups of afferents are relayed through the vestibular nuclei from which second order afferents synapse on motor nuclei for driving the muscles of the eyes, the neck and the limbs. A feature, which appears to be common to all the reflex pathways, is that some process of integration with respect to time takes place between the vestibular nuclei and the motoneurones. Where and how this integration process is achieved is a research topic currently attracting a lot of interest.

The vestibulo-ocular reflexes, which are essentially open loop in the absence of vision, provide a fairly simple mechanism for inducing eye movements which compensate for head movement. In the vestibulo-spinal reflexes it is more difficult to envisage the dynamic response which will be produced by the recorded EMG activity since the reflex has the possibility of operating as a closed loop system through proprioceptive feedback mechanisms. In contrast to the eye the dynamic load on the limb muscles may vary considerably, although it is possible that head control operates in open loop since its load is not likely to vary except when modern man is required to wear cumbersome protective headgear! It remains to be shown what functional role the reflex eye and limb movement evoked by dynamic otolith stimulation may play, particularly in the limbs where there appears to be a complex interaction with canal afferent information.

The research which has been carried out in recent years has given rise to many new and important techniques for the clinical diagnosis of the vestibular system and other associated areas, particularly that of eye movement control. In particular, the various experimental results implicating the vestibular nuclei and the cerebellum in the integration of visual and vestibular oculomotor control mechanisms have provided means of differentiating between some peripheral and central disorders of the vestibular system.

In aerospace medicine too, the investigation of the vestibular system continues to play an important role and provides much of the impetus for research, particularly with regard to the effect on visual acuity when the head and body are subjected to vibration and to the problems of disorientation and motion sickness associated with stimulation of the vestibular system.

ACKNOWLEDGEMENTS

This chapter was originally published as a review article in Clinical Physics and Physiological Measurement (Vol 1:3–40) and is reproduced by permission of the Institute of Physics.

REFERENCES

Abrahams V C, Richmond F, Rose P K 1975 Absence of monosynaptic reflex in dorsal neck muscles of the cat. Brain Research 92:130–131
Anderson J H, Soechting J F, Terzuola C A 1977a Dynamic relations between natural vestibular inputs and activity of forelimb extensor muscles in the decerebrate cat. 1. Motor output during sinusoidal linear accelerations. Brain Research 120:1–15
Anderson J H, Soechting J F, Terzuola C A 1977b Dynamic relations between natural vestibular inputs and activity of forelimb extensor muscles in the decerebrate cat. II. Motor output during rotations in the horizontal plane. Brain Research 120:17–33
Bach-Y-Rita P 1975 Structural-functional correlations in eye muscle fibres. Eye muscle proprioception. In: Bach-Y-Rita P (ed) Basic Mechanisms of Ocular Motility and their Clinical Implications. Pergamon Press, Oxford, pp 91–111
Baker R G, Mano N, Shimazu H 1969 Intracellular recording of antidromic responses from abducens motoneurons in the cat. Brain Research 15:573–580
Baker R, Precht W, Berthoz A 1973 Synaptic connections to trochlear motoneurons determined by individual vestibular nerve branch stimulation in the cat. Brain Research 64:402–406
Barmack N H 1974 Saccadic discharges evoked by intracellular stimulation of extraocular motoneurons. Journal of Neurophysiology 37:395–412
Barmack N H, Bell C C, Rence B G 1971 Tension and rate of tension development during isometric responses of extraocular muscle. Journal of Neurophysiology 34:1072–1079
Barnes G R 1971 A theoretical model of the utricular otolith and its response to angular motion with respect to an acceleration in shear. FPRC Rep 1315 London MOD (Air)
Barnes G R 1973 The mechanism for saccadic eye movement generation in the vestibulo-ocular system. FPRC Rep 1325 London MOD (Air)
Barnes G R 1974 The role of the vestibular system in head-eye coordination. Journal of Physiology 246:99–100P
Barnes G R 1976a The role of the vestibulo-ocular reflex in visual target acquisition. Journal of Physiology 258:64–65P
Barnes G R 1976b Vestibulo-ocular responses to head turning movements and their functional significance during visual target acquisition. Ph. D. Thesis, University of Surrey, Guildford, Surrey, UK
Barnes G R 1977 The role of the saccadic mechanism in head-eye coordination: The development of a theoretical model. RAF Institute of Aviation Medicine, Farnborough, Hants, UK Report No 570

Barnes G R 1979a Head-eye co-ordination in normals and in patients with vestibular disorders. Advances in Oto-Rhino-Laryngology, Vol 25 : pp 197–201 Karger, Basel

Barnes G R 1979b Vestibulo-ocular function during co-ordinated head and eye movements to acquire visual targets. Journal of Physiology, 287 : 127–147

Barnes G R, Benson A J 1973 A model for the prediction of the nystagmic response to angular and linear acceleration stimuli. The Use of Nystagmography in Aviation Medicine. NATO AGARD, CP-128, pp A23 1–13

Barnes G R, Benson A J 1978 Adaptation in the caloric response. In: Hood J D (ed) The vestibular system in health and disease. Academic Press, London, pp 254–262

Barnes G R, Forbat L N 1979 Cervical and vestibular afferent control of oculomotor response in man. Acta Oto Laryngologica 88 : 79–87

Barnes G R, Benson A J, Prior A R J 1978 Visual-vestibular interaction in the control of eye movement. Aviation, Space and Environmental Medicine 49 : 557–564

Barr C C, Schultheis L W, Robinson D A 1976 Voluntary, non-visual control of the human vestibulo-ocular reflex. Acta Oto-Laryngologica 81 : 365–375

Bartz P E, 1966 Eye and head movements in peripheral vision: Nature of compensatory eye movements. Science, 152 : 1644–1645

Belcher S J 1964 Ocular torsion. British Journal of Physiological Optics, 21 : 1–20

Bender M B, Shanzer S 1964 Oculomotor pathways defined by electric stimulation and lesion in the brainstem of monkey. In: Bender M B (ed) The Oculomotor System, Harper & Row, New York and London, pp 81–140

Benson A J 1959 Effect of labyrinthine stimulation on reflex and postural activity in gastrocnemius-soleus muscle group in man. Journal of Physiology 146 : 37–38P

Benson A J 1968 Lateral eye movements produced by a rotating linear acceleration. Journal of Physiology 197 : 85–86P

Benson A J 1979 Interactions between semicircular canals and gravireceptors. In: Busby D E(ed) Recent Advances in Aerospace Medicine, D. Reidel, Dordrechty Holland, pp 249–261

Benson A J 1972 Effect of angular oscillation in yaw on vision. Proceedings of the Aerospace Medical Association Scientific meeting 43 : 43–44

Benson A J 1974 Modification of the response to angular accelerations by linear accelerations. In: Kornhuber H H (ed) Handbook of Sensory Physiology, Springer-Verlag, Berlin pp 281–230

Benson A J, Barnes G R 1973 Responses to rotating linear acceleration vectors considered in relation to a model of the otolith organs. 5th NASA Symposium on the Role of the Vestibular Organs in the Exploration of Space, Pensacola Fla. SP-314. Washington DC. NASA pp 221–236

Benson A J, Barnes G R 1978 Vision during angular oscillation: The dynamic interaction of visual and vestibular mechanisms. Aviation, Space and Environmental Medicine

Benson A J, Bodin M A 1966a Interaction of linear and angular accelerations on vestibular receptors in man. Aerospace Medicine 37 : 144–154

Benson A J, Bodin M A 1966b Comparison of the effect of the direction of the gravitational acceleration on post rotational responses in yaw, pitch and roll. Aerospace Medicine 37 : 889–897

Benson A J, Burchard E 1973 Spatial Disorientation in Flight. NATO AGARD-AG-170

Benson A J, Guedry F E 1971 Comparison of tracking performance and nystagmus during sinusoidal oscillation in yaw and pitch. Aerospace Medicine 42 : 593–601

Benson A J, Guedry F E, Melvill Jones G 1970 Response of semicircular canal dependent units in vestibular nuclei to rotation of a linear acceleration vector without angular acceleration. Journal of Physiology 210 : 475–494

Berthoz A, Anderson J H 1971a Frequency analysis of vestibular influence on extensor motoneurons. I. Response to tilt in forelimb extensors. Brain Research 34 : 370–375

Berthoz A, Anderson J H 1971b Frequency analysis of vestibular influence on extensor motoneurons. II. Relationship between neck and forelimb extensors. Brain Research 34 : 376–380

Berthoz A, Pavard B, Young L R 1975 Perception of linear horizontal self-motion induced by peripheral vision. Experimental Brain Research 23 : 471–489

Biemond A, De Jong J M B V 1969 On cervical nystagmus and related disorders Brain 92 : 437–458

Bizzi E, Polit A, Morasso P 1976 Mechanisms underlying achievement of final head position. Journal of Neurophysiology 39 : 435–437

Bizzi E, Kalil R E, Morasso P, Tagliasco V 1972 Central programming and peripheral feedback during eye-head coordination in monkeys. In: Dichgans J, Bizzi E (eds) Cerebral control of eye movements and motion perception Karger, Basel pp 220–232

Blanks R H I, Estes M S, Markham C H 1975 Physiologic characteristics of vestibular first-order canal neurons in the cat. II. Response to constant angular acceleration. Journal of Neurophysiology 38 : 1250–1268

Breuer J 1889 Neue Versuche an den Ohrbogengangen. Pflügers Archiv für die gesamte Physiologie des Menschen und der Tiere 44 : 135–152

Brindley G S, Merton P A 1960 The absence of position sense in the human eye. Journal of Physiology 153 : 127–130

Brindley G S, Goodwin G M, Kulikowski J J, Leighton D 1976 Stability of vision with a paralysed eye. Journal of Physiology 258 : 65–66P

Brodal A, 1974 Anatomy of the vestibular neclei and their connections. In 'Handbook of Sensory Physiology'. Vol VI/1. Vestibular System. Ed. Kornhuber H H, Berlin. Springer-Verlag pp 239–352

Brodal A, Hoivik B 1964 Site and mode of termination of primary vesti bulocerebellar fibres in the cat. An experimental study with silver impregnation methods. Archives italiennes de biologie 102 : 1–21

Brodal A, Pompeiano O, Walberg F 1962 The vestibular nuclei and their connections, anatomy and functional correlations. Ramsay Henderson Trust Lectures. Edinburgh and London: Oliver & Boyd

Carpenter R H S 1972 Cerebellectomy and the transfer function of the vestibulo-ocular reflex in the decerebrate cat. Proceedings of the Royal Society of London. Series B. 181 : 353–374

Carpenter R H S 1977 Movements of the Eyes. (London: Pion)

Chun K S 1977 Mathematical model of the vestibulo-ocular reflex. Naval Surface Weapons Centre, Dahlgren Lab, Dahlgren, Virginia, US Report: NSWC/DL TR-3669

Cohen B, Henn V 1972 The origin of quick phases of nystagmus in the horizontal plane. In: 'Cerebral control of eye movements and motion perception'. Karger Basel, pp 36–55

Cohen B, Komatsuzaki A 1972 Eye movements induced by stimulation of the pontine reticular formation: Evidence for integration in oculomotor pathways. Experimental Neurology 36 : 101–117

Cohen B, Komatsuzaki A, Bender M B 1968 Electro-occulographic syndrome in monkeys after pontine reticular formation lesions. Archives of Neurology (Chic) 18 : 78–92

Cohen B, Suzuki J, Bender M B 1964 Eye movements from semicircular canal nerve stimulation in the cat. Annals of Otology, Rhinology and Laryngology (St. Louis) 73 : 153–169

Cohen B, Suzuki J, Bender M B 1965 Nystagmus induced by electric stimulation of ampullary nerves. Acta Oto-Laryngologica 60 : 422–436

Cohen L A 1961 Role of eye and neck proprioceptive mechanisms in body orientation and motor co-ordination. Journal of Neurophysiology 24 : 1–11

Collins W E, Crampton G H, Posner J B 1961 Effects of mental activity on vestibular nystagmus and the electroencephalogram. Nature, 190 : 194–195

Correia M J, Guedry F E 1966 Modification of vestibular responses as a function of rate of rotation about an earth horizontal axis. Acta Oto-Laryngologica 62 : 297–308

Correia M J, Landolt J P 1973 Spontaneous and driven responses from primary neurons of the anterior semicircular canal of the pigeon. Advances in Oto-Rhino-Laryngology 19 : 132–148

Correia M J, Money K E 1970 The effect of blockage of all six semicircular canal ducts on nystagmus produced by dynamic linear acceleration in the cat. Acta Oto Laryngologica 69 : 7–16

Dichgans J, Brandt T 1972 Visual-vestibular interaction and motion perception. In 'Cerebral control of eye movements and motion perception'. Karger Basel, pp 327–338

Dichgans J, Brandt T 1973 Optokinetic motion sickness and pseudo-coriolis effects induced by moving visual stimuli. Acta Oto-Laryngologica 339–348

Dodge R 1903 Five types of eye movements in the horizontal meridian plane of the field of regard. American Journal of Physiology 8 : 307–329

Dodge R, Cline T 1901 The angle velocity of eye movements. Psychological Review 8 : 125–157

Dow R S, Moruzzi G 1968 The Physiology and Pathology of the Cerebellum. (Minneapolis: Univ. Minnesota Press)

Duensing F, Schaefer K P 1957 Die Neuronenaktivitat in der Formatio reticularis des Rhombencephalons beim vestibularen Nystagmus. Archiv für Psychiatrie und Nervenkrankheiten, vereinigt mit Zeitschrift für die gesamte Neurologie und Psychiatrie 196 : 265–290

Dunlap K, Mowrrer O H 1931 Head movements and eye functions of birds. Journal of Comparative Psychology 11 : 99–112

Van Egmond A A J, Groen J J, Jongkees L B W 1949 The mechanics of the semicircular canals. Journal of Physiology 110 : 1–17

Estes M S, Blanks R H I, Markham C H 1975 Physiologic characteristics of vestibular first-order canal neurons in the cat. 1. Response plane determination and resting discharge characteristics. Journal of Neurophysiology 38 : 1232–1268

Fernandez C, Frederickson J M 1963 Experimental cerebellar lesions and their effect on vestibular function. Acta Oto-Laryngologica Suppl. 192 : 52–62

Fernandez C, Goldberg J M 1971 Physiology of peripheral neurons innervating semicircular canals of squirrel monkey. II. Response to sinusoidal stimulation and dynamics of peripheral vestibular system. Journal of Neurophysiology 34 : 661–675

Fernandez C, Goldberg J M 1976 Physiology of peripheral neurons innervating otolith organs of the squirrel monkey. Parts 1, 2 and 3. Journal of Neurophysiology 39:970–1008

Fernandez C, Goldberg J M, Abend W K 1972 Response to static tilts of peripheral neurons innervating otolith organs of the squirrel monkey. Journal of Neurophysiology 35:978–997

Fluur E, Mellstrom A 1971 The otolith organs and their influence on oculomotor movements. Experimental Neurology 30:139–147

Fuchs A F, Kimm J 1975 Unit activity in vestibular nucleus of the alert monkey during horizontal angular acceleration and eye movement. Journal of Neurophysiology 38:1140–1161

Fuchs A F, Kornhuber H H 1969 Extraocular muscle afferents to the cerebellum of the cat. Journal of Physiology 200:713–722

Fujita Y, Rosenberg J, Segundo J P 1968 Activity in cells of the lateral vestibular nucleus as a function of head position. Journal of Physiology 196:1–18

Gernandt B E 1949 Response of mammalian neurons to horizontal rotation and caloric stimulation. Journal of Neurophysiology 12:173–184

Gilson R D, Benson A J, Guedry F E 1970 Influence of vestibular stimulation and display luminance on the performance of a compensatory tracking task. Pensacola, Fla. Naval Aerospace Medical Institute Rep 1097

Goldberg J M, Fernandez C 1971 Physiology of peripheral neurons innervating semicircular canals of the squirrel monkey. Journal of Neurophysiology 34:635–684

Goldberg J M, Fernandez C 1975 Vestibular mechanisms. Annual Review of Physiology 37:129–162

Gonshor A, Melvill Jones G 1976 Short-term changes in the human vestibulo-ocular reflex arc. Journal of Physiology 256:361–379

Gresty M A 1974 Coordination of head and eye movements to fixate continuous and intermittent targets. Vision Research 14:395–403

Groen J J, Lowenstein O, Vendrick A J H 1952 The mechanical analysis of the responses from the end-organs of the horizontal semicircular canal in the isolated elasmobranch labyrinth. Journal of Physiology 117:329–346

Grillner S, Hongo T, Lund S 1970 The vestibulospinal tract. Effects on Alpha-motoneurones in the lumbosacral spinal cord of the cat. Experimental Brain Research 10:94–120

Guedry F E 1968 Relations between vestibular nystagmus and visual performance. Aerospace Medicine 39:570–579

Guedry F E, Harris C S 1963 Labyrinthine function related to experiments on the parallel swing. Pensacola, Fla, US Naval School of Aviation Medicine Report No 86

Guedry F E, Lauver L S 1961 Vestibular reactions during prolonged constant angular acceleration. Journal of applied physiology 16:215–220

Hallpike C S, Hood J D 1953 The speed of the slow component of ocular nystagmus induced by angular acceleration of the head: Its experimental determination and application to the physical theory of the cupular mechanism. Proceedings of the Royal Society. Series B 141:216–230

Henn V R, Young L R, Finley C 1974 Vestibular nucleus units in alert monkeys are also influenced by moving visual fields. Brain Research 71:144–149

Highstein S M 1971 Organisation of the inhibitory and excitatory vestibulo-ocular reflex pathways to the IIIrd and IVth nuclei in rabbit. Brain Research 32:218–224

Highstein S M, Ito M, Tsuchiya T 1971 Synaptic linkage in the vestibulo-ocular reflex pathway of rabbit. Experimental Brain Research 13:306–326

Hikosaka O, Maeda M 1973 Cervical effects on abducens motoneurons and their interaction with vestibulo-ocular reflex. Experimental Brain Research 18:512–530

Hikosaka O, Igusa Y, Nakao S, Shimazu H 1978 Direct inhibitory synaptic linkage of pontomedullary reticular burst neurons with abducens motoneurons in the cat. Experimental Brain Research 33:337–352

Hixson W 1974 Frequency response of the oculovestibular system during yaw oscillation. NAMRL-1212 Pensacola, Fla

Igarashi M 1966 Dimensional study of the vestibular end organ apparatus. In: Second Symposium on the Role of the Vestibular Organs in Space Exploration. Washington DC: NASA SP-115 pp 47–54

Janeke J B 1968 On nystagmus and otoliths. A vestibular study of responses as provoked by a cephalo-caudal horizontal axial rotation. Doctoral Thesis: Univ. of Amsterdam

De Jong P T V M, De Jong J M B V, Cohen B, Jongkees L B W 1977 Ataxia and nystagmus induced by injection of local anaesthetics in the neck. Annals of Neurology 1:240–246

Jongkees L B W 1967 On the otoliths: their function and the way to test them. In: 3rd Symposium on the Role of the Vestibular Organs in Space Exploration. NASA SP-152 pp 307–330

Keller E L 1974 Participation of medial pontine formation in eye movement generation in monkey. Journal of Neurophysiology 37:316–332

Keller E L 1978 Gain of the vestibulo-ocular reflex in monkey at high rotational frequencies. Vision Research 18:311–315

De Kleijn A 1921 Tonische labyrinth-und halsreflexe auf die augen. Pflügers Archiv für die gesamte Physiologie des Menschen und der Tiere 186:82–97

Landers P H, Taylor A 1975 Transfer function analysis of the vestibulo-ocular reflex in the conscious cat. In: Lenerstrand G, Bach-y-Rita P (eds) Basic mechanisms of ocular motility and their clinical implications. Pergamon Press, Oxford, pp 505–509.

Lau C G Y, Honrubia V, Jenkins H A, Baloh R W, Yee R D 1978 Linear model for visual-vesticular interaction. Aviation, Space and Environmental Medicine 49:880–885

Lee D N, Lishman J R 1975 Visual proprioceptive control of stance. Journal of Human Movement Studies 1:87–95

Lindsay K W, Roberts T D M, Rosenberg J R 1976 Asymmetric tonic labyrinth reflexes and their interaction with neck reflexes in the decerebrate cat. Journal of Physiology 261:583–601

Loe P R, Tomko D L, Werner G 1973 The neural signal of angular head position in the primary afferent vestibular nerve axons. Journal of Physiology 230:29–50

Lorente De No R 1933 Vestibulo-ocular reflex arc. Archives of Neurology and Psychiatry Chicago 30:245–291

Lowenstein O, Roberts T D M 1950 The equilibrium function of the otolith organs of the Thornback Ray Raja Clavata. Journal of Physiology 110:392–415

Lowenstein O, Sand A 1940 The mechanism of the semicircular canal. Study of the responses of single-fibre preparations to angular accelerations and to rotation at constant speed. Proceedings of the Royal Society. Series B London 129:256–275

Lowenstein O, Saunders R D 1975 Otolith-controlled responses from the first-order neurons of the labyrinth of the bullfrog (Rana Catesbeina) to changes in linear acceleration. Proceedings of the Royal Society of London. Series B 191:475–505

Lowenstein O, Wersall J 1959 A functional interpretation of the electron-microscopic structure of the sensory hairs in the cristae of the elasmo branch Raja Clavata in terms of directional sensitivity. Nature 184:1087–1808

Lund S, Pompeiano O 1968 Monosynaptic excitation of alpha motoneurons from supraspinal structures in the cat. Acta physiologica scandinavica 73:1–29

Luschei E, Fuchs A F 1972 Activity of brain stem neurons during eye movements of alert monkeys. Journal of Neurophysiology 35:445–461

McCabe B F 1965 The quick component of nystagmus. Laryngoscope 75:1619–1646

McCouch G P, Deering I D, Ling T H 1951 Location of receptors for tonic neck reflexes. Journal of Neurophysiology 14:191–195

McMasters R E, Weiss A H, Carpenter M B 1966 Vestibular projections to the nuclei of the extraocular muscles. Degeneration resulting from discrete partial lesions of the vestibular nuclei in the monkey. American Journal of Anatomy 118:163–194

Maeda M, Shimazu H, Shinoda Y 1972 Nature of synaptic events in cat abducens motoneurons at slow and quick phase of vestibular nystagmus. Journal of Neurophysiology 35:279–296

Maekawa K, Simpson J I 1973 Climbing fibre responses in vestibulocerebellum of rabbit from visual system. Journal of Neurophysiology 36:649–666

Maffei L, Fiorentini A 1977 Oculomotor proprioception in the cat. In: Baker R, Berthoz A (eds) Control of gaze by brainstem neurons. Elsevier, Amsterdam, pp 477–481

Malcolm R 1971 Human responses to vestibular stimulation and some implications to the flight environment. Ph D Thesis. McGill University, Montreal, Canada

Malcolm R 1974 A mechanism by which the hair cells of the inner ear transduce mechanical energy into a modulated train of action potentials. Journal of General Physiology 63:757–772

Manni E, Giretti M L 1970 Central eye nystagmus in the pontomesencephalic preparation. Experimental Neurology 26:342–353

Meiry J 1965 The vestibular system and human dynamic space orientation. Cambridge, Mass: MIT Report T-65-1

Melvill Jones G 1964 Predominance of anti-compensatory oculomotor response during rapid head rotation. Aerospace Medicine 35:965–988

Melvill Jones G 1971 Organisation of neural control in the vestibulo-ocular reflex arc. In: Bach-y-Rita P et al (eds) The control of eye movements. Academic Press, New York, pp 497–516

Melvill Jones G, Milsum J H 1970 Characteristics of neural transmission from the semicircular canal to the vestibular nuclei of cats. Journal of Physiology 209:295–316

Melvill Jones G, Milsum J H 1971 Frequency response analysis of central vestibular unit activity resulting from rotational stimulation of the semicircular canals. Journal of Physiology 219:191–215

Melvill Jones G, Sugie N 1972 Vestibulo-ocular responses in man during sleep. Electroencephalography and Clinical Neurophysiology 32:43–53

Melvill Jones G, Watt D G D 1971a Observations on the control of hopping and stepping movements in man. Journal of Physiology 219:709–727

Melvill Jones G, Watt D G D 1971b Muscular control of landing from unexpected falls in man. Journal of Physiology 219:729–737

Melvill Jones G, Barry W, Kowalski N 1964 Dynamics of the semicircular canals compared in yaw, pitch and roll. Aerospace Medicine 35:984–989

Melvill Jones G, Rolph R, Downing O M 1976 Human subjective and reflex responses to sinusoidal vertical accelerations. McGill Univ, Montreal. DRB Medical Research Unit Report. Vol 5, pp 256–270

Merton P A 1956 Compensatory rolling movements of the eye. Journal of Physiology 132:25–27P

Miller E F 1962 Counter-rolling of the human eyes produced by head tilt with respect to gravity. Acta Oto-Laryngologica 54:479–501

Milsum J H, Melvill Jones G, 1967 Trigonometric resolution of neural responses from the vestibular otolith organ. Digest 7th International Conference of Medical Biology Eng. Stockholm, p 203

Mishkin S, Melvill Jones G 1966 Predominant direction of gaze during slow head rotation. Aerospace Medicine 37:897–901

Nashner L M 1970 Sensory feedback in human posture control. Sc D. Thesis. Cambridge, Mass, Massachusetts Institute of Technology Report MVT-70-3

Niven J I, Hixson W C 1961 Frequency response of the human semicircular canals: I. Steady-state ocular nystagmus response to high level sinusoidal angular rotations. BuMed Project MR005. 13–6001 Subtask I Report No 58 US Naval School of Aviation Medicine, Pensacola, Fla

Niven J I, Hixson W C, Correia M J 1965 Elicitation of horizontal nystagmus by periodic linear acceleration. US Naval Aerospace Medical Institute Report No NAMI-953

Oman C M, Young L R 1972 The physiological range of pressure difference and cupula deflections in the human semicircular canal. Acta Oto-Laryngologica 74:324–331

Outerbridge J S, Melvill Jones G 1971 Reflex vestibular control of head movements in man. Aerospace Medicine 42:935–940

Partridge L D, Kim J H 1969 Dynamic characteristics of response in a vestibulomotor reflex. Journal of Neurophysiology 32:485–495

Peterson B W 1970 Distribution of neural responses to tilting within vestibular nuclei of the cat. Journal of Neurophysiology 33:750–767

Petrov A P, Zenkin G M 1973 Torsional eye movements and constancy of the visual field. Vision Research 13:2465–2477

Precht W, Baker R 1972 Synaptic organisation of the vestibulo-trochlear pathway. Experimental Brain Research 14:158–184

Precht W, Grippo J, Richter A 1967 Effect of horizontal acceleration on neurons in the abducens nucleus. Brain Research 5:527–531

Precht W, Richter A, Grippo J 1969 Responses of neurons in cat's abducens nuclei to horizontal angular acceleration. Pflügers Archiv für die gesamte Physiologie des Menschen und der Tiere 309:285–309

Precht W, Llinas R, Clarke M 1971 Physiological responses of frog vestibular fibers to horizontal angular rotation. Experimental Brain Research 378–407

Purdon-Martin J 1967 The Basal Ganglia and Posture. (London: Pitman)

Raphan R, Cohen B, Matsuo V 1977 A velocity-storage mechanism responsible for optokinetic nystagmus (OKN), optokinetic after nystagmus (OKAN) and vestibular nystagmus. Control of Gaze by Brain Stem Neurons. Ed: Baker R, Bethoz A (Amsterdam; Elsevier) pp 37–42

Rashbass C 1961 The relationship between saccadic and smooth tracking eye movements. Journal of Physiology 159:326–338

Reinhart R J, Zuber B L 1970 Horizontal eye movements from abducens nerve stimulation in the cat. IEEE Transactions on Bio-Medical Engineering Vol BME-17. No 1. pp 11–14

Richter A, Precht W 1968 Inhibition of abducens motoneurons by vestibular nerve stimulation. Brain Research 11:701–705

Roberts T D M 1978 Neurophysiology of Postural Mechanisms, 2nd Edition. (London: Butterworths)

Robinson D A 1964 The mechanics of human saccadic eye movement. Journal of Physiology 174:245–264

Robinson D A 1970 Oculomotor unit behaviour in the monkey. Journal of Neurophysiology 33:393–404

Robinson D A 1971 Models of oculomotor neural organisation. In: Bach-y-Rita P et al (eds) The control of eye movements. Academic Press, New York

Robinson D A 1976 Adaptive gain control of vestibulo-ocular reflex by the cerebellum. Journal of Neurophysiology 39:954–969

Robinson D A, Fuchs A F 1969 Eye movements evoked by stimulation of frontal eye fields. Journal of Neurophysiology 32:637–648

Ron S, Robinson D A, Skavenski A A 1972 Saccades and the quick phase of nystagmus. Vision Research 12: 2015–2022

Rosenthal N P, McKean T A, Roberts W J, Terzuolo C A 1970 Frequency analysis of stretch reflex and its subsystems in triceps surae muscles of the cat. Journal of Neurophysiology 33: 713–749

Rubin A M, Liedgren S R C, Odkvist L M, Milne A C, Fredrickson J M 1977 Labyrinthine input to the vestibular nuclei of the awake cat. Acta Oto-Laryngologica 84: 328–337

Rubin A M, Young J M, Milne A C, Schwarz D W F, Fredrickson J M 1975 Vestibular-neck integration in the vestibular nuclei. Brain Research 96: 99–102

Sasaki K 1963 Electrophysiological studies on oculomotor neurons of the cat. Japanese Journal of Physiology 13: 287–302

Schaefer K P 1965 Die Erregungsmuster einzelner Neurone des Abducens-Kernes beim Kaninchen. Pflügers Archiv für die gesamte Physiologie des Menschen und der Tiere 284: 31–52

Schiller P H 1970 The discharge characteristics of single units in the oculomotor and abducens nuclei of the unanaesthetised monkey. Experimental Brain Research 10: 347–362

Schmid R 1973 Systems analysis of the vestibulo-ocular system. NASA 5th Symposium on the Role of the Vestibular Organs in Space Exploration; Naval Aerospace Medical Centre, Pensacola, Fla. USA NASA SP-314

Schmid R, Lardini F 1976 On the predominance of anti-compensatory eye movements in vestibular nystagmus. Biological Cybernetics 135–148

Schneider L W, Anderson D J 1976 Transfer characteristics of first and second order lateral canal and vestibular neurons in gerbil. Brain Research 112: 61–76

Schwindt P C, Richter A, Precht W 1973 Short latency utricular and canal input to ipsilateral abducens motoneurons. Brain Research 60: 259–262

Shimazu M, Precht W 1965 Tonic and kinetic responses of cats vestibular neurons to horizontal angular accelerations. Journal of Neurophysiology 28: 989–1013

Shimazu H, Precht W 1966 Inhibition of central vestibular neurons from the contralateral labyrinth and its mediating pathway. Journal of Neurophysiology 29: 467–492

Shimazu H, Smith C 1971 Cerebellar and labyrinthine influences on single vestibular neurons identified by natural stimuli. Journal of Neurophysiology 34: 493–508

Shinoda Y, Yoshida K 1974 Dynamic characteristics of responses to horizontal head angular acceleration in vestibulo-ocular pathway in the cat. Journal of Neurophysiology 37: 653–673

Skavenski A, Robinson D A 1973 Role of abducens neurons in vestibulo-ocular reflex. Journal of Neurophysiology 36: 724–738

Sparks D L, Travis R P Jr 1971 Firing patterns of reticular formation neurons during horizontal eye movements. Brain Research 33: 477–481

Spoendlin H H 1965 Ultrastructural studies of the labyrinth in squirrel monkey. 1st Symposium on the Role of the Vestibular Organs in the Exploration of Space. NASA SP-77: 7–22

Sathle J 1958 Electro-nystagmography in the caloric and rotary tests. Acta Oto-Laryngologica Supplement 137

Steer R W Jr 1967 The influence of angular and linear acceleration and thermal stimulation on the human semicircular canal. Sc D Thesis. Massachusetts Institute of Technology (MIT-67–63)

Steinhausen W 1931 Uber den Nachweis der Bewegnung der Cupula in der intakten Bogengangs-ampulle des Labyrinthes bei der naturlichen rotatorischen und calorishen Reszung. Pflügers Archiv für die gesamte Physiologie des Menschen und der Tiere 228: 322

Stockwell C W, Turnipseed G T, Guedry F E 1971 Nystagmus responses during rotation about a tilted axis. Pensacola, Fla, Naval Aerospace Medical Research Laboratory Report NAMRL-1129

Sugie N, Melvill Jones G 1965 A mathematical model of the vestibulo-ocular system. Digest 6th International Conf. Med. Elec. Biol. Eng. Tokyo. Pp 422–423

Sugie N, Melvill Jones G 1971 A model of eye movements induced by head rotation. IEEE Trans. Syst. Man Cybern. SMC-1, 251–260

Szentagothai J 1950 The elementary vestibulo-ocular reflex arc. Journal of Neurophysiology 13: 395–407

Szentagothai J 1952 Die Rolle der einzelnen Labyrinthrezeptoren bei der Orientation von Augen und Kopf in Raume. Budapest: Akademiai Kiado

Szentagothai J 1964 Pathways and synaptic articulation patterns connecting vestibular receptors and oculomotor nuclei. In: Bender M B (ed) The Oculomotor System, Harper & Row, New York, pp 205–223

Takemori S, Cohen B 1974 Visual suppression of vestibular nystagmus in rhesus monkeys. Brain Research 72: 203–224

Takemori S, Suzuki J R 1971 Eye deviations from neck torsions in humans. Annals of Otology, Rhinology and Laryngology (St. Louis) 80: 439–444

Taylor A 1965 The role of sensory feedback in the vestibulo-ocular reflex in cats. Journal of Physiology 179: 76P

Vidal J, Jeannerod M, Lifscitz W, Levitan H, Rosenberg J, Segundo J P 1971 Static and dynamic properties of gravity-sensitive receptors in the cat vestibular system. Kybernetik 9: 205–215

DeVries H 1950 The mechanics of the labyrinth otoliths. Acta Oto-Laryngologica 38: 262–273

Waespe W, Henn V 1977 Neuronal activities in the vestibular nuclei of the alert monkey during vestibular and optokinetic stimulation. Experimental Brain Research 27: 523–538

Wall C, O'Leary D P, Black F O 1978 Systems analysis of vestibulo-ocular system response using In: Hood J D (ed) Vestibular mechanisms in health and disease, Academic Press, London, p 157–164 (London: Academic Press) pp 157–164

Wersall J, Lundquist P 1966 Morphological polarisation of the mechano-receptors of the vestibular and acoustic systems. In: Second Symposium on the Role of the Vestibular System in Space Exploration. Washington DC NASA SP-115, 57–72

Westheimer G 1954 Mechanism of saccadic eye movements. AMA Archives of Ophthalmology 52: 710–724

Whitteridge D 1960 Central control of eye movements. In: Handbook of Physiology, Neurophysiology 2, Williams and Wilkins, Baltimore, p 1089

Wilson V J, Maeda M 1974 Connections between semicircular canals and neck motoneurons in the cat. Journal of Neurophysiology 37: 346–357

Wilson V J, Peterson B W 1978 Peripheral and central substrates of vestibulospinal reflexes. Physiological Reviews 58: 80–105

Wilson V J, Yoshida M 1969 Comparison of the effects of stimulation of Deiters' nucleus and medial longitudinal fasciculus on neck, forelimb, and hindlimb motoneurons. Journal of Neurophysiology 32: 743–758

Wilson V J, Yoshida M, Schor R M 1970 Supraspinal monosynaptic excitation and inhibition of thoracic back motoneurons. Experimental Brain Research 11: 282–295

Wilson V J, Gacek R R, Maeda M, Uchino Y 1977 Saccular and utricular input to cat neck motoneurons. Journal of Neurophysiology 40: 63–73

Wolfe J W, Engelken E J, Kos C M 1978 Low frequency harmonic acceleration as a test of vestibular function: basic methods and illustrative cases. Transactions of the American Academy of Ophthalmology and Otolaryngology 86, ORL 130–142

Yamanaka Y, Bach-Y-Rita P 1968 Conduction velocities in the abducens nerve correlated with vestibular nystagmus in cats. Experimental Neurology 20: 143–155

Yasui S, Young L R 1975 Eye movements during after-image tracking under sinusoidal and random vestibular stimulation. In: Lennerstrand G, Bach-y-Rita P (eds) Basic mechanisms of ocular motility and their clinical implications, Pergamon Press, Oxford, p 509–513

Young L R 1969 The current status of vestibular system models. Automatica 5: 369–383

Young L R, Meiry J L 1967 A revised dynamic otolith model. In: The Third Symposium on the Role of the Vestibular Organs in Space Exploration. NASA SP-152, pp 363–368

Young L R, Oman C M 1969 Model for vestibular adaptation to horizontal rotation. Aerospace Medicine 40: 1076–1080

Young L R, Stark L 1963 Variable feedback experiments testing a sampled data model for eye tracking movements. IEEE Tans. on Human Factors in Electronics. Vol 1. HFE-4 No. 1, pp 28–51

Yules R B, Gault F P 1966 The relationship of nystagmus to lateral vestibular nucleus stimulation. Experimental Neurology 15: 475–483

Zacharias G L, Young L R 1977 Manual control of yaw motion with combined visual and vestibular cues. (Abstract). Proc. 13th Annual Conference on Manual Control. Massachusetts Institute of Technology. June 15–17

Zuber B L 1968 Sinusoidal eye movements from brain stem stimulation in the cat. Vision Research 8: 1073–1079

Investigation of balancing function

INTRODUCTION

As Caird and Judge (1974) point out, the neurological examination and assessment of the elderly may differ appreciably from that of young and middle aged patients. The same statement applies to the neuro-otological examination of the elderly. There are six reasons for this difference:

1. There may be problems of communication and cooperation. As Isaacs points out in Chapter 14, and Luxon in Chapter 16, there are particular problems with regard to falls and dizziness respectively.
2. Disease patterns (Ch. 14–16) are different in the elderly.
3. Multiple pathologies are a common occurrence. In Chapter 14 Isaacs points out the difficulty, particularly in respect of falls, of deciding which is (or are) relevant to the balance disorder.
4. The examination must be conducted, and the results interpreted, in the light of the different physiological 'norms' for the elderly, as indicated by Oosterveld in Chapter 13. In connection with this point, it should be noted that physical signs which may be invaluable in the diagnosis of balance disorders in younger subjects may be of less value in the elderly. For example, Rai and Elias-Jones (1979) found the corneal reflex absent in about 23 per cent of elderly subjects. Although this was particularly the case in patients with cerebrovascular disease, this areflexia was also found in many patients without other evidence for neurological disease. A more general study of changes in neurological functioning was undertaken by Potvin, Sydulko and Tourtellotte (1980). 61 men aged 20 to 80 years were studied. Significant age-related linear decreases were found in almost all neurological functions. For the lower extremities, the largest decline was in one-legged balance with eyes closed.
5. The objectives of the neuro-otological assessment in the elderly may be somewhat more extensive than is frequently needed in the case of younger subjects. It is thus important not only to make an accurate aetiological, anatomical and pathological diagnosis, but also to assess the functioning disability, the contribution of this to the overall disability, and the psychological and sociological impact of the dysfunction.
6. The standard, let alone extended, neuro-otological examination may have to be restricted because of the frailty of the subject and/or lack of cooperation; thus,

apart from the general medical (but particularly cardiovascular and neurological) examination, the doctor may have to be content with a simple examination of posture, an otoscopic examination and an examination of eye movements with or without Frenzel glasses.

Nevertheless, the principles underlying the neuro-otological investigation of younger subjects (Hinchcliffe, 1976) apply equally well to the elderly. In particular, there is the basic principle that the investigation of the disorder of balance constitutes an exercise in general medicine (Hinchcliffe, 1970). Indeed, this principle applies more so to the elderly. As Wilcock (1980) points out, the question 'Why did this patient fall?', may be elucidated not by any neuro-otological examination but by a general medical investigation.

The investigation of balancing function comprises the anamnesis and an examination of gait, stance and eye movements, including both spontaneous and provoked. The procedures used for provoking eye movements are particularly devised for the generation of both physiological and pathological nystagmus. In particular, there is the generation of optokinetic nystagmus, postural (both static and dynamic) tests and the caloric test. It would therefore be convenient to discuss these topics in the order: anamnesis, gait, stance, upper limb posture tests, eye movements, optokinetic nystagmus, visual pursuit tests, postural vestibular tests, caloric test, other nystagmogenic tests, other investigations.

ANAMNESIS

Although dizziness, oscillopsia, ataxia, falls and frank immobility associated with balance disorders embrace many aetio-pathological entities, different conditions may be associated with each of these particular symptoms (Ch. 14–16).

Consequently, the medical history taking will be moulded primarily to the particular manifestations of the balance disorder.

As pointed out in Chapter 16, a complaint of *dizziness* may be associated with the dysfunction of body system other than the vestibular system. Moreover, multiple sensory deficits will often be found to be the basis of complaints of dizziness in the elderly (Drachman and Hart, 1972). Such patients, who are often diabetic, complain of light-headedness when walking, particularly when turning. Bezold (1906) pointed out that dizziness due to a vestibular disorder can be differentiated from that due to a non-vestibular disorder by the effect of eye closure. Closing the eyes abolishes dizziness due to the latter disorder.

If the patient's complaint of dizziness or giddiness is found to be equatable with a hallucination of movement, then he (or she, which is more likely) is considered to have vertigo. The occurrence of vertigo, especially when a rotatory sensation is experienced, is more likely to indicate a disordered vestibular system. Schuknecht and Kitamura (1981) have examined the temporal bones from elderly patients who had sustained one or more episodes of acute vestibular failure (marked vertigo associated with nausea, and sometimes, vomiting) unassociated with other vestibular deficits. The results indicated that the pathological basis was a discrete degenerative neuropathy of the vestibular nerve. Moreover, these authors consider that the aetiology in their cases was viral. Nevertheless, an acute cerebellar infarct may mimic acute vestibular labyrinthine disease (Guiang and Ellington, 1977). However, a central lesion producing vertigo is diagnosed by evaluating the paraphenomena associated with the vertigo rather than by the characteristics of the vertigo itself (Levy and O'Leary, 1947).

The direction of the vertigo may or may not have lateralising value in respect of the site of the lesion. It would appear that only in the case of cerebellar tumours is the relationship constant (Stewart and Holmes, 1904). With unilateral tumours, the sense of movement of the individual or of external objects is towards the unaffected side.

Oscillopsia is the term given to the symptom of an apparent visual oscillation of a fixed stationary target. Various types of oscillopsia exist (Fig. 12.1). Oscillopsia which is experienced only on walking or riding is more likely due to bilateral dysfunction (and, more likely, afunction) of the vestibular end organ, nerve or nucleus. This symptom reflects the primary function of the vestibular labyrinths, i.e. to permit man to walk and see. Bender (1965) cites the case of a 70-year-old man who had had a five-week course of streptomycin therapy for a bacterial endocarditis. The man complained of an unsteady gait and blurred vision. He noticed that, as he walked towards his sister, her features became blurred and indistinct. When he stopped walking, she again became clear. There was no oscillopsia when the eyes moved from side to side or up and down, provided the head was held still and there was no body motion. Examination failed to disclose any nystagmus either on naked eye observation or on fundoscopy. The caloric test produced no response from either side.

Bender also reported that he had observed a case of periodic alternating oscillopsia as an adverse reaction to phenytoin. The patient experienced oscillopsia which alternated between horizontal and vertical movements; the horizontal phases lasted for between 100 and 200 seconds and the vertical for between 15 and 30 seconds.

A constant oscillopsia which persists even when the patient's head and body are at rest is more likely to be due to a brain lesion. If the oscillopsia is localised to homonymous visual fields, then it indicates an occipital lobe lesion. Bender reported a 68 years old man with a vascular lesion of the right occipital lobe who complained that objects viewed in the left field of vision moved to and fro but not in any particular plane. Ophthalmological examination disclosed scotomas in the left homonymous quadrants near the macular region. No nystagmus was detectable.

Both monocular and asymmetric oscillopsia are associated with disease of the basal ganglia, cerebellum or midbrain.

A spontaneous nystagmus can probably be observed in about two-thirds of patients with oscillopsia. In half the remainder, it is probably possible to detect ocular oscillations by ophthalmoscopic observation of the retina.

Just as the patient uses the umbrella term dizziness to cover a variety of dysfunctions other than those referable to the vestibular system, so he will use difficulty in walking to cover a variety of dysfunctions other than ataxias. The complaint of difficulty in walking, or with one leg, may, after examination, be shown to due not to a coordination disorder but to a motor or sensory neurological disorder, or even a non-neurological disorder.

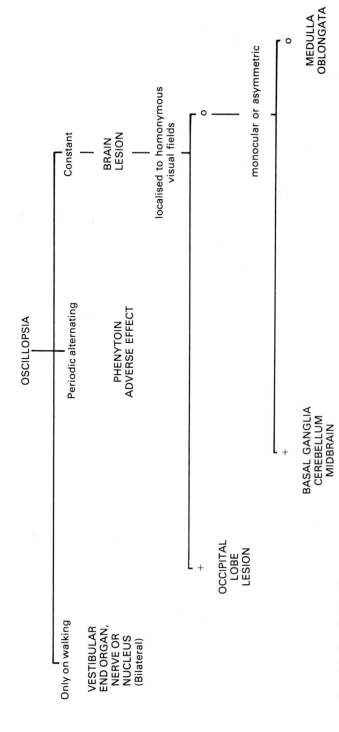

Fig. 12.1 Classification of oscillopsia

GAIT

The examination of gait begins with the observation of unstressed, natural walking. If this is normal, the examiner will then proceed to use various tests which are designed to show up balance disorders when walking. Finally, in certain centres, sophisticated electronic equipment may be available for the recording and analysis of gait.

As Adams (1978) points out, a description of a difficulty in walking in an older patient must always be checked by personal observation of the gait, allowing the patient to walk freely and, if possible, negotiate a few steps. Such an examination may be much more informative than a neurological examination since older people frequently have no ankle jerks, 'equivocal' plantar reflexes, no vibration sense, and show willing, but unhelpful, responses to other sensory testing.

In Chapter 15, Obeso and his colleagues describe the nature and patterns of gait control disorders in the elderly. The first task of the examiner will be to distinguish these and other neurological disorders from other causes of gait defect (Fig. 12.2).

As Hodkinson (1980) says, gait abnormalities due to deformities usually present no diagnostic difficulties. Abnormal posture may call attention to spinal deformities, i.e. kyphosis and scoliosis. A dipping gait may be due to shortening of a leg due to an old fracture or severe osteoarthritis of the hip. Bizarre gaits, where one grossly externally rotated leg leads and the other follows behind it, may result from bilateral osteoarthritis of the hips. An unsteady wobbling gait, where the affected knee is stabilised in a knock-kneed apposition to its healthy fellow, will result from the lateral instability of a grossly disorganised knee incurred either by advanced osteoarthritis or, less frequently, a Charcot joint.

A gait which Hodkinson likens to walking a pair of protractors, i.e. progression by small limited rocking movements, characterises hip stiffness due to severe osteoarthritis.

The anamnesis will have indicated if an intermittent limp is due to pain or intermittent claudication.

Hobbling gaits are the consequence of painful feet due to corns, bunions or just ill-fitting shoes. As Jahss (1971) points out, of the entire musculoskeletal system, the foot is perhaps the foremost in showing the ravages of time, abetted by the static stresses imposed by weight-bearing and by shoes. Longstanding deformities whether congenital or acquired are often at first flexible and asymptomatic but gradually become fixed and rigid. Consequently, painful exostoses and callouses ultimately develop.

Limping may be due to bone pain from Paget's disease, metastases or an undiagnosed fracture.

Marked lurching and staggering without the patient falling and hurting herself, and especially when the patient is knowingly being observed, points to a psychological cause.

More sensitive tests are indicated if the subject appears to walk normally. Fregly and Graybiel (1967) developed a battery of such tests. This battery is termed the Floor Ataxia Test Battery (FATB). The battery incorporates a number of tests— and all with assigned acronyms. Perhaps the most useful for clinical purposes is WOFEC (Walk on Floor Eyes Closed). The task requires a subject to walk as

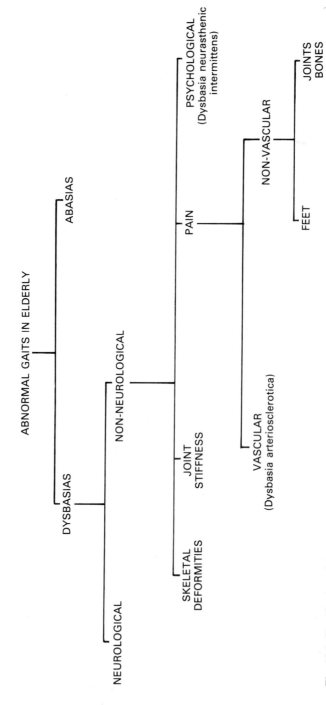

Fig. 12.2 Classification of abnormal gaits in the elderly

straight as possible with ten steps heel-to-toe beyond the first two starting steps. The results for this heel-to-toe test with the eyes closed should be compared with the results for the heel-to-toe test with the eyes open.

Drachman and Hart (1972) report a useful test for patients with dizziness due to multiple sensory defects. They say that the dizziness in patients with this syndrome is most closely reproduced by walking, or by walking and turning quickly. Touching the examiner's finger lightly provides sufficient additional sensory information to relieve symptoms markedly in most patients.

Electrical systems for investigating gait are used broadly for two types of measurement. First, there are foot-force measuring devices. Secondly, there are devices for recording the movement of one or other part of the body.

For example, Miyazaki and Iwakura (1978) describe a device for the continuous measurement of the vertical component of the forces exerted by the foot during walking. The device consists of two pairs of force transducers, an amplifier-transmitter unit and a receiver processing unit. A pair of force transducers are attached to the soles of a pair of shoes and adjacent to the posterior region of the metatarsals. The signals detected by the transducers are amplified, telemetered and summed to give the total force acting on each foot. For measuring the shearing forces on the sole of the foot, Tappin, Pollard and Beckett (1980) use a centre-tapped magneto-resistor in a bridge configuration, with a magnet placed centrally above it. Thus any lateral movement of a magnet will unbalance the bridge and give an electrical signal which is proportional to the movement of the magnet. By applying an elastic self-centering force to the magnet, the degree of movement can be made proportional to the shearing force applied.

To obtain virtually on-line trajectories of moving parts of the body, Brügger and Milner (1978) have developed a ccd (charge-coupled device)—image sensor. The labels (markers) whose motions are to be tracked may be reflecting material, small incandescent light sources or infra-red leds (light emitting diodes). Interfacing circuitry was developed to link the ccd-image sensors to a PDP 11/10 minicomputer to enable virtual on-line tracking of the labels. There are a number of advantages of the ccd system over other systems for tracking body motion. In particular, the digital nature of ccd-devices considerably simplify the design of the required computer-interface since no analogue-to-digital conversion is required for extraction of the data coordinates.

Imms and Edholm (1979) record and analyse gait by means of a metal walkaway on which the subject walks in shoes with metal-foil contacts on the heels and soles. Each time that a heel or sole is in contact with the walkaway a circuit is completed and the event recorded on ultraviolet paper. In addition, there are light beams crossing the walkaway which activate photocells. The velocity of walking may be; calculated from the interval between the subject breaking the two beams. Symmetry of gait may be examined by comparing the times of contact with the two feet, the swing phases of the two legs or the half-pace times for the legs.

STANCE

A psychological cause should be suspected where the patient cannot stand let alone walk and where there appears to be no neurological or other cause for the condition

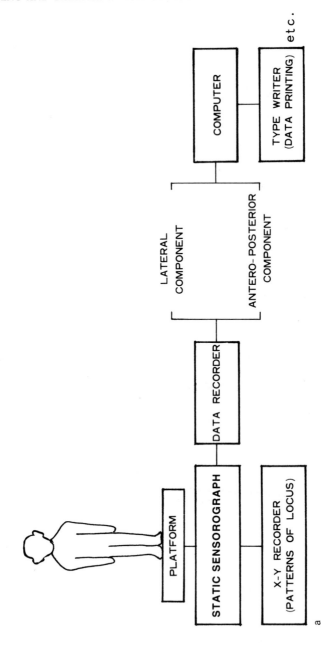

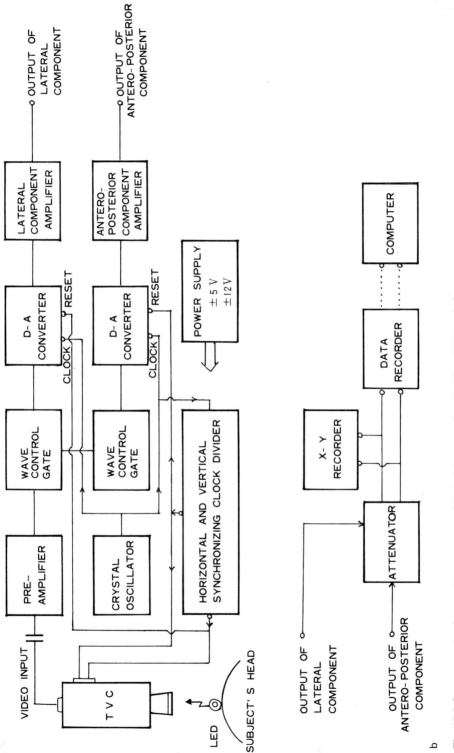

Fig. 12.3 Instrumentation for recording movement of the body's centre of gravity (Fig. 12.3a) and of the head (Fig. 12.3b) (after Taguchi, 1980).

(abasia-astasia). The terms abasia and astasia have tended to be restricted to inabilities to walk or stand respectively where no neurological or other organic defect can be demonstrated. However, it is more convenient, and etymologically correct, to use these terms in their literal interpretation. Thus the terms will cover the 'gone off legs' syndrome, which is usually used to describe the condition of immobility in the elderly.

Like dizziness, falls and difficulty in walking, the term 'gone off legs', as Wilcock and Middleton (1980) point out, embraces a multitude of diseases. Moreover, as with these other symptoms in the elderly, it is not uncommon for there to be a multiple aetiology, with one factor as the final straw. Coni, Davison and Webster (1980) give a more detailed account of immobility. The causes include pain in the bones, joints muscles and soft tissues, weakness due to endocrine, haemodynamic and neurological conditions, as well as psychological factors arising from inertia, anxiety, depression and dementia, together with iatrogenic factors related to over-sedation or the adverse effects of drugs.

If the patient is able to stand with the eyes open the Romberg (1846) test should be performed. As Rogers (1980) has pointed out, the nature and purpose of this simple test is frequently misunderstood. A subject's ability to stand erect with the eyes closed is compared with his ability to do so with the eyes open. If, on closing his eyes, he immediately becomes unstable and falls to the ground, then the test is positive. Such a result indicates a spinal cord posterior column lesion, e.g. tabes dorsalis.

As with all tests, there is the need, as specifically pointed out by Edwards (1973) for this test, to properly explain the test and gain the patient's confidence. When this is done, a normal subject may sway slightly with the eyes open and somewhat more with the eyes closed. Conversely if it is suggested to the patient that he may well fall, then he will frequently do so. Indeed, this forms the basis of Hull's (1933) body sway test for suggestibility. Thus the Romberg test can be linked to other balancing tests for purposes other than diagnosing a posterior column lesion. In particular, as mentioned in Chapter 11, quantitative measures of body sway, when the subject is standing with the feet set apart, provide an index of postural stability. In addition, the subject's ability to stand with the feet in tandem (heel-to-toe) would be influenced, *inter alia*, by the integrity of the vestibular mechanism (Fregly and Graybiel, 1968).

Electrical systems for investigating postural stability (*posturography*) may employ a variety of techniques. Head movement may be measured using an accelerometer, particularly a strain-gauge type linear accelerometer (Kitahara, 1965), or a television camera recording the movements of an LED (light emitting diode) which is fixed to a helmet worn by the subject (Taguchi, 1980). Kitahara and Taguchi refer to their systems as acceleration registrography and cephalography respectively (see Figs. 12.3 and 12.4).

Apart from television, other optoelectronic techniques are now available which exploit optical remote sensing to record body sway (Lindholm, 1974; Woltring, 1974).

Stabilography (statokinesimetry) entails measuring the displacement of the line of gravity within the area of support by means of a force platform. Such devices typically employ strain gauge techniques. Some systems provide an instantaneous

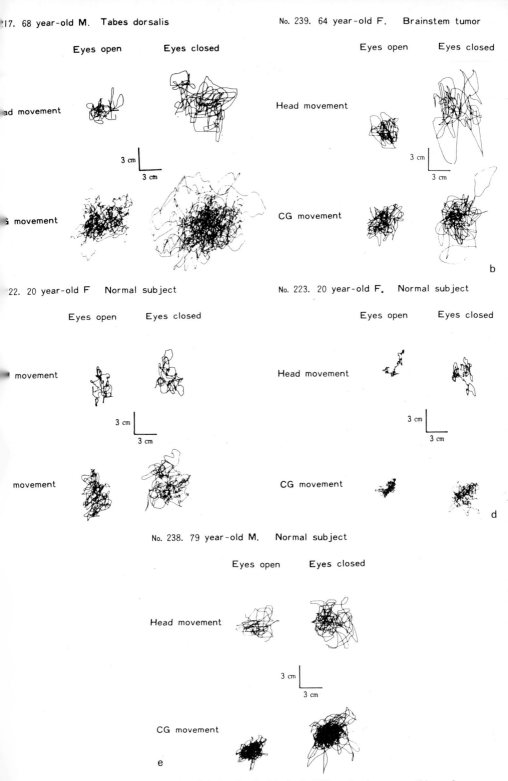

Fig. 12.4 Loci traced by movement of the head and of the body (CG) under the two conditions of eyes open and eyes closed for a 68-year-old man with tables dorsalis (Fig. 12.4a) and a 64-year-old woman with a brain stem tumour (Fig. 12.4b). For comparison, Figs. 12.4c and 12.4d show the recordings for two normal 20-year-old women and Fig. 12.4e the recordings for a normal 79-year-old man (after Taguchi, 1980 and Personal Communication.

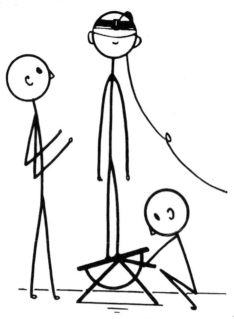

Fig. 12.5 Technique for performing tilting platform test of balance. The subject stands erect on the platform which is inclined by an assistant. Another assistant stands at the side of the platform to support the subject if and when he falls. Movement of the subject's head is recorded by acceleration registrography (Kitahara, 1965).

display on a television screen of the force distribution under a subject's feet (Chodera, 1960: Brull and Arcan, 1974).

Additional information can be provided by employing a tilting platform (Kitahara, 1965) (Fig. 12.5).

Taguchi found that, using combined cephalography and stabilography, the locus traced by the head closely resembled that traced by the centre of gravity, though shorter in overall length. The head moved more slowly than the centre of gravity. A phase delay was observed during standing with eyes closed. These results thus indicated that the movement of the head is controlled by the body's centre of gravity and the latter moves in order to keep the head steady, maintaining the eyes in the normal position.

The results of stabilography on 100 healthy subjects have been reported by Njiokiktjien and De Rijke (1972). The line of gravity for most people is situated to the right of the centre of the area of support. The antero-posterior amplitude is greater than the lateral one. An analysis of the frequency spectrum showed two clearly visible peaks, i.e. at 300 mHz and at 1 Hz to 2 Hz. The lower frequency peak was not always seen; it was considered to have a vestibular origin. The same authors also examined 300 neurological patients. The amplitude of sway increased considerably when the proprioceptive system was defective. Patients with verte-brobasilar insufficiency showed high amplitude slow movements. In vestibular disorders, the ratio of the antero-posterior amplitude to the lateral amplitude fell to less than unity. In brain stem and cerebellar disorders, the energy in the 0·2 to 2·5 Hz band is accentuated (De Wit, 1973; Tokita, 1976). Cases of cerebellar atrophy (mainly alcoholic) are characterised by a 3 Hz tremor superimposed on slower movements in the antero-posterior direction. Stabilography also provides a convenient means of monitoring the effects of drugs. Studies have shown that the serum concentration of carbamazepine is correlated with the amplitude of postural sway.

Using his tilt table, Kitahara showed that more than 90 per cent of Ménière's patient had an imperfect head righting reflex. These tilt test results were correlated with the caloric test results.

LIMB POSTURE TESTS

There are a number of versions of a test, variously attributed to Bárány, Güttich, Hautant and Quix, in which the spontaneous deviation of the outstretched upper limb (or limbs) is observed. Depending on the particular version employed, the test is conducted with the subject lying in bed, sitting, standing with the feet apart or standing with the feet together. The subject is asked to extend his arms in front of him with the hands closed but the index fingers also extended so that they nearly touch those of the examiner, who assumes a mirror image posture. The subject is then asked to close his eyes and the deviation of the limb(s) is observed. Quix's (1925) version, where the subject stands with the feet apart, has been studied extensively by Hart (1980) on 100 neuro-otological patients. Hart observed that the arms deviated to the left in 39 out of 47 left-sided peripheral balance disorders, and to the right in seven out of 17 right-sided peripheral balance disorders. No arm deviation was observed in eight left peripheral lesions and six right peripheral lesions. In eight out of 10 left-sided central lesions, the arms deviated to the left, but in three right-sided central lesions, the arms also deviated to the left. Hart's results would thus suggest that, with this method of testing, arm deviation to the right would be indicative of a right peripheral lesion. Arm deviation to the left would indicate that, with a peripheral lesion, a left-sided affection is most likely, and, with central lesions a left-sided affection is more likely than a right one. The emergence and pattern of the sinistrality phenomenon in Hart's study is of considerable interest. One wonders whether or not these intriguing results would be substantiated by further studies.

In a group of 33 cases of unilateral acute cerebellar injuries, Holmes (1917) observed that, in all except one case, the homolateral arm swung out and came to rest slowly. The exception was a case where the limb was so asthenic that it could not be raised. In slight injuries when deviation was not observed, it could be brought out by shaking or tapping the affected limb. In a few patients who suffered from extensive unilateral lesions, the contralateral arm tended to deviate inwards, but this deviation was always slight and neither constant nor regular. Holmes found that the tendency to deviation of the lower limbs was less common, but when this occurred, the homolateral leg swung inwards. Thus not only the direction, but also the pattern of spontaneous deviation of the limbs can be of diagnostic value.

These spontaneous extended arm deviation tests can be combined with Bárány's past-pointing test. If there is no deviation of the outstretched hands, the patient is then asked to bring his hands slowly down to his side and then back to the original position. In some cases, the test is positive when there has been no spontaneous deviation of the upper limb. Normally, a subject can regain his target relatively well on each attempt. When the test is positive, the patient's index finger deviates constantly to one side; if the test is repeated, the deviation initially increases with each attempt. The test can be quantified and, at the same time, the subject 'reassured', by the use of a tape-measure, which the examiner holds horizontally in front of the patient. By doing this, the error of each movement can be measured and, by allowing the patient's finger to touch the tape-measure, he is unable to ascertain whether or not there has been an error. This test will also disclose any dysmetria, i.e. overshooting, which is indicative of cerebellar dysfunction.

In association with these arm deviation tests, it is convenient to perform the 'finger-to-nose' test and look for tremor. Findley, Gresty and Halmagyi (1981) have reported a technique of using a Schottky barrier photodetector to record abnormal movements of the arms. Measurements can be made quickly and simply so that information on the frequency and waveform of movements is readily available. Six types of abnormal patterns are described. The different results between, for example, cerebellar atrophy and post-encephalitic Parkinsonism, are illustrated. The records of a 73-year-old man with cerebral and cerebellar atrophy showed marked intention tremor during flexion and extension, but when 'imagining' his target, i.e. with the eyes closed, the limb movements were within normal range. The records for a 62-year-old woman with post-encephalitic Parkinsonism showed more marked tremor with the eyes closed.

Fukuda's (1959) vertical writing test is another way of detecting an imbalance affecting the upper limbs. The square drawing test of Sekitani and his colleagues (1975) is perhaps a more convenient development of this test (Fig. 12.6). With these tests, the examiner must not allow any part of the patient's upper limb to come in contact with the writing surface, otherwise the results are vitiated.

The stepping tests of Unterberger (1938, 1962) and others form a group of tests which are intermediate between those for testing stance and those for testing gait.

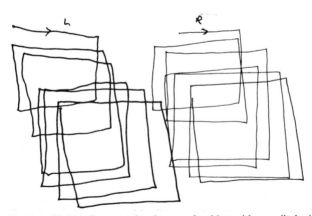

Fig. 12.6 A modification of Sekitani's square drawing test. A subject with a vestibular imbalance (arm deviation to the right) has drawn, simultaneously, a square with each hand and repeated this five times (eyes closed).

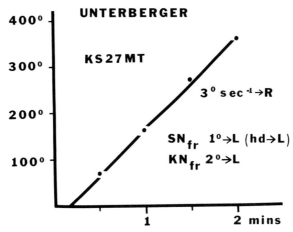

Fig. 12.7 Method for recording graphically the results for Unterberger's test. The angular deviation of the body (as indicated by the outstretched upper limbs) is recorded as a function of time. The patient turns to the right. The patient had a 1° spontaneous vestibular nystagmus to the left, which was accentuated by the head shaking manoeuvre. SN_{fr} denotes spontaneous nystagmus as observed with Frenzel glasses. KN_{fr} denotes head shaking nystagmus (*Kopfschüttelnystagmus*). The patient had a right unilateral vestibular lesion (after Hinchcliffe, 1973).

They are, however, an extension of the deviation test since this is what they are designed to measure (Fig. 12.7). As performed by Scherzer (1968) and others, the test is performed by asking the subject to mark time on the spot (the examiner demonstrates) with the arms outstretched in front of him and the hands clasped together. The subject is asked to close his eyes. The direction and degree of rotation is then noted. In addition to measuring the angular rotation in degrees in the stepping test, Peitersen (1967) measures the linear displacement of the patient from the starting position and conducts the test in a quiet, darkened room with the patient blindfolded and with arms hanging by the sides.

Previous criticisms of the invalidity of these deviation or turning tests regarding lateralising vestibular lesions was partly because of the failure to recognise the existence of recovery phenomena (central compensation). In this state it is possible to have a nystagmus, termed a recovery nystagmus (*Erholungsnystagumus*), which is directed towards the affected vestibular labyrinth or nerve (Stenger, 1959). Thus, in assessing the validity of these limb deviation and stepping tests, the results should be compared not with the side suspected to be involved, but with the direction of any spontaneous or provocation nystagmus.

EYE MOVEMENTS

As Uemura and his colleagues (1977) point out, before searching for nystagmus, the eye movements themselves should be examined for conjugate movements, limitation of gaze and vergence. But before these examinations are made, the resting position of the eyes should be observed. Observations should then be made of each eye during both conjugate gaze and uniocular gaze, i.e. when the other eye is covered.

Yap, Loong and Nei (1975) found that 44 per cent of stroke patients seen within 48 h of admission showed an ocular motor abnormality. The mortality rate of such patients appeared to be double that of patients without ocular motor abnormalities.

Conjugate deviation of the eyes towards the side of unilateral hemisphere lesion may be observed in stuporose patients. Unlike other motor phenomena, this defect disappears within a few hours of the patient regaining consciousness (Cogan, 1970). In acute unilateral cerebellar lesions, the eyes at rest are initially deviated away from the side of the lesion. Although this deviation is also more marked in unconscious patients, it may be observed in conscious patients (Holmes, 1917).

Squint (strabismus) is the pathological condition of chronically misaligned visual axes. This is frequently genetically determined and is rare in coloured races. Minor degrees of squint may be recognised clinically from the asymmetric positions of the bright corneal light reflections relative to their respective pupil margins. There are two principal types of squint, i.e. concomitant and paralytic squints. Concomitant squints are so named because the eyes retain their relative positions in all directions. In paralytic squints the difference in eye positions is greatest when gaze is in the direction of the normal action of the paralysed muscle. Concomitant squints are due to a disorder of the sensory component of the reflex arc or its central connection; paralytic squints are due to damage to the motor component of the arc. Persistent squints can result in an amblyopia ('lazy eye'). Experimental studies on monkeys have shown this to be due to shrinkage of cells in the lateral geniculate neuclei (von Noorden, 1974).

Robinson (1975a) has presented a static eye position model. The model offers, for the first time, a quantitative estimate of the multitude of ways in which muscles can interact and interfere with each other when they hold the globe. The results are quite interesting. Because muscles have different lengths and sizes, their innervational participation in a movement can appear to be quite different from their mechanical participation. From an innervational standpoint, the vertical recti and obliques participate equally in vertical gaze. Muscles interfere with each other a good deal and necessitate changes of innervation to counteract these cross-couplings.

Skew deviation of the eyes is characterised by a deviation of gaze of one eye above the other, the angle of which may or may not be fixed for all directions of gaze and is due to lesions other than those involving the extraocular muscles, their motor neurones or local mechanical factors in the orbit. The eye on the side of the lesion is usually hypotropic, i.e. the lower one. Holmes (1917) observed skew deviation in five cases of unilateral gunshot wounds of the cerebellum. The homolateral eye was directed downwards and inwards whilst the other looked upwards and outwards. This lack of parallelism in the optic axes disappeared however on fixation when this could be obtained; consequently diplopia did not result. Skew deviation was observed only during the first week or so after an injury of the cerebellum except in two cases in which rapid destruction and compression of the structure occurred owing to abscess formation. Skew deviation is thus seen in patients with acute asymmetrical cerebellar disease and represents a dysfunction of the vertical vergence mechanism. Although rare in demyelinating disease, it has been reported in cerebellar and pontine artery thromboses, in platybasias and in vestibulocochlear schwannomas ('acoustic neuromas'). It has also been produced experimentally in animals with lesions of the vestibular nuclei and their connections with the oculomotor nuclei (Oloff and Korbsch, 1926). Intermittent skew deviation is associated with intermittent vertebro-basilar insufficiency (Walsh and Hoyt, 1969).

Having considered eye deviations at rest, squint and skew deviations, the examiner can then consider abnormal eye movements in general. A broad classification is shown in Figure 12.8.

After muscular and neuromuscular causes of ocular motor nerve pareses have been excluded, it will be found that vascular disease is the commonest assignable cause of such pareses (Rucker, 1958). The next commonest cause in the elderly will be a neoplasm. In considering individual ocular motor nerves, a neoplasm will be the commonest assignable cause of abducent palsies, an aneurysm of oculomotor and vascular disease of trochlear palsies. An isolated trochlear palsy is unlikely to be due to a neoplasm. In the case of abducent palsies due to a neoplasm, the most likely lesion would be a primary other than a meningioma or one involving the hypophysis (pituitary). In the case of oculomotor palsies due to a neoplasm, the most likely lesion would be a metastasis or a hypophyseal tumour.

Of particular interest to the neuro-otologist is an internuclear ophthalmoplegia. This condition is characterised by adductor palsy on attempted conjugate lateral gaze. In the primary position of gaze, the eyes are usually directed straight ahead. There is usually an associated predominantly uniocular nystagmus of the abducted eye. The condition is due to a lesion of the medial longitudinal bundle ipsilateral to the adductor palsy. With lesions of the posterior part of the bundle (medullary part), convergence is unimpaired; with anterior bundle lesions (midbrain part), convergence is impaired (Cogan, 1970). Bilateral internuclear ophthalmoplegias, which are almost pathognomonic of disseminated sclerosis, are commoner in younger patients; unilateral internuclear ophthalmoplegias in older patients. Four out of eight patients with unilateral internuclear ophthalmoplegia reported by Cogan, Kubik and Smith (1950) were 60 years of age or more. All four cases presented with diplopia, although one had vertigo in addition, and another had a reeling gait. Three of the four cases were observed to have skew deviation. In each case, the cause was considered to be an infarct of the medial longitudinal bundle (two patients suffered from atrial fibrillation; the other two from diabetes mellitus).

In pseudo-ophthalmoplegia (supranuclear palsy), command eye movements are absent but eye position deviation occurs with head movements (oculocephalic manoeuvre—see later) or with vestibular stimulation.

Ocular dysmetria is best demonstrated by having the subject look from an eccentric position of gaze back to the midline position (Cogan, 1954). This movement is normally executed with remarkable precision but, in the presence of cerebellar disease, there is a characteristic overshoot (occasionally undershoot) with several pendular excursions of the eyes before final fixation is attained. One of the six cases described by Cogan was a 62-year-old woman who had complained of progressive difficulty in walking over the previous 22 years. Nine other members of the family were similarly affected. The condition was due to primary cerebellar atrophy. Goldstein and Cogan (1961) reported that saccadic (fast eye movement) overshoot dysmetria sometimes occurred only with saccades towards the side of the cerebellar lesion.

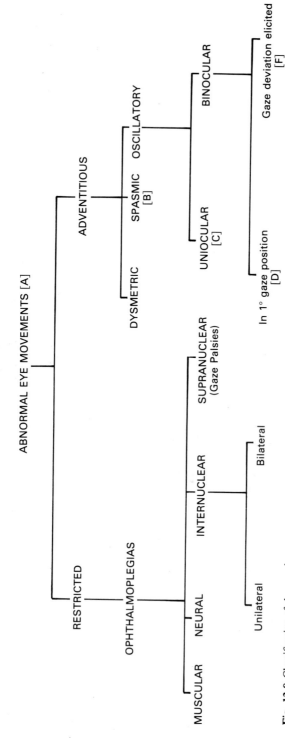

Fig. 12.8 Classification of abnormal eye movements.

Clinical evidence indicates that this dysmetria is due to dysfunction of the cerebellar vermis. The control system abnormality in saccadic overshoot dysmetria is an abnormally high gain in the brain's feed-forward path. Selhorst, Stark, Ochs and Hoyt (1976a) suggest that the cerebellum continuously modulates saccadic gain, although it may not lie directly on the visual ocular motor (feed-forward) path.

Ocular spasms

As Figure 12.9 indicates, ocular spasms may be classified into those of an oculomotor nerve or an extraocular muscle, those of conjugate gaze and those of convergence.

The features of muscle spasm, or overaction, are basically the converse of those of palsy. If the sound eye is used for fixation, the affected eye shoots beyond it in the direction of action, its movement being quicker and its total excursion greater than those of its fellow. As Duke-Elder and Scott (1971) point out, the differential diagnosis between a spasm and palsy of the contralateral synergist may be difficult and may not be necessary since the two conditions frequently coexist.

The spasm of conjugate gaze which has perhaps been most studied is that which characterizes oculogyric crises (chronic eye fits). These consist of conjugate spasmodic deviations of the eyes, usually upward. The eyes remain open and there are usually associated movements such as rhythmic contractions of levator palpebrae superioris and of orbicularis oculi, as well as head and neck movements. Although commonly a sequal of post-encephalitic Parkinsonism (Hohman, 1925), the phenomenon has also been reported in neurosyphilis (Krabbe, 1931; de Nigris, 1933) and following trauma (Käslin, 1936). Ablation and electrical stimulation studies indicate that the motor and premotor cortex are involved in the generation of these crises (Klemme, 1941). The crises can be abolished by coagulative lesions of the posterior limb (pathway of the corticospinal tract) of the internal capsule (Gillingham and Kalyanaraman, 1965).

As Guiloff, Whiteley and Kelly (1980) say, *convergence spasm* is not always a hysterical manifestation. They point out that this condition may be associated with organic disease affecting the cerebral hemispheres, the brain stem or both. In order of probability, these organic disorders are: head injury (de Mosier and Balavoine, 1949), labyrinthine lesion (Borries, 1926), encephalitis (Margulis and Model, 1926), tumours (including epidermoid cysts, pinealomas and schwannomas) (de Morsier and Balavoine, 1948), Wernicke's encephalopathy (Thompson and Lynde, 1969) and ocular muscle imbalance (Bagshaw, 1963), as well a various other disorders.

Uniocular oscillations

Abnormal spontaneous uniocular oscillations (Fig. 12.10) encompass not only nystagmus proper but also pseudo-nystagmus, which is represented by superior oblique myokymia (Susac, Smith and Schatz, 1973). This condition is characterised by intermittent, small amplitude, uniocular torsional eye movement in otherwise healthy adults. The disorder reflects phasic contraction of the superior oblique muscle. Affected subjects suffer from oscillopsia. The condition usually responds to carbamazepine.

Uniocular nystagmus is a rare condition (Duane, 1905; Cogan, 1963). There is a varied pathological basis. In the elderly, the more likely cause is a medial

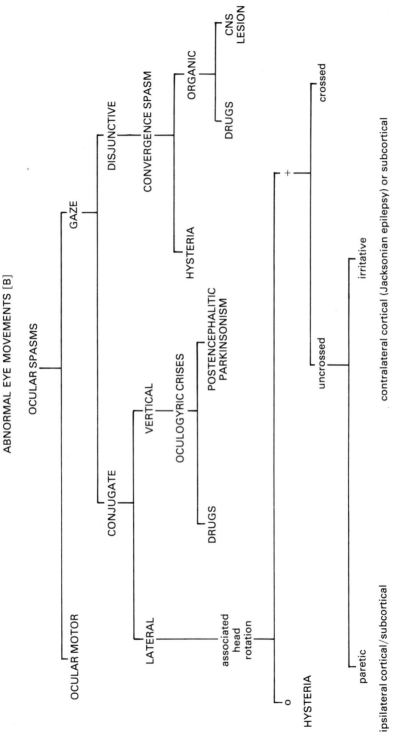

Fig. 12.9 Classification of ocular spasms.

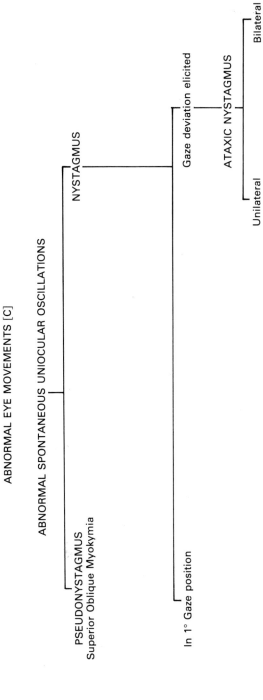

Fig. 12.10 Classification of abnormal spontaneous uniocular oscillations.

longitudinal bundle lesion with a vascular basis. As mentioned previously, this produces a predominantly uniocular nystagmus of the abducting eye.

Binocular pseudonystagmus

Apart from the searching movements of the blind, binocular pseudonystagmus comprises six conditions, viz. opsoclonus, ocular flutter, macrosaccadic oscillations, macrosquare wave jerks, ocular myoclonus and ocular bobbing (Fig. 12.11).

Opsoclonus. As Daroff (1977) points out, opsoclonus is characterised by most bizarre and dramatic ocular oscillations. The name was first suggested by Orzechowski (1927) who referred to the phenomenon a 'chaotique'. The term saccadomania (Daroff and Hoyt, 1971) is perhaps more descriptive. The eyes exhibit involuntary, rapid, unpredictable saccades which are multivectorial: horizontal, vertical, diagonal or circular. One of two cases reported by Cogan (1954) was that of a 61-year-old man who was referred to hospital complaining of twitching of the eyes, fever, difficulty in swallowing and difficulty in phonating. Examination was reported to show disorientation, continuous but irregular conjugate dancing of the eyes in horizontal, rotatory and vertical directions, and extensor plantar reflexes. The diagnosis was encephalitis. Other pathological bases which should be considered for opsoclonus in elderly subjects are vascular conditions and non-metastatic effects of visceral carcinoma. There have been clinical reports of opsoclonus in association with ocular dysmetria and ocular flutter (Ross and Zeman, 1967; Ellenberger, Keltner and Stroud, 1972). Ellenberger and his colleagues therefore consider that these three ocular movement disorders are related and represent dyskinesias of the saccadic oculomotor system. The morphological basis for opsoclonus is damage to the dentate nucleus (Ross and Zeman, 1967) or its connections (Gilbert, McEntee and Glaser, 1963).

Ocular flutter. Although Daroff (1977) says that ocular flutter is a wastebasket term to cover many diverse types of oscillation which clinically have similar appearances, Cogan (1954) restricts the term to episodes of three or four rapid pendular oscillations of the eyes in the horizontal plane which lasts no more than a few seconds. Affected subjects complain of momentary blurring of vision during attacks.

Two of eleven cases of ocular flutter reported by Cogan were over the age of 60 years. The first of these was a 61-year-old man who was awakened with severe vertigo and a left-sided headache. He then went into a stupor for eight days. Examination subsequently showed an intention tremor of the right hand and a coarse tremor of the left hand. Attempts to fixate an object were associated with pendular oscillations at 3 Hz over an arc of about 100 mrad* (about 6°). The eyes were stationary if no attempt was made to fixate. Although command eye movement were full, oscillation was observed on final fixation. In addition, the patient was unable to make smooth following eye movements; attempts at following eye movements were characterised by a series of quick cogwheel movements.

---

* It is unfortunate that the abbreviation of the SI unit for a plane angle is the same as that of a former unit of absorbed dose of ionising radiation; with the establishment of an SI unit (gray) for the latter measurement there should be no confusion in the future.

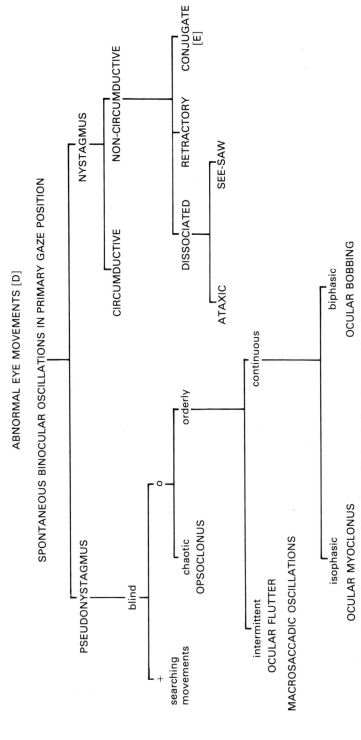

Fig. 12.11 Classification of spontaneous binocular oscillations in the primary position of gaze.

The second case was that of a 68 years old man who complained of difficulty in walking and a feeling of lightheadedness over a period of three or four months. More recently there had been right-sided seizures. Examination showed incoordination of both the right limbs and intermittent flutter-like oscillations of the eyes in all directions of gaze. Investigations indicated a renal carcinoma with a metastasis to the right cerebellar hemisphere.

Macrosaccadic oscillations are characterised by to-and-fro horizontal oscillations of the eyes of large amplitude (Daroff and Hoyt, 1971). The amplitude of the oscillations is in the range of a half to one radian. One of four cases reported by Selhorst, Stark, Ochs and Hoyt (1976b) was that of a 64 years old hypertensive woman who experienced sudden occipital headache and vomiting. Examination showed, *inter alia*, ataxia of the left limbs, hypotonia and a stiff neck. Following lumbar puncture, a diagnosis of acute cerebellar haematoma was made. Initially, the eyes tended to deviate to the right and there was a $1°$ vestibular nystagmus to the left. Subsequently, the conjugate deviation of the eyes diminished but the patient developed instability of fixation. Each saccadic shift of gaze initiated bursts of symmetrical horizontal macro-oscillations with an amplitude of 600 mrad and lasting about 4 seconds. The ataxia and other neurological signs regressed over a period of a few weeks; regression of the macro-oscillations followed.

Using electrical recordings of eye movements Selhorst and his colleagues studied a case of macrosaccadic oscillation in detail. Oscillation began with saccades that progressively increased in magnitude, often stabilising at about 700 mrad for several cycles and then progressively decreasing. Intersaccadic intervals averaged 260 ms. The overall impression was of a 2 Hz square wave oscillation. The oscillation stopped abruptly in complete darkness. Neither saccades as large as 700 mrad performed in the dark on command towards previously illuminated targets nor slow pursuit movements precipitated oscillations. However, gaze-holding nystagmus continued in the dark. Selhorst and his colleagues interpret macrosaccadic oscillations as due to a disruption of the normal feed-forward gain of the visual-ocular motor system. This normally fluctuates about a nominal value of 1·0. High level adaptive control is required to maintain this value. It is suggested that the cerebellum continually adjusts saccadic gain, acting as a calibrator organ (Gauthier, 1970). Because it does not lie directly in the feed-forward path, the cerebellum performs this adaptive gain control without interposing its own computational delays into the control loop. Acute disruption of this cerebellar function (a) removes cerebellar adjustment of saccadic gain, (b) allows for the accumulation of normal drifts and shifts in gain and (c) permits the development of runaway macrosaccadic oscillation. The parallel evolution of macrosaccadic oscillation and other cerebellar signs supports this view of cerebellar function.

Macrosaccadic oscillation must be distinguished from Kippdeviationen (Jung and Kornhuber, 1964; Kornhuber, 1966) and macrosquare wave jerks (Dell' Osso, Troost and Daroff, 1975).

Kippdeviationen (seesaw like swings of the eyes) are found only when optic fixation has been suppressed. They consist of huge amplitude (200 mrad to 900 mrad) oscillations in the range 1 Hz to 3 Hz. Nevertheless, Kippdeviationen have a similar anatomico-pathological basis (chronic cerebellar disease and myeloencephalitis) to macrosaccadic oscillations.

Macrosquare wave jerks are characterised by eccentric oscillations away from a point of fixation and back again, i.e. the intended fixation point is at one end of the oscillations. This phenomenon has been observed in advanced cerebellar and brain stem involvement in multiple sclerosis. These macrosquare wave jerks must be distinguished from square wave jerks with an amplitude of less than 200 mrad but of similar frequency (2 Hz) which may be observed in otherwise normal subjects when using Frenzel glasses (see p. 326) or when recording electro-oculographically with optic fixation abolished. Such movements are associated with mental alertness, particularly in apprehensive subjects. They are also to be found frequently at the termination of caloric-induced nystagmus.

Ocular myoclonus is characterised by continuous, pendular oscillations which are synchronous with the rhythmical movements of other midline structures (soft palate, tongue, facial muscles, pharynx, larynx) which are involved in the disorder. The frequency of the eye movements is in the range 1·5 Hz to 5 Hz and the direction is usually vertical. Only the coexisting movements of the other structures distinguishes ocular myoclonus from a pendular nystagmus (Tahmoush, Brooks and Keltner, 1973). The pathological basis for the myoclonus is pseudohypertrophy of the inferior olivary nucleus which follows an acute lesion of the dentate nucleus or its associated structures.

Ocular bobbing (Fischer, 1961; Susac, Hoyt, Daroff and Lawrence, 1970) is characterised by spontaneous abrupt, erratic downward jerks of the eyes followed by a slow return to the mid-position. Typically, affected individuals also have absent spontaneous or reflex horizontal eye movements.

Fischer and Susac and his colleagues classify ocular bobbing into binocular bobbing and monocular bobbing. The binocular bobbing is further subdivided into typical and atypical bobbing. Susaac and his colleagues illustrate each of the three types of ocular bobbing by, *inter alia*, the case histories of three older patients.

Typical binocular bobbing was evidenced by a 66-year-old woman who was admitted to hospital with vertigo, diplopia and generalized weakness. Examination showed her to be mildly confused and drowsy. The only neurological signs were dysarthria and a horizontal gaze-evoked nystagmus to either side. On the fourth day, the patient lapsed into coma and showed signs of decerebrate rigidity together with typical ocular bobbing. The latter was characterised by conjugate spontaneous downward jerks of the eyes together with a slow return to mid-position. The rate was unpredictable but increased with caloric stimulation. The patient died on the eighth day and postmortem examination revealed extensive haemorrhagic infarcts of the right cerebellar hemisphere.

Atypical binocular bobbing was exhibited by a 69-year-old male diabetic who, after operation for an abdominal aortic aneurysm, developed acute renal failure and required haemodialysis. He then developed intermittent ocular bobbing which was atypical in that conjugate horizontal eye movements were present in one direction. Postmorten examination showed small cystic infarctions of the left cerebellar hemisphere and the left caudate nucleus.

Monocular bobbing was illustrated by a 63 years old male diabetic and hypertensive who was found in a confused state at home. After admission to hospital, examination showed a profound right-sided hemiplegia and a left hemiparesis. The left pupil was dilated and unreactive. There was bilateral ptosis and paralysis of upward gaze. Voluntary and reflex eye movements were absent in the horizontal plane but the patient was able to move his right eye downwards. During attempts to execute the latter movement, the left eye only intorted. At irregular intervals, it was observed that the right eye would abruptly ascend; at the same time the left eye intorted. It was considered that this was a typical ocular bobbing picture that had been modified by unilateral oculomotor nerve palsy.

Ocular bobbing may occur in Wernicke's encephalopathy and be responsive to thiamine medication (Luda, 1980).

Binocular nystagmus

Typically spontaneous nystagmus is an involuntary, sustained quasi-periodic, symmetrical and conjugate eye movement with a frequency in the range 1 Hz to 5 Hz, and where the excursions of the centre of the cornea are observed to be linear. As indicated previously, exceptions to this pattern occur. Other patterns include voluntary nystagmus, circumduction nystagmus, dissociated nystagmus, retraction nystagmus and periodic alternating nystagmus.

Voluntary nystagmus is typically a high frequency (16 Hz to 23 Hz), horizontal, pendular, conjugate oscillation of the eyes initiated and maintained by willed effort (Blair, Goldberg and von Noorden, 1967). Uniocular cases may occur.

Shults, Stark, Hoyt and Ochs (1977) have shown that voluntary nystagmus consists of a series of to-and-fro saccadic eye movement. To explain this pattern of eye movement, Zee and Robinson (1979) postulate that the saccadic pulse generator in normal subjects is inherently unstable. In physiological terms, they consider it conceivable that some subjects may learn to generate voluntary nystagmus by inhibiting their pause cells which would, in turn, permit their burst neurons to oscillate.

Circumduction nystagmus is characterised by the centre of a cornea describing a circular or an elliptical path. This rare condition has been reported in multiple sclerosis and degenerative cerebellar lesions (Strubel, Eber, Monjour, Rohmer and Collard, 1980). It was also said to be the pattern of nystagmus in some cases of that rapidly disappearing occupational disorder, Miners' nystagmus, where it could also be of the dissociated type (Duane, 1905).

Dissociated nystagmus. The term dissociated nystagmus is used to designate rhythmic oscillations that are different in the two eyes. The range of movement may be detectably greater in one eye than the other but in the same direction, or it may be heterodirectional, or differ in both respects.

Dissociated nystagmus is a sign of a posterior cranial fossa lesion. Two of the fourteen cases which Cogan (1963) reported were 55 years of age or more. The first of these cases, a 55-year-old woman, had been admitted to hospital with nausea, vomiting, vertigo, unsteadiness and a right-sided hearing loss. The symptoms had all developed two weeks previously over a period of 24 hours. Examination disclosed cerebellar ataxia of the right limbs, weakness of the right facial muscles and a 1° spontaneous nystagmus directed upwards and in both directions of horizontal gaze; the vertical nystagmus was more marked in the right eye. Basilar artery disease was diagnosed. The patient was also suffering from diabetes.

The second of these two cases, a 63 years old man, had been awakened with dizziness. This was associated with clumsiness and dysphagia. He had previously suffered from an unequal oscillopsia since a stroke 3 years previously. Examination disclosed an unsteady gait, coarse ataxia of the right arm and conjugate rotary nystagmus in all directions of gaze. The nystagmus was, however, more marked in the right eye. A vascular disorder involving the right cerebellum was diagnosed.

Seesaw nystagmus is a special type of dissociated nystagmus. Characteristically this is a conjugate, pendular, torsional oscillation with a superimposed disconjugate vertical vector in which the intorting eye rises and the extorting (opposite) eye falls. Repetition of the sequence in the reverse direction provides the seesaw effect (Daroff, 1965). The most likely site of the causative lesion is in the parasellar region or suprasellar region anterior to the third ventricle. Most commonly the lesion is a tumour. Schurr (1963) described such a case in a 51-year-old woman which was due to a chromophobe adenoma of the hypophysis cerebri. Sano and his colleagues (1972) have reported abolition of this nystagmus by stereotactic destruction of the interstitial nucleus of Cajal on one side (this nucleus is a collection of cells situated in the lateral wall of the third ventricle immediately above the cranial end of the cerebral aqueduct; it also lies at the cranial end of the medial longitudinal bundle).

Cogan (1963) also considered that uniocular nystagmus is a special case of dissociated nystagmus. The syndrome of uniocular nystagmus and impaired lateral conjugate deviation due to contralateral adductor palsy was termed ataxic nystagmus by Harris (1944). As mentioned previously this is due to a medial longitudinal bundle lesion.

Abducting eye nystagmus. Stroud (1974) has described an abducting eye nystagmus in older people. This nystagmus is observed in lateral gaze and can either be diminished or increased by tonic deviations such as those caused by vestibular stimuli whether produced by rotatory or caloric stimulation.

Retraction nystagmus (Koerber, 1903; Salus, 1910; Elschnig, 1913) is characterised by irregular jerks of the eye backwards into the orbit when the patient attempts to look in one direction or the other.

Gay, Brodkey and Miller (1963) reported retraction nystagmus on attempting upward gaze in a 59-year-old man. The man had experienced pain in the neck of sudden onset. Although conscious, he was unable to see, speak, swallow or move his extremities. Recovery subsequently occurred. Basilar artery insufficiency was diagnosed as the cause of the disorder. Poission, van Effentere and Mashaly (1980) reported a 75-year-old woman with retraction nystagmus which disappeared after the removal of an adenoma of the hypophysis. Smith, Zieper, Gay and Cogan (1959) observed retraction nystagmus evoked by command upward eye movements in a 72-year-old man who had complained of intermittent diplopia and dizzy spells. Examination showed total paralysis of upward gaze (command, pursuit, passive, lid closure and optokinetic movements) and a left homonymous hemianopia. The patient was hypertensive. A right posterior cerebral artery occlusion was diagnosed.

The paralysis of upward gaze, which was observed in the last case, is termed Parinaud's (1883) syndrome. One of Parinaud's cases was a 67-year-old man who had paralysis of both upward and downward gaze, together with paralysis of convergence; horizontal movements were intact. This syndrome, together with retraction nystagmus and dissociated or total pupillary areflexia, make up the Koerber-Salus-Elschnig cerebral (Sylvian) aqueduct syndrome.

Daroff (1977) explains retraction nystagmus as due to anomalous cofiring of extraocular muscles. If medial rectus firing is greater than external rectus firing, a convergence retraction nystagmus is observed; the converse firing pattern produces a divergence retraction nystagmus.

Periodic alternating nystagmus (PAN) is the term applied to a spontaneous nystagmus that alternates in direction and does so in regularly recurring cycles. The period of these cycles is usually in the range 200 s to 300 s.

Baloh, Honrubia and Conrad (1976) reported the case of a 56 years old man with a long standing pain in the left shoulder and numbness and weakness of the left arm. Examination showed weakness and wasting of the distal left upper limb musculature together with absent tendon reflexes. There was hypalgesia and hypaesthesia on the left for C2 and T12 and for the face, together with a diminished left corneal reflex. Electrical recordings of eye movements (see later) showed a periodic alternating nystagmus with cycles of equal amplitudes and with a period of about 220 s; the mean duration of the left beating phase was 90 s, and of the right beating phase, 100 s. Null switchovers from left to right (average 20 s) were consistently longer than those from right to left (average 10 s). An Arnold-Chiari malformation was diagnosed by pneumo-encephalography.

Only three cases of periodic alternating nystagmus have been studied postmortem. In each case, multiple lesions of the brain stem were found (Towle and Romanul, 1970; Towle, 1971; Keane, 1974).

Baloh and his colleagues postulate that periodic alternating nystagmus represents firing between reciprocally connected groups of inhibitory neurons within the vestibular and oculomotor nuclei. The cyclical firing is initiated by a critical imbalance of tonic input to either group of normally functioning neurons. Leigh, Robinson and Zee (1980) base their explanation for PAN on instability in the central vestibular-optopkinetic pathways.

Halmagyi, Rudge, Gresty, Leigh and Zee (1980) report that both acquired PAN and it associated oscillopsia, but not congenital PAN, respond to baclofen medication.

After these atypical and infrequent pattern of nystagmus have been sought, we are left with the major body of spontaneous binocular nystagmus (Figs. 12.12 and 12.13), which may be variously classified as congenital or acquired, or occurring in the primary gaze position or gaze-deviation elicited. In addition, one may have rebound nystagmus and, perhaps, even rebound-rebound nystagmus.

Finally, mention will have to be made of physiological nystagmus.

Congenital nystagmus (CN). This type of nystagmus, which is typically asymptomatic, persists throughout life and may generate some initial confusion when it is first observed in an adult who is coincidentally afflicted with a disorder of balance.

Barber and Stockwell (1980) point out that CN (congenital nystagmus) shows three features; (i) nystagmus on upward gaze is virtually always horizontal and not vertical, (ii) it is reduced, if not abolished, on convergence, and (iii) it is observed only at, or very near, the primary position of gaze. However, a vertical congenital hereditary nystagmus has been reported (Jung and Kornhuber, 1964). Characteristically, CN is unaffected by abolishing optic fixation (Hood, 1967).

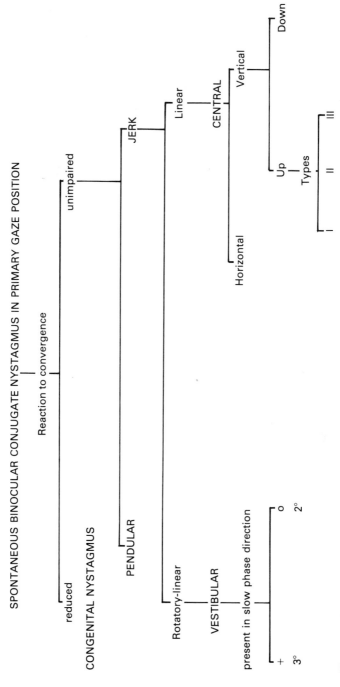

Fig. 12.12 Classification of spontaneous binocular conjugate nystagmus in the primary position of gaze.

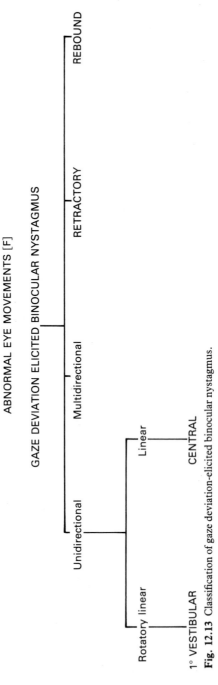

Fig. 12.13 Classification of gaze deviation-elicited binocular nystagmus.

Many subjects with CN show, on electrical recordings of eye movements, both pendular and jerk (i.e. a slow and a fast phase) waveforms. Daroff and Dell'Osso (1979) explain this on the basis of a high-gain instability of the slow eye movement subsystem (Dell'Osso, Gauthier, Lieberman and Stark, 1972; Dell'Osso, 1973). Alterations in the CN waveform and rate (6 Hz to about 2 Hz) have been associated with a need to permit foveal fixation which is associated with a change from a resting to an attentive situation (Gresty, Halmagyi and Leech, 1978). The vestibulo-ocular reflex is basically normal in patients with congenital nystagmus with or without associated ocular lesions (Yee, Baloh, Hornrubia and Kim, 1981).

Fixation nystagmus. There is considerable variation in what is meant by fixation nystagmus. Holmes (1917) defined fixation nystagmus when describing the signs of acute cerebellar injuries. This nystagmus is seen as a rule only when the patient fixes an object. 'It is on looking towards the injured side that the nystagmus is most pronounced; then it consists of wide, slow deviations towards the middle line, or more correctly, towards the rest point, and forcible jerks of large amplitude, slow in rate (2·3 Hz to 3 Hz) and fairly regular in rhythm, towards the point to which the eyes should be voluntarily directed . . . Both movements are as a rule strictly horizontal'. The rest point is the point to which the eyes, when at rest, tend to deviate. It is usually at 175 mrad to 525 mrad (10° to 30°) to the unaffected side of the midline. In such a position, no nystagmus is observed. Associated with this nystagmus towards the affected side is a 'nystagmus on fixing an object to his unaffected side, but it is more rapid, finer in range and less regular. Here too, the slow deviation is towards the rest point and the movements are most commonly horizontal . . . On convergence, both eyes often tend to deviate away from the side of the lesion and are brought back to their proper position by irregular jerks of small range . . . Spectacles with high, convex lenses . . . were placed in front of the patient's eyes and it was then found that when he moved them to order the oscillations were considerably less marked, or did not occur on deviation in certain directions.'

Nowadays, the term fixation nystagmus is often used to refer to any nystagmus which disappears or changes direction or form after optic fixation has been abolished. Moreover, the nystagmus which Holmes described in cerebellar lesions is frequently referred to as gaze paretic nystagmus.

Pendular nystagmus. This is an oscillatory eye movement in which fast and slow phases cannot be distinguished; the waveform is sinusoidal, with a frequency of about 4 Hz. Pendular nystagmus is also a fixation nystagmus. Congenital nystagmus may or may not be pendular. Pendular nystagmus may result from central vision being lost in early life. Acquired pendular nystagmus is probably due to a lesion of the cerebellar nuclei or their connections in the brain stem (Nashold, Slaughter and Gills, 1969; Aschoff, Conrad and Kornhuber, 1974). This acquired form is manifest as oscillopsia.

Vestibular nystagmus. This type of nystagmus exhibits both a slow and a quick phase; the waveform is thus like a sawtooth. There is usually a rotatory as well as a linear (usually horizontal) component to this nystagmus. It is most marked when the patient looks in the direction of the quick phase, and least marked on looking in the direction of the slow phase. Indeed, the nystagmus may be visible only when the patient's gaze is directed towards the side of the quick phase. This type

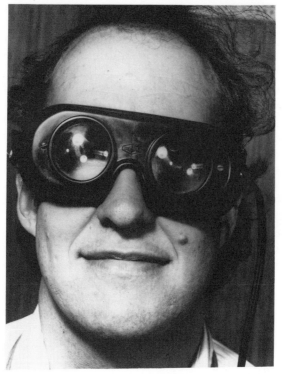

Fig. 12.14 Frenzel glasses.

of vestibular nystagmus is termed 1° (first degree) nystagmus. If the nystagmus is observed whilst in the primary gaze position also, it is termed 2° (second degree). If the nystagmus is also evident with gaze in the direction of the slow component, it is termed 3° (third degree).

A peripheral vestibular nystagmus is enhanced by abolishing optic fixation whether by the use of Frenzel glasses* (Fig. 12.14) or recording with the eyes closed or eyes open in darkness using electrical methods (see later). A central type vestibular nystagmus is diminished or abolished by removing optic fixation.

Gaze-deviation elicited nystagmus. In many instances, a SN (spontaneous nystagmus) may not be observed in the primary position of gaze. The nystagmus becomes evident only when the patient looks in one or other direction of gaze. Gaze-deviation elicited nystagmus comprises various types of nystagmus (Fig. 12.13). A mild degree (1°) of vestibular nystagmus may be present only when the patient looks in the direction of gaze of the quick component. Other types of nystagmus are elicited only when the gaze is shifted from the primary position.

* Frenzel (1925) glasses (Fig. 14) consist of a pair of +20 dioptre biconvex lenses. These not only interfere with fixation by the patient but also, by magnifying, assist observations by the observer. The source of illumination further interferes with fixation by the subject and improves conditions for observing the subject's eyes. Unfortunately the source of illumination may also provide some facility for the subject to fixate. Frenzel glasses are therefore not as effective in this respect as observing eye movements in complete darkness, e.g. by means of an infra-red viewer or by electrical registration methods.

Rebound nystagmus. This type of nystagmus was first reported by Bárány (Kornhuber, 1975) and was subsequently clearly demarcated by Hood, Kayan and Leech (1973). Hood and his colleagues point out that the features are such that, in the initial examination of the eyes in the primary position of gaze, no nystagmus is observed. With a subsequent gaze deviation to, say, the right, a brisk nystagmus with its fast component to the right appears. After about 20 s, the nystagmus fatigues and may even reverse direction. If at this time, the eyes are returned to the primary position, nystagmus to the left, not present initially, occurs and this too fatigues with time. Hood and his colleagues reported that this type of nystagmus is associated with chronic cellebellar disease and was found in 6 per cent of neurological patients referred for a neuro-otological examination.

Halmagyi and his colleagues (1979) have reported a rebound-rebound nystagmus which replaced a PAN treated with baclofen.

Physiological nystagmus. Daroff and Dell'Osso (1979) point out that there are three types of spontaneous physiological (normal) nystagmus, i.e. unsustained end-point nystagmus, sustained end-point and fatigue nystagmus.

Unsustained end-point nystagmus is the most common type of physiological nystagmus. This occurs with gaze deviations of 500 mrad (about 30°) or more. On initially attaining gaze deviations in excess of this angle, a few beats of nystagmus may occur. This nystagmus is typically a horizontal jerk nystagmus, with a quick and a slow component and with the quick component directed in the direction of gaze. Unsustained end-point nystagmus is frequently bilateral and commonly symmetrical.

Sustained end-point nystagmus again starts immediately the eyes attain an extreme lateral gaze position, or within a few seconds of attaining such a position. This nystagmus is again typically horizontal, bilateral and symmetrical. Under illuminated conditions the amplitude is within the range 15 mrad to 50 mrad (about 1° to 3°) and with a frequency in the range 1 Hz to 3 Hz. Changes occur in this pattern under conditions of darkness. Moreover, there is a distinct intra-subject variability (Schmidt and Kammerell, 1976). Of eleven normal subjects studied by Daroff and Dell'Osso using an infrared recording technique, six developed a sustained gaze-evoked nystagmus within gaze deviations of 700 mrad (40°); one subject developed the nystagmus at a gaze-deviation of only 350 mrad. In all cases, the slow phase shape was linear.

Fatigue nystagmus begins during extended maintenance of an extreme gaze deviation. This type of nystagmus becomes increasingly rotary with more pro-longed and extreme gaze deviations (Nylén, 1922). Bárány (1906b) reported that the condition occurred in 60 per cent of normal subjects with maximally deviated gaze maintained for periods in excess of 30 s. It would appear that the occurrence of this nystagmus is a function of the duration of the maintenance of extreme gaze deviation. Schmidt and Kammerell reported one subject where the nystagmus began after a latency of 90 s.

There is probably a continuum between many forms of physiological nystagmus and forms of pathological nystagmus. For example, both types of end-point nystagmus show remarkable similarities to gaze-evoked spontaneous nystagmus. The nystagmus of myasthenia gravis is probably an exaggeration of fatigue nystagmus.

Electrical registration of eye movements

A number of electrical techniques are now emerging for recording eye movements. The principal electrical technique, termed electro-oculography, depends on the fact that the eyeball behaves as a dipole, i.e. it is positively charged at one point with respect to a negative charge at another (Fig. 12.15). In man, the posterior pole is negatively charged with respect to the cornea and, fortunately, the electrical axis

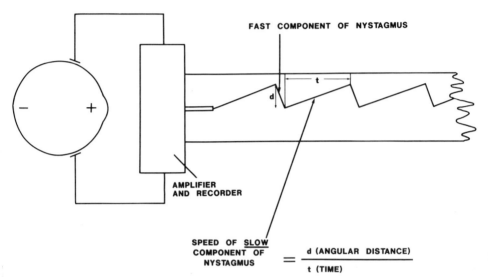

Fig. 12.15 Schematic showing the principles of electro-oculography in which the corneo-retinal potential is used to record deviations of the eyes from the primary gaze position. In this case the diagram shows how this electrical method will record a vestibular nystagmus as a saw-toothed wave because of the slow and the quick speed phases.

coincides with the anatomical and optic axes. Thus a pair of electrodes placed on either side of an eye will register a difference in potential whenever there is a movement of the eye in the plane of the electrodes. Since the eyeball acts as a dipole, potential differences produced by rotation of the eyeball in the plane of the electrodes will be proportional too the sine of the angle of rotation. However, in practice, because of the relatively small angles associated with nystagmus, this relationship between the voltage produced and the angular eye deviation is not significantly different from a linear one.

Vertical movements of an eye will be registered with one electrode above, and one below, the eye. A pair of vertical electrodes across each eye will be required to register a see-saw nystagmus. A patient with a spontaneous ataxic nystagmus shows a dissociated nystagmus on lateral gaze, where the abducting eye has greater amplitude. To detect and record this would require a *pair* of horizontal electrodes across each eye.

Controversy has raged over whether d.c. (direct current) or a.c. (alternating current) amplification should be used. If one requires to know the gaze position of an eye, when individual eye movements are registered, or the concomitant gaze position of the two eyes when their movement is recorded by a single pair of electrodes, then d.c. amplification must be used. Frequently, the examiner is prepared to forego knowledge of gaze direction, particularly when he is concerned only with recording the induced nystagmus which occurs with a caloric test. He will therefore frequently be content with a simple and electrically more stable a.c. amplifying system. Unfortunately, the characteristics of equipment for recording nystagmus are far from being standardised but some desirable features have been listed by Rubin (1968).

Optokinetic nystagmus and slow pursuit eye movements

Purkinje is said to have observed a nystagmus in bystanders who were watching passing cavalry. A nystagmus may also be observed in passengers in railway trains who gaze at the passing countryside (hence the term 'railway nystagmus'). This nystagmus is similar to vestibular nystagmus in that, although of optical origin, it shows a fast and a slow component.

Robinson (1975b) has sought to distinguish between OKN (optokinetic nystagmus) and pursuit nystagmus. The optokinetic system has little or nothing to do with following moving targets. It is concerned, phylogenetically, with estimating self-rotation and the generation of eye movements appropriate to self-rotation. Robinson illustrates the biological need for such a system to supplement the vestibular system by citing a fish which would swim around its territory every 10 s. This would give an angular velocity of 630 mrad s^{-1}. Accepting a cupular time constant of 4 s, there would be no vestibulo-ocular reflex left after 12 s, so that retinal images would slip at 630 mrad s and the fish would be unable to see anything. Thus the real purpose of the optokinetic system is not to track a moving visual environment whilst the object is stationary, but to use vision to help the vestibular system to assess self-rotation within the environment and generate appropriate eye movements. (As Robinson points out, one of the major conceptual advances in recent years has been the realisation that the semicircular canals are basically velocity transducers; they are not designed by nature to transduce head acceleration).

Vestibular and optokinetic signals are probably combined in the vestibular nuclei (Henn, Young and Finley, 1974) or in the prepositus hypoglossi nuclei of the dorsal medullary reticular formation (Baker and Berthoz, 1975; Uemura and Cohen, 1975).

Stimulation of the entire visual field is the appropriate stimulus for generating OKN. The subject should therefore be within a rotating cylinder. If the subject does not perceive self-rotation, the optokinetic system is probably not being stimulated. Robinson argues that rotating hand drums or moving stripes in front of the subject test the visual pursuit system and not the optokinetic system. However, for a number of years clinicians have used Bárány's vertically striped hand drum to elicit a nystagmus which has provided diagnostic information.

In 1926, Fox and Holmes showed that a DP (directional preponderance) of this optically-induced nystagmus occurred with lesions of the inferior part of the parietal lobe. In these patients where the DP occurs, the fast component of the nystagmus that is directed towards the side of a lesion is relatively more marked than that directed to the contralateral side. The actual change is a suppression of the nystagmus which is directed away from the side of the lesion. Gassel and Williams (1963) considered that the basic disturbance which is observed in these deep posterior hemisphere lesions is impaired slow visual pursuit function.

Baloh, Yee and Honrubia (1979) go further and say that the foveal pursuit system is impaired. The integrity of the slow pursuit system for objects going away from the side of a lesion would permit the fast phase of this nystagmus to be retained towards the side of a lesion.

Since Fox and Holmes' initial observation, this optically induced nystagmus has been shown to be disturbed by pathological processes in a variety of locations in the brain (Enoksson, 1956). Thus, even if the localising value is less specific than Fox and Holmes thought, the test has lateralising value, a DP being directed towards an involved cerebral hemisphere. Bárány (1907) first reported the abolition of the quick phases of both optically induced and vestibular nystagmus in supranuclear lesions. Dix and Hood (1971) reported that two cases (a man aged 62 years and a woman aged 64 years) of progressive supranuclear palsy showed abolition of the fast components both of this optically-induced nystagmus and of vestibular nystagmus (induced by simultaneous bilateral caloric stimuli) in the vertical plane in both cases. Tonic deviations of the eyes occurred in the direction of the slow component of both optically-induced nystagmus and vestibular nystagmus in both cases. Doll's head movements were intact in both cases in both vertical and horizontal planes.

The first and only sign of an internuclear ophthalmoplegia may be dissociation of this optically-induced nystagmus (Smith and David, 1964).

Hood and Leech (1974) and others have shown that, depending upon the condition of the test, it is possible to elicit two types of nystagmus with this so-called optokinetic drum. If the patient is instructed to count the stripes ('active' OKN), angular eye velocity is found to equal the drum angular velocity. Thus, under this condition, slow pursuit eye movement is being measured. However, despite conscious efforts of the patient, this 'active' type of response repeatedly lapses into the 'passive' type. This is the condition that is attained in clinical practice by asking the subject to 'just look at the drum'. Under this condition, angular eye velocity is not equal to drum angular velocity. A nystagmus induced by this method is usually considered to represent a true OKN. However, there is considerable variability in OKN responses (Abel and Barber, 1981).

In peripheral vestibular lesions, a DP may be observed with the 'passive' stimulation but not with the 'active' optical stimulation.

OKAN (optokinetic after nystagmus) is considered to be a response solely of the optokinetic system and not of the visual pursuit system. OKAN is a nystagmus which persists after an optokinetic stimulus has ended. Unlike a post-rotatory nystagmus (rotary after-nystagmus), the fast component of an OKAN beats in the same direction as the preceding OKN.

Since OKAN is usually completely suppressed with the eyes open in the light, it must be observed under conditions of darkness. This will require electrical registration of eye movements. The effective OKN stimulus is stopped by either switching off the room lights or covering the patient's eyes, at the same time instructing the patient to keep his eyes open. OKAN recorded with the eyes closed is usually less active or different to OKAN recorded with the eyes open (Suzuki, 1971).

OKAN is attributed to the brain extrapolating from the previous optokinetic stimuli (Robinson, 1975). It would appear, however, that tonic vestibular labyrinthine activity is required to permit optokinetic stimuli getting through to generate nystagmus. Labyrinthectomy in the rabbit abolishes, or almost nearly abolishes, both OKN and OKAN (Collewijn, 1975). There is also a complete loss of OKAN in patients with bilateral loss of semicircular canal function (Zee, 1975).

As with OKN a DP of OKAN may also occur with peripheral vestibular lesions.

Slow pursuit eye movements are usually examined by the PETT (pendulum eye tracking test) (Corvera, Torres-Courtney and Lopez-Rios, 1973). The subject is instructed to follow a moving pendulum and the consequent eye movements are recorded electrically. The pattern of pendulum movement is that of simple harmonic motion. Thus a sinusoidal recording will be observed from the eyes which faithfully follows such a movement. This is the normal finding. The visual amplitude of the pendulum swing is usually in the range 260 mrad (15°) to 520 mrad (30°). The period of pendulum is usually arranged to be in the range 2 s to 5 s, i.e. corresponding to a frequency range of 0.5 Hz to 0.2 Hz. Above a frequency of 0.5 Hz, saccadic (fast eye) movements begin to replace smooth (pursuit) eye movements (von Noorden and Preziosi, 1966).

Corvera and his colleagues reported that a normal sinusoidal curve with superimposed fast movements is associated with cerebellar disease and a deformed curve occurs with more widespread brain lesions. In brain stem lesions with a gaze nystagmus, impairment of pendular following movements is usually more marked than defects in optically-induced nystagmus (Jung and Kornhuber, 1964). Conversely, in peripheral vestibular lesions with a spontaneous vestibular nystagmus, the pendular following eye movement is esentially normal. Disappearance of the sinusoidal curve is associated with lesions of the ocular motor pathways in the tegmentum of the mesencephalon and of the pons. The following eye movement is also impaired by drugs, e.g. barbiturates (Rashbass and Russell, 1961), chlordiazepozide, ethanol and phenytoin (Corvera et al, 1973). Pendular eye tracking is also impaired with organic mercurial compound intoxication (Mizukoshi, Watanabe, Kato, Koike and Ino, 1975). Mizukoshi and his colleagues use a computerised system to subtract the basic sinusoidal wave from the eye movement trace.

Umeda, Ohtsu and Sakata (1975) have introduced a circular eye tracking test (CETT) to encompass the examination of vertical pursuit eye movements also. Umeda and his colleagues reported the use of this method on fifty-five patients with central vestibular disorders. Twenty-three of these patients showed eye movement abnormalities. The CETT abnormalities were classified into three types: (1) abnormalities principally with the horizontal component, (2) abnormalities principally with the vertical component, and (3) abnormalities in both the horizontal and vertical components. *Inter alia*, post-traumatic normal pressure hydrocephalus was associated with impaired horizontal slow pursuit movements, Wernicke's encephalopathy with impaired vertical pursuit movements, and late cortical cerebellar atrophy with abnormalities in both horizontal and vertical directions. The optimum parameters of the stimulus are: amplitude 700 mrad, frequency 0.33 Hz, target velocity 730 mrad s^{-1} (Umeda, 1980).

The obvious disadvantage of both the PETT and the CETT is the strong influence of the predictability of object motion (Dallos and Jones, 1963). In man, the pursuit eye movement system is able to predict future positions of a target up to 300 ms a head. It would thus appear that the present system for investigating eye tracking should be replaced by a more nearly random target movement in respect of both velocity and (at least in a two dimensional plane) of motion. This necessitates some type of large oscilloscope screen with a programmed target movement. Nevertheless, such a technique would enable one to study both the saccadic and the slow pursuit eye control systems and to do this not only with the horizontal gaze direction but with all gaze directions. At the Royal National Throat, Nose and Ear Hospital, a microprocessor-controlled television system is operating to produce such a visual stimulus.

Recent studies by Guedry and his colleagues (1979) and by Hood (1980) have shown that the nature of the background influences the ETT response. In cerebellar disorders, visual backgrounds improve response.

Oculocephalic reflex
The Roth-Bielschowsky or Doll's head phenomenon (*Puppenkopfphänomen*) refers to compensatory eye movements in response to passive turning of the head. The phenomenon is also termed the oculocephalic reflex and the method of inducing it, the oculocephalic manoeuvre. The manoeuvre is performed by (a) briskly turning the subject's head from side to side, and then (b) flexing and extending the neck. In each case, conjugate deviations of the eyes in the direction opposite to the direction of movement constitute a positive (normal) oculocephalic reflex. In such a case, the nuclear and infranuclear oculomotor pathways must be intact. When a conscious patient is examining, he should be told to fix his gaze on an object in the primary position of gaze. In such a case, the manoeuvre tests the fixation mechanism (position maintenance system), the slow pursuit (following mechanism) and the vestibular mechanism. With comatosed patients, only the last system is tested. Roth (1901) and Bielschowsky (1903) reported the occurrence of a phenomenon in patients who had lost the ability to make conjugate deviations of the eyes in one or other direction. This pattern of ocular response is referred to as the Roth-Bielschowsky syndrome. Vertical eye movements are preferentially affected. The syndrome is associated with lesions of the basal ganglia or tectum of the mid-brain. As mentioned previously, Dix and Hood (1971) reported preservation of Doll's head movements, but abolition of the fast components of both optically-induced nystagmus and of vestibular nystagmus, in older patients with progressive supranuclear palsy. In a series of 100 stroke patients seen within 48 h of admission, Yap and his colleagues (1975) observed that five had an absent oculocephalic reflex. Four of these five were dead within 4 weeks.

Counter-rolling
The phenomenon of counter-rolling of the eyes was first observed by John Hunter in 1786, and subsequently described, under the name *Gegenrollung*, by Bárány (1906a). In the French literature, this phenomenon is referred to as *la contrerotation oculaire*. Nelson and Cope (1971) refer to it as the ocular countertorsion reflex (OCR). Normally, static head tilts of up to 785 mrad (45°) produce compensatory

counter-rolling of the order of only 90 mrad (about 5°) (Miller, 1962). Vestibular disorders may be associated with either a reduction in the degree of counter-rolling or an accentuation, with rotations of up to 400 mrad (23°).

Ocular counter-rolling is absent in 'deaf mutes' (Miller and Graybiel, 1963) but may be preserved in cases of streptomycin intoxication where both caloric and rotatory stimuli failed to elicit a vestibular response. Nelson and House (1971) reported that the degree of counter-rolling was halved in subjects who had undergone unilateral labyrinthectomy or a vestibular nerve section.

Counter-rolling may be augmented during vertiginous episodes (Bárány, 1906a).

Ocular counter-rolling is frequently associated with skew deviation of the eyes and head tilting. This postural abnormality is termed the ocular tilt reaction (Rabinovitch, Sharpe and Sylvester, 1977). Halmagyi, Gresty and Gibson (1978) have reported the occurrence of this reaction following inadvertent destruction of a vestibular labyrinth during stapedectomy.

Halmagyi and his colleagues offer the most likely explanation for ocular counter-rolling never being fully compensated, i.e. the failure to realign the visual with the earth-fixed axes. They point out that, if there were full oculomotor compensation for head tilt, then the visual and earth-fixed axes will be matched despite the fact that the head might no longer be vertically aligned in space. A mismatch of visual, vestibular and proprioceptive information could be a disadvantage during natural movements. However, an incompletely compensatory response generates a continuous visual error signal to stimulate correct realignment of the head with respect to the earth-fixed axes.

Ocular counter-rolling is best observed by fundoscopy. Actual measurement of the torsion can be made with Lingwong and Herman's (1971) photographic method.

Positioning nystagmus and positional nystagmus

There are a group of tests, sometimes referred to as the positional tests for nystagmus, in which the nystagmus is elicited by means of a variety of either cervical posture or head positioning tests. In the routine examination for nystagmus, nystagmus should be sought not only with the head in the primary position but also when flexed, extended, laterally inclined or rotated. These constitute the cervical posture tests. Nystagmus produced, or accentuated, by these manoeuvres is due to the operation of cervical proprioceptors and/or vertebral artery compression.

The positional test described by Dix and Hallpike (1952) to elicit a nystagmus consists of firmly grasping the head of a patient, who is sitting on a couch, and then briskly taking the patient back into the critical position (Fig 12.16). This position is one in which the head is rotated 785 mrad (45°) to one side and extended 500 mrad (nearly 30°) over the edge of the couch. The test has consequently been criticised in that at least three nystagmogenic factors are operated. These are what are referred to in the French literature as *l'élément cinétique* (kinetic factor), *l'élément cervical* (cervical factor) and *l'élément spatial* (truly positional factor). It is, however, precisely because of these multiple factors that the test, performed in this manner, is a convenient screening test for 'positional nystagmus': thus in the French it is referred to as *une épreuve de dépistage* (Aubry and Pialoux, 1957). It is

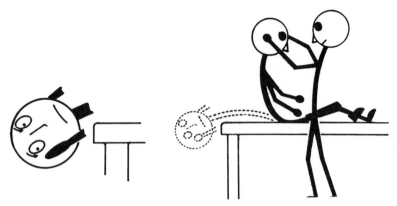

Fig. 12.16 Manoeuvre designed to elicit both positioning and positional nystagmus (courtesy of Dr M.R. Dix).

nevertheless doubtful whether the cervical factor is important in the production of nystagmus under these conditions, especially when the nystagmus is sought either by the naked eye or by Frenzel glasses. Dix and Hallpike retested a group of subjects who demonstrated nystagmus with this procedure by examining them on a tilt table; this would abolish any cervical factor. There was no appreciable change in the findings. In any case, subsequent manoeuvres can be conducted to eliminate one or other potential nystagmogenic factors. One can, as Nylén (1950) and others have reported, perform the positional test by asking the subject to assume the critical position slowly of his own accord. Thus any nystagmus produced by this procedure will be truly *positional* (*Lagenystagmus*) and not *positioning* (*Lagerungs-nystagmus*). The latter type of nystagmus broadly corresponds to the 'benign paroxysmal positional nystagmus' of Dix and Hallpike, and the former type, to the central type of positional nystagmus'. The paroxysmal type is much more common than the central type. The term 'benign' has been objected to by Lindsay (1962) and others because some of the cases, albeit a small proportion (probably less than 1 per cent), are associated with an intracranial tumour (Cawthorne and Hallpike, 1957; Riesco McClure, 1957; Harrison and Ozsahinoglu, 1972). Thus these cases are not representative of the clinical condition. Similarly, because of the paucity of histological material available, it is doubtful if this material is representative of positioning nystagmus in general. Moreover, there is disagreement among the experts regarding the interpretation of the histological material (compared Cawthorne and Hallpike, 1957; Schuknecht, 1962; Lindsay, 1962). Nevertheless, the histopathological studies of Schuknecht (1969) indicate that at least one pathological basis for positioning nystagmus is a condition termed cupulolithiasis. Cupulolithiasis encompasses the prevalence of an inorganic deposit on the cupula of the posterior semicircular duct; this renders the organ sensitive to gravitational force and therefore subject to stimulation with changes in head position. In some cases the cupulolithiasis may be due to dislodged otoliths (otoconia). These are minute crystalline bodies (calcite) which normally occur in the gelatinous otolithic membrane of the maculae of the utricle and saccule.

Dayal and his colleagues (1977) point out that paroxysmal positional nystagmus is the most frequently seen nystagmus prior to its disappearance in end-organ-induced nystagmus. Following a study of stapedectomised patients and drug-induced nystagmus, these authors consider that the type of spontaneous or provoked vestibular nystagmus was of little diagnostic value in localising the site of a lesion; the various types reflected different degrees of vestibular compensation that occurred.

A possible pathophysiological explanation for positioning nystagmus is that it represents an imbalance of a pair of vertical semicircular duct systems. Thus it would be analogous to the nystagmus *Nystagmusbereitschaft* (state of nystagmus 'readiness') which occurs in respect of the horizontal semicircular duct system, and which is indicated by a horizontal head-shaking (see later) nystagmus or a directional preponderance of the caloric test. It would be noted that, in the positional test, the head of taken back in a position wherein the head is rotated 785 mrad, i.e. the movement is in the plane of a pair of vertical semi-circular ducts (Stenger, 1955; Frenzel, 1960; Hallpike, 1967). Specifically, the ipsilateral posterior and the contralateral superior (anterior vertical) ducts are implicated. Stimulation of this pair of ducts would be expected to produce a nystagmus with a rotatory component when the eyes are viewed by the observer facing the patient. This is the usual finding. It is to be noted that Ledoux (1958), in animal experimental studies, demonstrated that the resting action potential discharges in the nerves from the vertical semicircular ducts were appreciably affected by head positioning. Duensing (1967) found that cells in the lateral vestibular nucleus, which received vertical duct signals also show a marked interaction with gravity receptor mechanisms. Baloh, Sakala and Honrubia (1979) analysed the electrically recorded eye movements associated with paroxysmal positional nystagmus. They concluded that the characteristics were consistent with a burst of excitatory activity originating in the posterior duct of the ear that is undermost at the end of the positioning manoeuvre.

Patients with persisting paroxysmal vertigo usually respond to a system of head and balance exercises (Dix, 1979). The *modus operandi* for this treatment is by an habituation mechanism. Intractable paroxysmal vertigo not responding to this method of physical treatment may be treated by transection of the posterior division of the vestibular nerve in the foramen singulare (Gacek, 1974). If there is no useful hearing in the involved ear, labyrinthectomy may be performed. Schuknecht (1962) reported performing the operation for this purpose on a 77 years old woman. She continued to be free from vertigo as long as six years later.

Head-shaking nystagmus

Kopfschüttelnystagmus is provoked by rapid side-to-side movements of the head (Vogel, 1932). Twenty such movements provide a suitable stimulus. The eyes are then observed for nystagmus immediately after this manoeuvre. In the case of peripheral lesions this nystagmus is usually directed to the contralateral side. This may be the case even when a recovery nystagmus is present (Frenzel, 1961). If such a discordance is evident, it may be due to the influence of neck cervical proprioceptors in the head-shaking procedure. However, it is equally (perhaps more) likely that such a discordance can be explained on the basis of the existence, within a deranged vestibular system, of something analogous to 'recruitment' in the auditory system.

Kamei and Kornhuber (1974) failed to demonstrate any head-shaking nystagmus in a group of forty normal subjects. However, in a group of patients with central vestibular lesions, head-shaking nystagmus under Frenzel's glasses was the only nystagmus detectable. The test is contraindicated in cases of raised intracranial pressure and retinal detachment.

Caloric tests
If a patient with a suspected vestibular disorder has not shown any spontaneous or provocation nystagmus in a examination conducted so far, he may then be investigated with rotatory tests (Bárány, 1907; van Egmond, Groen and Jongkees, 1948; Greiner, Conraux and Collard, 1969; Wall, O'Leary and Black, 1978; Wolfe, Engelken and Olson, 1979). However, the major problem with rotation tests is that both vestibular labyrinths are stimulated.

The caloric test (Fig. 12.17) is an attempt to stimulate a one-sided rotatory stimulus. Thermal stimuli applied to the ear under test tends to produce

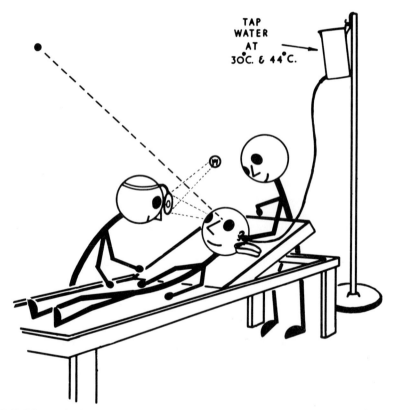

Fig. 12.17 Diagram indicating the general principles of the bithermal caloric test as standardised by Fitzgerald and Hallpike (1942) and as employed throughout the majority of ENT, and Neuro-otology clinics in Britain. Water at the appropriate temperature is mixed in, and delivered from, a douche can. One experimenter is delivering water to the ear under test. The other is observing induced nystagmus, if any, by means of light reflected from a head mirror (the room is in semi-darkness). The illumination is, however, sufficient for the subject to see a spot on the ceiling on which he fixes his gaze (by courtesy of Dr M.R. Dix).

convection currents in the semicircular ducts, i.e. a tendency to move the fluid relative to the walls of the duct, so exerting a deflecting force on the cupula concerned. On each side, the lateral semicircular duct lies more laterally than the other ducts so it is more convenient to attempt to stimulate this duct with thermal stimuli, i.e. fluids (usually air or water) above or below body temperature. Since this duct is inclined 520 mrad (30°) to the horizontal plane, the head must be tilted back about one radian to place the duct in the optimum (vertical) position for setting up convection currents. If the patient is recumbent, which is the usual position for conducting the conventional caloric test, this means the head will be flexed 520 mrad with the subject in the supine position. In order to have equally strong but opposite, i.e. equipollent ampullopetal and ampullofugal stimuli, the temperature of the warm stimulus should be the same number of degrees above body temperature as the cold stimulus is below it. Since 317 K (44°C) is the threshold of uncomfortable warmth, this is usually used as the temperature of the warm stimulus. Correspondingly, 303 K (30°C) is used as the temperature of the cold stimulus. The use of these two temperatures for caloric test stimuli forms the basis of the so-called bithermal caloric test which was first reported by Thornval (1971) and subsequently standardised for clinical use by Fitzgerald and Hallpike (1942). More recently, the Vestibular Laboratory of the Royal National Throat, Nose and Ear Hospital has been using temperatures at ±4 K re body temperature.

The use of air in lieu of water to provide the thermal stimuli has been reported by Capps, Preciado, Paparella and Hoppe (1973) and others.

With the patient in the prone position, the warm stimulus becomes an ampullofugal, and the cold an ampullopetal, stimulus. There is no significant difference in the nystagmic response to the caloric test stimulus in the prone compared with the supine position. (Lee, 1969).

The physics of the caloric test has been considered by Schmaltz (1932) who concluded that the observations regarding the latency and time course of the nystagmic response agreed with theoretical predictions. More recently, Chalabi (1981) has studied the transfer function of the caloric test using more sophisticated mathematical techniques and with more detailed biophysical considerations.

Two principal patterns of caloric test response are recognised, i.e. *canal paresis (CP) and directional preponderance (DP)*. In addition to these two principal patterns of response, there are a number of mixed patterns (Fig. 12.18).

A CP pattern of response, unassociated with a DP, occurs when one or both ears are completely, or partially, unresponsive to both the warm and the cold stimuli. A DP means that they nystagmus is more easily elicited, or shows a more marked activity, in one direction than the other. A DP pattern of response shows, for each ear, a difference in response to the two thermal stimuli; for the one ear, the warm stimulus gives a better nystagmic response, for the other ear, the cold stimulus elicits a greater response. The particular ear which gives a better response to the warm stimulus depends on the direction of the DP; if the DP is to the right, a warm stimulus applied to that right ear elicits a better response than a cold stimulus applied to that same ear, or a warm stimulus applied to the opposite (left) ear. In practice, caloric response patterns indicate a mixture of CP and DP. For unilateral vestibular lesions, this combined pattern is characterized by little or no

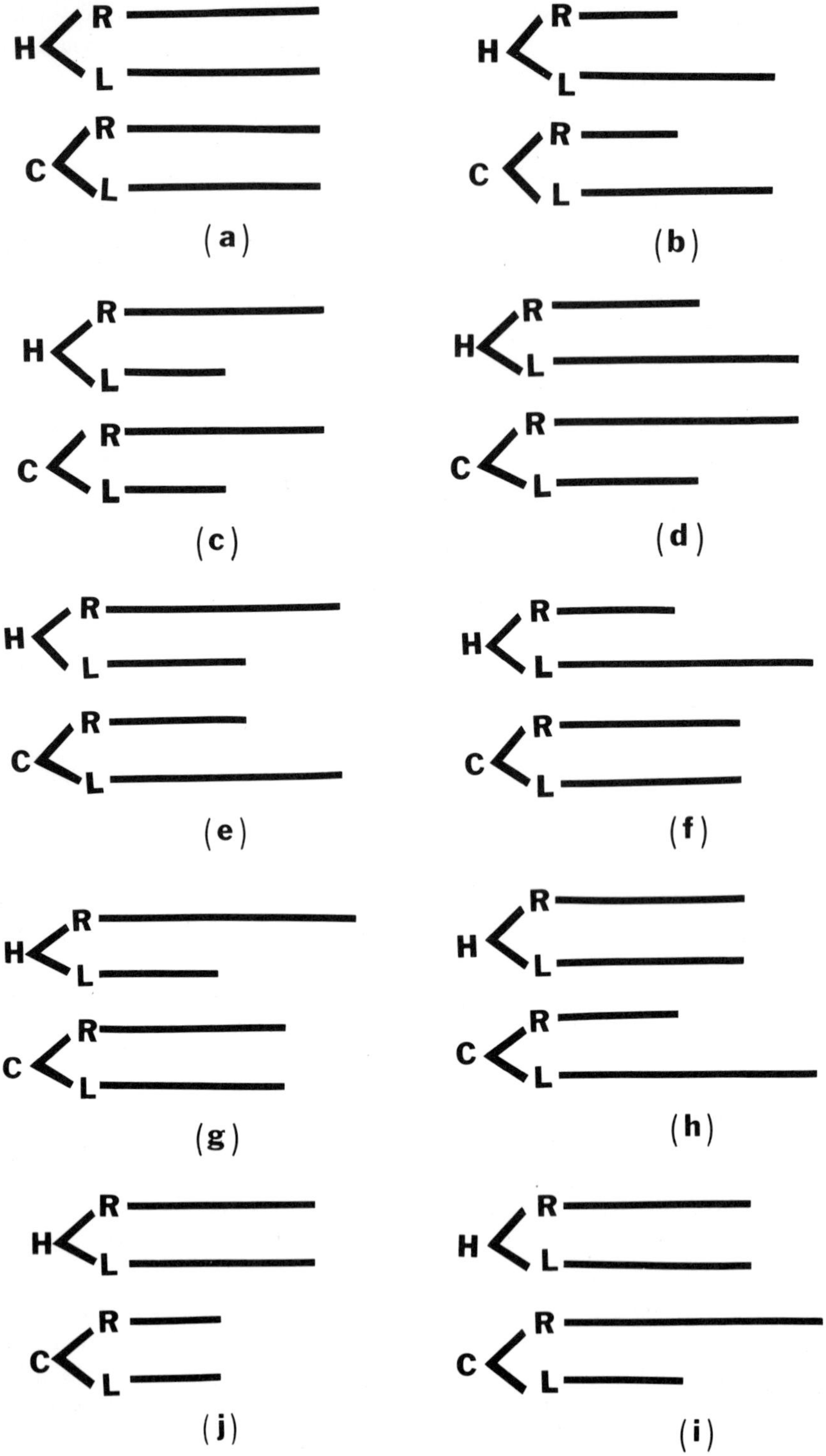

(a)

(b)

(c)

(d)

(e)

(f)

(g)

(h)

(j)

(i)

difference in response of the two ears in respect of one temperature, but a significant difference in the response of the two ears for the other temperature. For DPs away from the side of the paresis, the two ears show a significant difference in response to the warm stimulus, but little or no difference in respect of the cold reaction; for DPs directed towards the side of the paresis, the converse is true. One should remember that, in the interpretation of these responses, a warm caloric stimulus produces nystagmus to the same side as the stimulus, a cold caloric stimulus to the opposite side. A mnemonic which has been suggested to remember these directions is COWS (cold opposite; warm same). The direction of a nystagmus is always designated according to the direction of the fast phase. 'Warm' and 'cold' stimuli refer to caloric stimuli whose temperatures are above or below body temperature respectively.

The magnitude of nystagmic response (duration, total number of beats or maximum velocity of slow phase) in the caloric test can be specified by expressing either CP or DP as a percentage. Thus the percentage CP, E, can be expressed as

$$E = [\{(B + D) - (A + C)\}/(A + B + C + D)]\ 100 \qquad (1)$$

where   A = response to warm stimulus applied to the right ear,

B = response to warm stimulus applied to the left ear,

C = response to cold stimulus applied to the right ear,

and   D = response to cold stimulus applied to the left ear,

and the percentage directional preponderance, F, as

$$F = [\{(A + D) - (B + C)\}/(A + B + C + D)]\ 100 \qquad (2)$$

Thus, if F is positive, a RCP is the case, if negative a LCP is the case. If D is positive, the DP is to the right, if negative, to the left.

Equation (1) is a measure of the preponderance of one vestibular labyrinth, or, more specifically, the lateral duct, ampullary crest and nerve, over the contralateral corresponding structures. Consequently, Jongkees (1973) prefers to use the term labyrinthine preponderance instead of canal paresis. He also points out that the use of the term 'canal paresis' might lead to irrational utterances in certain cases, e.g. in demyelinating disorders, where the patient may have completely

---

Fig. 12.18 Method of recording the results of the caloric test. 'H' denotes responses to the hot thermal stimulus; 'C' results from the cold thermal stimulus and 'R' and 'L' refer to the right and left ears respectively. A bar is drawn against each stimulus and the length of this is proportional to the magnitude of the nystagmic response. Thus Fig. 12.18a, where the responses are the same, or a little different, would be a normal response. Fig. 12.18b, where the responses to irrigation of the right ear are reduced compared with the left ear, would be a right 'canal paresis'. Fig. 12.18c would indicate a left 'canal paresis'. Fig. 12.18d shows a pattern where one of the responses to each thermal stimulus is diminished compared with the other response, but the pattern of response is different for the two temperatures. This pattern of response is termed directional/preponderance since, in the case illustrated, the two stimuli providing greater responses are those where nystagmus is, in each case, produced in the same direction, i.e. to the left. This then is the pattern of a left 'directional preponderance (DP)'. Fig. 12.18e shows a directional preponderance to the right. Fig. 12.18f shows a combined RCP (right canal paresis) associated with a DP to the left; Fig. 12.18g, a combined LCP and a DP to the right; Fig. 12.18h, a combined RCP and a DP to the right; and Fig. 12.18i, a combined LCP and a DP to the left. Fig. 12.18j shows a poor response to the cold stimuli. If, in this test, the cold stimuli had followed the hot stimuli, this would be an index of vestibular habituation.

normal labyrinths. Most importantly, a semicircular canal, being a bony structure, cannot be paralysed. However, the term 'labyrinthine preponderance' is itself not free from criticism since 'labyrinth' is a synonym for the internal ear, and cochlear function in so-called labyrinthine preponderance cases may be entirely normal. Objections would also arise in respect of the terms 'duct preponderance' or 'ampullary preponderance'; abbreviation of the former would give confusion with directional preponderance and the abbreviation of the latter would give confusion with action potential. The matter must therefore rest until vestibulometric terminology has been standardised. Nevertheless, the term lateral ampulloneural preponderance (LAP) might be suggested since the term would (a) emphasise a relative caloric response in respect of the two ears and (b) emphasise that the test is primarily one of the lateral semicircular duct and its sensor (ampullary crest) together with its pathway (nerve). Thus an impaired response (to both warm and cold stimuli) for the left ear would be designated a RLAP (equals right lateral ampulloneural preponderance); a converse response would be termed a LLAP (left lateral ampulloneural preponderance).

The relative, rather than the absolute, response of the two ears is important; this is indicated by the animal experiments of McCabe and Ryu (1969). These authors showed that, after unilateral labyrinthectomy, cerebellar inhibitions shuts down the resting activity of tonic neurons of the medial vestibular muclei of the intact side. This would explain observations of diminished caloric reactivity of contralateral ears in a period subsequent to a unilateral vestibular labyrinthine damage.

Irrespective of whether we accept CP as an absolute or as a relative measurement, it is the sole measurement of vestibular function which can be used to lateralise the dysfunction. A DP due to a peripheral vestibular lesion may be directed away from or towards the involved side. A DP reflects the degree of vestibular imbalance so that, if a spontaneous nystagmus is present, it will be in the same direction as this nystagmus. If, during the course of recovery from a peripheral vestibular lesion, the spontaneous nystagmus disappears, then it will be replaced by a DP. This DP will, initially, at least, continue to be in the same direction as the antecedent nystagmus. Later, however, with the passage of time, it may reverse direction and be directed towards the affected ear. This condition is not infrequently found in chronic vestibular disorders. This reversed DP is analogous therefore to Stenger's (1959) *Erholungsnystagmus* (recovery nystagmus). A further complication is that if the caloric test has been conducted under conditions of optic fixation a DP may have arisen as the result of a hemisphere lesion, especially of the posterior half of the temporal lobe. The DP in such cases is directed towards the side of the lesion (Fitzgerald and Hallpike, 1942).

A recovery DP towards the side of a peripheral vestibular labyrinthine lesion (indicated by a 'canal paresis') is the basis for caloric test results which show a difference between the response to the cold but not to the warm stimuli. That such a condition is not uncommon is indicated by Norré's (1975) findings that the use of a warm caloric test as the sole vestibular screening test would not only miss cases of vestibular dysfunction, but would be just as bad as using the cold caloric test as the sole screening test. The use of a warm caloric test as a screening test must be conducted with other procedures, e.g. a search for spontaneous or provocation vestibular nystagmus using Frenzel glasses or electrical measurements, to detect the vestibular imbalance, which as Koch and his colleagues (1959) have indicated, can be termed a DPSN (directional preponderance/spontaneous nystagmus). In the event that these tests fail to indicate the presence of a vestibular imbalance, then a caloric test is required only to provide evidence for the existence (or otherwise) of a 'canal paresis'. A DP showing up in the caloric test results in the absence of any other evidence for a vestibular imbalance should not be considered to be of pathological significance.

The importance of testing sequence is evident in data presented by Van der Laan and Oosterveld (1974). Caloric test responses were clearly much more age dependent when a cold-warm sequence of testing was used than when a warm-cold sequence was used.

Influence of test conditions

The caloric test may be performed (a) with the eyes open and fixating, (b) with the eyes open in darkness, and (c) with the eyes closed. Not only might these three conditions influence the relative *intensities* of the *observed nystagmus* (or even whether it is present or not) (Hood 1967; Hinchcliffe 1971; Haciska 1973) but the *pattern* of the *caloric test results* may also be different (Carmichael et al, 1961; Dix and Leech, 1974). Consequently, caloric testing should, if possible, encompass these three conditions. The evidence which is now available (Hood and Dix, 1973) suggests that abolishing optic fixation may reduce the chance of detecting an abnormal caloric pattern not only in cerebral hemisphere disorders, but also in peripheral vestibular disorders. It might therefore seem appropriate, until the matter is further elucidated (including measurement of the reliability of the various tests and of the ability of a test to differentiate normal from abnormal), to employ screening caloric tests under conditions of optic fixation.

One of the perceptions associated with response to the caloric test (and many other vestibular stimuli) is the sensation that a particular point in visual space is moving. This illusion is termed the oculogyral illusion (OGI). The use of this as an index of caloric test response was suggested by van Dishoeck and Nijhoff in 1953. A clinical caloric test based on this method has been shown to be both simple and reliable (Arroyo and Hinchcliffe, 1977). These authors concluded that, when used in conjunction with other tests for detecting vestibular imbalance, e.g. examination for spontaneous and provocation nystagmus using Frenzel glasses, the OGI caloric test should provide a convenient procedure for the clinical examination of vestibular function.

The OGI caloric test has the supreme advantage that not only does it not require any special apparatus for the recording and registration of nystagmus but it can be done without requiring the examiner to be able to recognise nystagmus. However, it does require the availability of thermostatically controlled water baths which are used to fill the 50 ml syringes used to deliver the stimuli. A simpler test, but one which does require the observer to be able to recognise nystagmus, involves the use of, initially, 0·2 ml of ice water (Linthicum, 1964). Linthicum reported the endeavour to identify a 'threshold' by doubling the amount of ice water if no nystagmic response was found with the lower volume. Nelson (1969) has modified this method by using Frenzel glasses to abolish optic fixation and so enhance the induced vestibular nystagmus. Nelson points out that the features of his test which recommend it for clinical use include the universal availability and portability of the test materials since only a paper cup with water, three ice cubes, a plastic tuberculin syringe, a watch and the Frenzel glasses are required.

Caloric test with and without optic fixation
In 1963, Hart and Riesco-MacClure modified the conventional caloric test to encompass the effect of both optic fixation and absence of optic fixation on the induced nystagmus (Hart, 1967). The precise pathological significance of the findings were, however, not clarified until the studies of Ledoux and Demanez (1967) and Haciska (1970). It would appear that, as with normal subjects (e.g. Sokolovski, 1965), patients with peripheral vestibular disorders show a more marked caloric response when optic fixation has been abolished. Patients with central lesions may show a more marked response in the presence of optic fixation (Fig. 12.19). Demanez (1968) observed that this phenomenon was sometimes the only abnormal vestibular sign in patients with vertebrobasilar insufficiency. Moreover, with some central lesions, e.g. vestibulocochlear schwannomas, the effect was a function of the magnitude of the disease process. The phenomenon may be observed on the side opposite to a vestibulocochlear schwannoma when there is no ipsilateral caloric response (Hinchcliffe, 1971). As well as observing the phenomenon in brain stem lesions, Haciska found the phenomenon to be produced by drugs acting on the reticular formation of the brain stem.

Attempts have been made to quantify the phenomenon both by Demanez (1968) and by Hood and Korres (1979). Demanez proposed an ocular fixation index which is the percentage ratio of the product of the amplitude of induced nystagmus and its frequency with the eyes open to the product of the amplitude of the nystagmus and its frequency with the eyes closed. The fixation index proposed by Hood and Korres is the ratio of the maximum slow phase speed with the eyes open in darkness with the maximum slow phase speed with optic fixation. The two indices

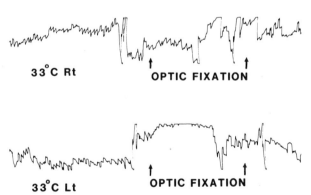

33°C Rt   OPTIC FIXATION

33°C Lt   OPTIC FIXATION

Fig. 12.19 Caloric responses to 306 K (33° C) for the right and left ears of a 56-year-old man with a suspected tumour involving the right vestibulocochlear nerve. On each occasion the test is commenced with optic fixation abolished. A period of optic fixation is indicated on the recording. The upper recording shows that the caloric-induced nystagmus is not inhibited by optic fixation, whereas that in the lower recording is. This reflects the operation of two phenomena: (i) the failure of optic fixation to inhibit vestibular nystagmus in centreal lesions, and (ii) the accentuation of abnormal caloric response patterns under conditions of optic fixation.

are therefore somewhat different, not only in respect of the measures taken but also the conditions under which responses are observed.

Nystagmic responses under conditions of eye closure are frequently different to when optic fixation is abolished by the eyes being kept open, e.g. in darkness. The state of arousal, as Sokolovski and others have shown, has a greater influence on the eye-closure condition. Moreover, elevation of the eyes behind closed lids (Bell's phenomenon) operates in the eye closure condition (Takemori, Moriyama and Totsuka, 1979; Tjernström, 1973).

Hart (1967) described the University of Chicago method of performing the 'fixation and non-fixation' caloric test as follows: The caloric test proceeds first under the condition of optic fixation being inhibited (either by Frenzel glasses or by eye closure—if electro-oculography is available)*. The particular ear is irrigated with water at the appropriate temperature for 40 s. The maximum response (under conditions of absence of optic fixation) is recorded during the period 60 s to 75 s after the onset of aural irrigation. At 75 s, optic fixation is ensured and the subsequent response over the period 75 s to 90 s is recorded. As soon as the nystagmus stops under this condition of optic fixation, fixation is again abolished. Any further nystagmic response is recorded.

Simultaneous binaural caloric testing
If, with the subject supine, the two ears are irrigated simultaneously with water at the same temperature, a nystagmus will result which, at least in theory, will reflect the difference in response to the two stimuli given separately. Thus, if a response of the same magnitude is obtained with water at 303 K (30°C) when the ears are separately stimulated, then the responses will cancel out when the ears are simultaneously stimulated. No nystagmus would then be observed. If water at 303 K produces, when given monaurally, a greater response from the right ear than from the left ear, simultaneous (binaural) stimulation with water at the same temperature should produce nystagmus to the left. This technique of bilateral calorisation was introduced into neuro-otology by Ruttin and by Brunner many years ago but it is only recently that Brookler (1971) has reported a satisfactory procedure where the test is performed and recorded electro-oculographically. For judging an abnormal response to binaural stimulation, Brookler now looks for three clearcut beats in a 3 s period and occurring within 30 s after the end of an irrigation. Unfortunately, the absence of any observable nystagmus following both warm and cold bilateral stimulation could mean not only that the labyrinth (specifically the ampullary cristo-neural system) was normal but also that there was no vestibular function whatsoever. Moreover, in the absence of any vestibular imbalance, the absence of any nystagmus following bilateral stimulation could also mean that the two labyrinths showed equal degrees of hyporeflexia (bilateral vestibular nerve or labyrinth lesion) or equal degrees of hyperreflexia (central release). In clinical practice, equal degrees of hyporeflexia or hyperreflexia without vestibular imbalance should be infrequent so that the only pathological condition to guard against would be bilateral non-functioning vestibular labyrinths.

---

* The Vestibular Laboratory of the Institute of Laryngology and Otology and other centres have shown that it is convenient to use both Frenzel glasses and record eye movements electrically.

Simultaneous bilateral caloric stimulation may also be used to test cristo-neural function in respect of the vertical semicircular canals. For such purposes, the subject's head is placed in the vertical position. Downward directed nystagmus occurs with binaural warm caloric stimuli; upward directed nystagmus occurs with binaural cold caloric stimuli. Dix (1970) has used this procedure in the investigation of patients with supranuclear ophthalmoplegias.

Measures of caloric test response

Using electro-oculographic recording techniques, it is possible to measure a number of indices of the nystagmic response to the caloric test. A quarter of a century ago, in extensive studies, Henriksson (1956) demonstrated the diagnostic value of the slow phase speed. A multivariate analysis of caloric test measurements, including duration and slow phase speed of the responses to both warm and cold stimuli has been done using electrical recordings of eye movements. The results showed that the slow phase speed of nystagmus induced by the warm stimulus was the most valid of these measures of vestibular function (Hinchcliffe, 1967). Subsequent studies have indicated that the interbeat interval is a more stable, yet better discriminatory, measure than either the slow phase or the quick phase speed (Sayers and Hinchcliffe, 1976; Sayers, Hinchcliffe and Hamid, 1978; Hamid, 1979) (Fig. 12.20).

The implementation of a computer-based electro-oculographic analysis system has been reported by Hamid, Sayers, Vickery and Hinchcliffe (1979).

Finally, mention should be made of an interesting experiment by Barnes and Benson (1978). The left ear of eight subjects was irrigated with water at 317 K for 30 s. The stimulus was administered with the subject in the conventional caloric position, i.e. in the near supine position, with the coronal plane of the head at about one radian to the vertical. Each subject was exposed to two experimental conditions separated by a period of at least 24 hours. One condition was a control in which the subject remained in the classical clinical caloric position. The other (reorientation) condition involved the subject's head being brought forward through a right angle; in this position the effective stimulus to the cupula attributable to the density gradient is reduced to zero. The subject was then moved back and forwards between the two positions at intervals of 60 s for 540 s. With these conditions of testing, nystagmus was observed for at least the period of the test (Fig. 12.21). Fortunately, with the usual conditions of clinical testing (when the head is kept in the one position), no significant interaction have been detected when the next thermal stimulus is given as soon as the nystagmus generated by the preceding stimulus has finished.

CONCLUSIONS

It is clear that there are a multiplicity of diverse tests for the investigation of balancing function in the elderly. Clearly not all of these will be needed in a given case. A selection of tests will be governed by many factors, including not only what aspects of balancing function are deranged but also what the general psychological and medical condition of the patient appears to be, as well as the availability of particular apparatus. Nevertheless, it will be clear that much can now be done in the way of characterising the disorders of balance in the elderly.

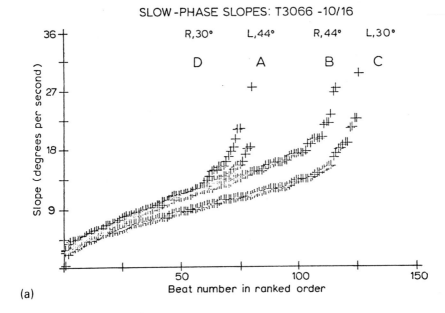

(a)

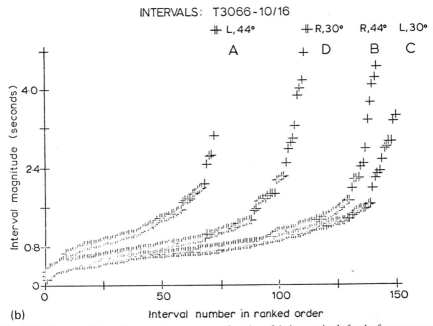

(b)

Fig. 12.20 Graphs of the rank ordered measures as a function of their magnitude for the four responses in a single caloric test. No nystagmus beats have been rejected. Fig. 12.20a shows the sequence of slow-phase speeds of successive beats re-ordered according to their absolute magnitude. Fig. 12.20b shows a similar display of the interbeat interval sequences. The pattern is that of a DP to the right. Note that the pattern is brought out better with the rank-ordered interbeat interval sequences than with the slow phase speed.

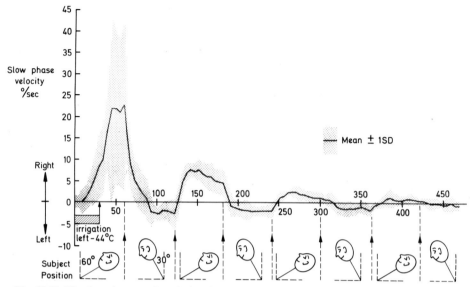

Fig. 12.21 The slow phase angular velocity of the eye (mean of eight subjects) following irrigation of the left ear canal with water at 317 K for 30 s. Subjects were moved as indicated in the sagittal plane between the initial classical clinical caloric position and the forward position at regular 6 s intervals. Note not only the persistence of nystagmus over a much longer time span than recorded when the subject remains in the near-supine position but also reversal of direction when the head is brought forwards (Barnes and Benson, 1978).

REFERENCES

Abel Sharon M, Barber H O 1981 Measurement of optokinetic nystagmus for otoneurological diagnosis. Annals of Otology, Rhinology and Laryngology, 90: Suppl. pp 1–12

Adams G 1978 Essentials of geriatric medicine. Oxford Medical Publications, Oxford

Arroyo J A, Hinchcliffe R 1977 Caloric test with oculogyral illusion as response. Journal of Laryngology and Otology 91: 309–321

Aschoff J C, Conrad B, Kornhuber H H 1974 Acquired pendular nystagmus with oscillopsia in multiple sclerosis: a sign of cerebellar nuclei disease. Journal of Neurology, Neurosurgery and Psychiatry 37: 570–577

Aubry M, Pialoux P 1957 Maladie de l'oreille interne et otoneurologie. Masson, Paris

Bagshaw J 1963 Secondary convergence spasm following primary failure of accommodation. British Orthoptics Journal 20: 112–113

Baker R, Berthoz A 1975 Is the prepositus hypoglossi nucleus the source of another vestibulo-ocular pathway? Brain Research 86: 121–127

Baloh R W, Honrubia V, Konrad H R 1976 Periodic alternating nystagmus. Brain 99: 11–26

Baloh R W, Sakala Susan M, Honrubia V 1979 Benign Paroxysmal Positional Nystagmus. American Journal of Otolaryngology 1: 1–6

Baloh R D, Yee R D, Honrubia V 1980 Optokinetic nystagmus and Parietal Lobe Lesions. Archives of Neurology 7: 269–276

Bárány R 1906a Über die vom Ohrlabyrinth ausgelöste Gegenrollung der Augen bei Normalhörenden, Ohrenkranken und Taubstummen. Archiv für Ohrenheilkunde 68: 1–30

Bárány R 1960b Untersuchungen über den vom Vestibularapparat des Ohres reflektorisch augelösten rhythmischen Nystagmus und seine Begleiterscheinungen. Monatsschrift für Ohrenheilkunde 40: 191–297

Bárány R 1907 Die Untersuchungen der reflektorischen vestibulären und optischen Augenbewegungen und ihre Bedeutung für die topische Diagnostik der Augenmuskellähmungen. Münchener medizinische Wochenschrift 54: 1072–1074, 1132–1135

Bárány R 1921 Diagnose von Krankheitserscheinungen im Bereiche des Otolithenapparates. Acta otolaryngologica (Stockholm) 2: 434–437

Barber H O, Stockwell C W 1980 Manual of Electronystagmography. Mosby, London
Barnes G R, Benson A J 1978 Adaptation in the Caloric Response. In Vestibular Mechanisms in Health and Disease. J D Hood (ed). Academic Press, London
Bender M B 1965 Oscillopsia. Archives of Neurology 13:204–213
Bezold F 1906 Lehrbuch der Ohrenheilkunde. Bergmann, Wiesbaden
Bielschowsky A 1903 Das klinische Bild der assoziierten Blicklähmung und seine Bedeutung für die topischen Diagnostik. Münchener medizinische Wochenschrift 50:1666–1670
Blair C J, Goldberg M F, Noorden G K von 1967 Voluntary Nystagmus. Archives of Ophthalmology 77:349–354
Borries G V T 1926 Konvergenzspasmus und Labyrinthleiden. Monatschrift für Ohrenheilkunde 60:736–755
Brookler K H 1971 Simultaneous bilateral bithermal caloric stimulation in electronystagmography. Laryngoscope 81:1014–1019
Brügger W, Milner M 1978 Computer-aided tracking of body motions using a ccd-image sensor. Medical and Biological Engineering and Computing 16:207–210
Brull M A, Arcan M 1974 A method and instrument for recording the pressure distribution between the foot and the ground. Proceedings of the Second World Congress of ISPO, Montreux
Caird F I, Judge T G 1977 Assessment of the Elderly Patient. Pitman Medical. Tunbridge Wells
Capps Mary J, Preciado M C, Paparella M M, Hoppe W E 1973 Evaluation of the air caloric test as a routine examination procedure. Laryngoscope 83:1013–1021
Cawthorne T E, Cobb W A 1954 Temperature changes in the perilymph space in response to caloric stimulation in man. Acta oto-laryngologica (Stockholm) 44:580–588
Cawthorne T C, Hallpike C S 1957 A study of the clinical features and pathological changes within the temporal bone, brain stem and cerebellum of an early case of positional nystagmus of the so-called benign paroxysmal type. Acta oto-laryngologica (Stockholm) 48:89–105
Chalabi Z 1981 Stochastic signal analysis of thermally induced vestibular electronystagmograms. PhD Thesis. London University
Chodera J 1960 Pedobarograph—apparatus for the visual demonstration of the clinging surfaces of the irregularly shaped objects. CZS Patent 104 514 30d. Quoted by Nayak, 1979
Cogan D G 1954 Ocular dysmetria; Flutter-like oscillations of the eyes, and opsoclonus. Archives of Ophthalmology 51:318–335
Cogan D G 1963 Dissociated nystagmus with lesions in the Posterior Fossa. Archives of Ophthalmology 70:361–368
Cogan D G 1970 Neurology of the ocular muscles. Thomas, Springfield, III
Cogan D G, Kubik C S, Smith W L 1950 Unilateral Internuclear Ophthalmoplegia. Archives of Ophthalmology 44:783–796
Collewijn H 1976 Impairment of Optokinetic (After-) Nystagmus by Labyrinthectomy in the Rabbit. Experimental Neurology 52:146–156
Coni N, Davison W, Webster S 1980 Lecture Notes on Geriatrics. Blackwell, Oxford
Corvera J, Torres-Courtney Gabriela, Lopez-Rios G 1973 The Neurotological significance of alterations of pursuit eye movements and the pendular eye tracking test. Annals of Otology, Rhinology and Laryngology 82:855–867
Daroff R B 1965 See-saw nystagmus. Neurology 15:874–877
Daroff R B 1977 Ocular oscillations. Annals of Otology 86:102–107
Daroff R B, Dell'Osso L F 1979 Nystagmus—a contemporary approach. In: Thompson HS (ed) Topics in neuro-ophthalmology. Williams Wilkins, Baltimore
Daroff R B, Hoyt W F 1971 Supranuclear disorders of ocular control systems in man. In: The control of eye movements. Bach-y-Rita P, Collins C C (eds) Academic Press, London
Davis D G, Smith J L 1971 Periodic alternating nystagmus. American Journal of Ophthalmology 72:757–762
Dayal V S, Tarantino L, Farkashidy J, Thibert R 1977 End-organ and drug-induced vestibular nystagmus. Annals of Otology 86:89–93
Dell'Osso L F 1973 Fixation characteristics and hereditary congenital nystagmus. American Journal of Optometry 50:85–90
Dell'Osso L F, Troost B T, Daroff R B 1975 Macro square wave jerks. Neurology 25:975–979
Dell'Osso L F, Gauthier G, Lieberman G, Stark L 1977 Eye movement recordings as a diagnostic tool in a case of congenital nystagmus. American Journal of Optometry 49:3–13
Demanez J P 1968 L'influence de la fixation oculaire sur le nystagmus postcalorique. Sa mesure. Son importance sémiologique. Acta oto-rhino-laryngologica Belgica 22:739–754
De Morsier G, Balavoine C 1948 Spasms de la Convergence. Ophthalmologica 116:248–253
De Morsier G, Balavoine C 1949 Encephalopathie traumatique et spasm de la convergence. Revue oto-neuro-opthalmologie 21:400–403

Dishoeck H A E van, Nijhoff P 1953 Proceedings of the Vth International Congress of Otolaryngology, Amsterdam

Dix M R 1970 Clinical Observations upon the Vestibular Responses in Certain Disorders of the Central Nervous System. Advances in Oto-rhino-laryngology 17:118–128

Dix M R 1979 The rationale and technique of head exercises in the treatment of vertigo. Acta oto laryngologica Belgica 33:370–384

Dix M R, Hallpike C S 1952 Pathology, symptomatology and diagnosis of certain disorders of the vestibular system. Proceedings of the Royal Society of Medicine 45:341–354

Dix M, Hood J D 1971 Further observations upon the neurological mechanism of optokinetic nystagmus. Acta otolaryngologica (Stockholm) 71:217–226

Drachman D A, Hart C W 1972 An approach to the dizzy patient. Neurology 22:323–334

Duane A 1905 Unilateral and unusual forms of nystagmus. New York State Journal of Medicine 5:245–249

Duensing F 1967 Quoted by Hallpike 1967

Duke-Elder S, Scott G I 1971 System of Ophthalmology. Vol. XII Neuro-ophthalmology. Kimpton, London

Edwards C H 1973 Neurology of Ear, Nose and Throat Diseases. Butterworths, London

Egmond A A J Van, Groen J J, Jongkees L B W (1948) The turning test with small regulable stimuli. Journal of Laryngology and Otology 62:63–69

Ellenberger C Jr, Campa J F, Netsky M G 1968 Opsoclonus and parenchymatous degeneration of the cerebellum. Neurology 18:1041–1046

Elschnig A 1913 Nystagmus retractorius, ein cerebrales Herdsymptom. Medizinische Klinik 9:8–11

Enoksson P 1956 Optokinetic nystagmus in brain lesions. Acta ophthalmologica 34:163–184

Findley L J, Gresty M A, Halmagyi M G 1981 A Novel Method of recording arm movements. Archives of Neurology 38:38–42

Fisher C M 1961 In: Fields W S (ed) Pathogenesis and treatment of cerebrovascular disease. Thomas, Springfield. III

Fitzgerald G, Hallpike C S 1942 Studies in Human Vestibular Function I Observations on the Directional Preponderance ('Nystagmusbereitschaft') of Caloric Nystagmus resulting from cerebral lesions. Brain 65:115–137

Fox J C, Holmes G 1926 Optic nystagmus and its value in the localisation of cerebral lesions. Brain 49:333–371

Fregly A R, Graybiel A 1968 An ataxic test battery not requiring the use of rails. Aerospace Medicine 39:277–282

Frenzel H 1960 Pathologisch-Anatomische und Pathologisch—Physiologische Grundlagen des Lagenystagmus. Acta oto-laryngologica (Stockholm) Suppl. 159:73–77

Frenzel H 1961 Zur Systematik, Klinik und Untersuchungsmethodik der Vestibularisstörung. Springer, Berlin

Fukuda T 1959 Vertical writing with eyes closed. Acta otolaryngologica (Stockholm) 50:26–36

Gacek R R 1974 Transection of the Posterior Ampullary Nerve for the relief of Benign Paroxysmal Positional Vertigo. Annals of Otology, Rhinology and Laryngology 83:596–605

Gassel M M, Williams D 1963 Visual Function in Patients with Homonymous Hemianopia. Part II. Oculomotor Mechanisms. Brain 86:1–36

Gauthier G M 1970 Bio-engineering studies of cerebellar influences on oculomotor control. PhD Thesis. University of Illinois, Chicago. Quoted by Selhorst, Stark, Ochs & Hoyt 1976

Gay A J, Brodkey J, Miller J E 1963 Convergence retraction nystagmus. Archives of Ophthalmology 70:456–461

Gilbert G J, McEntee W J, Glaser G H 1963 Familial Myoclonus and ataxia: Pathophysiologic implications. Neurology 13:365–372

Gillingham F J, Kalyanaraman S 1965 The Surgical treatment of Oculogyric Crises. Confinia neurologica 19:237–245

Goldstein J E, Cogan D G 1961 Lateralising value of ocular motor dysmetria and skew deviation. Archives of Ophthalmology 66:517–518

Greiner G-F, Conraux C, Collard M 1969 Vestibulométrie Clinique. Doin, Paris

Gresty M, Halmagyi G M, Leech J 1978 The Relationship between Head and Eye movement in Congenital Nystagmus with Head Shaking: Objective Recordings of a single case. British Journal of Ophthalmology 62:533–535

Guedry F E, Davenport K S, Brewton C B, Turnispeed G T 1979 The Pendular Eye Tracking Test under two background viewing conditons. Naval Aerospace Medical Research Laboratory Report, NAMRL, Pensacola, Florida, USA

Guiang R L Jr, Ellington O B 1977 Acute pure vertiginous dysequilibrium in cerebellar infarction. European Neurology 16:11–15

Guiloff R J, Whiteley A, Kelly R E 1980 Organic convergence spasm. Acta neurologica scandinavica 61:252–259

Güttich A 1913 Beitrag zur Physiologie des Vestibularapparates. Beitrage zur Physiologie, Pathologie und Therapie des Ohres 7:1–18

Haciska D T 1973 The influence of drugs on caloric-induced nystagmus. Acta oto-laryngologica (Stockholm) 75:477–484

Hallpike C S 1967 Some types of Ocular Nystagmus and their Neurological Mechanisms. Proceedings of the Royal Society of Medicine 60:1043–1054

Halmagyi G M, Gresty M A, Gibson W P R 1978 Ocular Tilt Reaction with Peripheral Vestibular Lesion. Annals of Neurology 6:80–83

Halmagyi G M, Rudge P, Gresty M A, Leigh R J, Zee D S 1980 Treatment of Periodic Alternating Nystagmus. Annals of Neurology 8:609–611

Hamid M A 1979 Statistical Signal Analysis of Induced Vestibular Nystagmus in Man. Ph.D Thesis. University of London

Hamid M A, Sayers, B McA, Vickery J C, Hinchcliffe R 1979 Implementing a computer-based electro-oculographic analysis system. Clinical Otolaryngology 4:163–167

Harris W 1944 Ataxic Nystagmus: A Pathognomonic Sign in Disseminated Sclerosis. British Journal of Ophthalmology 28:40–42

Harrison M S, Ozsahinoglu C 1972 Positional Vertigo: Aetiology and Clinical Significance. Brain 95:369–372

Hart C W 1967 Ocular fixation and the caloric test. Laryngoscope 77:2103–2113

Hart C W 1973 The ocular fixation index. Annals of Otology, Rhinology and Laryngology 82:848–851

Hart C W 1980 The Quantified Quix Test. Proceeding of the Precongress Symposium 'Basic Aspects of Electronystagmography', Bad Kissingen, West Germany, March 6

Henn V S, Young L R, Finley C 1974 Vestibular nucleus units in alert monkeys are also influenced by moving visual scenes. Brain Research 71:144–149

Henriksson N G 1956 Speed of the slow component and duration in caloric nystagmus. Acta oto-laryngologica (Stockholm) Supplement 125

Hinchcliffe R 1967 Validity of Measures of Caloric Test Response. Acta oto-laryngologica (Stockholm) 63:69–73

Hinchcliffe R 1970 Investigation du Vertige. Cahiers d'ORL 5:861–872

Hinchcliffe R 1971 Examen otoneurologique pour le diagnostic des neurinomes acoustiques. Acta oto-rhino-laryngologica Belgica 25:770–783

Hinchcliffe R 1973 Investigation of vertigo. In: Ransome J, Holden H, Bull T R (eds) Recent Advances in Otolaryngology. Churchill Livingstone, Edinburgh

Hinchcliffe R 1976 Neuro-otology. Scienctific foundations of otolaryngology. In: Hinchcliffe R, Harrison D F N (eds) Heinemann. London, Ch 28

Hinchcliffe R, Voots R J 1962. An electronystagmographic technic for the examination of vestibular function. Neurology 12:686–697

Hodkinson H M 1980 Common Symptoms of Disease in the Elderly. Blackwell, Oxford.

Hohman L B 1925 Forced conjugate upward movements of the eyes in postencephalitic Parkinson's syndrome. Journal of the American Medical Association 84:1489–1490

Holmes G 1917 The symptoms of acute cerebellar injuries due to gunshot injuries. Brain 40:461–535

Hood J D 1967 Recent advances in the electronystagmographic investigation of vestibular and other disorders of ocular movement. In: de Reuck AVS, Knight J (eds) Myotatic, Kinesthetic and Vestibular Mechanisms. Churchill, London

Hood J D 1980 Unsteadiness of cerebellar origin. An investigation into the cause. Journal of Laryngology and Otology 94:865–876

Hood J D, Dix M R 1973 The significance of optic fixation in tests of vestibular function. Equilibrium Research 3:95–101

Hood J D, Korres S 1979 Vestibular suppression in peripheral and central vestibular disorders. Brain 102:785–804

Hood J D, Leech J 1974 The significance of peripheral vision in the perception of movement. Acta Otolaryngologica (Stockholm) 77:72–79

Hood J D, Kayan A, Leech J 1973 Rebound Nystagmus. Brain 96:507–526

Hull C L 1933 Hypnosis and suggestibility. Appleton Century Croft, New York

Imms F J, Edholm O G 1979 The assessment of gait and mobility in the elderly. Age and Ageing 8:261–267

Jahss M H 1971 Geriatric aspects of the foot and ankle. In: Rossman I (ed) Clinical geriatrics. Lippincott, Philadelphia

Jung R, Kornhuber H H 1964 Results of electronystagmography in man: The value of optokinetic, vestibular and spontaneous nystagmus for neurologic diagnosis and research. In: Bender MB (ed) The oculomotor system Harper and Row, New York, Ch 19

Kamei T, Kornhuber H H 1974 Spontaneous and head shaking nystagmus in normals and in patients with central lesions. Canadian Journal of Otolaryngology 3 : 372–380

Käslin W 1936 Postencephalitische und sonstige Parkinsonismen nach Trauma (an Hand der in den Jahren 1930–1934 bei der Suva angemeldeten Fälle). Zentralblatt für die gesamte Ophthalmologie 36 : 477

Keane J R 1974 Periodic alternating nystagmus with downward beating nystagmus. A clinico-anatomical case study of multiple sclerosis. Archives of Neurology 30 : 399–402

Kitahara M 1965 Acceleration Registrography. A new method of examinations concerned with the labyrinthine righting reflex. Annals of Otology, Rhinology and Laryngology 74 : 203–214

Klemme R M 1941 Oculogyric crises: A Therapeutic Approach. American Journal of Ophthalmology 24 : 1000–1004

Koch H, Henriksson N G, Lundren A, Andrén G 1959 Directional Preponderance and Spontaneous Nystagmus in Eye-speed Recording. Acta oto-laryngologica (Stockholm) 50 : 517–525

Koerber H 1903 Uber drei Fälle von Retraktionsbewegungen des Bulbus (Nystagmus retraktorius) Ophthalmologishe Klinik 7 : 65 : 67

Kornhuber H H 1975 In: Proceedings of the Fifth Extraordinary Meeting of the Bárány Society, Kyoto. Supplement to International Journal of Equilibrium Research, p 240

Krabbe K H 1931 Crises oculogyres et Parkinsonisme dans la syphilis cérébrospinale. Acta psychiatrica et neurologica 6 : 457–467

Ledoux A 1958 Les Canaux Semicirculaires Brussels, p 73

Ledoux A, Demanez J P 1967 Nystagmographie les yeux ouverts our fermés au cours del'épreuve calorique. Acta oto-rhino-laryngologica Belgica 21 : 31–40

Lee M D 1969 The caloric test in the supine and the prone positions. Journal of Laryngology and Otology 83 : 797–801

Levy I, O'Leary J L 1947 Incidence of vertigo in neurologic conditions. Transactions of the American Otologic Society 35 : 329–347

Lindsay J R 1962 Discussion of Schuknecht's paper on Positional Vertigo. Transactions of the American Academy of Ophthalmology and Otolaryngology 66 : 331–332

Lingwong M, Herman S J 1971 Cycloduction of the Eyes with head tilt. Archives of Ophthalmology 85 : 570–573

Margulis M S, Model M M 1926 Zur Pathologie der Assozierten Bewegungen der Augenmuskeln in Zusammenhang mit Vestibulären Symptomenkomplex bei Encephalitis. Deutsche Zeitschrift für Nervenkranke 93 : 80–92

Miller F F 1962 Counter-rolling of the human eyes produced by head tilt with respect to gravity. Acta oto-laryngologica (Stockholm) 54 : 479–501

Miller E F, Graybiel A 1963 A comparison of Ocular counter-rolling movements between normal persons and deaf subjects with bilateral labyrinthine defects. Annals of Otology, Rhinology and Laryngology 72 : 885–893

Miyazaki S, Iwakura H 1978 Foot-force measuring device for clinical assessment of pathological gait. Medical and Biological Engineering and Computing 16 : 429–436

Mizukoshi K, Watanabe Y, Kato I, Koike Y, Ino H 1975 Computer analysis of the Eye-Tracking Test. Proceedings of the Fifth Extraordinary Meeting of the Bárány Society, Kyoto. M. Morimoto (ed.) International Journal of Equilibrium Research Suppl. p 158

Nashold B S Jr, Slaughter D G, Gills J P 1969 Ocular reactions in man from deep cerebellar stimulation and lesions. Archives of Ophthalmology 81 : 538–543

Nayak U S L 1979 Measurement Techniques. Research Seminar on Falls in Old People. University of Birmingham. UK Feb. 1st

Nelson J R 1969 The Minimal ice-water caloric test. Neurology 19 : 577–585

Nelson J R, Cope D 1971 The Otoliths and the Ocular Countertosion Reflex. Archives of Otolaryngology 94 : 40–50

Nelson J R, House W F 1971 Ocular Countertorsion as an indicator of otolith function: Effects of Unilateral Vestibular Lesions. Transactions of the American Academy of Ophthalmology and Otolaryngology 75 : 1313–1321

Nigris G de 1933 Sindrome oculocefalogira in soggetto neuroluetica. Rivista Oto-neuro-oftalmologica 10 : 73–75

Njiokiktjien C J, Rijke W De 1972 The recording of Romberg's Test and its application in neurology. Agressologie 13 : C : 1–7

Noorden G K von 1974 Factors involved in the production of amblyopia. British Journal of Ophthalmology 58 : 158–164

Noorden G K von, Preziosi T J 1966 Eye movement recordings in neurological disorders. Archives of Ophthalmology 76 : 162–171

Norré M E 1975 Evaluation of a screening-procedure by hot-water caloric tests. Acta oto-rhino-laryngologica. Belgica 29: 632–638

Nylén C O 1922 A nystagmus phenomenon. Acta otolaryngologica (Stockholm) 3: 502–503

Nylén C O 1950 Head Posture Test. Journal of Laryngology and Otology 64: 295–318

Oloff H, Korbsch H 1926 Uber das Hertwig—Magendiesche Phänomen (Vertikaldivergenz der Augen) Klinische Monatsblätter für Augenheilkunde 77: 618–627

Orzechowski K 1927 De l'ataxie dysmétrique des yeux: Remarques sur l'ataxie des yeux dite myoclonique (opsoclonie, opsochorie). Journal für Psychologie und Neurologie 35: 1–18

Parinaud 1883 Paralysie des mouvements associés des yeux. Archives de Neurologie 5: 145–172

Peitersen E 1967 Vestibulospinal Reflexes. Archives of Otolaryngology 85: 192–198

Potvin A R, Syndulko K, Tourtellotte W W 1980 Human neurologic function and the ageing process. Journal of the American Geriatric Society 28: 1–9

Quix F H 1925 The Function of the Vestibular Organ and the Clinical Examination of the Otolithic Apparatus. Journal of Laryngology and Otology 40: 425–511

Rabinovitch H E, Sharpe J A, Sylvester T O 1977 The Ocular Tilt Reaction. Archives of Ophthalmology 95: 1395–1398

Rai G S, Elias-Jones A 1979 The corneal reflex in elderly subjects. Journal of the American Geriatric Society 27: 317–318

Rashbass C, Russell G E M 1961 Action of a Barbiturate Drug (Amylobarbitone Sodium) on the vestibulo-ocular reflex. Brain 84: 329–335

Riesco McClure J S 1957 Es el vertigo aural de origen exclusivamente periferico? Revista otorrinolaringologica 17: 42–54

Robinson D A 1975a A quantitative analysis of extraocular muscle cooperation and squint. Investigative Ophthalmology 14: 801–825

Robinson D A 1975b How signals are processed in the vestibulo-ocular reflex. Proceedings of the Fifth Extraordinary Meeting of the Bárány Society, Kyoto. M. Morimoto (ed). International Journal of Equilibrium Research. Suppl

Rogers J H 1980 Romberg and his test. Journal of Laryngology and Otology 94: 1401–1404

Romberg M H 1846 Lehrbuch der Nerven Krankheiten des Menschen. Dunker, Berlin

Ross A T, Zeman W 1967 Opsoclonus, Occult Carcinoma and Chemical Pathology in Dentate Nuclei. Archives of Neurology 17: 546–551

Roth W 1901 Demonstration von kranken mit Ophthalmoplegie. Neurologisches Centralblatt 20: 921–923

Rucker C W 1958 Paralyses of the third, fourth and sixth cranial nerves. American Journal of Ophthalmology 46: 787–794

Salus R 1913 On Acquired Retraction Movements of the Eyes. Archives of Ophthalmology 42: 34–40

Sano K, Sekino H, Tsukamoto Y, Yoshimasu N, Ishijima B 1972 Stimulation and destruction of the region of the interstitial Nucleus in cases of Torticollis and See-saw Nystagmus. Confinia Neurologica 34: 331–338

Sayers B McA, Hinchcliffe R 1976 Signal analysis of neuro-otological measurements. In: Stephens S D G (ed) Disorders of auditory function II. Academic Press, London

Sayers B McA, Hinchcliffe R, Hamid M A 1978 Parameter variability of the post-caloric EOG response. In: Hood J D (ed) Vestibular mechanisms in health and disease. Academic Press, London

Scherzer E 1968 Die Störungen des Gleichgewichtssystems nach Unfällen. Wiener Medizinsche Akademie. Vienna

Schmaltz G 1932 The Physical Phenomena occurring in the semicircular canals during rotatory and thermic stimulation. Proceedings of the Royal Society of Medicine 25: 359–381

Schuknecht H F 1962 Positional Vertigo: Clinical and Experimental Observations. Transactions of the American Academy of Ophthalmology and Otolaryngology 66: 319–332

Schunknecht H F 1969 Cupulolithiasis. Archives of Otolaryngology 90: 765–778

Schuknecht H F, Kitamura K 1981 Vestibular Neuritis. Annals of Otology, Rhinology and Laryngology. Vol. 90, Suppl. 78. pp 1–19

Schuknecht H F, Ruby R 1973 Cupulolithiasis. Advances in Otorhinolaryngology 20: 434–443

Schurr P H 1963 See-saw nystagmus. Proceedings of the Royal Society of Medicine 56: 808–810

Sekitani T, Honjo S, Kobayashi T, Shimamoto K 1975 Square Drawing Test—a Quantitative evaluation for Ataxia. Proceedings of the Fifth Extraordinary Meeting of the Bárány Society, Kyoto. M Morimoto (ed). International Journal of Equilibrium Research. Suppl

Selhorst J B, Stark L, Ochs A L, Hoyt W F 1976a Disorders in Cerebellar Ocular Motor Control. I Saccadic overshoot dysmetria: An oculographic, control system and clinico-anatomical analysis. Brain 99: 497–508

Selhorst J B, Stark L, Ochs A L, Hoyt W F 1976b Disorders in Cerebellar Ocular Motor Control. II

Macrosaccadic oscillation: An oculographic, control system and clinico-anatomical analysis. Brain 99:509–522

Shults W T, Stark L, Hoyt W F, Ochs A L 1977 Normal saccadic structure of voluntary nystagmus. Archives of Ophthalmology 95:1399–1404

Smith J L, Zieper I, Gay A J, Cogan D G 1959 Nystagmus Retractorius. Archives of Ophthalmology 62:864–867

Sokolovski A 1966 The influence of mental activity and visual fixation upon caloric-induced nystagmus in normal subjects. Acta oto-laryngologica (Stockholm) 61:209–220

Stenger H H 1959 Erholungsnystagmus nach einseitigem Vestibularisausfall, ein dem Bechterew-Nystagmus verwandter Vorgang. Archiv für Ohren-Nasen-und Kelkopfheilkunde 175:545–547

Stewart T G, Holmes G 1904 Symptomatology of cerebellar tumours: a study of forty cases. Brain 27:522–591

Stroud M H 1974 The vestibular system and abducting eye nystagmus in old age. Canadian Journal of Otolaryngology 3:363–366

Strubel D, Eber A M, Monjour A, Rohmer E, Collard M 1980 Le nystagmus de circumduction. Revue d'oto-neuro-ophtalmologie 52:433–438

Susac J O, Hoyt W F, Daroff R B, Lawrence W 1970 Clinical spectrum of ocular bobbing. Journal of Neurology, Neurosurgery and Psychiatry 33:771–775

Susac J O, Smith J L, Schatz N J 1973 Superior oblique myokymia. Archives of Neurology 29:432–434

Suzuki J-I 1971 Examination of Eye Movements. In: Uemura T, Suzuki J-I, Hozawa J, Highstein S M (eds) Neuro-otological Examination. University Park Press, London, p 106

Taguchi K 1980 Relationship between the head's and the body's center of gravity during normal standing. Acta oto-laryngologica (Stockholm) 90:100–105

Tahmoush A J, Brooks J E, Keltner J L 1972 Palatal myoclonus associated with abnormal ocular and extremity movements. Archives of Neurology 27:431–440

Takemori Setsuko 1977 Visual Suppression Test. Annals of Otology 86:80–85

Takemori Setsuko, Moriyama H, Totsuka G 1979 The Mechanism of Inhibition of Caloric Nystagmus by Eye Closure. Advances in Oto-Rhino-Laryngology 25:208–213

Tappin J W, Pollard J, Beckett E A 1980 Method of measuring 'shearing' forces on the side of the foot. Clinical Physical and Physiological Measurement 1:83–85

Thompson R A, Lynde R H 1969 Convergence spasm associated with Wernicke's encephalopathy. Neurology 19:711–712

Thornval A 1917 Funktionsundersøgelser af Vestibularorganet og Cerebellum. Busck, Copenhagen

Tjernström O 1973 Nystagmus inhibition as an effect of eye-closure. Acta oto-laryngologica (Stockholm) 75:408–418

Towle P A 1971 Quoted by David and Smith, 1971

Towle P A, Romanul F 1970 Periodic Alternating Nystagmus: first pathologically studied case. Neurology 20:408

Uemura T, Cohen B 1975 Loss of optokinetic afternystagmus (OKAN) after dorsal medullary reticular formation (Med RF) lesions. Proceedings of the Fifth Extraordinary Meeting of the Bárány Society, Kyoto. M Morimoto (ed). International Journal for Equilibrium Research: Suppl p 168

Uemura T, Suzuki J-I, Hozawa J, Highstein S M 1977 Neuro-otological Examination. University Park Press, London

Umeda Y 1980 The Eye-Tracking Test. Annals of Otology, Rhinology and Laryngology, vol 89 Suppl 71 p 1–12

Umeda Y, Ohtsu K, Sakata E 1975 The circular eye tracking test: A new approach to the analysis of vertical eye movements. Proceedings of the Fifth Extraordinary Meeting of the Bárány Society, Kyoto. M Morimoto (ed). International Journal for Equilibrium Research: Suppl p 168

Unterberger S 1938 Neue objective registrierbare Vestibularis-Drehreaktion, erhalten durch Treten auf der Stelle. Der 'Tretversuch' Archiv für Ohren-, Nasen- und Kehlopfheilkunde 145:478

Unterberger S 1962 Neue objective registrierbare Vestibularis-Korperdrehreaktion erhalten durch Treten auf der Stelle. Der Tretversuch. Archiv fur Ohren-, Nasen-und Kehlkopfheilkunde 179:273–282

Van Der Laan F L, Oosterveld W J 1974 Age and Vestibular Function. Aerospace Medicine 45:540–547

Vogel K 1932 Uber den Nachweis des latenten Spontannystagmus. Zeitschrift für Laryngologie und Rhinologie 22:202

Wall C, O'Leary D P, Black F O 1978 Systems analysis of vestibulo-ocular system response using white noise rotational stimuli. In: Hood J D (ed) Vestibular mechanisms in health and disease. Academic Press, London

Walsh F B, Hoyt W F 1969 Clinical Neuro-ophthalmology. Williams and Wilkins, Baltimore, p 236
Wilcock G K, Middleton A M 1980 Geriatrics. Grant McIntyre London
Wolfe J W, Engelken E J, Olson J E 1979 A Low-frequency harmonic acceleration in the evaluation of
    surgical treatment of Ménière's disease. Advances in Otorhinolaryngology 25 : 192–196
Woltring H D 1974 New possibilities for human motion studies by real-time light spot position
    measurements. Biotelemetry 1 : 132–146
Yap M H-L, Loong S C, Nei I P 1975 Eye signs in strokes. Annals of the Academy of Medicine of
    Singapore 4 : 133–137
Yee R D, Baloh R W, Honrubia V, Kim Y S 1981 A study of congenital nystagmus: vestibular
    nystagmus. Journal of Otolaryngology 10 : 89–98
Zee D S 1975 Quoted by Robinson, 1975
Zee D S, Robinson D A 1979 A hypothetical explanation of saccadic oscillations. Annals of Neurology
    5 : 405–414

Changes in vestibular function with increasing age

INTRODUCTION

Age provides an indication of the various stages of development, the psychosomatic functioning and the medical and physiological status of man at a certain moment. Age is the product of the inherent growth potential (Meyer 1970), the ability to react against disease, and the accumulation of all previous diseases and traumata. The chronological age is not a valid measure of the functional age. At most one can speak of an age for a function but not of an age for a complex of physical, physiological and psychological functions all together.

These functions change, partly independently of each other, and in a different tempo (Heron and Chown, 1967).

A useful standard will be retained longer by those capacities that are used in a daily life. Tasks that call for a one-sided functioning could lead to a decline in the capacity of other functions. This was called by Smith and Greene (1962) the 'work-feedback concept of ageing'.

Ageing concerns a complex of alterations encompassing a decrease in vitality, a progressive drop in biological efficiency and a blunting of the power of the organism to maintain itself as an efficient machine. The tempo of ageing varies from organ to organ (Shock, 1962).

In clinical medicine one has to distinguish between alterations in physiological functions as a result of ageing and a decline as a result of pathological processes.

SENSORY ORGANS IN GENERAL

The decline in visual and auditory performance with advancing age is well known. A similar regression is shown by the sense of taste as described by Hinchcliffe (1958), Zilstorff Pedersen (1962, 1972) and Feldmann (1962).

The function of the sense of smell decreases too (Boccuzzi, 1962; Matzker, 1965; Zilstorff Pedersen, 1962). Krmpotić-Nemanić (1969) described diminished ability in old age of the vestibular and olfactory function and considered this to be caused by analogous biological processes. Histological studies have shown a decrease in the number of taste buds (Allara, 1939; Kranz, Berndt and Wagner, 1968; Hughes, 1969).

It is reasonable to expect that the performance of the vestibular organ also deteriorates with increasing age. Age-dependent losses of sensory and nervous elements in the auditory system are known. Presbyacusis is the term that describes the effect of ageing on hearing and points to changes in histological structures.

Zwaardemaker (1894) described atrophic changes in the basal turn of the cochlea and suggested this to be the cause of presbyacusis, Mayer (1920) found an increasing rigidity of the basilar membrane in ageing people and Saxén (1937) described an atrophy of the spiral ganglion and marked changes in the cochlear duct causing flattening of the strial epithelium, hyalinisation of blood vessels in the stria vascularis, collapse of the spiral organ of Corti and adhesions of the vestibular (Reissner's) membrane to the strial epithelium. These changes are equally present in all parts of the cochlea and are caused by capillary sclerosis in the stria vascularis. Schuknecht (1955, 1964) found degeneration of the spiral organ with loss of hair cells and supporting cells. In the basal part of the cochlea this atrophy was most severe. Fleischer (1956) described the loss of ganglion cells in the basal part of the cochlea, between the 3rd to the 4th decade as the only change.

In presbyacusis Van Dishoeck (1966) found a loss of ganglion cells in the basal turn of the spiral ganglion, the part of the cochlea where high tones are preceived. The spiral organs shows degenerative changes as a result of angiosclerosis. Noise is another important cause of high frequency hearing loss. Rosen and his colleagues (1962) found no presbyacusis in elderly people who had lived all their life in a practically noise-free environment. However, Glorig and Nixon (1962) described only a slight effect of noise on the development of presbyacusis.

The role of noise in presbyacusis should not be over-estimated, since, with increasing age, metabolic changes as well as physical changes take place in all tissues, particularly the connective tissues. All structures of the internal ear may be affected. Atherosclerotic changes could also affect the internal ear circulation. Atrophy of the spiral ganglion and associated nerve fibers, angiosclerotic degeneration of the internal ear, loss of elasticity of the basilar membrane, atrophy of the centres and pathways in the central nervous system and bony deposits at the base of the internal acoustic meatus resulting in stenosis at the beginning of the foraminous spiral tract (Krmpotić-Nemanić 1963, 1969) have all been named as causes for presbyacusis.

Independently of local arteriosclerosis, senile atrophy of the spiral ganglion becomes more pronounced with advancing age. Ganglion cell atrophy and haircell degeneration in the spiral organ are two different entities which are not exclusively caused by ageing.

As indicated by Bergman in Chapter 6 of this volume, there is evidence for contributory central factors in the occurrence of presbyacusis (Beyermann-Gösser 1964; Matzker, 1954). Matzker found a pronounced decrease in central synthesis of two binaurally applied acoustic signals after the 4th decade of life. The progressive bone apposition at the fundus of the internal acoustic meatus, beginning rather early in life, as described by Serćer and Krmpotić (1958) is similar to the bone apposition in the lamina cribosa leading to the loss of smell. These conditions cause compression closure of the canaliculi, resulting in nerve fibre and spiral ganglion cell atrophy. Most pronounced are the pathological changes in the basal turn of the cochlea, the corresponding ganglion cells and nerve fibres. It has been established that there is a decrease in the number of fibres of the vestibular nerve, that the sensory cells show atrophy, and that the semicircular canal walls show osteoporosis (Haas, 1964).

VESTIBULAR ORGANS

It can be expected that the performance of the vestibular organ will deteriorate with increasing age. At the two poles of life, infancy and old age, great differences exist in structure and function. These differences give reason to speak of the anatomy and physiology of infancy and the anatomy and physiology of old age. The semicircular canals are formed during the 5th or 6th week of embryonic life; first the superior and posterior canals, followed by the lateral canals after a short time. The parts of the labyrinth which control the equilibrium functions are ready to operate at this stage. The vestibular apparatus of the fetus and newborn is completely developed and differs only from the vestibular apparatus of adults in size and situation. Galebsky (1927) found that all three semicircular canals react immediately after birth to rotation and calorisation, giving the appropriate type of nystagmus. However, the reaction of the new-born during rotation differs from rotatory reaction in adults in its intensity, and in the absence, or very weak character, of the quick component. In 1918 Bárány stated that the slow component of nystagmus originates in the vestibular nuclei, whereas the quick component is the result of cerebral function.

However, Galebsky (1927) assumed that the quick component does not originate in the brain, but in the region of the vestibular nuclei. In new-born infants the cerebellum is still underdeveloped and incompletely myelinised (Vogt 1905). From the fact that the vestibular apparatus is well developed early in intrauterine life, and that all components are functioning in the first extrauterine hours, even during intrauterine life when it seems of no use whatsoever, it is suggested that the function of the vestibular apparatus in the new-born infant, and also in the fetus, is a repetition of a very old stage in the evolution of the nervous system, which in its time was of great importance. This hypothesis is supported by the fact that the centres where nystagmus is elicited in the new-born are embedded in the palencephalon. The palencephalon is the oldest portion of the brain that already exists in fishes and here the semicircular canals are well developed.

The membranous and bony labyrinths (Dayal et al, 1973), the number of myelinated vestibular nerve fibers (Bergstöm, 1973) and the vestibular hair cells (Rosenhall, 1972) are mature at birth.

It is well known that the compensations following damage to the vestibular system are much greater than those following damage to the acoustic apparatus (Ferreri, 1954; De Vido and Pagnini, 1956). The absence of clinical manifestations related to the aged vestibular apparatus is one of the reasons why no specific interest has been taken by researchers in the consequences of its senile degeneration.

The posterior labyrinth is well preserved throughout the advancing years (Ferreri, 1954) and old people less frequently manifest vestibular symptoms, although a diminution of hearing occurs. Vestibular disorientation in aged people is more often the result of uncertainty and blurring of vision than of true vertigo. Droller and Pemberton (1953) found vertiginous disturbances in 47 per cent of men over the age of 67 years and in 61 per cent of women over 62 years of age. Those authors attributed this to arteriosclerotic lesions in the vestibular end-organ receptors. Aubry (1955) found slight vertigo common; this was often accompanied by an unpleasant tinnitus in elderly patients. Vestibular signs in these cases were rare, and, at the most, a slight degree of vestibular hyporeflexia was present.

Comel (1932) examined the vestibular function (by means of the caloric test) in a group of patients over 70 years of age. He saw a relationship between the anatomical condition of their nose and the function of the cochleo vestibular apparatus. An increase of vestibular reflexes was clear on the side where a nasal obstruction existed as a result of a nasal septum deviation. Scuderi (1947) found an increase in vestibular reflexes in some old people, normal reflexes in others, but sometimes a diminution of reflexes. He also found different results on different occasions in the same people and considered this to be due to the blood circulation at the times of examination. It is obvious that the blood circulation of the internal ear in elderly subjects is not normal, and depends on the degree of atherosclerosis.

Pallestrini (1933) assumed two stages in the occurrence of atherosclerosis of the labyrinth, i.e. angioneurosis (vasospasm) followed by angiosclerosis. Scuderi (1947) reported, similar to Pallestrini, that, in most cases belonging to the angioneurotic stage, an increase occurs in vestibular reflexes, whilst a decrease appears in the angiosclerotic stage.

A post-rotatory hyper-reactivity was found by Zelenka and Kozak (1963) in 132 patients with various stages of arterial degenerative disease, ranging from vasospasm to frank atherosclerosis.

Vestibular neurons which mediate inhibitory functions are the first to suffer from age-related ischaemia or other diseases.

Changes in the cochlear apparatus have been investigated more often than those of the vestibular and olfactory apparatus. This can be explained by the fact that the changes in hearing become manifest earlier than those of the vestibular and olfactory organs. The vestibular system has a greater possibility of being compensated, whilst slight changes in the olfactory apparatus cannot easily be recognised so that they remain hidden for a long time. The cochlear nerve, the vestibular nerve, and the fila olfactoria are sensory nerves and they conduct stimulations from the corresponding sensory organs. These nerves pass through a system of tiny holes in a thin bony plate on their way from the sensory epithelium to the central nervous system. In these tiny holes a piling up of bony substance takes place from the fetal period until the end of life. Krmpotić (1969) found, on examining one hundred skulls, that the number of holes in the spiral tract (tractus spiralis foraminosus) as well as in the vestibular area (of the internal acoustic meatus) is progressively reduced with advancing age. The reduction in the number of holes was greater in the basal turn than in the modiolar region. Cross-sections through the spiral tract established that the endosteal bone which forms the tractus, increases in thickness from the fetal to the adult period of life. Analogous thickening of the bony substance and reduction of the number of openings in the vestibular, saccular and utriculo-ampullar area were more obvious when present, because the number of holes being fewer from the beginning could be more easily counted. This piling up of the bony substance develops progressively. At the end of the 6th or beginning of the 7th fetal month, the openings in the spiral tract are large. By the apposition of bony substance in the region of the tractus, the holes become smaller and the bony substance between them thicker. In the fetus the number of holes varies from 100 to 140, but diminishing in adults by a third. Krmpotić described bony cuffs surrounding the artery in 13 specimens (64–78 years) in the region of the entrance of the cochlear branch of the labyrinthine (internal auditory) artery. According to Schwartze the branches of the labyrinthine artery enter the cochlea through the central canal or through one of the openings in the spiral tract. The cuffs were found in these cases at the beginning of the basal coil only. Histological sections were made through the vestibulocochlear nerve, near the fundus of the internal acoustic meatus, in order to demonstrate the consequences of these changes on the nerve fibers in the fundus. The nerve in the region of the fundus is divided into small bundles and has a sheath of connective tissue up to a length of 2 mm. From that point centrally, Krmpotić found glial elements in the nerve. In cadavers of elderly people the nerve was cut very close to the fundus in the region where the number of holes in the tract is reduced, and it was found that the number of fibres in this area was also reduced. The number of nerve fibres in the cochleas and the vestibular nerves was not counted systematically, but, from the number counted, the findings of Rasmussen (1940) could be substantiated. According to Rasmussen the number of cochlear fibres is reduced with increasing age by more than a half, but the vestibular fibres to a far lesser extent. The absolute number of cochlear fibres is greater than that of the vestibular fibres. The reduction with increasing age of fibres is in general symmetrical and so is the reduction of the number of openings in the spiral tract. Unfortunately no audiograms of the examined cases were available.

Engström and his colleagues (1974, 1977) reported age-dependent changes in electron microscopic studies of vestibular sensory cells in rhesus monkeys. Bergström (1973abc) found a reduction in the number and calibre of the vestibular nerve fibers in aged people when compared to young people. In analogy with presbyacusis the changes of vestibular and olfactory functions due to ageing are called presbyastasia and presbyosmia. Naumann (1968) tested different age groups in connection with the olfactory sense. He found a decline with increasing age. Krmpotić (1969) proposes that the apposition of bone comes first, followed by the degeneration of the nerve, and that the vascular element is of less importance than the bony changes.

The vestibular mechanism is sensitive to local changes in arterial blood supply and can also be affected easily by circulatory changes of a more remote origin. A decrease in the blood supply through the basilar artery leads to ischemia of brain-stem structures. This condition causes a syndrome which includes vestibular, visual, auditory, as well as somatic motor and sensory disturbances. Vertigo is the most common symptom (Denny-Brown 1949, 1952, 1953; Millikan and Siekert 1955; Sillevis Smit 1965; Fields, 1968). Most disturbances in the vertebrobasilar circulation are seen in aged people. This fact suggests that atherosclerosis, like mechanical compression in cervical arthrosis (Brain 1965), is a causative factor. An important symptom is postural dizziness. Other clinical findings are high blood-sugar values, sometimes heart failure but, surprisingly, no hypertension (Orma and Koskenoja 1957). As a result of atherosclerosis the labyrinth is subjected to degeneration. Williams (1963) found degenerative changes in the macula and cristae with advancing years caused partly by inadequate nutrition. The entire condition cannot be explained on this basis. An important part of degenerative changes can be termed 'the process of ageing'.

Fields (1968) did 2000 bilateral angiographies to screen the entire arteriolar tree, to ascertain whether occlusive lesions were present in the cervical and cranial arteries, and to determine the quality of the collateral circulation. Patenostre (1912) introduced the term 'senile mastoid' and distinguishes, according to Depoutre (1912) two different types: the ivory type (rarely seen) and the pneumatic type (frequently seen). He compared the results of audiometric and caloric tests, and concluded that the vestibular part of the labyrinth shows a decrease in reactions to these tests in elderly people (60 to 70 years age-group) when compared to the results found in younger age groups. Similar findings were obtained in the cochlear part, but to a more severe degree. Zelenka and Slaninová (1964) came to a similar conclusion, i.e. that senile changes have their effect on the entire labyrinth. The predominance of auditory symptoms is due to the greater sensitivity of the cochlear part of the labyrinth to harmful agents like noise, trauma, and toxic agents. The vestibular organ seems to be much more resistant to senile changes; spontaneous symptoms are only rarely found. Their experiments proved that at about the age of 20 years the reactivity of the vestibular system begins to increase with age, attaining maximal reactivity in the forties and fifties. After the age of 60, responsiveness tends to decline, and the authors called this senile hyporeactivity. The authors further propose that hyporeflexia in children is due to a still imperfect connection between the vestibular and oculomotor pathways. Normal functioning is only possible when linkage of both pathways is accomplished. This process is enhanced by personal experience and individual training at different ages. The reflexes then become normal.

Malkevick (1963) subjected 97 humans, aged from 50 to 90 years, to rotation tests and caloric tests and observed changes that were of central vestibular origin. These findings can be explained on the assumption of an increased inhibitory effect of the cortical part of the central nervous system which controls the labyrinth.

Habituation and adaptation are not clearly separated in the literature. Whereas adaptation means a decrease in reaction during one stimulus, habituation is the decrease of the reaction after repeated stimuli. The ability not to react on biological meaningless stimuli is a very important phenomenon, which, for vestibular reactions, was already described many years ago by Abels (1906). Habituation is a process of learning, with the typical characteristics: acquisition (the learning phase), the phase of transfer (of this habituation) to certain other vestibular stimuli, and the phase of storage, i.e. retention ('keep it in mind') for a certain time after the phase of learning. Vestibular habituation of course is an important part of the insensitivity to motion sickness, and therefore important to seamen (De Wit, 1953), pilots (Krijger, 1954; Aschan, 1954), figure skaters (McCabe, 1960; Collins, 1966) and ballet dancers (Dix and Hood, 1968).

With habituation the genuine natural habituation is meant, i.e. the changing of the vestibular status as the person grows, develops, and learns; the ability to adapt himself to new different, sometimes whirling situations. There should be a peak performance of this phenomenon during the physically active periods of life, when occupation or sport demands a lot of the sense of equilibrium. The greater loss of reaction rates in older subjects originates from a reduction or loss of natural habituation. A decrease of central inhibition would seem the likely neural correlate of this process.

Experimental habituation means that a temporary habituation develops as a result of a series of artificial vestibular stimuli. It is a 'getting used' to event, in the vestibular apparatus; it is also called, though incorrectly, adaptation: the vestibular apparatus adapts itself to this one and only series of stimuli.

Fatigue is a phenomenon that stands on its own when a decrease in reaction is observed after application of a certain stimulus, mostly a repeated stimulus, and it depends on various factors such as the time of the day or night, the amount of stimuli given, the constitution and nutritional status of the test person and his age. It is well known that older people are more quickly tired than younger ones, when repeated stimuli are given.

Vestibular tests demonstrate the reaction of the peripheral vestibular apparatus to the application of appropriate stimulation. The role of the CNS is to conduct, to process and to interpret the information collected by the peripheral organs. It is not possible to determine the effect of an isolated stimulus in the intact organism since the vestibular message undergoes strong influence on its way to the CNS, due to fresh external influences, before it can evoke a response (Gernandt, 1967). The purely mechanical function of the peripheral vestibular labyrinth (cupulo-endolymphatic system) can only be demonstrated in an isolated vestibular labyrinth.

Vestibular tests are the only available way to obtain insight into changes in vestibular function. Spontaneous signs and symptoms such as dizziness and vertigo in aged people do not necessarily indicate a decrease in vestibular function. The most commonly used tests performed to evaluate vestibular function are the rotation test and the caloric test.

ROTATORY TESTS

Minnigerode and Grohmann (1966) described typical features in the electro-nystagmograms recorded in response to rotatory acceleratory stimuli of healthy test subjects of different ages (0–65 years). They found that the total amplitude (the sum-total of all individual amplitudes of the recorded nystagmus beats during a nystagmus period) decreases with increasing age. They considered the amplitude of all beats of the induced nystagmus to be a quantitative measure and a good standard for the intensity of a limited nystagmus event. This decrease in total amplitude with age was described earlier by Dohlman (1935), by Jung and Tönnies (1948), and Mittermaier (1954).

Bartels (1910) was the first to examine the reaction of the vestibular apparatus in neonates by means of rotation. He noticed nystagmus during and after rotation. The strongest reaction occurred on the seventh day after birth. He also noted that if the head were suddenly flexed, the upper eye lid was elevated and the forehead puckered via a vestibular reflex. This phenomenon was later confirmed by Bárány who also agreed with the statements of Bartels (1910) and of Alexander (1911) that the head movements evoked by stimulation of the vestibular apparatus are more pronounced in newborns than in adults. The reaction of the new-born to rotation also differs from the one in adults both in intensity and in the prominence of the slow component. In sleeping infants the quick component was absent after rotation. Optokinetic nystagmus cannot be provoked in new-born infants.

The changing reaction of the growing infant to rotation reflects maturation of the subcortical nuclei. Vestibular responses in newborns are considered to come from the 'archaic' motor system (Ford, 1944), which is free from cerebral inhibition. According to Lawrence and Feind (1953) the vestibular system of the new-born is capable of functioning entirely on its own. This is because the involved neurons are amongst the earliest to become myelinated, starting at a fetal age of 20 weeks. The neurons involved in nystagmus provoked by stimulation of the semicircular canals are the third, fourth, sixth cranial nerves, the vestibular part of the eighth (vestibulocochlear) cranial nerve, and the median longitudinal fasciculus.

Pendleton and Paine (1961) described rotatory and post-rotatory nystagmus in new-borns and very young infants. The presence of a response to rotational stimuli in neonates is explained on the assumption that the response originates at the brainstem level if there is little or no cerebral cortical activity.

Silverstein (1965) studied rotatory and post-rotatory nystagmus in 35 infants aged from 1 to 12 months old. They all had a per-rotatory nystagmus. Nineteen infants from 1 to 5 months old showed a clear post-rotatory nystagmus, but from the 16 older infants (over six months old) only two showed a post-rotatory nystagmus, and 14 failed to show such a nystagmus. He stated that 'inhibitory' corticofugal fibres (from cortex to the vestibular nuclei) are known to be underdeveloped in new-born and young infants. This causes a bilateral facilitation of the vestibular nystagmus, as proved by post-rotational nystagmus following a vestibular stimulus. At the age of six months, enough inhibitory cortico-vestibular fibres have developed to raise the threshold, and weak vestibular stimuli do not elicit a post-rotational response anymore. Meadow (1968) also studied nystagmus in babies during and after rotation and found that the post-rotational nystagmus disappeared after the age of four to six months.

Tibbling (1969) examined 84 children (from new-borns to fifteen years of age) and obtained similar results to Rossberg (1964), and to Minnigerode and Grohmann (1966). She found that both the amplitude and the eye speed of rotatory nystagmus were most intense in very young children and tended to decrease with age up to 15 years, which was the oldest age studied in her group. The older children in Tibbling's sample presumably correspond to the children over seven years old in Zelenka and Slaninová's sample who were considered hyporeflexive. The duration of nystagmus, however, is a poor measure of the strength of vestibular activity. This explains why Zelenka and Slaninová (1964) reported that children over seven years of age had vestibular hyporeflexia since they only took the duration of the nystagmus into consideration. The newborns in the study of Tibbling responded to acceleration with the eyes deviating in the expected direction of the slow component. The fast component, with its probable pontine origin (Cohen, 1972), did not always occur. Groen (1963) examined the vestibular function of a new-born with cupulometry on the 9th day after birth and on several occasions up to the age of three months, and found a decrease in vestibular action developing 25 to 60 days postpartum; at that time inhibitory tendencies are fully developed.

Mitchell and Cambon (1969) conducted rotational tests on 45 neonates (1–4 days old) and found per- and post-rotational nystagmus in the majority of cases. At the age of six weeks most infants showed a vestibular response to rotatory and caloric stimuli, and this response was fully developed at 16 weeks of age. Bartels (1932) studied eye movements in new-borns, the so-called Doll's eye movements (head downwards → eye movements upwards; head upwards → eye movements downwards) and eyelid reflexes (when the baby lies on his back, his eyes are closed, but, when he is turned over, he opens the eyes). These reflexes disappear during the first two months and may have nothing to do with the vestibular system.

Several authors observed post-rotatory nystagmus durations in six to nine month old (Kantner et al, 1976), in three to five year old (Steinberg et al, 1976) and in three to seven year old children (Ornitz et al, 1974).

Rotation tests and caloric tests in very young infants, less than two months old, were recorded by Eviatar and his colleagues (1974).

Michishita (1967) examined—with rotatory and caloric tests—children who were aged from new-born up to 15 years. In agreement with other authors he found very faint reactions in children the age of four years. In children from four to six years old, the reaction values increased remarkably to almost the same level as in adults. The reactions of the children between seven and nine years were the highest of all.

The shape of the age-function for vestibular reactivity is thus very complex. Beginning with infants and young children, the curve reveals a rather high reactivity level and decreases to a lower point in the second decade, followed by an increase to peak response in the higher middle aged groups and finally regaining hyper-reactivity again in old age when inhibitory influences from the brain get smaller again, another instance where senescence recapitulates childhood.

Galebsky confirmed the findings of Bartels that, in new-borns, the reflex of the upper eyelid is elicited by bending the head downwards. Under certain conditions Bárány could arouse a definite optical nystagmus in the new-born, i.e. the child should be awake, not crying and with no intense lighting present.

Guerrier and his colleagues (1970) performed the pendular test on 80 children aged from 0 to 12 years and tried to find the threshold of vestibular stimulation. They defined the threshold of the nystagmus as the moment when it became impossible to see an organised nystagmus (i.e. with an alternating slow and quick phase). Until the age of six weeks no organised nystagmus in babies was found, but merely a 'vestibulo-ocular reflex'. From the sixteenth day after birth, with the maturation of the vestibular apparatus, the nystagmus became more organised, but showed a very high threshold. When the child grows older the threshold becomes lower and at the age of twelve the adult pattern seems to be established. McGraw (1941) studied the changing postural and ocular behaviour of infants (0–2 years) to bodily rotation and concluded that the function of the vestibular apparatus is so complex and interwoven with other receptors that developmental factors are difficult to appraise. The changing reaction of the infant indicates an adaptation of the neural system involved. Another expression used in this respect is habituation.

Ornitz and his colleagues (1979) measured the amplitudes, durations and velocities of the slow and fast phases of both the primary and secondary nystagmus induced by constant angular acceleration in 46 normal children aged from 1 month to 11 years. Significant changes were found in nystagmus parameters with respect to maturation. During both the primary and secondary nystagmus, young infants had larger amplitudes and higher eye speeds than older children.

Camarda (1959), using angular rotation, found that, under similar circumstances, vestibular stimuli give less vegetative reactions in elderly people when compared to younger ones. This is easily explained by the fact that the sensation of rotation is a perceptive phenomenon and old people show a delay in recording nervous and perceptive sensations. Rossberg (1964) studied post-rotatory nystagmus in a group of people from 20 to 80 years of age and found reduction of the excitability of the vestibular system with advancing age.

Meyer zum Gottesberge and Maurer (1950) found a reduction of the vestibular regulatory function in elderly people. They explained this by assuming a depression in the activities of the vestibular centres where co-ordination takes place. They concluded that there is a reduction of peripheral vestibular excitability with increasing age, as well as a reduction in the regulation of vestibular co-ordination.

The rotatory threshold was determined by Haas (1964) in 104 subjects aged from 15 to 80 years. He found a diminishing function of the vestibular system with increasing age.

Chladek (1966) made cupulograms of 51 subjects aged 60 to 75 years (27 with pure presbyacusis, 24 with a more severe defect of hearing) and obtained normal results in the group with presbyacusis. In the other group the supra-threshold post-rotational excitability was raised in many cases. They revealed a post-rotational hyper-reactivity but a reduced caloric excitability.

Van der Laan and Oosterveld (1974) examined the rotational nystagmus provoked by means of a torsion swing in a group of 395 subjects, who according to their age, were subdivided into nine groups, each representing a 10-year period. The quantitative measures were the nystagmic frequency, the amplitude, the speed of the slow phase and the speed of the fast phase as well as the nystagmic threshold. The nystagmus frequency showed variations depending on age (increase in response up to age 60). After 60 years of age, there was a decrease (Fig. 13.1). The nystagmus amplitude was examined in another group of 77 subjects between one and 80 years of age. Here again variations appeared in the size of the amplitude depending on the age, mostly the reverse of the frequency, but very clearly marked, especially in the two extreme age-groups, so that the amplitude seems a very good measure when looking for age differences in nystagmograms (Fig. 13.2).

Testing another group of 113 test-subjects between two and 91 years old, the speed of the slow phase was measured during an increasing stimulation on a torsion swing. An age-dependency was found when the results in the different age-groups were compared. The best vestibular reaction appeared in the young groups, with a decline thereafter (Fig. 13.3). More or less the same results were found after testing a different group of 72 subjects between two and 80 years, and, measuring the speed of the quick phase in the different age-groups, it became clear that the quick phase is the measure least affected by age-changes.

CALORIC TEST

Thornval (1921) performed the caloric test on 74 babies, aged from four hours to eight days, and obtained a good response in all. The induced nystagmus appeared clear and instantaneous. He also noticed spontaneous eye movements in all babies

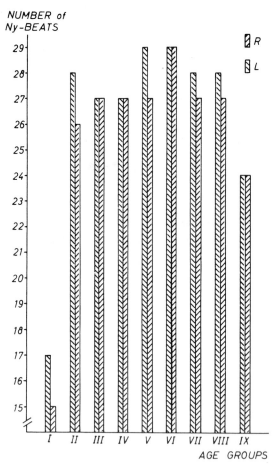

Fig. 13.1 Torsion-swing induced nystagmus and age. Age related changes in nystagmus provoked by a torsion swing. A group of 395 subjects from 2 to 90 years of age subdivided into nine age groups, each covering a ten year period. The swing was allowed to move freely from a position of 180° to the zero-point. The first swing-movement was always to the left. The total number of nystagmus beats to the left and to the right during the first ten swings was counted. The mean values for each age group are represented by the two contiguous hatched columns in the figure.

prior to the test, similar to the nystagmoid eye movements of people under general anaesthesia. As already mentioned, Michishita (1967) found only faint caloric reactions in children younger than four years.

Bartels (1932) reported that, in response to caloric stimulation, the semi-circular canals of new-borns give responses of much longer durations when compared to adults. This could be expected to happen because habituation has not yet developed. According to Mulch and Petermann (1979), the studies of Zelenka and Slaninová (1964, 1966) on caloric tests in children under the age of 10 years concerned mainly the behaviour of nystagmic reactions and the latency time. Arslan (1957), Chládek (1966) and Reichold (1969) found a relatively small excitability of the vestibular organs in elderly people, while Schöder (1973) described hyperexcitability. Zelenka and Slaninová (1964) found the highest values for the duration of the caloric nystagmus in the age groups between 26 and 45

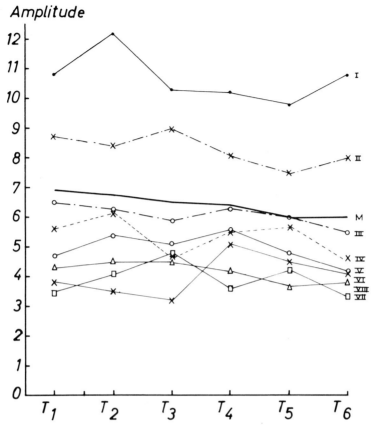

Fig. 13.2 Amplitude of torsion-swing induced nystagmus and age. Variations in the total amplitude of nystagmus with increasing age in 77 subjects between 1 and 80 years of age subdivided into eight age groups, each covering a ten year period. The nystagmus was measured during the first three excursions, i.e. 6 half turns (T1–T6) of the swing. The mean total amplitude in each group for every semi-turn is given. M is the mean of the total amplitudes for all subjects together. Amplitude is given in mm.

years. The highest values for the maximum velocity of the slow phase were observed in the 31 to 40 age group by Van der Laan and Oosterveld (1974), coinciding with the findings of Mulch and Petermann (1979) with regard to the cold irrigations.

However, Bruner and Norris (1971) calculated the highest values for the maximum speed of the slow component and for the nystagmus frequency in the age group 60–70 years.

Mulch and Petermann found the maximum frequency in the age group from 50–60 years. Forgacs (1957) could not detect differences in excitability between middle aged and elderly people.

Gramowski and Unger (1973) and Lämmli (1972) have also reported age related differences in nystagmus measures.

Kotyza (1939) reported the strongest nystagmus reaction in people aged from 45 to 51-years-old.

Arslan (1957) conducted a study with the aid of electronystagmography. He examined 50 people between 49 and 84 years of age and found 30 cases with

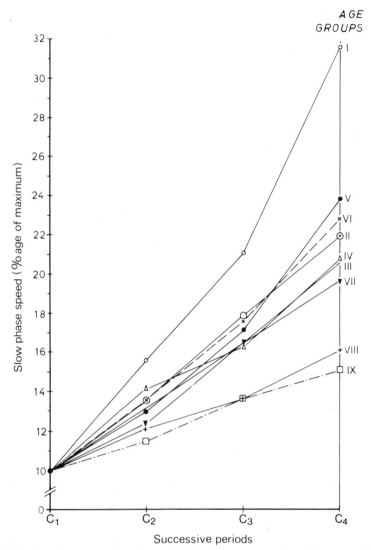

Fig. 13.3 The slow phase speed of a torsion-swing induced nystagmus and age. The course of the slow phase speed of the nystagmus measured on 113 subjects between 2 and 91 years of age, subdivided into nine age groups, each covering a ten year period. Increasing stimulation was given on a torsion swing. C_1, C_2, C_3 and C_4 indicate the 4 successive periods.

decreased, six with increased, and 14 with normal caloric reflexes. His middle-aged subjects appeared hyper-reactive and the subjects over 70 years hypo-reactive. The reaction was in most cases better on the side with the better hearing. There was, however, an inconsistent relationship between hypoacusis and vestibular reactivity. Arslan explained the hyperreflexia after caloric stimulation in subjects affected by atherosclerosis as due to a greater or lesser degree of decreased inhibition which is normally exercised by the supra-nuclear structures in the cortex, cerebellum and mesencephalon.

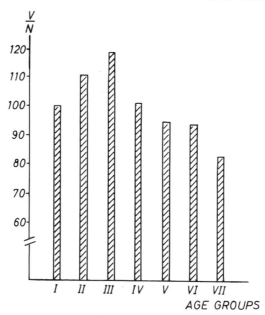

Fig. 13.4 Caloric induced nystagmus and age. Caloric nystagmus measured on a group of 250 subjects from 10 to 90 years of age, subdivided into seven age groups, each covering a ten year period. The sequence of irrigation was Left Cold-Right Cold-Right Warm-Left Warm. V is the total value of the four responses, representing the maximum speed of the slow phase after syringing with water of 30°C and 40°C, for all the members of one group together. N is the number of individuals in each group. V/N represents the mean maximum eye-speed of the slow component for each age group.

With regard to the response changes following repeated caloric tests in relation to age, Gramowski and Unger (1969) noticed a more marked decline in response in 60 to 70-year-old subjects than in 15 to 25-year-old receiving five cold irrigations at eight-minute intervals. All subjects in this study showed some response decline upon repeated testing. The authors, however, expected a greater decline in re-actions in young persons, because they supposed that this decrease in reaction to repeated stimuli was the result of training (process of learning) which, according to them, should be better in young people. They explained these findings on the assumption that older people are more quickly tired than young ones, when repeated stimuli are given (fatigue), and that old people have a deficient natural habituation or a complete loss of natural habituation. This natural habituation develops and grows in young people, where stimuli from every-day life, such as sport, dancing, cycling, and skating, build up a changed vestibular status.

People with bilateral presbyacusis were compared to people with normal hearing by Lämmli (1972). He found an increased duration of the caloric nystagmus in aged people and a decreased velocity of the slow phase of nystagmus.

Mulch and Petermann (1979) found the greatest caloric reaction, with regard to total number of beats and maximum frequency per 10 seconds in people aged 51 to 60 years. For the maximum velocity of the slow phase the cold calorisation showed the greatest response in the age group 31 to 40 years old and the warm irrigation in the age group 41 to 50 years.

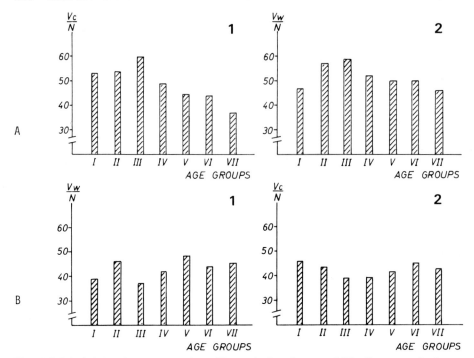

Fig. 13.5 Caloric induced nystagmus and age. Changes in slow phase speed. The diagrams under A represent the results when the cold stimulation was given first, followed after an interval of 20 minutes by a warm stimulation. The diagrams under B represent the results when the warm stimulation was given first, followed after an interval of 20 minutes by a cold stimulation. The diagrams A1 and B2 therefore show the results for cold stimulation (sequence A1 : left cold-right cold, sequence B2 : right cold-left cold). The diagrams A2 and B1 show the results for warm stimulation (sequence A2 : right warm-left warm, sequence B1 : left warm-right warm). Vc is the total value of the two cold responses, representing the maximum speed of the slow phase after syringing with water of 30°C, for all the members of one group together. Vw is the total value of the two warm responses, representing the maximum speed of the slow phase after syringing with water of 44°C, for all members of one group together. Vc/N and Vw/N represent the mean maximum eye-speed of the slow component per group for cold and warm stimulation respectively. Each successive ten year age group is indicated by a Roman numeral.

Van der Laan and Oosterveld (1974) reported that responses to cold calorisation showed a greater age dependency than responses to warm calorisation. They administered caloric tests to 250 healthy test subjects ranging in age from 10 to 90 years. The sequence of irrigation was left cold, right cold, right warm, left warm. The temperature of the irrigation water was 30°C and 44°C. The nystagmus measure used (maximum speed of the slow phase) revealed an increased response with age up to 40 years followed by a decline (Fig. 13.4).

Age increments in nystagmus were more pronounced for warm stimuli than for cold (Fig. 13.5). A possible explanation of the observed age effects is based on habituation, vascular influences, and vestibular nerve degeneration. This review of the literature conclusions that age dependent differences exist in the results of vestibular tests. The pattern of change is complex. The most intense reactions occur in subjects of middle age and late middle age; the least intense reactions are found in neonates. A possible explanation of the reported age affects may be based on habituation, vascular influences and vestibular nerve degeneration.

REFERENCES

Abels H 1906 Ueber Nachempfindungen im Gebiete des kinästhetischen und statischen Sinnes. Zeitschrift für Psychologie, Physiologie und Sinnesorgane 43 : 268–347

Alexander G 1911 Die Reflexerregbarkeit des Ohrlabyrinthes am menschlichen Neugeborenen. Zeitschrift für Psychologie, Physiologie und Sinnesorgane 45 : 153–197

Allara E 1939 Ricerche sull'organo del gusto dell'uomo. I. La struttura delle papille gustative nelle varie età della vita. Archivio italiano di anatomia e di embriologia 42 : 506–564

Arslan M 1957 The senescence of the vestibular apparatus. Pract oto-rhino-laryng. (Basel) 19 : 475–483

Aschan G 1954 Response to rotatory stimuli in fighter pilots. Acta otolaryngologica (Stockh.) Suppl 116

Aubry M 1955 La sénescence auriculaire. In: Précis de Gérontologie par L. Binet et al F, Bourlière (Ed Masson & Cie, Paris)

Bartels M 1910 Ueber Regulierung der Augenstellung durch den Ohrapparat. Graefes Archiv für Ophthalmologie 76 : 1–97

Bartels M 1932 Ueber Augenbewegungen bei Neugeborenen. Deutsche medizinische Wochenschrift 36 : 1477–1478

Bergström B 1973a Morphological studies of the vestibular nerve. Acta Universitahs Uppsala 159 : 1–41

Bergström B 1973b Morphology of the vestibular nerve. II. The number of myelinated vestibular nerve fibres in man at various ages. Acta Otolaryngologica (Stockh.) 76 : 173–179

Bergström B 1973c Morphology of the vestibular nerve. III. Analysis of the calibers of the myelinated vestibular nerve fibers in man at various ages. Acta Otolaryngologica (Stockh.) 76 : 331–338

Beyermann-Grösser P 1964 Altersschwerhörigkeit und Binauraltest: Studie über die bisherigen Auffassungen der Altersschwerhörigkeit, sowie eigene Untersuchungen mit einem neuen Verfahren. Archiv für Otolaryngologie 79 : 28–29

Boccuzzi V 1962 Fenomeni di senescenza nell'olfatto. Bolletino delle malattie dell'orecchio della gola e della naso 80 : 654–665

Brain R W 1965 In: Duizeligheid bij oudere mensen door P G Gerlings. Nederlandsch tijdschrift voor geneeskunde 109 : (43) 2023–2024

Bruner A, Norris T W 1971 Age-related changes in caloric nystagmus. Acta otolaryngologica (Stockh.) Suppl 282

Camarda V 1959 La reazioni vegetative da stimolazione vestibolare dell'uomo in età senile (ricerche elettronistagmografiche). Giornale di gerontologia 7 : 525–531

Chádek V 1966 Changes in the vestibular apparatus in old age. Ces Lék Ces 105 : (1) 15–18

Cohen B 1972 Origin of quick phases of nystagmus. In: Brodal A, Pompeiano O (eds) Basic Aspects of Central Vestibular Mechanisms. Progress in Brain Research 37 : 1–649, 1972

Collins W E 1966 Vestibular responses from figure skaters. Aerospace Medicine 37 : 1098–1105

Comel G 1932 Sullo stato funzionale cochleo-vestibolare nei vecchi. Otorinolaringologia italiana 32 : 97

Dayal V S, Farkashidy J, Kokshanian A 1973 Embryology of the ear. Canadian Journal of Otolaryngology 2 : 136–142

Denny-Brown D E 1949 Neurological aspects of vertigo. New England Journal of Medicine 241 : 144–145

Denny-Brown D E 1952 Recurrent cerebrovascular symptoms of vasospasm. Archives of Neurology and Psychiatry 67 : 117–118

Denny-Brown D E 1953 Basilar artery-syndromes. New England Medical Center 15 : 53–60

Depoutre 1912 Examen fonctionnel du labyrinthe chez le vieillard. Annales des Maladies de l'oreille et du larynx 38 : 159–160

Dishoeck H A E van 1966 Presbyakusis. In: Berendes J (ed) Hals-Nasen-Ohren-Heilkunde Bd III, Teil 3 Stuttgart

Dix M R, Hood U D 1968 Vestibular habituation, its clinical significance and relationship to vestibular neuronitis. Proceedings of the Bárány Society Vestibular Symp. Uppsala

Dohlman G 1935 Some practical and theoretical points in labyrinthology. Proceedings of the Royal Society of Medicine 28 : 1371–1380

Droller H, Pemberton J 1953 Vertigo in a random sample of elderly people living in their homes. Journal of Laryngology 67 : 689–695

Engström H, Bergström B, Rosenhall U 1974 Vestibular sensory epithelia. Archives of Otolaryngology 100 : 411–418

Engström H, Ades H W, Engström M B et al 1977 Changes in the vestibular epithelia in elderly monkeys and humans. Advances in Otorhinolaryngology 22 : 93–110

Eviatar L, Eviatar A, Naray I 1974 Maturation and neurovestibular responses in infants. Developmental Medicine and Child Neurology 16 : 435–446

Feldmann H 1962 Die Geschmackprüfung. Deutsche medizinische Wochenschrift 87 : 1732–1740

Ferreri G 1954 The senile labyrinth. Giornale di gerontogia 1 : 389–399

Fields W S 1968 Vertigo related to alteration in arterial blood flow. In: Wolfson R J (ed) The vestibular system and its diseases, Philadelphia

Fleischer K 1956 Histologische und audiometrische Studie der altersbedingten Struktur- und Funktionswandel des Innenohres. Archiv für experimentelle Ohren- Nasen- und Kehlkopfheilkunde 170:142–168

Ford F R 1944 Diseases of nervous system in infancy, childhood and adolescence. Thomas, Springfield

Forgacs P 1957 The cochlea and vestibular function at advanced age. Fül-orr-gégegyógyászat 1:5–10

Galebsky A 1927 Vestibular nystagmus in new-born infants. Acta otolaryngologica (Stockh.) 11:409–424

Gernandt B E 1967 Central regulation of the vestibular system. Archives of otolaryngologica 115:521–520

Glorig Nixon J 1962 Hearing loss as a function of age. Laryngoscope (St. Louis) 72:1596–1611

Gramowski K H, Unger E 1969 Experimentelle vestibuläre Habituation bei jungen und älteren Versuchspersonen. Zeitschrift für Laryngologie, Rhinologie und Otologie 3:207–214

Gramowski K H, Unger E 1973 Ober die Altersabhängigkeit thermischer Labyrinthreaktionen. Zeitschrift für Laryngologie, Rhinologie und Otologie 52:541–547

Groen J J 1963 Postnatal changes in vestibular reactions. Acta otolaryngologica (Stockh.) 56:390–398

Guerrier Y, Dejean Y, Basseres F, Denise 1970 Le seuil vestibulaire de l'enfant normal (Methode pendulaire). Revue de Laryngologie, otologie, rhinologie (Bordeaux) 23:881–900

Haas E 1964 Zur Frage der Alterabhängigkeit der Drehreizschwelle. Zeitschrift für Laryngologie, Rhinologie und Otologie 43:238–246

Heron A, Chown S 1967 Age and function. Churchill, London

Hinchcliffe R 1958 Clinical quantitative gustometry. Ata otolaryngologica (Stockh.) 49:453–466

Hughes G 1969 Changes in taste sensitivity with advancing age. Gerontologica Clinica 11:224–230

Jung R, Tönnies J F 1948 Die Registrierung und Auswertung des Drehnystagmus beim Menschen. Klinische Wochenschrift 26:513–515

Kantner R M, Clark D L, Allen L C, Chase M F 1976 Effects of vestibular stimulation on nystagmus response and motor performance in the developmentally delayed infant. Physical Therapy 56:414–421

Kotyza F 1939 Vestibular reaction at various ages. Československá otolaryngologie 78:755–756

Kranz D, Berndt H, Wagner H 1968 Untersuchunger zur Altersveränderung der Geschmacksschwelle. Archiv für klinische experimentelle Ohren- Nasen- und Kehlkopfheilkunde 192:258–267

Krmpotić-Nemanić J 1963 Presbykusis und Presbyosmie als Folgen eines analogen biologischen Prozesses. Bulletin scientifique 8:135

Krmpotić-Nemanić J 1969 Presbyacusis, presbystasis and presbyosmia as consequences of the analogous biological process. Acta otolaryngologica (Stockh.) 67:217–223

Krijger M W W 1954 The significance of the labyrinth in aviation. Thesis, Utrecht

Laan F L van der, Oosterveld W J 1974 Age and vestibular function.Aerospace Medicine 45:540–547

Lämmli K 1972 Die Altersveränderungen der Labyrinthfunktion im Elektronystagmogramm. ORL 34, 62

Lawrence M M, Feind C R 1953 Vestibular responses to rotation in the new-born infant. Pediatrics 12:300–307

MaCkevick, L K 1963 The vestibular apparatus in elderly people. Mekhanizmy Stareniya (Kiev) 271–275

Matzker J 1954 Untersuchungen über die zentrale Synthese differenter Schallbilder beider Ohren. Zeitschrift für Laryngologie und Rhinologie 33:296–304

Matzker J 1965 Riochen und Lebensalter—Riechen und Rauchen. Archiv für Ohren- Nasen- und Kehlkopfheilkunde 185:755–760

Mayer D 1920 Das anatomische Substrat der Altersschwerhörigkeit. Archiv für klinische und experimentelle Ohren- Nasen- und Kehlkopfheilkunde 105:1–13

McCabe B F 1960 Vestibular suppression in figure skaters. Transactions of the American Academy of Ophthalmology and Otolaryngology 64:264–268

McGraw M B 1941 Development of rotatory-vestibular reactions of human infant. Child Development 12:17–19

Meadow S R 1968 Vestibular nystagmus in infants and the effect of streptomycin in the neonatal period. Developmental Medicine and Child Neurology 10:317–321

Meyer zum Gottesberge A, Maurer W 1950 Das Ewaldsche Gesetz. Zeitschrift für Laryngologie und Rhinologie 29:532–543

Meyer B J 1970 Fisiologie van veroudering. Publ Univ Pretoria

Michishita K 1967 Studies of normal vestibular reaction in children. Journal of Oto-laryngology (Japan) 70:37–60

Millikan C H, Siekert R G 1955 Studies in cerebrovascular disease. IV. The syndrome of intermittent insufficiency of the carotid arterial system. Proceedings of the Mayo Clinic 30: 186–191

Minnigerode B, Grohmann R 1966 Untersuchungen zur Bestimmung des massgebenden Charakteristika des Elektronystagmograms gesunder Versuchspersonen verschiedenen Lebensalter bei rotatorischen Beschleunigungsreizen. Acta otolaryngologica (Stockh.) 61: 101–113

Mitchell T, Cambon K 1969 Vestibular responses in the neonata and infant. Archives of Otolaryngology 90: 556–558

Mittermaier R 1954 Ueber systematische nystagmographische Untersuchungen des kalorischen und rotatorischen Nystagmus. Acta otolaryngologica (Stockh.) 44: 574–579

Mulch G, Petermann W 1979 Influence of age on results of vestibular function tests. Annals of Otology, Rhinology and Laryngology, Suppl 85

Naumann H H 1968 In: Presbyacusis, presbyastasis and presbyosmia. Acta oto-laryngologica (Stockh.) 67: 217–223

Orma E J, Koskenoja M 1957 Postural dizziness in the aged. Geriatrics 12: 49–59

Ornitz E M, Brown M B, Manson A, Putnam N H 1974 The effect of visual input on postrotatory nystagmus in normal children. Acta otolaryngologica (Stockh.) 77: 418–425

Ornitz M, Atwell C W, Walter D O, Hartmann E E, Kaplan A R 1979 The maturation of vestibular nystagmus in infancy and childhood. Acta otolaryngologica 88, 244–256

Pallestrini E 1933 Arteriosclosi o funzione labirintica. Acta Societatis O R L Latina 2: 166–177

Patenostre H 1912 Examen fonctionnel du labyrinthe chez le vieillard. Annales des maladies de l'oreille et du larynx 38: 158–178

Pendleton M E, Paine R S 1961 Vestibular nystagmus in newborn infants. A study by visual, photographic and electro-oculographic methods. Preliminary report. Neurology (Minneap.) 11: 450–459

Rasmussen A F 1940 Studies in the VIIIth cranial nerve of man. Laryngoscope (St. Louis) 50: 67–83

Reichold J 1969 Die altersbedingten Veränderungen der Labyrinthfunktion. Inaugural-dissertation, Zürich

Rosen S, Bergman M, Plester D, El-Mofty A, Satti M H 1962 Presbyacusis study of a relatively noise-free population in the Sudan. Annals of Otolaryngology (St. Louis) 71: 727–743

Rosenhall U 1972 Vestibular macular mapping in man. Annals of Otology, Rhinology and Laryngology 81: 339–351

Rossberg G 1964 Die Altersabhängigkeit der vestibulären Leistungsfähigkeit. Ein Beitrag zur Regulations funktion des Vestibularissystems. Archiv für klinische und experimentelle Ohren-, Nasen- und Kehlkopfheilkunde 181: 475–490

Saxén A 1937 Pathologie und Klinik der Altersschwerhörigkeit usw. Acta oto-laryngologica (Stockh.) Suppl 23

Schöder H J 1973 Zur Reaktionsweise des Vestibularysystems im Alter. Verkehrsmedizin, Ihre Grenzgebiete 20: 180–183

Schuknecht H F 1955 Presbyacusis. Laryngoscope (St. Louis) 65: 402–419

Schuknecht H F 1964 Further observations on the pathology of presbyacusin. Archives of Otolaryngology 80: 369–383

Scuderi R 1947 Aspetti anatomo-clinici della arteriosclerosi labirintion. Archivio italiano di otologia 58: 278–316

Serćer A, Krmpotić J 1958 Ueber die Ursache der progressiven Altersschwerhörigkeit (Presbyakusis). Acta otolaryngologica (Stockh.) Suppl 143

Shock N W 1962 The physiology of ageing. Science 206: 100–112

Schöder H-J 1973 Zur Reaktionsweise des Vestibularsystems im Alter. Verkehrsmedizin: Ihre Grenzgebiete 20: 180–183

Sillevis Smit H H 1965 In: Duizeligheid bij oudere mensen door P G Gerlings. Nederlandsch Tijdschrift voor geneeskunde 109 (II) 43, 2022

Silverstein H 1965 Induced rotational nystagmus in normal infants. Journal of Pediatrics 67: 432–438

Smith K U, Greene D 1962 Scientific motion study and ageing processes in performance. Ergonomics 5: 155–164

Steinberg M, Rendle-Short J 1977 Vestibular dysfunction in young children with minor neurological impairment. Developmental Medicine and Child Neurology 19: 639–651

Thornval A 1921 L'épreuve calorique chez les nouveau-nés. Acta otolaryngologica (Stockh.) 2: 451–455

Tibbling L 1969 The rotatory nystagmus response in children. Acta otolaryngologica (Stockh.) 68: 459–467

Vido G de, Pagnini G 1956 Problems of gerontology in oto-rhinolaryngology. IXth Nat. Congress of the Gruppo Otologico Ospedaliero Italiano. Salsomaggiore

Vogt O 1905 Die myelogenetische Gliederung des Cortex cerebelli. Journal für Psychologie und Neurologie 5: 235–250

Williams H L 1963 Dizziness in the older age group. Postgraduate Medicine 33:606–610

Wit G de 1953 Seasickness (Motion sickness). Acta oto-laryngologica (Stockh.) Suppl 108

Zelenka J, Kozak P 1963 Vestibular findings in hypertension and arteriosclerosis. Ceskoslovenska otolaryngologie 12:112–117

Zelenka J, Slaninová B 1964 Changes of labyrinth function due to age. Československá otolaryngologie 13:21–26

Zilstorff-Pedersen K 1962 Die quantitative und qualitative Olfactometrie. HNO (Berl) 10:97–103

Zwaardemaker H 1894 The range of hearing at various ages. Zeitschrift für Psychologie 7:10–28

Falls in old age

INTRODUCTION

Falls in old age lie in a zone of rapidly expanding ignorance. The population at risk of enduring falls is increasing faster than knowledge of their prevention. There have, however, been a number of recent significant advances. Much is now known about the who, where and when of falling; but little as yet about the how and why. The changes which succeed falls are better understood than are those which precede them. Many mechanisms may be at fault, but in individual cases diagnosis depends on conjecture. There is no policy for prevention and no system for treatment. But at least there is a beginning awareness in the medical, nursing and rehabilitation professions that falls in old age are not adequately described as a 'social problem'. The symptom of Instability is recognised as one of the 'Giants of Geriatrics' (Isaacs, 1976)—gigantic in terms of the number of sufferers afflicted and the severity of their disability, but gigantic also in its challenge to medical science.

DEFINITION

This chapter deals with those incidents in which the conscious subject suffers displacement and comes to rest unintentionally on the floor. Excluded from consideration are falls resulting from syncope with loss of consciousness, or as a result of epilepsy or the onset of a stroke. Also excluded are episodes of staggering in which the victim falls against a wall or into a chair but not on to the ground.

BARRIERS TO PROGRESS

Limitations of sampling

One reason for slow progress in elucidating the causes of falls in old age is an inherent limitation on the acquisition of knowledge. A fall, like a street accident, is a momentary event which cannot be studied until it has happened; and in which the testimony of independent witnesses is required but is not always available.

Falls come to medical attention if they are atypical in location or consequences. The best observed cases come from the abnormal population of hospitals and residential homes. Referrals from the community are mostly of those who have sustained injury or whose families have experienced stress. Falls lacking these consequences are often dismissed as 'normal for age'; and the victims are not interrogated or examined at a stage when the mechanism of the fall might be more readily elucidated and further falls prevented.

History taking

Falls in old people, apart from those occurring in institutions, are often unwitnessed. The sole source of information is the faller, who may be bemused by the unexpectedness of the event and bewildered by questioning. Previous falls may be forgotten; or recent and remote events confused. Repeated interrogation may result in the formulation of a consistent but not necessarily accurate story.

Limitations of language

The faller faces difficulty in putting into words the experiences which accompanied the fall. This can lead to errors in interpretation. Wild and her colleagues (1980), studying old people who had fallen at home, found discrepancies between their responses to the instruction 'Tell me what happened' and their replies to direct questions. Spontaneous descriptions rarely included the words 'dizzy' and 'giddy'; instead the word 'just' figured frequently, in such phrases as 'I just fell', or 'my legs just gave way'. Another common usage was the phrase 'must have', e.g. 'I must have tripped' or 'I must have slipped'. These expressions convey the unexpectedness of the fall and the absence of presenting symptoms or external hazards. The phrase 'I must have tripped' was interpreted as meaning 'I fell . . . falls are caused by trips . . . I do not recall having tripped . . . but I suppose . . . *I must have tripped'*.

A direct question such as 'Did you feel dizzy?' often produced an affirmative reply, sometimes after a short delay, in subjects who had not used this term in their spontaneous description. It seemed as though subjects were willing to accept these familiar words as approximations to the sensation which they had experienced. The impression was gained that the patients were seeking for words to describe some sort of conflict between visual, vestibular and proprioceptive information which had given them a sense of instability but which had none of the connotations of rotation or lightheadedness usually associated with the words 'dizziness' and 'giddiness'.

A few fallers used the expression, 'I had a blackout'; or 'I went out like a light'; or 'I found myself on the floor'; but denied loss of consciousness. To one or two the word 'blackout' had a visual connotation—a sort of clouding or graying of the field of vision.

The word 'dizziness' may be translated by doctors into 'vertigo', focussing attention on the vestibular apparatus, which may be wholly innocent, and leading to the inappropriate prescription of so-called vestibular sedatives. A 'blackout' may be interpreted as a syncopal attack, and attributed to disturbance of the carotid sinus, the heart rhythm, the postural control of blood pressure or flow through the vertebral and basilar arteries.

Drachman and Hart (1972), in their 'Dizziness Clinic', claimed some success in reproducing the patients' symptoms by subjecting them to a range of perturbing motions—an unpleasant substitute for verbal interpretation.

Linguistic uncertainty is not confined to patients. Doctors too use imprecise expressions. The term 'drop attack' is widely used and variously defined (Kremer, 1958; Sheldon, 1960; Lund, 1963; Stevens and Mathews, 1973; Kubala and Millikan, 1964). Little is gained by treating this as a separate entity: it is an unexpected fall while walking. Tumarkin (1936) and Ethelberg (1950) introduced some colour into the terminology when they described the tendency to sudden unexpected falls as 'otolithic catastrophe' and 'symptomatic cataplexy' or 'chalastic fits' respectively. Their views on pathogenesis have not been confirmed, and their terms never established themselves.

'Loss of balance' is sometimes included among the causes of falls. This is tautological (Isaacs, 1978); one cannot very well fall without losing balance. Doctors should beware of translating statements about symptoms into assumptions about causes. For example falls on standing up are not necessarily due to postural hypotension; and the experience of a sense of rotation is not necessarily due to disordered vestibular function.

Limitations of physical examination
Physical examination reveals disabilities present at the time of the fall which may have contributed to the fall, such as an old hemiplegia or Parkinson's disease. It may demonstrate physiological changes such as disturbance of cardiac rhythm, drop in blood pressure on standing, abnormality of gait or balance, states of fear or anxiety; without any certainty that these were present at the time of the fall or that they contributed to the fall. Examination cannot reproduce the exact circumstances of the fall; and cannot detect the presence of inattention or pre-occupation which may have made important contributions.

Limitations of multiple pathology
The balance function employs many pathways, and is susceptible to damage at many points. The discovery of abnormalities along the pathway is insufficient evidence that these caused the fall. Many popular diagnostic labels attached to fallers, such as postural hypotension, cervical spondylosis and vertebro-basilar insufficiency, are almost equally common among non-fallers. Evaluating the causes of falls requires epidemiological methods; or else assumptions have to be made about the possible contribution of a variety of extrinsic and intrinsic factors.

EPIDEMIOLOGY

Recent epidemiological studies make it possible to offer some estimate of the number of falls in old people and of some of the factors which are associated with them.

In any one year in the United Kingdom, with its population of fifty-five million, of whom nearly 6 per cent are aged seventy-five and over, there are approximately:-
Three million falls in old people in the community (Wild et al, 1980);
Three hundred thousand falls in old people in institutions (Wild et al, 1980);
Thirty thousand falls resulting in fracture of the proximal part of the femur (Evans et al, 1979);

Three thousand deaths certified as due to falls (Registrar-General, 1978).

Epidemiological studies of falls have taken the following form:

1. Surveys of accidents in the home (Seiler and Ramsay, 1954; Droller, 1955; Gray, 1966; Berfenstam et al, 1969; Lucht, 1971; Akhtar et al, 1973; de Fonseka and Roberts, 1972; Roberts et al, 1974; Waller, 1974).
2. General community surveys (Sheldon, 1948; Droller, 1955).
3. Analysis of accident reports routinely submitted in hospitals (Parrish and Weil, 1958; Fine, 1959; Leitch et al, 1964; Scott, 1976; Hanton and Leopoldt, 1978; Tinker, 1979; Morris and Isaacs, 1980).
4. Prospective surveys of residents in special facilities (Ashley et al, 1977; Gryfe et al, 1977; Kalchthaler et al, 1978).
5. Admissions to or attendances at hospital for fractures (Over, 1965; Lucht, 1971; Campbell, 1976; MacDonald and MacDonald, 1976; D.P.C.P., 1978;* Brocklehurst et al, 1978; Evans et al, 1979).
6. Statistics of fractures (Knowelden, 1964; Eddy, 1972; 1973; Gallanaugh et al, 1976).
7. Analysis of death certificates (Eddy, 1972; 1973).

The information derived from these studies can be summarised as follows:

1. The incidence of falls and of fractures rises steeply with increase of age (Sheldon, 1948; Knowelden et al, 1964; Gray, 1968).
2. At all ages the incidence of falls and fractures is higher in females than in males (Droller, 1955; Knowelden et al, 1964; Lucht et al, 1964; Gray, 1966; Stevens and Mathews, 1973; Brocklehurst et al, 1978).
3. The proportion of falls which are followed by fractures is low (Gray, 1966; Iskrant, 1968; Scott, 1976; Gryfe et al, 1977; Morris and Isaacs, 1980).
4. The proportion of fractures which are caused by falls in the home rather than by accidents and falls outside the home rises with increase of age and is higher at all ages in females than in males (Knowelden et al, 1964).
5. Fractures of the femur are more likely to occur after a first than a subsequent fall (Evans et al, 1979a).
6. A high proportion of falls occur in old people who live alone or with one other old person (Brocklehurst et al, 1976; Wild et al, 1980).
7. Most falls in old people at home occur at times and in places where activity occurs. Falls at night are relatively infrequent (Gray, 1966; Lucht, 1971; Wild et al, 1980).
8. There is an excess mortality after falls (Naylor and Rosin, 1970; Lucht, 1971; Evans et al, 1979b). The greatest excess occurs some months after the fall, rather than as a direct consequence of it (Wild et al, 1980).

MECHANISM OF FALLS

If a fall is thought of as failure to correct a displacement, the quest for causes can be resolved into seeking the cause of, first the displacement, and second, the failure to correct.

*Department of Prices and Consumer Protection

Table 14.1 Displacement causing falls

Extraordinary imposed	e.g. patch of ice, dog
Extraordinary initiated	e.g. fall from ladder, sudden head movement
Ordinary imposed	e.g. trip on carpet
Ordinary initiated	e.g. error on standing up

Displacements are of two types, which may be called 'initiated' and 'imposed'. The former is originated by the subject, the latter comes from without. Both types of displacement may be further subdivided into 'ordinary' and 'extraordinary' (Table 14.1).

Ordinary initiated displacements include getting up from a chair, walking, getting into or out of bed, or on or off the toilet. Falls attributed to 'loss of balance', 'drop attacks' and 'change of posture' are examples of this type.

Extraordinary initiated displacements include the above activities undertaken in haste or inattention. To these may be added the abnormal gait patterns associated with painful feet and joints; and with stroke, neurological deficits such as drop-foot or old hemiplegia; and structural abnormalities of the joints.

Ordinary imposed displacements are the encounters with unperceived hazards which are of common occurrence in daily life, e.g. tripping over a kerb, missing a step, slipping on a damp patch. These do not usually cause falls.

Extraordinary imposed displacements include these encounters at times of haste or inattention; or with greater displacing forces such as are caused by slipping on a patch of ice or being struck by a motor car.

In addition to these four types of displacement some falls seem to be caused by the 'correction' of a displacement which did not take place but which the victim believes took place. Such illusory percepts underlie the fear of falling expressed by victims of the 'post-fall syndrome' (Murphy, 1980), some of whom show disordered perception of the vertical (Tobis et al, 1981).

CORRECTION OF THE DISPLACEMENT

Correction of the displacement may be thought of as occurring in three phases, i.e. detection, processing and effecting. The greater the displacement the less time is available for its correction.

The displacement is perceived by visual, tactile, vestibular and proprioceptive receptors and transmitted to the central mechanism. Mechanoreceptors in the neck are an important source of information on the position and movement of the head (Wyke, 1979).

The central structures involved in the processing of the detection of displacement signals and the transmission of instructions to the muscles include large areas of the cerebral cortex, the cerebellum, the basal ganglia and their inter-connecting loops (Eccles, 1978).

The effecting of correction calls for the activation of very large numbers of motor units in the skeletal musculature, whose activity is monitored and corrected through feed-back loops (Granit, 1972).

AETIOLOGY

While many factors are involved in falls, there must always be an imbalance between the displacing force and the correcting mechanism. The less the displacing force which causes the fall then the greater is the disturbance of the correcting mechanism. An extraordinary imposed displacement most nearly earns the name of 'accidental' fall; while a fall during a normal initiated displacement implies serious disturbance of the correcting mechanism.

Defects of correction may result from momentary, temporary or permanent disturbances of the correction mechanism.

Momentary disturbances affect correction of displacement for just long enough for the fall to occur. Several mechanisms have been proposed, but none is susceptible of proof. The candidates include:

1. Transient disturbances of cardiac rhythm of sufficient duration to cause a reduction in cardiac output and reduced perfusion of the brain stem, cerebellum or spinal cord but without loss of consciousness. In a single case report, Gordon (1978) has demonstrated an infarction in the reticular formation of the brain stem in a patient with recent onset of 'drop attacks', in which the power seemed to leave her legs and she 'just fell'. This strengthens the view that transient ischaemia of this part of the brain may be responsible for 'drop attacks'.
2. Transient drop of blood pressure, for example on postural change, may cause reduction of cerebral perfusion resulting in falls without loss of consciousness.
3. There may be transient occlusion of the vertebral artery in the neck by osteophytes as a result of cervical spondylosis (Sheehan et al, 1960; Williams and Wilson, 1962; Kubala and Millikan, 1964; Kameyama, 1965).
4. Transient occlusion or reduction of flow in the spinal artery may cause momentary paraparesis, resulting in a fall (Silver and Buxton, 1974).
5. Unexplained failure of the gamma servo loop, possibly associated with loss of cerebellar Purkinje cells, has been postulated (Kremer, 1958; Sheldon, 1960).
6. An error of visual, vestibular or proprioceptive perception or interpretation may produce momentary displacement (Over, 1966).
7. An error in the initiation or completion of a synergistic movement, e.g. stepping, or transferring from sitting to standing may place the moving body in an unperceived position of instability (Guimaraes and Isaacs, 1980).
8. Transient loss of attention in the course of a displacing movement may result in delay in bringing the correcting mechanism into play.

Temporary disturbances

Temporary disturbances in the correcting mechanism may result from a wide range of systemic illnesses and intoxications including hypoxia, acute infections, muscle weakness especially after acute illness, and after alcohol and drugs which are discussed below.

Permanent disturbances

Permanent changes in the correcting mechanism can be inferred from physiological and pathological studies of the muscular and nervous systems of old people.

Though these have not been directly correlated with the occurrence of falls, it is reasonable to suggest that they pose a threat to the balance mechanism. Granit (1972) has explained how even healthy young subjects err frequently in their execution and appreciation of movement, and has identified the mechanisms which might be at fault. In a bold but successful experiment Greenwood and Hopkins (1976a; 1976b; 1977) demonstrated a failure of activation of pre-programmed muscular fall-breaking responses when old people were suddenly released from a parachute and dropped to the floor. Melvill Jones and Watt (1971) obtained similar results with more conventional experimental methods.

Structural changes in the ageing human brain which slow central processing are described by Brizzee (1977); and the neurophysiological and psychological features are summarised by Isaacs (1978). Hasselkus (1972) has reviewed the changes in muscle which might contribute to the slowing and weakness of responses to command; and the inadequate feeding of information back through the gamma linkages to monitor the progression of movement.

The presence of permanent deficiencies in the correcting mechanism produces unadventurous adaptive behaviour with limitation of mobility and changes in the stepping pattern (Guimaraes and Isaacs, 1980). To some extent these compensate for the instability, but insufficiently; so that permanent defects of the neuromuscular apparatus provide a constant background of uncertainty in the performance of bipedal locomotion.

MEASUREMENTS

Measurement of 'balance'

The clinician thinks of 'static balance' as the ability to maintain the standing position; and 'dynamic balance' as the ability to remain upright during locomotion. The difference is merely of degree, the 'dynamic' state making greater demands on the balance mechanism than are exerted during quiet standing. Static balance is more readily measured and seems to provide a good indication of gait performance (Murray, Seireg and Sepic, 1975).

Hellebrandt (1938) demonstrated that, during quiet standing, the line of pressure, the resultant of the ground forces acting on the body, falls somewhat in front of the line of gravity, which is the vertical line through the centre of mass. The upright posture is maintained by the aid of low intensity activity in the muscles of the calf (Basmajian, 1961; 1962). In healthy young people the upright stance is accompanied by barely perceptible sway, mostly in an anteroposterior direction, and is associated with firing of motor units in the calf muscles (Burke and Eklund, 1977). This is thought to represent either a means of safeguarding standing posture by maintaining the centre of gravity behind the centre of pressure (Murray et al, 1967) or, more speculatively, a mechanism of 'dynamic interrogation of proprioception' (Bonnet et al, 1976), which employs the alpha-gamma linkage to determine periodically the state of stretch of the structures acting around the ankle, and to apply instantaneous corrections. This 'central programme for postural fixation' is presumably vulnerable to damage in old age, reflecting uncritical processing of sensory input (Murray et al, 1975); and many investigators have linked increased sway to advancing years (Hellebrandt and Braun, 1939; Hasselkus and Shambes, 1975) and to postural instability and liability to falls (Sheldon, 1963; Overstall et al, 1977).

Measurement of 'sway'

Baron and his colleagues (1956) introduced the 'stabilograph' to register the position of the centre of pressure and the vertical, horizontal and transverse ground forces during standing. Many other investigators have employed similar instruments, using the output from strain gauges or piezo-electric crystals (O'Leary, 1970; de Wit, 1973; Snijders and Verduin, 1973; Terekhov, 1978). These platforms are however costly and not always reliable; and clinically useful data have been obtained by naked eye observation of enhanced sway; by a pen attached to the subject's forehead (Sheldon, 1963) or by a simple ataxiameter (Wright, 1971) which counts anteroposterior sway movements by a fine wire attached to the trunk and operating a ratchet (Overstall et al, 1977).

Using a force platform, Murray, Seireg and Sepic (1975) found in normal young subjects that the excursion of the line of pressure about its mean position during quiet standing was very small; and the area within which stability could be maintained on voluntary displacement was very large. However both measures of balance sharply deteriorated with increasing age of the subject. The excursion of the line of pressure during ordinary movements such as rising from a chair goes far beyond the support base (Murray et al, 1967), necessitating constant vigilance to maintain balance.

For clinical purposes the observation of excessive sway is readily made and can be taken as evidence of impaired function of the balance mechanism. In a series of studies Isaacs and his colleagues (Wild et al, 1980; Guimaraes and Isaacs, 1980; Murphy et al, 1980; Murphy, 1980) used the response to a simple tap on the sternum of a quietly standing subject as an indicator of balance. Abnormal responses were 'startle' movements of the upper limbs or backwards stepping. There were striking differences in the probability of further falls and in mortality in relation to the results of this simple test.

In patients who had undergone hip operations Murray and her colleagues (1975) found a good correlation between balance tests and walking performance. In general terms there appears to be a relation between the observable efficiency of comparatively simple measures of stability and the propensity to fall during complex movement.

MENTAL STATE

Old people who fall perform less well on tests of mental function than do control subjects (Brocklehurst et al, 1978; Wild et al, 1980); while disturbances of mobility and of mental state are also related (Waller, 1974). The interpretation of these findings is not clear. It is common experience that patients with quite severe dementia are able to venture out of doors and into traffic without falling. At present all that can be said is that those who fall do not perform well on tests.

DRUGS

Chalmers has said that it is often prescription rather than pride which goes before a fall. Evidence of the association between the consumption of drugs and falling is available for antihypertensives (Wild et al, 1980), barbiturates (MacDonald and MacDonald, 1977), other hypnotics, sedatives and tranquillisers (Brocklehurst et al, 1978; Wild et al, 1980); and alcohol (Waller, 1974; Wild et al, 1980). These presumably slow central nervous system conduction and impair the accuracy of corrective movements. Hypnotics go on acting for a long time in old people; and the falls are more likely during the day rather than during the night following their ingestion.

The phenothiazine drug, prochlorperazine, widely used for the treatment of 'dizziness' has been suspected as a cause of falls, but Wild and her colleagues (1980) found no difference between its consumption by fallers and by non-fallers. However the tricyclic antidepressant drugs imipramine and amitriptyline, are associated with falls, in consequence of their postural hypotensive effects (Glassman et al, 1979; Wild et al, 1980).

THE ROLE OF MUSCLES

Muscle disease in early and middle life frequently presents with an undue liability to fall. In old age many recurrent fallers have muscle wasting (Wild et al, 1980), usually caused by systemic diseases such as cancer, rheumatoid arthritis and malnutrition; while certain other diseases are associated with pathological changes in muscle, for example thyrotoxicosis, diabetes and osteomalacia.

THE NECK

In a series of important papers Wyke (1975, 1979) has drawn attention to the role played in human balance by the mechanoreceptors of the apophyseal joints and other structures of the cervical spine. With the assumption of the upright posture he believes that man has come to depend on this system, in preference to the vestibular labyrinth, for information about the position and the movement of the head in space. These structures are sensitive to tension in the joint capsule. Their afferents are connected to the spinal motoneurone pool, the brain-stem reticular system, the cerebellum, thalamus and parietal cortex. Lesions of the joints impose abnormal stress on the mechanoreceptors; and this is especially so in the presence of such common conditions in old age as reduction in height of the cervical intervertebral disc; or collapse or displacement of cervical vertebrae; and may be responsible for postural instability and unsteadiness of gait. Dizziness on head turning could, in Wyke's opinion, be caused by an imbalanced inflow of stimuli from deficient mechanoreceptors in the neck. This view of the relation between cervical spondylosis and balance disturbances is impressively documented. Its main value to the clinician at present is to direct his attention away from the over-medicated vestibular labyrinth. Unfortunately cervical spondylosis is an almost universal radiographic finding in the elderly; and immobilisation of the neck is an unpopular method of treatment.

FALLS AND GAIT

Many falls occur for no apparent reason while the subject is walking. This proved to be the largest single group encountered in a study of falls amongst old people at

Table 14.2 Activity at time of fall in 125 falls in persons aged 65 and over at home

	Number of Falls
Walking on the level	52
Turning while walking	5
Ascending or descending stairs	14
Into or out of bed	12
On or off chair	7
On or off toilet or commode	6
Dressing or washing	4
Standing at cooker or sink	7
Adventurous circumstances	3
Out of chair	5
Uncertain	10

home (Wild et al, 1980) (Table 14.2). Azar and Lawton (1964) attributed the higher incidence of falls in women than in men to differences in the stepping pattern of the female. Guimaraes and Isaacs (1980) compared the gait characteristics of old people who had been hospitalised after suffering a fall with other groups. They noted the slow speed and short step length of these subjects, together with the prolonged period of double support, wide range of frequency of stepping (Fig. 14.1) and high step-to-step variability (Table 14.3). These findings were interpreted as indicating that the gait had lost its automatic quality; and that each step was, as it were, individually constructed. Error in foot placement, if not adequately perceived, could place the walker in a position where the line of gravity fell outside the support base, so that an unavoidable fall would result. It is possible that some falls during walking (and this may include so-called 'drop attacks') are a consequence of errors in step production and are associated with focal or diffuse brain damage.

PROGNOSIS

Fractured neck of femur carries a high mortality (Evans et al, 1979b) but falls which do not result in fracture are also attended by high mortality. Wild and her colleagues (1980) found that one-quarter of people who fell in their own homes were dead within a year; this was four times as many as in an age-and sex-matched control group (Fig. 14.2). The excess mortality of fallers was not confined to the period immediately after the fall but continued throughout the ensuing year. Mortality was highest in those who had been housebound before falling; those who showed abnormal balance; and those who had suffered previous falls in which they lay for long periods on the floor. On the other hand the few subjects in this series who suffered fractures all survived for the full year. A possible explanation is that many who fall at home in late life are suffering from serious disease from which they are shortly likely to die. The fall may be no more than an indicator of forthcoming death; or else it may contribute to the probability of such an outcome.

Those who have fallen are liable to fall again, usually because the capacity to resist displacement remains permanently impaired. Two-thirds of old people who had fallen at home fell again in the ensuing year, many of these repeatedly. Recurrent falls were more likely in those with gait and balance abnormalities (Wild et al, 1980).

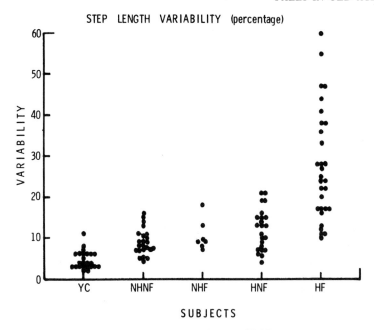

Fig. 14.1 Percentage Variability of Step-length in Five Groups of Subjects

FREQUENCY (steps/min)   FREQUENCY   SUBJECTS

160   140   120   100   80   60   40   20   0

YC   NHNF   NHF   HNF   HF

YC   : Young controls, mean age 28
NHNF : Non-hospitalised non-fallers, mean age 70
NHF : Non-hospitalised fallers, mean age 70
HNF : Hospitalised non-fallers, mean age 79
HF   : Hospitalised fallers, mean age 79.

Table 14.3 Parameters of gait in five groups of subjects.

	YC		NHNF		NHF		NHF		HF	
	Mean	SD	Mean	SD	Mean	SD	Mean	SD	Mean	SD
Step length (cm)	64·67	7·72	45·87	7·45	45·43	9·90	37·73	9·37	22·07	9·38
Stride width (cm)	11·38	4·46	13·70	3·35	16·86	3·18	13·55	4·30	14·30	4·50
Speed (m. s⁻¹)	72·21	9·84	42·62	13·06	44·00	11·80	34·39	12·26	21·27	9·75
Frequency (step/min)	111·96	10·18	94·30	14·16	96·50	11·64	89·91	19·07	94·63	39·51
Variability of step length (percentage)	4·63	2·14	8·98	3·2	10·5	3·80	12·20	5·36	27·60	13·61

YC   = Young controls, mean age 28
NHNF = Non-hospitalized non-fallers, mean age 70
NHF   = Non-hospitalized fallers, mean age 70
HNF   = Hospitalized non-fallers, mean age 79
HF   = Hospitalized fallers, mean age 79

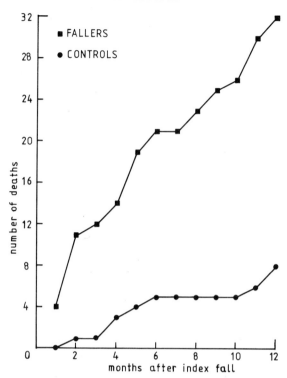

Fig. 14.2 Cumulative mortality in 125 fallers and 125 controls in 12 months after index fall. (*Reproduced by kind permission of the editor of the British Medical Journal*).

The experience of having fallen is sometimes followed by the development of a dread of further falls which limits the enjoyment of life. Fear of falling is expressed even before the subject rises from the chair, and is associated with an inveterate tendency to grab at any object in sight. This crippling disorder, which has been called the 'post-fall syndrome' (Murphy, 1982), may represent a pathological phobia (Marks and Bebbington, 1976) or it may be based on a disturbance or misinterpretation of sensory information.

SOCIAL ASPECTS

In Wild and Isaacs' (1980) study of old people who fell at home, three-quarters of the fallers lived alone or with a spouse only. Similar findings were reported by Sheldon (1960), Brocklehurst and his colleagues (1978) and Evans and his colleagues (1979a). Those living alone found methods of summoning help to be largely ineffectual. Whilst nearly half of the fallers lived in a house with a telephone, only one-third of those who lived alone or with a spouse had a telephone compared with two-thirds of those who lived with a son or daughter. Special alarms were provided in the homes of those who lived in sheltered housing; and a small number of privately housed old people had installed alarms. However very little use was made of these devices at the time of the fall. Either they proved inaccessible or the faller did not think of using them. Many alerting devices are appearing on the market (Hook and Lindberg, 1973), but more thought needs to be given as to how these are actually to be used in an emergency. In the United Kingdom, the Borough of Stockport has pioneered a scheme in which the homes of old people at risk are linked by short-wave radio to a central switchboard from which emergency calls can be transmitted to home-helps in radio-controlled cars. In the event of a fall the system can be activated from the floor, and help will arrive within minutes of the summons. The scheme is costly and elaborate but ingenious and effective, and has already been copied by several other Local Authorities. However the majority of fallers of the future will have to depend on personal contact with neighbours, and a less elaborate method of telephone and personal surveillance, if prolonged lies on the floor are to be avoided.

PREVENTION

Prevention of falls in old age has hitherto depended largely on propaganda to eliminate hazards in the home. This should now be supplemented by propaganda to eliminate hazards of medication, including the avoidance of inappropriate prescription of antihypertensive (Isaacs, 1979), sedative and 'antidizziness' drugs. Doctors should also be alerted to the value of treating heart rhythm disturbances and osteomalacia, thereby reducing two preventable causes of falls. Physiotherapists should provide guidance on the best exercise regimes for older people to maintain stability. Community nurses and health visitors, while remaining vigilant for the minimisation of environmental hazards in the home, should also direct attention to increasing the mobility and balance skills of their elderly patients.

CONCLUSION

The human body has developed an elaborate defence mechanism to enable it to maintain the upright posture safely through a wide range of activities, but the force of gravity is always present. The vulnerability of this mechanism in extreme old age offers to the elderly the choice of limiting activities or accepting instability. However, many of the factors which contribute to impaired correction of displacement are avoidable or correctable. The potential for maintaining and improving the efficiency of the correction mechanism has not yet been fully explored. Further research into the mechanism of falls may point to ways in which adaptive changes can be facilitated and falls avoided.

REFERENCES

Akhtar A J, Broe G A, Crombie A, McLean W M R, Andrews G R, Caird F I 1973 Disability and dependence in the elderly at home. Age and Ageing 2:102
Ashley M J, Gryfe C I, Amies A 1977 A longitudinal study of falls in an elderly population. II Some circumstances of falling. Age and Ageing 6:211–220
Azar G J, Lawton A H 1964 Gait and stepping as factors in the frequent falls of elderly women. Gerontologia 4:83–84
Baron J B, Bobot J, Bessineton J C 1956 Statokinésimètre Presse médicale 64:863
Basmajian J V 1961 Electromyography of postural muscles. In: Evans FG (ed) Biomechanical studies of the musculo-skeletal system. Thomas, Springfield, Ill., pp 136–160
Basmajian J C 1962 Muscles alive. Williams and Wilkins, Baltimore
Berfenstam R O, Lagerberg D, Smedby B 1969 Victim characteristics in fatal home accidents. Acta Sociomedica Scandinavica 1:145–164

Bonnet M, Gurfinkel S, Lipchits M-J, Popov K-E 1976 Central programming of lower limb muscular activity in the standing man. Aggressologie 17:35–42

Brizzee K R 1975 Aging changes in relation to diseases of the nervous system. In: Ordy J M, Brizzee K R (eds) Neurobiology of aging an interdisciplinary life-span approach. Plenum Press, New York, pp 545–574

Brocklehurst J C, Exton-Smith A N, Lempert Barber S M, Hunt L P, Palmer M K 1978 Fracture of the femur in old age: a two-centre study of associated clinical factors and the cause of the fall. Age and Ageing 7:7–15

Burke D, Eklund G 1977 Muscle spindle activity in man during standing. Acta physiologica Scandinavica 100:87–89

Campbell A J 1976 Femoral neck fractures in elderly women: a prospective study. Age and Ageing 5:102–109

Department of Prices and Consumer Protection 1978 The Home Accident Surveillance System: the first 12 months data. London, DPCP

Drachman D A, Hart C W 1972 An approach to the dizzy patient. Neurology 22:323–334

Droller H 1955 Falls among elderly people living at home. Geriatrics 10:239–244

Eccles J C 1977 Voluntary Movement In: Popper K R, Eccles J C (eds) The self and its brain: an argument for interactionism. Springer-Verlag International, London pp 275–294

Eddy T P 1972 Deaths from domestic falls and fractures. British Journal of Preventive and Social Medicine 26:173–179

Eddy T P 1973 Deaths from falls and fractures: Comparison of Mortality in Scotland and USA with that in England and Wales. British Journal of Preventive and Social Medicine 27:247–254

Ethelberg S 1950 Symptomatic 'cataplexy' or chalastic fits in cortical lesions of the frontal lobe. Brain 73:499–512

Evans J G 1979 Fractured proximal femur in Newcastle upon Tyne. Age and Ageing 8:16–24

Evans J G, Prudham D, Wandless I 1979a A prospective study of fractured proximal femur: factors predisposing to survival. Age and Ageing 8:246–250

Evans J G, Prudham D, Wandless I 1979b A prospective study of fractured proximal femur. Public Health 93:235–241

Fine W 1959 An Analysis of 277 Falls in Hospital. Gerontologia clinica 1:292–300

Gallanaugh S C, Martin A, Millard P H 1976 Regional survey of femoral neck fractures. British Medical Journal 2:1496–1497

Glassman A H, Bigger J T, Giardina E V, Kantor S J, Perel J M, Davies M 1979 Clinical characteristics of imipramine-induced orthostatic hypotension. Lancet 1:468–472

Gordon M 1978 Occult cardiac arhythmias associated with falls and dizziness in the elderly: detection by Holter monitoring. Journal of the American Geriatric Society 26:418–423

Granit R 1972 Constant errors in the execution and appreciation of movement. Brain 95:649–660

Gray B 1966 Home accidents among older people: report of a research carried out in the Birmingham area. Royal Society for the Prevention of Accidents, London

Greenwood R J, Hopkins A P 1976a Muscle responses during sudden falls in man. Journal of Physiology 245:507–518

Greenwood R, Hopkins A 1976b Landing from an unexpected fall and a voluntary step. Brain 99:375–386

Greenwood R, Hopkins A 1977 Monosynaptic reflexes in falling man. Journal of Neurology, Neurosurgery and Psychiatry 40:448–454

Gryfe C I, Amies A, Ashley M J 1977 A longitudinal study of falls in an elderly population. I. Incidence and morbidity. Age and Ageing 6:201–210

Guimaraes R M Isaacs B 1980 Studies of gait and balance in normal old people and in people who have fallen. Characteristics of the gait of old people who fall. International Rehabilitation Medicine 2:177–180

Hasselkus E R 1974 Aging and the human nervous system. American Journal of Occupational Therapy 28:16–24

Hasselkus B R, Shambes G M 1975 Aging and postural sway in women. Journal of Gerontology 30:661–667

Hawton K, Leopoldt H 1978 Accidents in a psychiatric hospital. British Journal of Psychiatry 133:224–227

Hellebrandt F A 1938 Standing as a geotropic reflex: the mechanism of the asynchronous rotation of motor correction. American Journal of Physiology 121:471–474

Hellebrandt F A, Braun G L 1939 The influence of sex and age on the postural sway of man. American Journal of Physical Anthropology 24:347–360

Höök O, Lindberg B 1973 Alarm telephone for handicapped and elderly living alone. Scandinavian Journal of Rehabilitative Medicine 5:18–22

Isaacs B 1976 The Giants of Geriatrics: a study of symptoms in old age. Inaugural lecture, University of Birmingham.

Isaacs B 1978 Are falls a manifestation of brain failure? Age and Ageing 7: (Suppl) 97–105

Isaacs B 1979 Should we treat hypertension in the elderly? Age and Ageing 8: 115–120

Iskrant A P 1968 The etiology of fractured hips in females. American Journal of Public Health 58: 485–490

Kalchthaler T, Bascon R A, Quintos V 1978 Falls in the instituionalised elderly. Journal of the American Geriatric Society 26: 424–428

Kameyama M 1965 Vertigo and drop attacks: with special reference to cerebrovascular disorders and atherosclerosis of the vertebral-basilar system. Geriatrics 20: 892–900

Knowelden J, Buhr A J, Dunbar O 1964 Incidence of fractures in persons over 35 years of age. British Journal of Preventive and Social Medicine 18: 130–141

Kremer M 1958 Sitting, standing and walking. British Medical Journal 2: 63–68; 121–126

Kubala M J, Millikan C H 1964 Diagnosis, pathogenesis and treatment of 'drop attacks'. Archives of Neurology 11: 107–113

Leitch I H, Knowelden J, Seddon H J 1964 Incidence of fractures, particularly of the neck of the femur, in patients in mental hospitals. British Journal of Preventive and Social Medicine 18: 142–145

Livesley B, Atkinson L 1974 Repeated falls in the elderly. Modern geriatrics 4: 458–467

Lucht U 1971 A prospective study of accidental falls and resulting injuries in the home among elderly people. Acta socio-medica Scandinavica 2: 105–120

Lund M 1963 Drop-attacks in association with Parkinsonism and basilar artery sclerosis. Acta Neurol, Scandinavica 39: (Suppl 4) 226–229

MacDonald J B, MacDonald E T 1977 Nocturnal femoral fracture and continuing widespread use of barbiturate hypnotics. British Medical Journal 2: 483–485

Marks I, Bebbington P 1976 Space phobia: syndrome or agaraphobic variant? British medical Journal 2: 345–347

Melvill Jones G, Watt D G D 1971 Muscular control of landing from unexpected falls in man. Journal of Physiology 219: 729–737

Morris E V, Isaacs B 1980 The prevention of falls in a geriatric hospital. Age and Ageing 9: 181–185

Murphy J 1980 The post-fall syndrome: a clinical study. In preparation

Murphy J, Obonyo T, Nayak U S L, Isaacs B 1980 The sternal pressure test of balance. In preparation

Murray M P, Seireg A, Scholz R C 1967 Center of gravity, center of pressure and supportive forces during human activities. Journal of Applied Physiology 23: 831–838

Murray M P, Seireg A, Sepic S 1975 Normal postural stability and steadiness: quantitative assessment. Journal of Bone and Joint Surgery 57A: 510–516

Murray M P, Brewer B J, Gore D R, Zuege R C 1975 Kinesiology after McKee-Fannon total hip replacement: a two-year follow-up of one-hundred cases. Journal of Bone and Joint Surgery 57A: 337–342

Naylor M B, Rosin A S 1970 Falling as a cause of admission to a geriatric unit. Practitioner 205: 327–330

O'Leary J P 1970 A strain-gauge platform for studying human movement. Perceptual and Motor Skills 30: 698

Over R 1966 Possible visual factors in falls by the old people. Gerontologist 6: 212–214

Overstall P W, Exton Smith A N, Imms F J, Johnson A L 1977 Falls in the elderly related to postural imbalance. British Medical Journal 1: 261–264

Parrish H M, Weil T P 1978 Patient accidents occurring in hospitals: epidemiologic study of 614 accidents. New York State Journal of Medicine 58: 838–846

Registrar-General for England and Wales, Annual Report, 1978. HMSO, London

Roberts J L, Fonzeka C P de 1972 Investigating Accidents in the Home. Bristol Medico-Chirurgical Journal 87: 37–51

Roberts J L, Payne V, Northover D, Simmons L, de Fonseka C P 1974 Home accidents and health education. Health Education Journal 33: 35–45; 67–78

Scott C J 1976 Accidents in hospital with special references to old people. Health Bulletin 18: 330–335

Seiler H, Ramsay C B 1954 Home Accidents. Practitioner 172: 628–631

Sheehan S, Bauer R B, Meyer J S 1960 Vertebral artery compression in cervical spondylosis: arteriographic demonstration during life of vertebral artery insufficiency due to rotation and extension of neck. Neurology 10: 968–986

Sheldon J H 1948 The social incidence of old age: report of an enquiry in Wolverhampton. Oxford University Press, London

Sheldon J H 1960 On the natural history of falls in old age. British Medical Journal 2: 1685–1688

Sheldon J H 1963 The effect of age on the control of sway. Gerontologia clinica 5: 129–138

Silver J R, Buxton P H 1974 Spinal stroke. Brain 97: 539–550

Snijders C J, Verduin M 1973 Stabilograph: an accurate instrument for sciences interested in postural equilibrium. Aggressologie 14 : 15–20

Stevens D L, Matthews W B 1973 Cryptogenic drop attacks: an affliction of women. British Medical Journal 1 : 439–442

Terekhov Y V 1978 Instrumentation for automatic measurement and real-time evaluation of man's postural equilibrium. Journal of Medical Engineering Technology 2 : 182–186

Tinker G M 1979 Accidents in a geriatric hospital. Age and Ageing 8 : 196–198

Tobis J S, Nayak L, Hoehler F 1981 Visual perception of verticality and horizontality among elderly fallers. Archives of physical medicine and rehabilitation 62 : 619–622

Tumarkin A 1936 The otolithic catastrophe: a new syndrome. British Medical Journal 2 : 175–177

Waller J A 1974 Injury in aged: clinical and epidemiological implications. New York State Journal of Medicine 74 : 2200–2208

Wild D, Isaacs B, Nayak U S L 1980 How dangerous are falls in old people at home? British medical Journal 282 : 266–268

Williams D, Wilson T G (1962) The diagnosis of the major and minor syndromes of basilar insufficiency. Brain 85 : 741–774

Wit G de 1973 The stabilometry as an auxiliary in investigations of patients with vestibular disturbances. Aggressologie 14 : 27–31

Wright B M 1971 A simple mechanical ataxiameter. Journal of Physiology 218 : 27–28P

Wyke B 1975 Structural and functional characteristics of receptor systems. Proceedings of 10th International Congress of Anatomy, Tokyo

Wyke B 1979 Cervical articular contributions to posture and gait: their relation to senile disequilibrium. Age and Ageing 8 : 251–258

15   *J. A. Obeso, M. M. Traub and C. D. Marsden*

Ataxia in the elderly

INTRODUCTION

Ataxia literally means 'lack of muscular coordination', but common usage has restricted application of the term to an 'unsteadiness of action'. Movement of the eyes or arms may be ataxic, but in keeping with the theme of this volume we will restrict discussion to a consideration of ataxia of gait.

When man stands, walks or runs the narrowness of his base would render him unstable were it not for equilibratory reactions which maintain him upright. We will concentrate on the imbalance caused by the breakdown of such mechanisms.

Imbalance causes falling, a common and distressing problem in old age. Isaacs (Ch. 14) deals with the problem of falls in the elderly, and it is inevitable that our own contribution will, to some extent, complement his discussion. But imbalance and falling are not synonymous. Ataxia or imbalance is a common cause of falls but, as Isaacs points out, there are many other reasons why the elderly collapse; for example, postural hypotension or cardiac dysrhythmias, and syncope due to cough, micturition or defaecation. We will not dwell on the many alternative causes of falling, but will confine our discussion to the problem of imbalance.

Both unsteadiness and falling are distressing, frightening and disabling. To no longer be able to trust one's stance leads to a loss of self-confidence, which in itself adds to the disability caused by the problem. Indeed, a number of psychological syndromes such as agoraphobia and space-phobia, commonly are grafted onto imbalance. The psychological and sociological impact of imbalance in the elderly are important but will not be covered in this chapter. Nor will we deal with the treatment and rehabilitation of elderly patients with disorders of balance, for this is the subject of Overstall's presentation (Ch. 18).

We will confine our task to a consideration of the mechanisms and differential diagnosis of imbalance, or ataxia of gait, with specific reference to the elderly patient.

DIFFERENTIAL DIAGNOSIS OF ATAXIA

By convention, the term ataxia is used to describe imbalance or unsteadiness due to cerebellar disease (cerebellar ataxia) or sensory loss (sensory ataxia).

All of the conditions shown in Table 15.1 may cause unsteadiness of gait and a tendency to fall.

Table 15.1 Main causes of imbalance

Weak legs	Especially in the elderly
Myopathy	Osteomalacia
Myasthenia gravis	Senile
Peripheral neuropathy	Diabetes
	Para-neoplastic
	Cyanocobalamin (B12) deficiency
Paraplegia	Cervical spondylosis
Hemiplegia	Stroke
Parkinsonism	
Akinetic-rigid syndrome	See Table 15.2
Sensory Ataxia	
Peripheral neuropathy	
Myelopathy	
Cerebellar Ataxia	See Table 15.3
Frontal Lobe Apraxia	Alzheimer's disease
	Cerebrovascular disease
	Hydrocephalus

Muscle weakness, especially if severe and proximal, occasionally confuses. A clumsy, unsteady gait may be the presenting complaint of the occasional patient with primary muscle disease, myasthenia gravis, peripheral neuropathy (especially Guillain-Barré's subacute polyneuropathy which tends to preferentially affect proximal limb muscles) and motor neurone disease.

Patients with a spastic paraplegia resulting from spinal cord damage also walk clumsily and unsteadily, but the spastic gait is unmistakable.

Certain abnormal involuntary movements may distort the gait. The sudden, unpredictable muscle jerks of chorea produce a typical lurching and staggering. Myoclonic jerks similarly may distort gait, particularly that form of myoclonus known as post-anoxic myoclonus, in which muscle jerking occurs on action. The prolonged muscle spasms of torsion dystonia likewise may cause bizarre gait disturbances and unsteadiness.

Postural abnormalities, alterations in gait and imbalance are typical of Parkinson's disease, and other rarer basal ganglia disorders causing an akinetic rigid syndrome.

Stroke usually causes the distinctive hemiplegia, but occasionally leads to disability in both legs when anterior cerebral arterial territories are involved. Bilateral damage to both frontal lobes, whatever the cause, causes a peculiar disturbance of walking, variously known as gait apraxia or frontal lobe ataxia. Typical conditions that may produce such a disturbance are diffuse brain diseases (for example, multi-infarct dementia or Alzheimer's disease), hydrocephalus of whatever cause (including normal pressure hydrocephalus) and frontal lobe mass lesions (for example, meningioma or even subdural haematoma).

The gait may be unsteady in all the conditions mentioned so far, but, by convention, it is not described as ataxic (with the possible exception of the gait disturbance otherwise known as apraxia). It can be difficult on occasion to distinguish the gait disturbance of a patient with an akinetic-rigid syndrome, or frontal lobe disease from that of someone with cerebellar damage, although other clinical signs usually decide the matter. Sensory ataxia is diagnosed on the basis of associated physical findings of dense posterior column sensory loss (of appreciation of vibration and joint position sense).

These introductory comments highlight the range of conditions that may produce unsteadiness of gait and imbalance, and the somewhat arbitrary conventional use of the word ataxia. For the purposes of the present article we intend to consider the range of conditions that may produce unsteadiness, with particular reference to the elderly.

UNSTEADINESS IN THE ELDERLY

Of the conditions listed in Table 15.1, some are of particular relevance in old age. Primary muscle disease and florid peripheral neuropathy are uncommon at that time of life, but a spastic ataxia due to spinal cord damage, resulting from degenerative changes in the cervical spine, is commonplace. Likewise, while restricted cerebellar degenerations rarely are present in the elderly, Parkinsonian syndromes are very common. So, too, are the gait disturbances characteristic of diffuse cerebral disease, for degenerations such as those attributable to Alzheimer's pathological change occur all too frequently. We will deal with each of these groups of causes in turn, but before doing so it is necessary to consider two other facets of the problem which are peculiar to the senium. Firstly we will discuss those changes in gait and balance that are considered to form a part of normal ageing. Secondly, we must discuss that peculiar problem of the elderly in whom slight, but multiple, deficits can add up to produce disability disproportionate to their individual contributions. We are talking here of that characteristic imbalance which may be caused by multiple sensory deficits and other slight disabilities in the elderly.

NORMAL AGEING AND GAIT

The degenerative changes that take place in the ageing nervous system often make the criteria of normality in younger patients inapplicable to the senium. This is so obvious with regard to man's higher functions that we take some loss of recent memory, for example, as a normal feature of ageing. Equally, certain physical signs have quite different connotations in the old compared to the young. For example, Prakash and Stern (1974) who examined 100 geriatric patients without a history of neurological disease found that 38 had absent ankle jerks and 31 lacked vibration sense at the ankles. These clinical changes have their electrophysiological correlates in the age-related changes in peripheral and central conduction velocity (e.g. Dorfman and Bosely, 1979).

A certain deterioration in posture and steadiness of gait occurs so commonly in the senium that it can be regarded as almost a normal attribute of ageing. Characteristically (Fig. 15.1) the attitude is flexed, steps are shortened (à petit pas) and more uncertain, whilst there is a generalised poverty and slowness of movements. Such changes are reminiscent of extrapyramidal disorders but differ from Parkinson's disease in the lesser severity of the signs and the absence of tremor at rest (Parkes et al, 1974). The pathological basis for age-related changes in posture and movements has not been established (Critchley, 1956), mainly because the widespread neuronal degeneration makes uncertain any clinico-pathological correlation. However, loss of striatal and substantia nigra neurons and a decline in

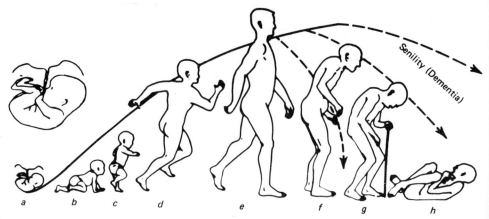

a   b   c   d   e   f   g   h

Fig. 15.1 Yakovlev's concept of the evolution of erect stance and gait, and its dissolution with ageing.

dopamine synthesis has recently been considered a major cause of the extra-pyramidal features in the elderly (McGeer et al, 1977).

MULTIPLE SENSORY DEFICIT

As underlined by Purdon Martin (1967), man normally relies on the integration of proprioceptive, labyrinthine and visual information for the maintenance of balance, but in most circumstances there is adequate compensation for the loss of any one of these modalities. In the elderly there is commonly some degree of disturbance in each of these systems. Typical are decreased visual acuity due to cataracts or retinal degeneration, and loss of proprioceptive sense secondary to changes in the peripheral nerves or to myelopathy causing interference with normal postural adjustments and preventing compensation for loss of sensory cues. For instance, a normal person can shut his eyes or walk easily into a darkening room, but many elderly people with subtle sensory deficit may not be able to walk steadily in the dark. In fact, multiple sensory deficit was found to be the third major cause of unsteadiness in a study of 125 patients (Drachman and Hart, 1972). The main abnormalities reported in these patients were peripheral neuropathy (85 per cent), cervical spondylosis (71 per cent), vestibular abnormalities shown as inadequate labyrinthic response (64 per cent) and visual loss secondary to cataracts (35 per cent). All subjects presented a combination of the above causes and most of them were said to be old and diabetic.

Vestibular damage, which is dealt with in detail elsewhere (Ch. 13), may play a much more important role in causing imbalance in the elderly than it does in the young. Loss of vestibular function in youth leads to dramatic vertigo and imbalance initially, but recovery occurs within weeks. Compensatory mechanisms are soon brought into action so that the patient with bilateral vestibular loss rapidly regains normal balance, except when blindfold and walking on uneven ground. Such compensation, however, is fragile and may break down if there is subsequent additional damage to any of the mechanisms responsible. Of course, this is just what happens in the elderly, in whom failure to compensate for vestibular deficit is common.

The problems of multiple sensory deficits in the elderly are compounded by other difficulties in old age. Joint disease in the young does not cause imbalance, for compensation is rapid and adequate. But in the old, a pattern of gait distorted by joint disease may provoke unsteadiness, because the elderly cannot compensate adequately for misalignment of joints, muscles and tendons, with consequent alterations of force vectors. Failure to compensate for joint disease in the elderly may be due to subclinical peripheral neuropathy, cord damage or vestibular abnormality, or even to damage to joint and capsular sensory receptors.

In summary, imbalance in the elderly commonly is multifactorial. Unsteadiness always represents a breakdown of compensation, and the mechanisms responsible for such compensation often are impaired in the elderly.

CERVICAL MYELOPATHY

In middle-age and later life there are often degenerative changes in the cervical spine, causing damage to the spinal cord. There are many mechanisms responsible for such spondylitic cervical myelopathy, including pressure by disc protrusions, osteophytes or infolding of the ligamentum flavum, as well as secondary vascular damage.

In a study of patients over the age of 50 who had no neurological complaints, Pallis, Jones and Spillane (1954) showed that some 75 per cent had radiological evidence of cervical spine canal narrowing. Impairment of vibration sense and pyramidal signs were found in nearly a half of their sample and were attributed to cervical myelopathy, since such 'cord signs' never occurred in the absence of radiological changes.

Although, as in the patients of Pallis and his colleagues, cervical myelopathy often causes little functional impairment, it is one of the most important causes of unsteadiness in the elderly. The predominant symptoms are usually those of a spastic paraplegia, in which hypertonia may be disproportionately severe in comparison to weakness and may be most obvious on walking (Clarke and Robinson, 1956). Interference with the spinocerebellar pathways may contribute to the unsteadiness, as may loss of position sense, but the incidence of the latter is debated. Spillane and Lloyd (1952) suggested that loss of proprioception is rare in cervical spondylosis, whilst Yuhl and his colleagues (1955) found loss of joint position sense in a quarter of their sample of patients with cervical myelopathy.

When there is cervical pain and limitation of neck movements, together with signs of root lesions in the upper limb (appropriate sensory loss, lower motoneurone weakness or reflex changes such as an inverted supinator jerk), diagnosis usually is simple. In the absence of such clinical data, cervical myelopathy may have to be differentiated from other causes of cord pathology such as compression by tumour or subacute combined degeneration of the cord. In cases in which the patient's decline is rapid or there is sphincter involvement, the matter may have to be resolved by myelography, a procedure which is only performed when surgery is contemplated. Usually a conservative approach is advocated, especially in the elderly, in view of the relatively benign prognosis in this condition (Lees and Turner, 1963).

SENSORY ATAXIA

Although minor sensory changes such as loss or decrement of vibration sense, absent ankle jerks and reduced nerve and spinal conduction velocity are commonplace in old age (Prakash and Stern, 1974) impairment of position sense is rarely by itself the cause of ataxia. Tabes dorsalis now is a rarity. Florid peripheral neuropathies are not common in old age, but, as already pointed out, subclinical peripheral neuropathy, mainly diabetic, may be an important conditioning factor in the elderly with multisensory deficit.

Pernicious anaemia usually can be diagnosed on the basis of associated clinical signs and the specific laboratory tests, provided it is remembered. The typical paraesthesiae that preface the illness may not be conspicuous in the elderly, and the combination of absent ankle jerks, loss of appreciation of vibration and joint position, with extensor plantar response, often is attributed to age, diabetes and cervical spondylosis. Haematological abnormality need not be present in patients with the neurological consequences of deficiency of vitamin B_{12}, which always should be measured in those with the typical neurological findings. The status of neurological deficit due to folic acid deficiency is not yet certain.

PARKINSONISM

Idiopathic Parkinson's disease is one of the most common neurological disorders in the elderly occurring in about 1 in 200 of the population over the age of 50. Postural instability is a feature of this illness, although it often occurs late in the course of the disease. The introduction of levodopa therapy has done much to alleviate the condition, but it may be harmful in similar disorders because of its side-effects, thus underlining the importance of a correct diagnosis.

Tremor is present in about two-thirds of patients with Parkinson's disease. Typically this tremor is a 4 Hz 'pill-rolling' movement present at rest. It is often more prominent in the upper limbs, but the legs and even the entire body can also be affected.

Benign essential tremor must be distinguished from Parkinson's disease (Marsden, 1980). This illness, frequently inherited as an autosomal dominant trait, is characterised by a tremor present when the limb is moved or a posture is maintained. Rigidity, akinesia and postural abnormalities are never present. Levodopa is not the correct treatment for this condition.

The rigidity of Parkinson's disease is classically described as plastic, in which resistance to passive movement is equal in both flexors and extensors and throughout the range of movement. The cogwheel phenomenon is a special sign of extrapyramidal hypertonia in which resistance to passive stretch is rhythmically interrupted at a rate of about 8 Hz. Rigidity must be distinguished from spasticity and *Gegenhalten*. Spastic hypertonia is most obvious in the flexors of the arms and in the extensors of the legs; the resistance to passive movement increases initially, then collapses, and spasticity is always associated with other pyramidal signs. *Gegenhalten*, or paratonia, is an increase of tone in both extension and flexion, but the resistance is much reduced when the limb is displaced slowly and, paradoxically, it is increased when the subject is actively asked to relax. Paratonia is characteristic of frontal lobe disease but is also commonly seen in widespread cerebral disorders (Plum and Posner, 1980).

Akinesia refers to a defect in the initiation and execution of a movement. It is clearly shown by the emotionless expression of the face or the lack of associated movements when walking. Akinesia is not a consequence of weakness or rigidity for much strength is normal in Parkinson's disease once a movement is initiated and rigidity can be entirely abolished by stereotatic surgery without modifying the speed of movement (Cooper, 1969).

As well as adopting a characteristic flexed attitude, patients suffering moderate or severe Parkinsonism suffer from postural instability. Purdon Martin (1967) found that patients with post-encephalitic Parkinsonism failed to exhibit normal equilibrating or protective reactions following a sudden tilt, and would often topple over. Such gross ataxia usually is a late feature of idiopathic Parkinson's disease, but often occurs earlier in other akinetic rigid syndromes that are discussed below.

OTHER AKINETIC-RIGID SYNDROMES

Akinesia and rigidity with postural abnormality are the most important features of many neurological illnesses other than Parkinson's disease. Among all the causes of an akinetic-rigid syndrome listed in Table 15.2 cerebrovascular disease probably is the most important differential diagnosis in the elderly. In this condition symptoms and signs sometimes are a consequence of cerebral infarctions in different vascular territories, secondary to atherosclerotic emboli from extracranial arteries or the heart, often with dementia, the so-called multi-infarct dementia described by Hachinski, Lassen and Marshall (1974).

Table 15.2 Differential diagnosis of Parkinsonism

Parkinson's disease (Idiopathic paralysis agitans)
Post-encephalitic Parkinsonism
Drug-induced Parkinsonism
Progressive supranuclear palsy
Multiple system atrophy (includes Shy-Drager syndrome, olivopontocerebellar disease and strionigral degeneration)
Parkinsonism in dementia — Alzheimer's disease
                             Cerebrovascular disease

In other patients, particularly those with hypertension, multiple small lacunar strokes cause a disabling akinetic-rigid syndrome, often with profound ataxia and speech disturbance due to a pseudobulbar palsy. In the akinetic-rigid syndrome of cerebrovascular disease, in contrast to Parkinson's disease, tremor is almost never present, pyramidal or other localised signs of cerebral lesions can be recognised and dementia is a major sign (Parkes et al, 1974). The EEG is normal in most patients with Parkinson's disease, while an excess of slow focal activity is frequently found in multi-infarct dementia. At present, CT scan provides the most reliable method to confirm the diagnosis of multi-infarct Parkinsonism.

Cerebrovasular disease is, of course, much less frequent as a cause of dementia than Alzheimer's disease, the pathology of which is responsible for the majority of those with senile dementia. Patients with Alzheimer's disease often develop obvious signs of basal ganglia damage, and exhibit akinesia, rigidity and instability (Pearce, 1974), but inevitably also are demented by the time such signs appear.

A word on dementia in Parkinson's disease is appropriate. Undoubtedly a proportion of those who start with symptoms quite typical of idiopathic Parkinson's disease eventually dement. In view of the age incidence of idiopathic Parkinson's disease, it is not surprising to find that the commonest cause of dementia in Parkinson's disease is the pathology characteristic of Alzheimer's disease (Boller et al, 1980). However, other treatable causes of dementia should be excluded whenever a patient with Parkinson's disease begins to dement. Conspicuous dementia early in the course of the illness should prompt a review of the diagnosis.

Most of the other causes of an akinetic-rigid syndrome can be suspected and correctly diagnosed on the basis of the history and accompanying neurological signs. Drug-induced Parkinsonism should be specifically considered before establishing the diagnosis of Parkinson's disease. Careful enquiry must be made about the possible intake of drugs such as phenothiazines and butyrophenones which, through blocking dopaminergic receptors, produce a typical Parkinsonian syndrome in about 20 to 40 per cent of patients (Marsden and Jenner, 1980). The incidence of drug-induced pseudo-Parkinsonism is known to increase with age (Ayd, 1961), in parallel with the incidence of idiopathic Parkinson's disease, and it may take as long as eighteen months after drug withdrawal for complete recovery to take place.

There also are a group of uncommon conditions which mimic Parkinson's disease fairly accurately, but which differ in their pathology in that they lack the characteristic Lewy body degeneration of pigmented brain-stem nuclei, and which are distinguished by other characteristic clinical features.

Progressive supranuclear palsy, viz. Steele-Richardson–Olzewski disease (Steele, 1972) presents as Parkinsonism, particularly in the form of axial rigidity with imbalance but without tremor, plus a distinctive paralysis of gaze. Voluntary and following vertical gaze is lost early, particularly up-gaze, but reflect eye movements and head posturing (doll's head manoeuvre) are preserved; subsequently lateral gaze also is lost. Of course, patients with Parkinson's disease also may lose up-gaze, so progressive supranuclear palsy can only be diagnosed when down-gaze and/or lateral gaze is lost.

Also there are a group of conditions now collectively referred to as the multiple system atrophies (Bannister and Oppenheimer, 1972), because individual patients frequently have an admixture of the pathology of each entity. Some individuals with multiple system atrophy innitially present with idiopathic orthostatic hypotension, and subsequently go on to develop a florid autonomic neuropathy with severe sphincter impairment and Parkinsonism (Shy and Drager, 1960). Others begin with a cerebellar syndrome (olivopontocerebellar degeneration) or pure Parkinsonism (strionigral degeneration), and may go on to develop the features of the other illnesses.

These various conditions that may mimic Parkinson's disease can be difficult to diagnose, particularly as postural hypotension, but not other features of autonomic neuropathy, may occur with Lewy bodies. However, failure to respond to levodopa may give the clue, and should always prompt a review of the diagnosis of simple Parkinson's disease.

CEREBELLAR ATAXIA

As described by Gordon Holmes (1922) a complete cerebellar syndrome includes gait and limb ataxia, hypotonia, disturbance of eye movement and slurred speech. While the diagnosis of a cerebellar lesion generally is clear, a few conditions can escape recognition unless they are specifically looked for. Truncal ataxia, in particular, may be the sole clinical feature of certain disorders affecting the midline of the cerebellum and will be missed if the patient is not got out of bed or chair to examine walking and balance.

An ataxia of gait, indistinguishable from that produced by cerebellar disease, can also be present in cerebral pathology not affecting directly the cerebellum, presumably by damaging the cortico-cerebellar pathway (Meyer and Barron, 1960). Focal frontal lobe lesions and occult hydrocephalus are particularly important in this regard.

Most of the causes of the cerebellar syndrome listed in Table 15.3 are not restricted to the senium. Some, however, are important in the elderly because the special effect of age on the incidence of these diseases.

Transient ischaemic attacks (neurological deficit lasting less than 24 hours) in the vertebrobasilar territory are a common cause of intermittent ataxia. Other clinical manifestations are variable, but dizziness, dysarthria, diplopia, blurred vision, and motor and sensory deficit of all four limbs are the most common. Every effort to detect a treatable cause should be made. Heart function, blood pressure, haemoglobin, erythrocyte sedimentation rate, blood glucose and lipids are particularly important.

Cerebellar signs are usually combined with brainstem signs in a completed stroke in the distribution of the basilar artery. Necropsy findings, however, have shown that cerebellar infarction is not associated with a brainstem stroke in about 50 to 65 per cent of the cases (Sypert and Alvord, 1975; Scotti et al, 1980). The introduction of the CT scan has allowed the separation of two different types of clinical evolution (Scotti et al, 1980). Progressive deterioration of consciousness or coma of sudden onset characterise the first group, while a typical cerebellar syndrome with ataxia (limb and trunk) and variable involvement of cranial nerves

Table 15.3 Differential diagnosis of cerebellar ataxia

Stroke	Transient ischaemic attacks
	Complete stroke
Tumour	Metastases
	Primary, e.g. vestibulocochlear schwannoma
	(acoustic neuroma)
Cerebella ectopia	
Metabolic	Myxoedema
	Alcohol
	Para-neoplastic
	Drugs, e.g. barbiturates
Cerebellar degeneration	Sporadic
	Hereditary

(mainly the vestibulocochlear) in patients with normal consciousness make up the second group. Cerebellar haemorrhages comprise 10 per cent of all intracranial haemorrhage. Although there is a higher incidence of headache in haemorrhages than in infarcts, the clinical distinction of both conditions at times may be impossible, but CT scan provides a most reliable diagnostic method.

A progressive history of cerebellar ataxia in the elderly should prompt the clinician to rule out a tumour by applying the appropriate tests. Unfortunately, metastases are common at this age, and it is rare to find a benign tumour such as a vestibulocochlear schwannoma ('acoustic neuroma') or other cerebello-pontine angle lesion. CT scan is the best non-invasive diagnostic technique, although false negative results occur with posterior fossa tumours. Neuro-radiological advances also have highlighted the frequency of cerebellar ectopia as a cause of ataxia and, in some cases, other symptoms of brainstem compression, syringomyelia and cough headache. However, the frequency of this condition in the elderly is unknown. A high proportion of patients with a progressive cerebellar syndrome have only cerebellar atrophy. Alcoholism, hypothyroidism and chronic intake of drugs such as phenytoin should be suspected for early diagnosis may lead to effective treatment. Cerebellar degeneration due to a remote neoplasm is another rare disease causing a progressive, chronic, or subacute, cerebellar syndrome. In about half of the cases the cerebellar signs are found before those of the associated neoplasm, which in most of the reported cases has been a lung carcinoma.

No cause for a progressive cerebellar syndrome due to atrophy with onset in middle or late life can be established in many cases. Such patients with cortical cerebellar atrophy of late onset have greater atrophy of the vermis than the hemispheres, with almost complete loss of Purkinje cells and in many cases degeneration of the inferior olives (Greenfield, 1975). The disease is familial in about a half of the cases reported.

APRAXIA OF GAIT

It has been known since the end of the 19th century that frontal lesions can lead to disorders of gait and balance (for review see Meyer and Barron, 1960; Denny Brown, 1958). In a number of cases where there is a large space occupying lesion of the frontal lobe, there is a true ataxia, caused by the compression of the cerebellum or its connections (Frazier, 1936), but localised damage may cause another characteristic disturbance, apraxia of gait. Gait apraxia caused by cerebral lesions is defined by Meyer and Barron (1960) as the loss of ability to properly use the lower limbs in the act of walking which cannot be accounted for by demonstrable sensory impairment or motor weakness. Although the patient's stance is broad-based and his gait is unsteady as in cerebellar disease, the leg movements are slow and hesitant similar to those seen in Parkinsonian syndromes. In addition, there are associated signs pointing to frontal lobe pathology such as grasp reflexes of the hands or feet, Gegenhalten and difficulties with imitative movements of the legs such as kicking an imaginary football. When the patient is examined on the couch, leg movements are often surprisingly normal, a finding which has led Denny Brown (1958) to suggest that some of the difficulty in walking is secondary to 'magnetic response' provoked by contact of the foot to the ground.

Such apraxia of gait may be responsible for the walking difficulties of a number of old people although there has been no formal study to confirm this. For instance, many elderly subjects appear relatively normal when examined in the recumbent posture, but when the patient attempts to walk he usually seeks support and then after some delay may take a few shuffling steps before stopping again or collapsing to the ground (Critchley, 1949). Such abnormalities may be ascribed to functional causes such as loss of confidence, both by the doctor and the patient, but are probably secondary to cerebral degenerative changes.

NORMAL PRESSURE AND OTHER HYDROCEPHALUS

The symptoms of hydrocephalus, as may occur with obstruction to CSF flow from any cause, have been known for many years, and a disturbance of gait is an integral part of that syndrome. In 1965 Hakim and Adams drew attention to the existence of this syndrome in the presence of normal CSF pressure, yet with an excellent response to ventricular shunting.

The typical triad is early disturbance of gait, loss of sphincter control and cognitive impairment leading to dementia. The abnormality of gait has never clearly been defined as ataxia or apraxia; indeed, it has features of both.

Such a clinical picture may be due to hydrocephalus caused by aqueduct stenosis, an intraventricular tumour, or by obstruction to CSF flow, either at the tentorial notch or over the hemispheres leading up to the arachnoid villi adjacent to the saggital venous sinus. Such communicating hydrocephalus may be caused by basal meningitis, sub-arachnoid haemorrhage due to a berry aneurysm, arterio-venous malformation or trauma, or may appear without evident cause.

The response to CSF shunting can be dramatic, but there are great difficulties in selecting those suitable for surgery. The main problem is to distinguish communicating hydrocephalus from cerebral atrophy. Both produce dilated ventricles evident on CT scan, in the former case due to extraventricular obstruction to CSF flow, in the latter to cerebral atrophy. However, dilated superficial cortical sulci may not be obvious in some patients with cerebral atrophy. In addition, many cases of communicating hydrocephalus may arrest, to produce equivocal radiological and CSF hydrodynamic changes. Such patients usually do not benefit from surgery. Frequently it is necessary to return to the clinical history to decide. Diseases causing cerebral atrophy produce dementia early; usually the gait disturbance and incontinence appear later in the illness. In hydrocephalus, an abnormality of gait and sphincter disturbance occur early in the illness, and dementia may be delayed.

Most investigations and treatment of established hydrocephalus have been undertaken in patients who are not elderly. The incidence of this condition in the elderly, and the practicality of surgical treatment, has not been established.

CONCLUSION

A number of factors conspire to make it difficult to diagnose the cause of ataxia of gait in the elderly. An adequate history may not be readily available and the patient's cooperation may be limited, especially when other incapacitating diseases such as hip or knee fractures or arthritis, are present. Such obstacles are typical of geriatric medicine as a whole and not specific to neurological diagnosis. There are, however, the added complications of ageing of the nervous system, in which the limit of normal involution and disease is not easy to establish. Such age-related changes tend to impair the mechanisms that compensate for defects in balance so that an illness, which in the young does not cause persistent unsteadiness, often produces much more disability in the elderly. Also, multiple deficits in many sensory systems, each of which individually is not sufficient to cause ataxia, may combine in the elderly to produce disabling imbalance.

REFERENCES

Ayd F J 1961 A survey of drug-induced extrapyramidal reactions. JAMA 175, 1054–1060
Bannister R, Oppenheimer D R 1972 Degenerative disease of the nervous system associated with autonomic failure. Brain 95:457–474
Boller F, Kizutani T, Roessmann V, Gambeti P 1980 Parkinson's disease: dementia and Alzheimer's disease. Clinicopathological correlations. Annals of Neurology 7:329–335
Clarke E, Robinson P K 1956 Cervical myelopathy: a complication of cervical spondylosis. Brain 79:483–510
Cooper I S 1969 Involuntary movement disorders. Harper and Row, New York
Critchley M 1949 On senile disorders of gait, including the so-called 'senile paraplegia'. Geriatrics 3:364–370
Critchley M 1956 Neurological changes in the aged. Journal of Chronic Diseases 3:459–477
Denny-Brown D 1958 The nature of apraxia. Journal of Nervous and Mental Disorders 126:9–31
Dorfman L, Boseley M J 1979 Age-related changes in peripheral and central nerve conduction in man. Neurology 29:38–44
Drachman D A, Hart C W 1972 An approach to the dizzy patient. Neurology 22:323–334
Frazier C H 1936 Tumor involving the frontal lobe alone. Archives of Neurology and Psychiatry 35:525–575
Greenfield J G 1976 In: Blackwood G, Corsellis JAN (eds) Greenfield's nueropathology. Arnold, London
Hachinski V C, Lassen N A, Marshall J A 1974 Multi-infarct dementia—a cause of mental deterioration in the elderly. Lancet 2:207–209
Hakim S, Adams R D 1965 The special clinical problems of symptomatic hydrocephalus with normal cerebrospinal fluid pressure: observations on cerebrospinal fluid dynamics. Journal of Neurological Science 2:307–327
Holmes G 1972 On the clinical symptoms of cerebellar disease and their interpretation. Lancet I:1177–1231; II:59–111
Lees F, Turner J W A 1963 Natural history and prognosis of cervical spondylosis. British Medical Journal 2:1607–1610
McGeer P L, McGeer E G, Suzuki J S 1977 Ageing and the extrapyramidal system. Archives of Neurology 34, 33–35
Marsden C D 1980 Involuntary movement disorders. Medicine 34:1766–1769
Marsden C D, Jenner P 1980 The pathophysiology of extrapyramidal side effects of neuroleptic drugs. Psychological Medicine 10:55–72
Martin J P 1967 The basal ganglia and posture. Pitman Medical, London
Meyer J S, Barron D W 1960 Apraxia of gait: a clinico-physiological study. Brain 83:261–284
Pallis C A, Jones A M, Spillane J D 1954 Cervical spondylosis. Brain 77:274–289
Parkes J D, Marsden C D, Rees J E, Curzon G, Kantamaneni B D, Knill-Jones R, Akbar A, Das S, Kataria M 1974 Parkinson's disease, cerebral arteriosclerosis and senile dementia. Quarterly Journal of Medicine 63:49–61
Pearce J 1974 The extrapyramidal disorder of Alzheimer's disease. European Neurology 12:94–103
Plum F, Posner J B 1980 The diagnosis of stupor and coma. Davis, Philadelphia
Prakash C, Stern G 1973 Neurological signs in the elderly. Age and Ageing 2:24–27
Scotti G, Spinnler H, Sterzi R, Vallar G 1980 Cerebellar softening. Annals of Neurology 8:133–140
Shy G M, Drager G A 1960 A neurological syndrome associated with orthostatic hypotension. A clinical pathologic study. Archives of Neurology 2:511–527

Spillane J D, Lloyd G H T 1952 The diagnosis of lesions of the spinal cord in association with osteoarthritic disease of the cervical spine. Brain 75: 177–225

Steele J C 1972 Progressive supranuclear palsy. Brain 95: 693–704

Sypert G W, Alvord E C 1975 Cerebellar infarction: a clinico-pathological study. Archives of Neurology 32: 357–363

Yuhl E T, Hanna D, Rasmussen T, Richter R B 1955 Diagnosis and surgical therapy of chronic midline cervical disc protrusions. Neurology 5: 494–509

Dizziness in the elderly

Dizziness is a non-specific term, which encompasses a number of symptoms of dysequilibrium, including lightheadedness, faintness, giddiness, sensations of 'swimming' or floating, vertigo, imbalance, ataxia, minor episodes of mental confusion and minor epileptic seizures. It is defined in an English dictionary as 'a feeling of being dazed, or in a whirl, or as if about to fall'. In clinical terms, it is a vague symptom of little value in establishing the underlying pathological process, whereas vertigo is 'an hallucination of movement' (Cawthorne, 1952) or 'a disagreeable sensation of instability or disordered orientation in space' (Agate, 1963) and is a cardinal manifestation of a disordered vestibular system (Dix, 1973). It is, however, unrealistic to expect the elderly patient, alarmed and confused by unfamiliar sensations of movement, either involving himself and/or his surroundings, to give precise and accurate descriptions of new and unphysiological experiences. For this reason, the following consideration of dizziness will ignore semantics and encompass all of the above complaints, which the patient may describe as 'dizziness'.

Despite the ubiquitous nature of the complaint of dizziness, in many branches of medicine (cardiology, neurology, psychiatry, haematology, ophthalmology and endocrinology), little interest has been shown in the evaluation of this symptom, except in the field of otology. Previous work has revealed a wide divergence of opinion as to the relative frequency of different causes of dizziness. In part, this may be due to the difficulties encountered in diagnosing the primary aetiology and hence, the same disorder being differently labelled by different clinicians (Torok, 1964; Clemis and Becker, 1973; Slater, 1979) and, in part, may merely reflect the interest, and thus referral pattern, of any particular author (Dix and Hallpike, 1952; Money, 1968; Drachman and Hart, 1972). Nonetheless, the conditions which cause dizziness in the young may also affect the elderly, although the frequency of certain disorders is greater in an elderly population.

AGEING AND VESTIBULAR APPARATUS

Ageing is a continual physiological process occurring throughout life; it is unacceptable to attribute certain symptoms of the elderly to this process alone. There is an extensive literature on the histo-pathology of the effects of ageing on the auditory system, in contrast to the relative paucity of information with respect to the vestibular system. This disparity is presumably related to the high incidence of hearing and tinnitus with advancing age, compared to the rarity of vestibular symptoms, as a direct result of senescence. Overt vestibular dysfunction results from an asymmetry of afferent information, and as ageing tends to be a bilateral phenomenon, vestibular symptoms may not be prominent.

Ageing produces well defined changes in the cochlea, the spiral ganglion, the auditory nerve and the cochlear nuclei (Saxén and Fieandt, 1937; Jorgenson, 1961; Schuknecht, 1964). It has been suggested, as a result of a pathological study on an 85-year-old male (Schuknecht et al, 1965) that the cochlea and saccule are more susceptible to the ageing process than the phylogenetically older part of the vestibular system, the utricle and the semicircular canals. The more recent work of Johnsson and Hawkins (1972), who have reported that, with ageing, there is a degeneration of the saccular macula, with severe loss of otoconia, and comparable, but less severe, degeneration of the utricular macula, would also support this hypothesis. Rosenhall (1973) and Rosenhall and Rubin (1975) have confirmed these findings, and have also described an age-dependent reduction of the hair cells of the cristae ampullares. Furthermore, Rosenhall (1974) has observed epithelial cysts in the sensory epithelium of the vertical cristae in advanced old age, which he interpreted as a sign of degeneration.

Although a severe loss of neurones has been reported in the spiral ganglion as a result of senescence, no such changes were found in the vestibular ganglion (Fleischer, 1972). However, Bergström (1973) has reported a significant reduction in the number and calibre of the vestibular nerve fibres in old people, compared with a control group of young people. Rasmussen (1940) reported this fall-out of nerve fibres in the vestibular portion of the vestibulocochlear nerve as a function of age, but noted that this phenomenon was more marked in the cochlear portion of the nerve.

Physiological studies of the effects of ageing on the vestibular system have been extensively discussed in Chapter 13 and the ensuing comments are intended only to put the ageing process into perspective in the clinical assessment of dizziness in the elderly. Some authors have described hypoexcitability of the vestibular system with advanced age (Arslan, 1957), while others have reported vestibular hyperexcitability (Schoder, 1973) and normal vestibular function (Forgacs, 1957). Other authors have investigated the effect of age on various measures of induced vestibular nystagmus (duration, maximum velocity of the slow and fast phase, maximum amplitude and maximum frequency). Van der Laan and Oosterveld (1974) found definite age dependent changes in both caloric and rotation test responses in large numbers of healthy people. Mulch and Petermann (1979) have shown that the absolute values of nystagmic measures in the caloric test are dependent upon age. They have established that the maximum nystagmic response, as judged by maximum slow phase velocity, maximum amplitude, maximum frequency and total number of beats, occurred in alert healthy subjects of middle and late middle age. Why this should be so, when definite age related degeneration of sensory and nerve cells has occurred, cannot be explained at the present time. The decline of all nystagmic measures after this age can be readily understood from the established, age-dependent, degenerative changes in the peripheral and central vestibular system.

The increase in frequency of vestibular vertigo with advancing age (Droller and Pemberton, 1953) is unlikely to be solely the consequence of degeneration of nerve and sensory cells, but is probably caused by associated age-dependent vascular changes. Indeed, these authors reported a significant correlation between the clinically diagnosed extent of arteriosclerosis and the frequency of vertigo.

CLINICAL ASPECTS

Dizziness is a very common symptom of the elderly, and yet considerable diagnostic and therapeutic skill is required to ascertain the underlying aetiology. A complete list of possible aetiologies would be unmanageable. Table 16.1 is merely intended to provide a background upon which it is possible to consider the more relevant causes of dizziness and vertigo in old age.

Man has developed the ability to control his balance by integrating, in the central nervous system, sensory information from the visual, superficial sensory, proprioceptive and vestibular systems. This information is further modulated by activity of the cortex, cerebellum, extrapyramidal system and reticular formation. Perfect equilibration thus requires a very complex and finely balanced system. Dysfunction, at any point, in the generation, integration or modulation of the sensory stimuli may result in dizziness or vertigo.

In subjects over 60 years of age, Bender (1975) has reported marked perceptual deficiencies of cutaneous and visual modalities. Two of the main sensory in-puts for maintenance of equilibrium may, therefore, be impaired in the elderly. Drachman and Hart (1972) have emphasised the importance of sensory deficits in the elderly and have postulated a syndrome producing dizziness when two or more of the following conditions are present: visual impairment (not correctable), neuropathy, vestibular deficits, cervical spondylosis and orthopaedic disorders interfering with ambulation.

Another important factor in the aged is the severe loss of cortical neurones (Brody, 1955), which may merely be one of the manifestations of central nervous system degeneration, but may, per se, impair modulation of sensory information. Furthermore, many pathologies common in the elderly (e.g. arthritis, cardiac disease, vascular disease and degenerative disorders) may result in dysfunction, not only of the vestibular system itself, but also of its multiple central connections. These observations emphasise how easily the fine balance, necessary for perfect equilibrium may be deranged.

In attempting to elucidate the individual problem, it is essential to obtain a detailed and accurate history (Table 16.2) and to perform a full medical examination, with special reference to the otological and neurological assessment in this instance. It has been emphasised (Drachman and Hart, 1972; Hinchcliffe, 1978) that it is only by bringing a multi-disciplinary approach to the problem of dizziness, that the many diverse medical disorders which may be identified with this complaint, will be correctly diagnosed. This is certainly the case in an elderly population in whom multiple pathologies and multi-system disease are almost the rule. Many different investigations may be indicated in the evaluation of dizziness, and it is necessary for the clinician to select the most appropriate investigations in

Table 16.1 Causes of dizziness in the elderly

General medical	Otological	Miscellaneous
1. Haematological (a) Anaemia (b) Polycythaemia rubra vera (c) Miscellaneous	1. Ménière's syndrome 2. Post-traumatic syndrome 3. Positional nystagmus 4. 'Vestibular neuronitis' 5. Infection 6. Otosclerosis and Paget's disease 7. Vascular accidents 8. Tumours 9. Auto-immune disorders 10. Drug intoxication	1. Ocular 2. Odontogenic 3. Cervical
2. Cardiovascular (a) Postural hypotension (b) Carotid sinus syndrome (c) Dysrhythmias, including sick sinus syndrome. (d) Mechanical dysfunction—ventricular hypokinesia —aortic stenosis (e) Shock		
3. Metabolic (a) Hypoglycaemia (b) Hyperventilation		

4. Neurological A. Supratentorial
(a) Epilepsy
(b) Syncope
(c) Psychogenic
B. Infratentorial
(a) Multiple sclerosis
(b) Vertebro-basilar insufficiency—subclavian steal syndrome
                    — Wallenberg's syndrome
                    —anterior inferior
                      cerebellar artery syndrome
(c) Infective disorders—Ramsay Hunt
                    —neurosyphilis
                    —tuberculosis
(d) Degenerative disorders
(e) Tumours, including those of the vertibulocochlear nerve
(f) Foramen magnum abnormalities		

Table 16.2 Essential detail from history

General	Specific
Age	Duration of symptoms
Occupations — noise / chemical exposure / weight exposure to neck, e.g. hodman	?Precipitating illness/accident/incident
Social conditions — marital status / ?living alone / house/flat / ?telephone / ?visitors	Dizziness/vertigo
Medical and surgical	Constant/intermittent
Past history — head neck injury — car accident / boxing / horse riding; Otologic	Duration of episodes — shortest / longest
Family history — cardiovascular / neurologic / otologic	Frequency of episodes
Smoking habits	Length of intervals — shortest / longest
Drug therapy — previous / present	?Clusters
Exposure toxic agents	Precipitating factors — cold weather / upper respiratory tract infection / changing posture or head position
Noise exposure — military / civilian: hobby/employment	Associated symptoms — otologic (hearing loss, tinnitus) / neurologic (headache, visual disturbance, dysarthria, loss of consciousness) / medical (palpitations, chest pains etc)
Travel — ?tropics	Interval symptoms
General health — vision, musculoskeletal and neurological function	

Table 16.3 Laboratory investigation of dizziness/vertigo

Blood	* Full blood count including sedimentation rate.
	Urea and electrolytes
	Liver function tests
	Random sugar and glucose tolerance test
	Fasting lipids and electrophoresis
	Thyroid function tests
	* Specific serological tests (FTA-ABS and TPHA)
*Urine	Sugar
	Protein
(C.S.F.	Cells, sugar, protein and culture)
Radiology	* Chest
	Skull
	Cervical Spine
	Tomography/Zonograms of internal acoustic meati
	(Myelography)
	(CAT scan)
Electrodiagnosis	* Electronystagmography
	(Electroencephalography)
	(Electromyography)
	* Electrocardiogram (and 24 hour ECG monitoring)
	(Electrocochleogram)
	(Acoustically evoked brainstem responses)
Audiometry	* Pure tone audiogram
	Tympanometry and stapedial reflexes
	* Tests of loudness recruitment
	Tests of abnormal auditory adaption
	Speech discrimination
Vestibular assessment	* Caloric test
	Rotational test

( )—Procedures not frequently used, only when specifically indicated.
*—Essential basic investigations in every elderly vertiginous patient.

each individual case. Table 16.3 lists the tests most frequently found to be of value by the author.

The remainder of this chapter will be devoted to a review of the causes of dizziness, which are particularly pertinent in an elderly population, in particular, vertebrobasilar ischaemia and the post-traumatic syndrome. The therapeutic options available for treatment will be considered.

GENERAL MEDICAL DISORDERS

Haematological abnormalities

Broadly speaking, haematological disorders may be divided into anaemias, disorders affecting lymph nodes and the spleen, myeloproliferative disorders and the haemorrhagic disorders.

In the elderly, anaemia and polycythaemia rubra vera are the two most important disorders to consider. Severe anaemia may be present with throbbing headache, dizziness, visual disturbance and fainting. Possible aetiological factors in this age group are:

1. Iron deficiency: dietary; partial gastrectomy; gastro-intestinal bleed (Beveridge et al, 1965) (e.g. occult carcinoma, chronic aspirin ingestion).

2. Cyanocobalamin (Vitamin B_{12}) deficiency: pernicious anaemia; postgastrectomy; terminal ileal resection.
3. Folate deficiency: dietary; iatrogenic (Stebbins and Bertino, 1976) (e.g. phenytoin, phenylbutazone).
4. Malignancies: reticulum cell sarcoma, lymphosarcoma, giant follicular lymphoma, chronic lymphatic leukaemia (Hallpike and Harrison, 1950).

Polycythaemia rubra vera occurs in the elderly and results in increased blood viscosity, with decreased flow. About one third of patients with this disorder complain of dizziness or vertigo. Secondary polycythaemia, as a result of acquired heart disease, respiratory disease or hyperventilation, associated with obesity or cerebral lesions, may produce similar symptoms. In the myeloproliferative group, myelomatosis and Waldenstrom's macroglobulinaemia, may also give rise to the hyperviscosity syndrome with associated dizziness or vertigo (Bloch and Maki, 1973). Any haemorrhagic disorder may result in labyrinthine haemorrhage and, in the elderly, this is particularly relevant in the context of head injury.

CARDIO-VASCULAR DISORDERS

Postural hypotension
As a result of a number of reflex mechanisms, a change in posture causes only minimal variation in blood pressure in the normal person. These reflexes incude (a) baroreceptor reflexes, which mediate constriction of peripheral vessels (b) carotid sinus reflex and Bainbridge reflex, which cause reflex alteration in heart rate and (c) increased cardiac output, as a result of increased venous return secondary to muscular activity in the limbs. It is of note that a marked diminution in baroreceptor sensitivity has been reported with increasing age (Gribben et al, 1971) and that the carotid sinus is one of the most common sites for development of atheroma (Sleight, 1978).

Idiopathic orthostatic hypotension is a relatively common disorder in the elderly and may be the result of impairment of the reflex control of circulation. In some elderly patients who have recovered from hypothermia, postural hypotension due to impaired baroreceptor reflexes is a common finding and Ferguson Anderson (1978) has postulated that a central lesion in the brain may cause a disturbance of both temperature regulation and vasomotor control. Orthostatic hypotension may result from venous pooling, associated with severe varicose veins, and may be secondary to surgical sympathectomy for peripheral vascular disease.

The Shy-Drager syndrome (1960) is a recently recognised condition that as yet can only be described as degenerative. Although there are many variations, the most common feature is degeneration of the autonomic nervous system, of which the most obvious symptom is postural hypotension. (Bannister, 1971). Usually it is possible to elicit a number of less dramatic symptoms that have been noticed but ignored for a number of years, for example the distribution of sweating, sexual impotence in the male, and fluctuating retention of urine. In some patients, more widespread involvement of the central nervous system does not occur. Others, however, develop cerebellar ataxia, loss of tendon reflexes or signs of Parkinson's disease. There is no curative treatment and the course of this disorder is progressive over many years. Some patients die as a result of hypotension, others from the usual terminal events associated with debilitating disorders. Diabetes mellitus, tabes dorsalis and syringomyelia may also be associated with an autonomic neuropathy and thus give rise to postural hypotension.

Iatrogenic disease is common in the aged, frequently as a result of polypharmacy, which may be necessary in the face of multiple pathologies. For this reason, acute drug induced orthostatic hypotension should be borne in mind. Hypotensive drugs, especially if associated with diuretic administration, anti-depressants, tranquillisers, levodopa, opiates and barbiturates may all produce postural hypotension with dizziness and/ or fainting.

The clinician should have a high index of suspicion of the possibility of postural hypotension as a cause of dizziness in the elderly. In every patient the blood pressure should be recorded both lying and standing. Symptomatic treatment may be of value and elastic stockings, together with an abdominal binder may reduce postural hypotension. If the symptoms are sufficiently severe, fludrocortisone may be of value.

Carotid sinus syndrome

Dizziness, or syncope, in the elderly may be the result of a hypersensitive carotid sinus reflex (Uesa et al, 1976) which is often found in association with coronary heart disease, diffuse atherosclerosis and hypertension. Carotid sinus hypersensitivity may result in a drop in blood pressure, cardiac slowing or heart block, with or without ventricular asystole, or reflex cerebral ischaemia. In the normal subject, only a slight reduction in pulse rate and blood pressure occur following stimulation of the carotid sinus. Occasionally, the sinus on one, or both sides, becomes over sensitive such that compression induced by turning the head, wearing a tight collar or even shaving may cause symptoms of giddiness, faintness or loss of consciousness.

If a hypersensitive carotid sinus is suspected, carotid sinus massage may confirm the diagnosis. Massage should be performed for no longer than ten seconds, with electrocardiographic monitoring, and if there is any ECG change, or, if the patient complains, should be discontinued instantly. In most patients with appropriate symptoms, however, carotid sinus massage produces only the normal bradycardia. It should be emphasised that carotid compression or vigorous massage must be avoided in view of the rare, but catastrophic complication of occlusion of the internal carotid artery.

The carotid sinus syndrome is a rare cause of dizziness, 3 per cent of a large series of patients presenting with syncope (Wayne, 1961), but is most commonly seen among the elderly. Relief may be obtained by denervating the sinus.

Dysrhythmias

Cardiac dysrhythmias are a common cause of dizziness and syncope in an elderly population (Tzivone and Stern, 1975). Ischaemic heart disease has assumed epidemic proportions in many prosperous countries, and it is with this disorder that dysrhythmias are commonly associated. The effect of a dysrhythmia upon cerebral circulation has been well documented (Corday and Irving, 1960; Samet

1973), and the importance of haemodynamically significant dysrhythmias, in patients presenting with symptoms of non-focal transient cerebral dysfunction, including dizziness and syncope, has recently been emphasised (Goldberg, Raftery and Cashman 1975). Their detection may be difficult, especially if the resting electrocardiogram is normal, but the development of prolonged, ambulatory electrocardiographic monitoring has enabled the detection of transient dysrhythmias (Harrison et al, 1976; Luxon et al, 1980).

A complete classification of dysrhythmias and their underlying aetiologies is beyond the scope of this presentation, but, certain aspects deserve some emphasis. In the elderly as has already been stated, polypharmacy is a serious problem. It is, therefore, important to recall that many drugs (digitalis, quinidine, betablocking agents, anti-depressants, nicotine, excess potassium) may cause cardiac dysrhythmias. In addition, certain disease states common in the elderly, for example myxoedema, thyrotoxicosis, intra-cranial pathologies, cardiomyopathies and autonomic degeneration, are associated with dysrhythmias.

In recent years, disease of the sino-atrial node has become of increasing clinical importance and the clinical states resulting from pathology of the human pacemaker have been grouped together as the *Sick Sinus Syndrome*. The pathologies which may produce this syndrome include ischaemia, sclerosis, rheumatic heart disease, pericarditis, cardiomyopathies, Friedreich's ataxia, progressive muscular dystrophy, collagen disease, surgical injury, metastatic disease, infiltrative diseases e.g. amyloidosis and haemochromatosis and isolated fibrosis of unknown cause. Although this condition may occur in the young, it is more common in the elderly. It is characterised by episodes of tachycardia, followed by sino-atrial block or sinus arrest (Kaplan et al, 1973; Ferrer, 1973) which may result in episodes of dizziness and Stokes-Adams attacks. If prolonged ambulatory monitoring fails to confirm the diagnosis, it may be necessary to undertake electro-physiological studies of the conducting system of the heart.

In the first instance, treatment of a dysrhythmia lies in excluding any causative disease process and reviewing all drug therapy. Specific anti-dysrhythmic therapy may then be commenced, although, it may be necessary, as for instance in the case of the Sick Sinus Syndrome, to consider permanent cardiac pacing.

The complaint of dizziness, and arrhythmias on 24 hour ambulatory monitoring, does not of course prove a cause and effect relationship unless they occur simultaneously. However, if asymptomatic dysrhythmias are detected on ambulatory monitoring and full neurological investigation is negative there may be an indication for further electro-physiological cardiac investigation, or a trial of anti-arrhythmic therapy, or both. Conversely, 24 hour monitoring may yield valuable negative information, if a patient's typical symptoms occur in the absence of a cardiac arrythmia.

Mechanical dysfunction

Any pathological state interfering with cardiac output may result in a reduction of cerebral blood flow with lightheadedness, dizziness or vertigo, and probably the commonest cause, in the elderly, is left ventricular dysfunction, as a result of *ischaemic heart disease* with ventricular hypokinesia or aneurysm formation.

Valvar aortic stenosis is another important cause of cardiac disability, particularly in elderly males. The classical symptoms are breathlessness, chest pain and syncope, but often these symptoms are only observed in the severe case. Dizziness, or syncope, in aortic stenosis probably reflects a number of different pathophysiological disturbances. In certain patients, the symptoms are clearly related to execise and appear to be due to hypotension, resulting from a combination of exercise induced vasodilatation, with a fixed cardiac output. In other cases, transient complete atrio-ventricular block due to involvement of the atrio-ventricular node by calcification, may result in a decreased cardiac output, while, in other instances, short periods of ventricular fibrillation or tachycardia are the precipitating factor.

Physical examination may reveal a slow rising pulse of reduced amplitude and a sustained apex beat on palpation. On auscultation, in the elderly patient with a calcified valve, a single second heart sound, due to lack of the aortic component, and the characteristic ejection systolic murmur, at the base of the heart, with radiation to the carotid artery, may be heard. A chest radiograph, electrocardiogram, echocardiogram and cardiac catheterisation may be necessary to confirm the diagnosis. Surgical treatment of this condition is extremely effective with a relatively low mortality and morbidity, even in the elderly. For this reason, the clinician seeing a patient with dizziness and/or syncope should carry out a full cardiovascular examination, especially in view of the increased incidence of sudden cardiac death in aortic stenosis.

Many other disorders which may result in the mechanical dysfunction of the heart e.g. primary atrial myxoma; myocardial infarction; myocarditis and pericardial effusion may also cause dizziness. However, the presentation and management of these conditions do not differ as a result of age.

Cardio-vascular shock
Any acute loss of circulating volume may result in the clinical syndrome of shock, with which dizziness and vertigo are common symptoms. It should, however, be emphasised that these symptoms are rapidly overshadowed by more lifethreatening problems and it is most unlikely that there would be any difficulty in the diagnosis of 'dizziness'.

METABOLIC DISORDERS

Hypoglycaemia of any cause may produce dizziness or vertigo (Currier, 1971). Hypoglycaemia is most commonly due to an excess of insulin, or hypoglycaemic agents, in a known diabetic. An elderly person who appears unusually confused, with lightheadedness or dizziness, should have an immediate estimation of the blood sugar level, followed by administration of oral sugar in an attempt to alleviate the symptoms.

Other endocrine disorders in which hypoglycaemia is a prominent feature are Addison's disease and hypopituitarism, but both these disorders are rare. Although hypothyroidism does not produce dizziness as such, it is well recognised that cerebellar ataxia and cerebellar syndromes may occur, as is fully discussed in

Chapter XVI. These symptoms may be described by the elderly patient as 'dizziness' and this diagnosis should be borne in mind.

Hypoglycaemia may occur in chronic alcoholism, either secondary to acute alcoholic ingestion, or as a result of cirrhosis. Neoplasia is common in the elderly and hypoglycaemia may be the result of a neoplasm of the β cells of the pancreas (lightheadedness was found in 30 per cent of group of patients with insulinomas (Crain et al, 1949)), but may also be associated with malignant tumours not derived from pancreatic islet cells, e.g. mesotheliomata, fibrosarcomata or bronchial carcinoma. Dizziness is also associated with salicylate overdose and, in this situation, may result from either hypoglycaemia, or as a direct effect of the drug together with pallor, sweating and tinnitus.

The *hyperventilation syndrome* has been reported as an important cause of dizziness (Drachman and Hart, 1972), but a recent, large survey revealed no patient over 60 years of age with this diagnosis (Pincus, 1978). However, in the presence of psychiatric disorders, the diagnosis should be considered even in the elderly. (See Psychogenic Disorders).

NEUROLOGICAL DISORDERS

Vertigo is a symptom of many neurological diseases, especially posterior fossa lesions, affecting the cerebellum and brain stem, and temporal lobe lesions. Cawthorne (1959) reported that in a large series of patients affected by vertigo, approximately 12 per cent had diseases of the central nervous system. These disorders are discussed in relation to their anatomical locality.

Supra-tentorial lesions

The temporal lobes are thought to exert a modifying influence upon the vestibular nuclei (Carmichael et al, 1954) and any disturbance of these corticospinal pathways may, therefore, result in vertiginous symptoms. The following conditions deserve mention in the context of an elderly population:

Epilepsy

In an elderly population, cerebrovascular disease and primary (Figs 16.1 and 16.2) and metastatic brain tumours are common pathologies, which may give rise to temporal lobe epilepsy (Nielsen, 1959), but vertigo may also occur as an aura to both temporal lobe seizures and other forms of epilepsy (Lennox, 1960). Vertigo is not a rare symptom of seizures (Schneider et al, 1968), and, indeed Gowers (1907) reported it in 90 of a series of 505 cases. The question of whether or not every patient who loses consciousness during a vertiginous attack is epileptic is open to controversy. Some authors (Boudin et al, 1959) state that loss of consciousness may be associated with labyrinthine episodes, whereas others (Cawthorne, 1959; Alpers, 1960) feel that when true vertigo, or dizziness, is the only symptom it may be extremely difficult to arrive at a diagnosis of epilepsy. In the presence of other stigmata of temporal lobe epilepsy (auditory hallucinations, automatic behaviour, absences, outbursts of rage, perceptions of *déjà vu* or *jamais vu* and unique motor abnormalities e.g. chewing, lip-smacking and facial grimacing), the diagnosis may be made with more certainty. Two thirds of patients with temporal lobe seizures

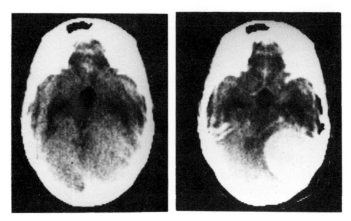

Fig. 16.1 Unenhanced and enhanced computerised axial tomographic scans of right meningioma producing temporal lobe epilepsy.

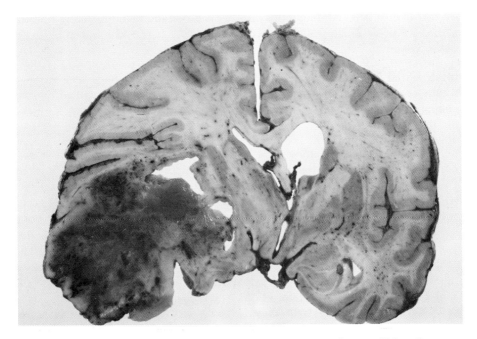

Fig. 16.2 Temporal lobe metastasis giving rise to vertigo as a component of temporal lobe epilepsy.

suffer grand mal seizures at some period in their life. In contra-distinction to the diagnosis of vertiginous epilepsy, is the entity of vestibular or vestibulogenic epilepsy which is considered to be a form of reflex epilepsy precipitated by, most frequently, paroxysmal vertigo of labyrinthine origin (Behrman, 1955), e.g. in association with Ménière's Disease or chronic middle ear disease.

Vasovagal syndrome or syncope
This is usually described as a short episode of loss of consciousness, associated with an acute reduction in cerebral blood flow. In the elderly, as in the young,

this is often of functional origin, but many cardiovascular disorders, which have already been discussed may give rise to this event.

Psychogenic disorders

Flemming (1960) reported that true vertigo could be emotional, and cases of vertigo are very common in psychiatric practice, expecially in anxiety neuroses (Sloane, 1967). Furthermore, it has been emphasised that organic vertigo may be influenced by emotional factors (Weiss and English, 1957) and, indeed, may produce extreme anxiety (Cawthorne, 1957). It is also of relevance that Hallpike and his colleague, (1951) reported a high incidence of caloric abnormalities in patients with schizophrenia and other mental disorders.

In the elderly population, in whom there is a high incidence of psychiatric disorders, as a result of organic brain disease, it is, therefore, especially important to consider the emotional, as well as the organic factors in the evaluation of dizziness. It is perhaps valuable to note that 60 per cent of patients studied by Drachman and Hart (1972) with the hyperventilation syndrome, had significant psychiatric disorders. Although this disorder is classically found in young women, in the face of psychiatric disturbances it should be borne in mind even in the elderly patient.

Infratentorial lesions

A number of the most important causes of dizziness in the elderly fall within this group.

Multiple sclerosis

Multiple sclerosis is predominantly a disease of young adults, but the onset may occasionally be delayed until the age of 60 or even older (Matthews, 1978). It is one of the most common diseases encountered in neurological practice and is characterised by single or multiple discrete lesions of demyelination, which may occur randomly thoughout the brain and spinal cord (Fig. 16.3). Late age of onset is a sign indicative of a poor prognosis. It is well recognised that patients with this disorder may present with vertigo and/or dizziness (Noffsinger et al, 1972). The vertigo may be severe and prostrating and characteristically persists for a week or longer. It does not occur in brief paroxysms and hearing is usually preserved. Remission of brainstem symptoms of this type is usually complete. Scattered signs throughout the nervous system, together with visual and auditory evoked responses and estimation of the protein level, IgG percentage and white cell count in the cerebrospinal fluid may help in reaching a diagnosis.

Vertebrobasilar insufficiency

Cerebrovascular disease is the third commonest cause of death in this country. In addition, labyrinthine disorders are very common and consideration of these two pathologies is frequently cited as the explanation of the high incidence of episodes of dizziness in many people over the age of 50. The overlap of dizziness of peripheral and central origin in an elderly population also becomes apparent.

The labyrinthine (internal auditory) artery, which supplies the peripheral apparatus of the auditory and vestibular systems, arises from the anterior inferior cerebellar artery in 83 per cent of individuals and directly from the basilar artery

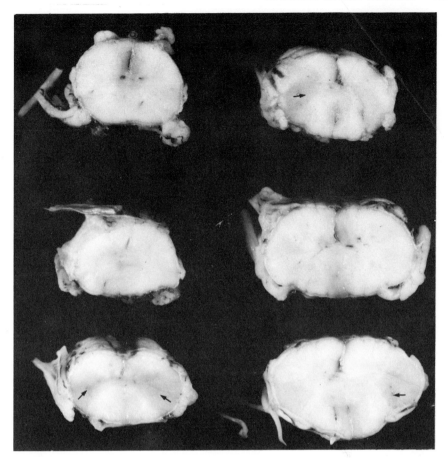

Fig. 16.3 Patchy demyelination (as arrowed) in sections of the spinal cord and lower medulla.

in 17 per cent (Sunderland 1945). The vestibular nuclei are supplied by penetrating branches of the anterior inferior cerebellar and vertebral arteries. The blood supply to the vestibular system may, therefore, be compromised in the tiny penetrating vessels of the labyrinth, or in the labyrinthine artery, the anterior inferior cerebellar artery, the basilar artery, one vertebral artery or both vertebral arteries (Fig. 16.4). The vestibular nuclei ocupy a greater area of space within the brainstem than any other neighbouring nuclei and, as Gillilan (1964) has pointed out, they lie in the area of the brainstem (lateral zone), which is most likely to be affected by a reduction of blood flow in the main basilar artery. Thus, vertigo and/or dizziness are reported in many series as the first and most frequent symptoms of vertebrobasilar insufficiency (Williams, 1964; Loeb and Meyer, 1965; Fisher, 1970). Furthermore, the incidence of vertigo is significantly higher in cases in which the basilar artery is stenosed greater than 50 per cent of its diameter (Kanejama, 1965). Conversely, vertebrobasilar ischaemia is the commonest cause of dizziness in an elderly population.

Vertebrobasilar insufficiency is defined as a state of transient decrease in the cerebral blood flow, without actual infarction, resulting in transient inability to

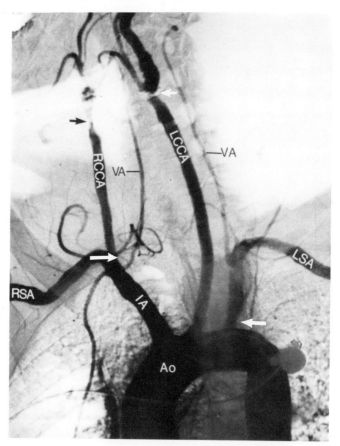

Fig. 16.4 Arch aortogram showing diffuse atheroma with complete occlusion of the right internal carotid artery, stenosis of the left common carotid artery (LCCA), stenosis of both sublcavian arteries (RSA and LSA) and both vertebral arteries (VA) are small.
IA = innominate (brachiocephalic) artery
Ao = Aorta
(Stenoses Arrowed)

meet the metabolic requirements of the brain (Millikan and Siekert, 1955). Such a fall in blood flow may result from primary disease of the vertebrobasilar system itself, or may be a secondary result of cardiac disorders, haematological disease or stenosis of extracranial cerebral vessels. Arteriosclerosis is the commonest cause of arterial insufficiency and usually occurs at arterial origins, with progressive narrowing and occlusion, producing distal arterial insufficiency, if collateral circulation is insufficient. Vertebral artery stenosis, *per se*, most often occurs at the origin from the subclavian artery, but 70 per cent of patients with basilar ischaemia have occlusive disease of the extracranial cerebral vessels.

Vertigo of central origin is often described as being insidious in onset and continuous in pattern, while it is commonly assumed that peripheral labyrinthine dysfunction gives rise to episodic attacks of vertigo or dizziness. Transient ischaemic attacks in the vertebrobasilar territory are the exception to this general rule, and it is important that they are diagnosed early for two practical reasons.

Firstly, they may herald an impending stroke and secondly, they may be amenable to treatment either medically, with anticoagulants, or surgically (DeBakey, 1962). The interpretation of dizziness is simple when it is part of an obvious stroke, but when it occurs alone, unaccompanied by any other aural or neurological symptom or sign, it presents a difficult diagnostic problem (Fisher, 1967; Barber and Dionne, 1971).

The symptoms and signs of brain stem ischaemia (Fig. 16.5) reflect the close proximity of many long tracts and cranial nerve nuclei. Fisher (1967) reported that in 112 patients with basilar occlusion, 77 per cent experienced dizziness, although under a quarter of these gave a history of true rotational vertigo. Nonetheless, of the 86 patients who experienced dizziness, in one quarter it was the first and unaccompanied symptom; in a further 50 per cent, dizziness was one of two or more initial symptoms and was accompanied by neurological phenomena, which allowed the disorder to be correctly interpreted as a transient ischaemic attack, rather than a labyrinthine disturbance. The same author also emphasised that dizziness, unaccompanied by any other symptom or sign, was unlikely to be of vascular origin, if a stroke had not declared itself within six weeks. He cites the symptoms and signs of ischaemia that follow most often after isolated vertigo, in order of frequency, as dysarthria, numbness of the face, hemiparesis, headache and diplopia. Other pointers of value, in reaching the diagnosis of vertebrobasilar insufficiency, are visual disturbances (field defects, oscillopsia, dimness of vision and transient blindness), dysphagia, drop attacks (often precipitated by neck

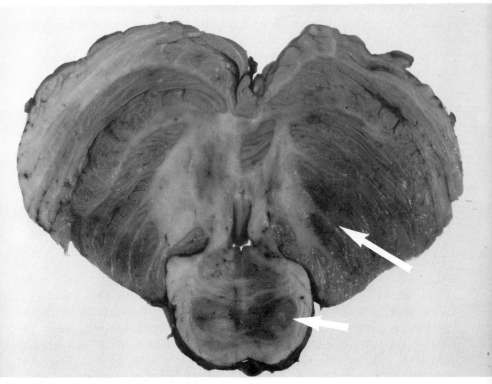

Fig. 16.5 Patchy ischaemia of the brainstem and cerebellum as a result of basilar insufficiency.

movement), alternating weakness of opposite sides of the body, diffuse dysaesthesia and cerebellar ataxia. Tinnitus and impairment of hearing are unusual manifestations of vertebrobasilar ischaemia (Barber and Dionne, 1971) and when they accompany vertigo, there are almost always other signs of brainstem deficit. Indeed, true vertigo, or dizziness accompanied only by vestibulocochlear nerve manifestations is less likely to be vascular in origin.

Attacks of vertebrobasilar insufficiency may last seconds, minutes or hours and have a variable frequency of recurrence. They may or may not be stereotyped in any one individual. Loeb and Meyer (1965) emphasised that only five out of 23 cases had the same clinical features in recurrent attacks and Millikan and Siekert (1955) emphasised the importance of the same symptoms on opposite sides of the body, in different attacks. The diagnostic probability of vertebrobasilar ischaemia is increased in the presence of hypertension, diabetes mellitus, hyperlipidaemia, ischaemic heart disease, other vascular disease, and polycythaemia. Furthermore, 80 per cent of the patients with this diagnosis are over the age of 50 years (Burns, 1973). In the absence of definitive neurological symptoms and signs, careful otoneurological examination reveals a high incidence of vestibular and oculomotor abnormalities, but there is no characteristic pattern of abnormalities associated with vertebrobasilar insufficiency (Corvera et al, 1980).

This is perhaps to be expected in a disease which may cause many different and widespread lesions both at the labyrinthine and neurological levels. Thus, a definitive diagnosis is only possible by arteriography which is an invasive procedure, carrying a significant mortality and morbidity especially in an aged population. Non-invasive methods of obtaining information about cerebral haemodynamics, e.g. plethysmography (Backlund et al, 1969), ophthalmodynamometry, and effects of vascular insufficiency e.g. computerised axial tomography, provide valuable adjuncts to diagnosis in this situation.

Atherosclerosis may be predominantly localised in the cerebral vessels (cerebrovascular disease), but is essentially a diffuse disorder. Most commonly vertebrobasilar ischaemia results from stenosis, or occlusion, of the vertebrobasilar system itself, but, more recently, Bergan and his colleagues (1967) and Fisher (1970) have reported that the functional equivalent of bilateral vertebral compromise may result from occlusion, or stenosis, of more proximal vessels, e.g. the innominate artery or the subclavian arteries. As early as 1951, Denny-Brown pointed out that extracranial arterial spasm might give rise to transient symptoms in the vertebrobasilar territory.

Total occlusion of the proximal subclavian artery may result in reversal of blood flow in the vertebral artery, which then acts as a collateral to the upper limb. (Irvine et al, 1965). As a result of the lower pressure and low peripheral resistance in the arm, blood is siphoned from the vertebrobasilar system, via the distal vertebral artery, into the distal subclavian artery (Fig. 16.6). This condition is known as the *subclavian steal syndrome* (Contorni, 1960; Reivich et al, 1961), and occurs in 3 per cent of patients with recurrent vertebrobasilar symptoms. The diagnosis may be considered when symptoms are precipitated by exercise of an upper limb, especially if there is claudication or fatigue of the limb itself. The characteristic physical signs are a systolic bruit in the supraclavicular fossa and a disparity in blood pressure between the two arms.

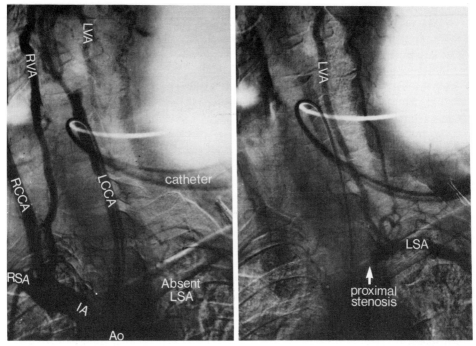

Fig. 16.6 Serial arteriograms following introduction of a catheter via the left common carotid artery (LCCA). Injection of dye outlines the brachiocephalic artery (BA), the right subclavian artery (RSA), right common carotid artery (RCCA) and right vertebral artery (RVA). Following the early injection (Fig. 16.5 A), the left vertebral artery (LVA) can be seen to be filling from above but no left subclavian artery (LSA) can be visualised. In the late film (Fig. 16.5b), the left vertebral artery has totally filled and the left subclavian artery is now clearly visualised.

Carotid artery insufficiency may also produce vertebrobasilar symptoms, in the presence of an anomalous circulus arteriosus (Circle of Willis), or insufficiency of the vertebral arteries, both of which may result in carotid collaterals supplying the base of the brain. (Fields and Weibel, 1964; Humphries, 1965). It has been reported that 50 per cent of patients with vertebral artery stenosis also have carotid artery stenosis. Other lesions of the extracranial circulation, which may result in flow changes in the vertebrobasilar system include anatomical abnormalities, e.g. an anomalous origin of the vertebral artery (Sheehan, 1960) and mechanical compression of vertebral arteries by skeletal e.g. cervical spondylosis, and/or muscular structures, e.g. fibrous band formation (Powers, Dirsland and Nevins, 1961). In this latter condition, it is postulated that there is intermittent vertebral artery compression by the thyrocervical trunk and the scalenus anterior muscle upon the vertebral artery, near its origin.

As vertebrobasilar ischaemia is only one aspect of diffuse cerebro-vascular disease, Fisher (1967) considered the incidence of dizziness, as a symptom in patients with intracranial arterial disease affecting other vessels. Dizziness occurred in 77 per cent of patients with basilar occlusion, 24 per cent of patients with posterior cerebral artery disease, and 8 per cent of patients with internal carotid and middle cerebral artery ischaemia.

Vertebrobasilar ischaemia usually results in scattered regions of ischaemia involving the brainstem, cerebellum, pons, medulla and occipital and/or temporal lobes. Less commonly individual branches of the vertebrobasilar system may be diseased and give rise to specific syndromes, often associated with dizziness.

The lateral medullary, or *Wallenberg's syndrome*, is the most frequently encountered brainstem syndrome. Dizziness, or imbalance, is a constant feature, together with ipsilateral dissociated sensory loss, in the distribution of the facial nerve, with contralateral truncal loss. Other ipsilateral signs include cerebellar ataxia, bulbar palsy and Horner's syndrome. Originally ascribed to occlusion of the posterior inferior cerebellar artery, it is now considered that this syndrome is secondary to disease of the vertebral artery (Fisher, 1967).

Vertigo is also described as occurring in the less common *anterior inferior cerebellar artery syndrome*, and in occlusion of the labyrinthine artery, which arises from the anterior inferior cerebellar artery. Furthermore, syndromes giving rise to dizziness have been ascribed to occlusion of two of the three terminal branches of the labyrinthine artery, namely the vestibular artery and the vestibulocochlear artery. However, there is little pathological confirmation of the existence of these latter syndromes. Fisher (1967) argues cogently against them.

Pontine and cerebellar haemorrhages may also present with dizziness. In the former, dizziness is never an isolated symptom and is usually a fleeting event before the patient becomes unconscious (Fig. 16.7). Cerebellar haemorrhage is of importance, as, if diagnosed early, it may be surgically remediable. The patient may present with acute vertigo, vomiting and inability to stand. The dizziness may be aggrevated by motion, or lying on one side. Without rapid treatment the patient will die in a few hours from brainstem compression. Computerised axial tomography and/or angiography may facilitate diagnosis.

Infective disorders
Viral encephalitis may be associated with vertigo and general malaise (Herbert, 1954). The clinical picture, together with cerebrospinal fluid findings of an elevated protein and white cell count, should leave the diagnosis in no doubt.

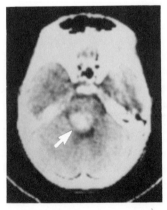

Fig. 16.7 Computerised axial tomographic scan of pontine haemorrhage (area of high attenuation arrowed).

Herpes zoster affecting the geniculate ganglion results in unilateral facial paralysis, accompanied by severe pain in and around the external acoustic meatus and throat. Occasionally, there is concomitant vertigo, tinnitus and some hearing loss from involvement of the vestibulocochlear nerve (otic herpes zoster). This is known as the *Ramsay Hunt syndrome.*

Neurosyphilis may cause vertigo and all stages of the disease are to be found in the vestibular labyrinth (Eggston and Wolff, 1947). In their classic work on this subject, Merritt and his colleagues (1946) reported dizziness as a symptom in 24 per cent of cases of cerebrovascular syphilis and 14 per cent of meningeal neurosyphilis. A recent review of neurosyphilis found that 30 per cent of patients were over the age of 60 years at the time of presentation and although the incidence of this disorder has fallen dramatically with the introduction of antibiotics, a high index of suspicion is necessary if rare cases are not to be missed (Luxon et al, 1979).

Although tuberculosis is no longer a common disorder in this country, the possibility of a tuberculoma in the brainstem, cerebellopontine angle or temporal lobe should be borne in mind, especially in elderly immigrants and in eldery debilitated, or alcoholic, patients. In addition, streptomycin used for the treatment of tuberculosis may result in vestibular paralysis, with associated dizziness and oscillopsia.

Degenerative conditions
Cerebellar degeneration may present with imbalance, nystagmus and vertigo, especially in the middle aged and elderly, but episodic vertigo, as opposed to sensations of unsteadiness, is uncommon in cerebellar disease. Degeneration may be suspected in association with malignancies, lymphoma, phenytoin intoxication, alcoholism, myxoedema, vitamin B deficiency and is fully discussed in Chapter 15 (Fig. 16.8).

Syringobulbia is the clinical syndrome characterised by cavities in the medulla oblongata. This disease is slowly progressive and may be heralded by paroxysmal vertigo, followed by disturbances of equilibrium and positional nystagmus. It is often associated with syringomyelia, in which the classical sensory dissociation facilitates diagnosis.

Tumours
'Vertigo is one of the most common symptoms of extracerebellar and intracerebellar tumours and it is especially frequent in the former' (Stewart and Holmes, 1904). Primary intramedullary tumours are rare in adults, but the possibility of a secondary deposit should be considered in the elderly. Before making the diagnosis of an intramedullary lesion in a patient over the age of 20 years, the possibility of an extrinsic compressive lesion should be excluded e.g. vestibulocochlear nerve tumours, a tumour of another cranial nerve, meningioma, keratoma, arachnoid cyst or vascular abnormality. Again, in the cerebellopontine angle a metastasis from a primary carcinoma, e.g. bronchus, must be borne in mind (Cawthorne and Hinchcliffe, 1961).

Brainstem turmours (Figs. 16.9 and 16.10) may often be diagnosed by the characteristic constellation of multiple cranial nerve palsies and long tract signs. Although dizziness and/or vertigo has been reported as an early or initial symptom

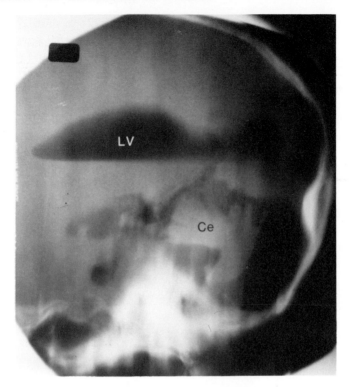

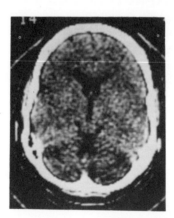

Fig. 16.8 Cerebellar atrophy as demonstrated by air encephalography (Fig. 16.8 A, LV = lateral ventricle, Ce = cerebellum), and computerised axial tomography (Fig. 16.8 B).

in 25 per cent of cases of brain stem tumours (Barnett and Hyland, 1952), it is, frequently, a minor symptom in comparison to some of the more life-threatening symptoms e.g. respiratory failure. Treatment of these lesions in the elderly is essentially symptomatic and, despite radiotherapy and steroids, the prognosis is extremely poor.

In tumours of the cerebellopontine angle, vertigo is most commonly seen in *vestibulocochlear schwannomas* ('acoustic neurinomas') (Fig. 16.11), but it should

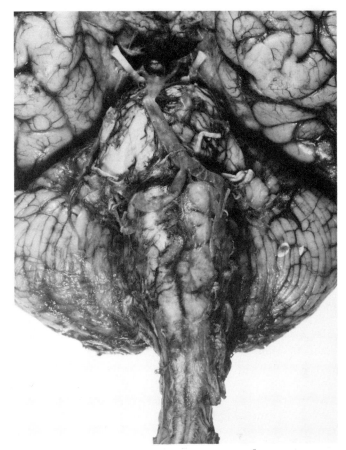

Fig. 16.9 Underside of brainstem with cerebellar and cerebral hemispheres in situ showing swelling of left side of medulla with distortion of vertebral and basilar arteries.

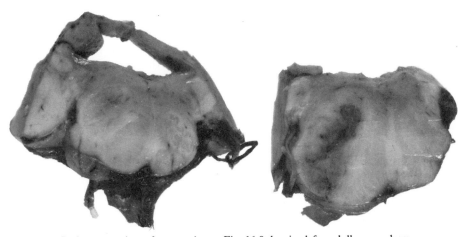

Fig. 16.10 Brainstem sections of same patient as Fig. 16.9 showing left medullary neoplasm.

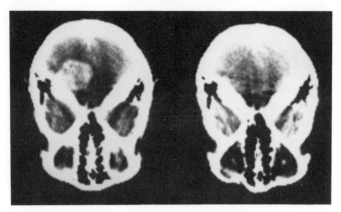

Fig. 16.11 Unenhanced and enhanced computerised axial tomography of a cystic right vestibulocochlear schwannoma.

be emphasised that the frequency of this disorder is very low in a random group of dizzy patients (Drachman and Hart, 1972). In a large series of vestibulocochlear schwannomas (Morrison, 1975), 20 per cent of patients were over the age of 60 at the time of presentation. In the same series, 10 per cent of patients complained of vertigo, dizziness and/or unsteadiness as the initial symptom. Generally, the patient describes a vague dizziness, although on occasions paroxysmal vertigo may occur and simulate Ménière's disease (Pulec et al, 1971). The diagnosis and management of vestibulocochlear schwannomas in the elderly is no different from that of the young patient. However, it is particularly necessary for a clinician to have a high index of suspicion with respect to this disorder, as mild giddiness and hearing loss may be dismissed in the elderly, whereas the symptoms in the young may prompt more aggressive investigation (Figs. 16.12 and 16.13).

In the otological stage of this disease, the pertinent features are a unilateral, or asymmetrical bilateral, sensorineural hearing loss, with evidence of abnormal auditory adaption. However, a typical cochlear pattern of hearing loss, or, indeed, inconsistent audiometric findings may be found, and are especially common in small tumours (Johnson, 1968). Caloric testing and electronystagmography may be of considerable value. Tomography of the internal acoustic meatuses and contrast studies, with or without air, may be necessary to outline a small tumour. Tumours larger than one centimetre should be visualised on computerised axial tomography.

In the neurological stage, the tumour expands from the internal acoustic meatus and begins to fill the cerebellopontine angle and involve the brainstem. This results in ipsilateral trigeminal disturbance with spontaneous nystagmus directed to the opposite side. Later, cerebellar involvement causes ataxia of the homolateral limbs and coarse, spontaneous nystagmus to the homolateral side. (Dix and Hallpike, 1966). As the disease progresses, pyramidal signs develop more usually contra-lateral to the lesion, but they may be bilateral, and gross ataxia of gait develops. Tumours of this size should be readily identified by computerised axial tomo-graphy.

The importance in reaching this diagnosis early, is based on the excellent surgical results, which may be achieved, especially with small vestibulocochlear nerve tumours (Morrison, 1978; House, 1978). In the past, especially in the elderly

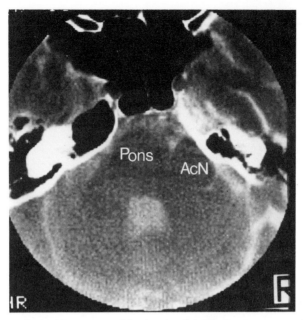

Fig. 16.12 Computerised axial tomograms following metrizamide, showing an acoustic neuroma, (AcN) compressing the pons to produce the characteristic features of a cerebellar pontine angle tumour.

patient, surgery has been delayed on the alleged slow rate of expansion of these tumours. This view is now strongly disputed and the increased risk of surgical mortality and morbidity, associated with operations on medium and larged sized tumours (Yasargil and Fox, 1974), emphasises the need to operate as soon as possible, unless the patient is an extremely poor anaesthetic risk.

For the sake of completeness, tumours of the cerebellum should be mentioned. They are rare in the elderly, but include astrocytomas, ependymonas, metastatic lesions, abscesses, tuberculomas, arteriovenous angiomas, sarcomas and gummas. Vertigo may occur with any of these disorders. *Brun's syndrome*, which consists of severe episodic vertigo, violent headaches and vomiting with changes in head posture, has been reported with cerebellar astrocytoma, varied lesions of the fourth ventricle and lesions of the third ventricle.

Foramen magnum abnormalities
Of importance in the elderly, Paget's disease giving rise to basilar impression (Fig. 16.14) has been reported to be accompanied occasionally by vertigo (Davis, 1968). The neurological symptoms produced by spinal cord and cerebellar compression, together with obstruction of the fourth ventricle, overshadow the vertigo. This condition may be recognised by radiological examination and surgical decompression is the treatment of choice.

OTOLOGIC CAUSES OF VERTIGO

Severe attacks of vertigo associated with nausea and vomiting are more frequently of labyrinthine than of central origin. Gowers (1892) wrote of his experiences at

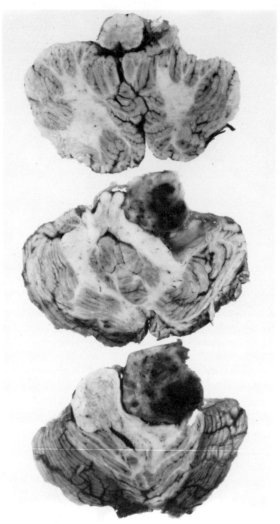

Fig. 16.13 Sections showing large vestibulocochlear schwannoma distorting the brainstem and cerebellum.

Queen Square 'of 106 consecutive cases in which definite vertigo made the patient seek advise, in no less than 94, ear symptoms were present. . . . It is exceedingly rare for definite vertigo to occur apart from aural symptoms and it is certain that in the majority of cases in which vertigo has been ascribed to other causes these have only had an exciting influence, and the symptom has been essentially due to the affect of unobtrusive labyrinthine disease.'

Ménière's disease
This condition was first described by Prosper Ménière in 1861, and is characterised by tinnitus, hearing loss and episodic vertigo. Although it usually presents between

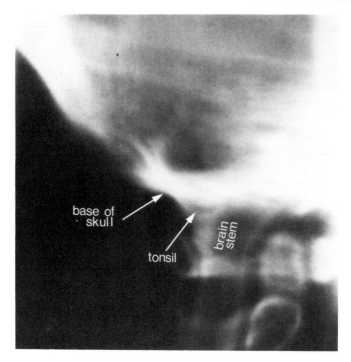

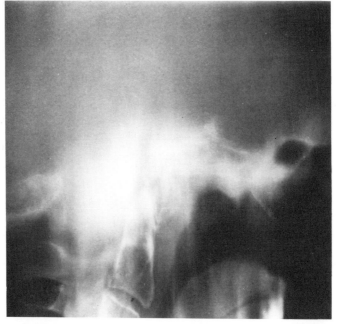

Fig. 16.14 (A) Metrizamide myelogram showing cerebellar ectopia as arrowed with forward compression of the brainstem (B) Basilar impression secondary to Paget's disease.

the ages of 30 to 40, it may rarely occur in the elderly (Cawthorne and Hewlett, 1954). In the absence of any underlying primary aetiology, the condition is defined as Ménière's disease, but in 36 per cent of patients with this symptom complex, Pulec (1973) has reported that careful evaluation reveals a causative pathological process and, in this situation, the symptom complex is called Ménière's syndrome. The possible aetiological factors cited include allergy, especially to food, (Williams, 1952), syphilis (Schuknecht, 1974), hypo-adrenalism and hypopituitarism, myxoedema, (Pulec, 1972) physical or acoustic trauma, emotional factors (Fowler and Zeckel, 1952) and vertebral artery insufficiency (Kristensen, 1963).

The clinical picture of Ménière's syndrome in the elderly is identical to that in the young patient. The onset is often insiduous, often with a sensation of dullness, or fullness, in one or both ears. The irregular, severe attacks of vertigo, which last less than 24 hours, and on occasions are associated with hearing loss and tinnitus, are common. An outstanding feature of Ménière's syndrome is the fluctuation in auditory acuity. The natural history of the disorder is that this fluctuation decreases and the hearing loss becomes permanent, with involvement of, not only, the low frequencies, but also the high.

The audiometric findings may be extremely valuable in the diagnosis of endolymphatic hydrops, which is the histopathological correlate of Ménière's disorder. Fluctuating, low tone, sensorineural hearing loss, with complete loudness recruitment (Dix et al, 1948) is a classical finding. Diplacusis may be present and vestibular function is frequently abnormal. In particular, caloric test abnormalities have been reported in 94 per cent of cases (Dix and Hallpike, 1952). The dynamic nature of Ménière's disease makes changes in vestibular function and test results commonplace (Stahle, 1968).

In the first instance, any specific underlying aetiology should be identified and treated. In the case of allergy, elimination of the allergens or desensitisation may result in improvement. The detection of syphilis, by specific antitreponemal tests, requires hospitalisation to enforce the administration of penicillin 20 million units intravenously daily for seven days. The presence of hypoadrenalism or hypopituitarism will require hormone replacement therapy. Patients with myxoedema are treated with thyroxine. Those in whom emotional factors are considered to be important, are treated with minor tranquillisers, as deemed necessary. In Ménière's disease, the therapeutic options are legion (Arenburg and Bayer, 1977). Encouraging reports have resulted from sodium restricting diet, diuretics, vasodilators, including nicotinic acid, antihistamines, including betahistine, and many surgical procedures, which have been advocated for the treatment of Ménière's disease. The role and value of these different modalities of therapy are considered in more detail at the end of this chapter.

The condition of delayed endolymphatic hydrops (Nadol, Weiss and Parker, 1975; Schuknecht, 1978) should be mentioned with respect to dizziness in the eldery. Ménière-like attacks of vertigo occur in a patient in whom there has been total or almost total loss of cochlear function, with preservation of vestibular function, usually about 20 years previously. As there is no useful auditory function, the treatment of choice is labyrinthectomy, but, if this is not indicated in an elderly patient drugs appropriate to the management of Ménière's disease will often control the symptoms.

Post-traumatic vertigo

It is well recognised that patients frequently complain of dizziness following closed head, or neck, injury (Hart, 1973; Pearson and Barber, 1973; Rubin, 1973). The current consensus of opinion is that this symptom is the result of vestibular dysfunction (Toglia et al, 1970), as opposed to an earlier view, that post-traumatic symptoms were often psychogenic in origin (Spector, 1967). The elderly are particularly prone to falls for a variety of reasons, as outlined by Isaacs in Chapter 14. Furthermore, rehabilitation of the elderly following trauma may be prolonged because of coincidental disease and socio-psychological stresses, for example, loneliness and loss of confidence.

Any external injury to the skull or neck may result in trauma to the labyrinth, or its central connections. In the elderly, the occiput is commonly injured, as a result of slipping on ice or falling downstairs. The physical impact may be transmitted directly through the skull to the temporal bones, or as a result of shearing, may indirectly produce damage to the brainstem and cerebellum.

Head injury, may broadly speaking, result in one of two post-traumatic syndromes. The first is the syndrome of sudden unilateral vestibular failure, in which function is suddenly and immediately lost in one labyrinth. In this situation, there is severe vertigo, nausea and vomiting, with spontaneous nystagmus to the normal side, and loss of balance, with the patient tending to fall towards the affected side. The symptoms and signs are most severe with the affected side down, and are aggravated by any rapid head movement. The clinical state gradually improves over the first few days and, over a six to twelve week period, the patient becomes asymptomatic. This clinical picture is most often seen following moderately severe head injuries, with or without fracture. Transverse fractures of the temporal bone usually result in permanent total unilateral loss of vestibulocochlear function (Pearson and Barber, 1973) and should be suspected in the presence of blood in the middle ear, the external acoustic meatus or retro-auricular ecchymoses.

The second clinical syndrome of benign positional vertigo, is the commonest type of vestibular disturbance following head injury, and is seen especially after longitudinal fractures of the temporal bone (Barber, 1964). Rubin (1973) has reported that it is also the most common abnormal finding in patients after whiplash injury, although Barber (1973) has disputed this. The symptoms develop after a symptom free interval of some days or weeks, and vertigo then occurs on change of posture. The features of benign paroxysmal vertigo are a latent period of a few seconds, severe vertigo which lasts for less than a minute, during which time the patient feels dizzy, unsteady and profoundly nauseated, and fatiguability upon repeated testing. These symptoms are usually accompanied by a paroxysm of rotatory nystagmus. The complaint may persist for months or even years following injury. In prognostic terms, the episodes gradually diminish in severity from the time of the accident, with complete resolution in three to six months, but they may persist at the same level of intensity for years after the incident (Rubin, 1973).

On occasions, other clinical syndromes may be seen following head injury, and furthermore, severe vestibular paresis may gradually evolve into the more common clinical picture of benign paroxysmal vertigo. In addition, Ménière's syndrome, secondary to trauma, has been reported (Pulec, 1972) and traumatic perilymph fistula (Fee, 1968) is being shown to be of considerable importance.

Pathologically, it is considered that with minor head injuries, the labyrinth probably bears the brunt of the damage, as vertigo is a very common complaint, without other neurological signs. Experimental work in animals has shown that haemorrhage may occur into the endolymph and perilymph, and there may be petechial haemorrhages of the vestibulocochlear nerve. In experimental animals, Wickstrom and his colleagues (1960) and Ommaya and his associates (1968) have demonstrated whiplash induced lesions from the level of the soft tissues, joints and nerves of the neck, to the brain stem and inner ear. As early as 1934, Voss coined the term 'Labyrinthine Concussion' to denote damage to the labyrinth, without any evidence of fracture. Schuknecht (1969) has postulated labyrinthine concussion as one of the aetiological factors leading to cupulolithiasis, which he proposes as a cause of post-traumatic positional nystagmus. In this condition, Schuknecht has suggested, on the basis of histological studies of the temporal bone, that post-traumatic degeneration of the utricular otolithic membrane may release otoconia, which then become deposited upon the cupula of the posterior semicircular canal, where they provoke rotatory nystagmus on change of position. Other aetiological factors suggested as responsible for the development of cupulolithiasis, include spontaneous degeneration of the utricular otolithic membrane and ischaemia, in the territory of the anterior vestibular artery. Both these latter conditions are more likely to occur in an elderly population, with pre-existing cervical spondylosis and vertebrobasilar insufficiency, thus making the elderly patient more susceptible to the effects of head and neck trauma.

As has been discussed earlier in this chapter, the symptom of dizziness is generally a result of failure of integration of sensory input (Bos, 1962). In craniocervical trauma, injury to the brainstem may result in dysfunction of the data storage and integrating centres which have been described by Henriksson (1970). This injury is superimposed on age-dependent defects in integration, possibily due to a reduction in the number of neurones, which has been observed by the same author (Henriksson, 1976). In addition, cerebrovascular disease often may have resulted in pre-existing central nervous system disease, and it may therefore, readily be understood that elderly patients do not compensate as well, or as quickly, from vestibular insults, as their younger counterparts. Furthermore, Pearson and Barber (1973) emphasise that in the majority of cases of head injury, there is an organic basis for the high incidence of emotional and intellectual disorders, which are much more important, than the cochlear or vestibular dysfunctions, in delaying recovery. These emotional and psychiatric consquences of head injury are particularly important in the elderly, in whom there is a higher prevalence of pre-existing mental dysfunction (Bender, 1975). Consideration of these factors underlines that compensation and habituation to vestibular injuries are age and motivation dependent. The elderly person who suffers craniocervical injury is, therefore, at a severe disadvantage.

It is clear that the site of the underlying pathological disturbance may be anywhere in the vestibular system from the peripheral labyrinth to the cerebral cortex and examination may therefore reveal both abnormal central and peripheral vestibular signs. The most crucial procedure however, is a briskly performed Cawthorne positional test (Ch. 12) as this may provide the only positive finding. The features which clinically distinguish nystagmus of benign paroxysmal type

Table 16.4 Characteristics of positional nystagmus

	Benign paroxysmal type	Central type
Latent period	2–20 seconds	None
Adaption	Disappears in 50 seconds	Persists
Fatiguability	Disappears on repetition	Persists
Vertigo	Always present	Typically absent
Direction of nystagmus	To undermost ear	Variable
Incidence	Relatively common	Relatively uncommon

from positional vertigo of more sinister central nervous system disease are listed in Table 16.4.

Positional nystagmus

There is a considerable controversy in the literature regarding the classification and interpretation of positional nystagmus, which is reported to occur predominantly in later life (Schuknecht, 1969; Spencer-Harrison and Ozsahinoglu, 1975). This disorder may result from trauma, as discussed above, but is also associated with aural pathology (Dix and Hallpike, 1952); spontaneous degenerative change in the vestibular labyrinth (Schuknecht, 1969); cervical spondylosis (Sandstrom, 1962); vertebrobasilar ischaemia (Spencer-Harrison and Ozsahinoglu, 1972); brainstem disorders, such as demyelination, ischaemia, e.g. occlusion of the anterior vestibular artery (Lindsay and Hemenway, 1956); posterior fossa tumours (Nylén, 1939; Cawthorne and Hinchcliffe, 1961); alcohol (Aschan et al, 1964) and drug intoxication, (Dix, 1973).

The work of Nylén (1939) and Hallpike (1967) have defined two clear cut types of positional nystagmus:

1. Nystagmus which persists as long as the critical head position is maintained, and in which vertigo is inconstant.
2. Transitory nystagmus with marked vertigo.

Aschan (1961) has sub-divided the first group into persistent nystagmus, which is direction-changing (commonly reversing in opposite head positions) and persistent nystagmus, which is direction-fixed, irrespective of head position. Spencer-Harrison and Ozsahinoglu (1972) have classified a third group of paroxysmal cases, in which the characteristics of the nystagmus are not clear cut, in that, although the vertigo may be severe, the direction and form of the nystagmus may be atypical. The same authors have reported that in 50 per cent of a large series of 476 patients, with all types of positional nystagmus, no underlying pathology could be identified despite prolonged follow-up. Nonetheless, 38 per cent of cases with persistent positional nystagmus were found to have central lesions, compared with only 4 per cent of patients with paroxysmal positional nystagmus.

Nylén (1950) found that 22 per cent of cases of brain tumour had positional nystagmus, which occurred more commonly with subtentorial tumours (69 per cent), than with supratentorial tumours (26 per cent). However, only 2 per cent of patients with positional nystagmus have been found to have intra-cranial tumours, (Schiller and Hedberg, 1960).

In the assessment of positional nystagmus, an attempt should be made to define a possible underlying aetiology, and in the elderly, vertebrobasilar insufficiency, cervical lesions and trauma should be particularly considered, and primary aural pathology must be excluded. The clinical features of the nystagmus may suggest whether or not a central disorder should be suspected. All cases of positional nystagmus should undergo full audiometric and vestibular testing, together with routine assessment of the cardiovascular and neurological systems. If abnormalities are detected, further investigation of the central nervous system may be indicated.

Positional vertigo of the benign paroxysmal type is now frequently attributed to the pathological state of cupulolithiasis (see above). It is generally self-limiting, especially following head injury, but, in the elderly, experience has shown that this is not always the case and, if the underlying aetiology is vertebrobasilar insufficiency, symptoms may persist for many months, or even years. Spencer-Harrison and Ozsahinoglu, (1972) have made the observation that 'a protracted recovery from positional vertigo is much more likely in the later years of life, when, indeed, the disability may be permanent.'

Patients are often alarmed by their attacks and considerable therapeutic benefit is derived from an understandable explanation. In the absence of any sinister symptoms or signs, it is valuable to explain that regardless of how symptomatically disturbing positional vertigo may be, it is essentially a benign condition. Most patients adjust to the disorder by a set of self-imposed restrictions to avoid precipitating their symptoms. Nonetheless, it is advisable to counsel patients to perform movements slowly, which they know will precipitate their symptoms and to avoid provocative positions. They should be reminded of the dangers of certain situations, for example climbing ladders, standing on the edge of station platforms. In most cases, patients may be allowed to continue to drive, as vertigo results very rarely from rotational neck movements alone. The symptoms are frequently exacerbated by loss of confidence, and rehabilitation may be accelerated by a system of re-educative vestibular exercises of the type devised by Cawthorne (1945) and Cooksey (1945). Drug therapy is, in general, ineffective, although diazepam 2 mg three times daily and at bed time may be helpful for an extremely over-anxious patient. Specific therapy, such as a cervical collar, for a limited period, in the case of cervical spondylosis may be helpful. Anti-coagulant therapy has been advocated for the relief of positional nystagmus of ischaemic origin (Barber, 1973), but the advantages of this therapy must be weighed against the disadvantages (overdosage, drug interaction, risk of cerebral haemorrhage), especially in an elderly patient, who may be hypertensive.

In very rare instances, when the disability is so severe as to interfere with the quality of life, it may be necessary to consider surgical labyrinthectomy to destroy the vestibular end organ; division of the vestibular portion of the vestibulocochlear nerve by the posterior fossa approach (Barber, 1973); or denervation of the posterior semicircular ampulla by section of its nerve (Gacek, 1978).

Vestibular neuronitis

'Vestibular neuronitis' is the term given to the entity of vertigo unaccompanied by cochlear symptoms or signs. Although this condition may be seen in the elderly, it is rare and, indeed in the definitive paper on this subject (Dix and Hallpike, 1952) only one patient out of the series of 100 was over 60 years of age. The vertigo is usually self-limiting, within seven to ten days, and treatment is symptomatic. Recent work has suggested that the term 'vestibular neuronitis' comprises a heterogenous group of disorders which require improved diagnostic methods to enable further classification (Clemis and Becker, 1973).

Infection

Any acute infective process may be associated with general malaise and dizziness. Specific viral neurolabyrinthitis often results in bilateral labyrinthine abnormalities, in which cochlear and vestibular derangements may occur on opposite sides (Cawthorne et al, 1969). Vertigo, as a consequence of bacterial infection of the middle ear cleft, develops more frequently from chronic destructive middle ear disease than from acute infection. Acute infective labyrinthitis, secondary to otitis media, should be recognised easily by the development of sensorineural hearing loss and severe rotatory vertigo. This condition demands immediate swabs for microbiological examination, followed by antibiotic therapy. Chronic middle ear disease is very prevalent condition in the elderly, and it cannot be over-stressed that, in any patient with vestibular symptoms, in whom there is the slightest suspicion of middle ear disease, the presumptive diagnosis must be of labyrinthine erosion (Fig. 16.15). Only if operative inspection fails to reveal such a cause should other explanations for the vertigo be sought. A spontaneous fistula of the labyrinth is almost always the result of bone erosion by cholesteatoma, but it may rarely occur in syphilitic osteitis, tuberculous otitis media, chronic perilabyrinthine osteomyelitis, or neoplasia, e.g. carcinoma or a glomus jugulare tumour.

Accidental destruction of the labyrinth, with total cochlear loss and severe vertigo may occur following middle ear operations. Vestibular symptoms usually abate in ten days to two weeks but this process takes longer and recovery may be

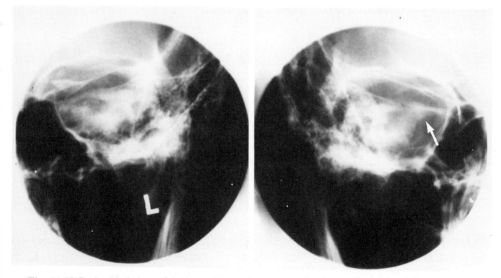

Fig. 16.15 Peri-orbital views of the internal acoustic meatuses showing erosion of the right petrous apex (as arrowed) in a case of cholesteatoma.

incomplete, in older patients. Furthermore, 'breakdown in compensation' may occur if the patient becomes unwell for some other reason or there is subsequent impairment of other sensory systems.

In the long term, after mastoid surgery, vertigo and imbalance may develop for many reasons, the most important of which include:

1. Persisting disease with further bone erosion.
2. 'Perilabyrinthitis'.
3. Delayed endolymphatic hydrops.
4. Compensation breakdown, after labyrinthine destruction.
5. Unrelated vestibular disease.
6. Cerebellar abscess.

Cawthorne (1975b) has described the condition of 'perilabyrinthitis', in which there is a fistula of one of the bony semicircular canals, caused either by injury or disease, but the activity of the end organ remains unimpaired. Pressure and temperature variations may create minor disturbances in the labyrinth and produce episodes of vertigo, or bizarre effects upon equilibrium and gait.

Even in the current era of antibiotic treatment, no consideration of infection is complete without some discussion of syphilis. It is well recognised that both congenital and late acquired syphilitic aural disease show a slow relentless progression to profound bilateral deafness, but vestibular disturbances may be the presenting feature, and certainly form an important part of the natural history in the majority of patients. Vestibular manifestations may present in episodes indistinguishable from Ménière's disease, or there may be slowly progressive bilateral destruction of the vestibular end organs resulting in progressive imbalance and unsteadiness of gait, especially in the dark. Morrison (1979) emphasises that 'the diagnosis of late acquired syphilitic ear disease is probably missed quite often, especially in elderly male patient.' Specific serological tests for syphilis (*Treponema pallidum* Haemoglutination Test and Flourescent Treponemal Antibody Test) are required to establish the diagnosis, and treatment requires hospitalisation to ensure adequate penicillin and steroid therapy (Pirozzi, 1973).

Otosclerosis and Paget's disease

Otosclerosis is a common hereditary, localised disease of the bone derived from the otic capsule. Morrison (1979) notes that in 4 per cent of patients with this disorder, hearing loss is first noted over 45 years of age. Paparella and Chasin (1966) have described a variety of vestibular symptoms in otosclerosis and Donaldson (1976) has reported vertigo in 4 per cent of his patients, making this an extremely rare cause of dizziness in the elderly. *Paget's disease* may also affect the otic capsule and may give rise to hearing loss and vertigo (Davis, 1968) (Fig. 16.16). In the presence of obvious skeletal changes (enlarged skull, short stature, kyphosis, bowing of the legs) the diagnosis is straightforward, but osteitis deformans may be symtomless, apart from the otological features and in these circumstances, the diagnosis is easily missed. The hearing loss may be conductive or mixed in type, and the diagnosis may be confirmed by skull radiographs, an elevated serum alkaline phosphatase, and by an increase in the total urinary hydroxyproline.

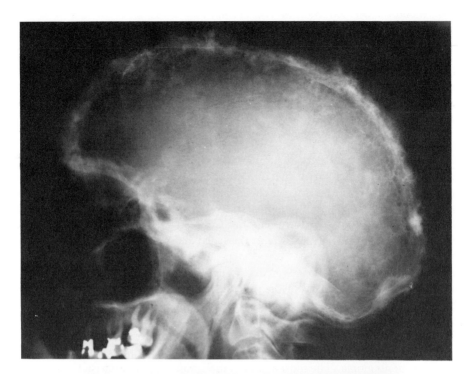

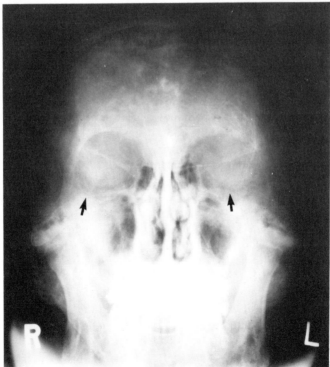

Fig. 16.16 Radiographs of the skull of a 63-year-old man presenting with drop attacks, episodes of dizziness and sensorineural hearing loss, showing gross Paget's disease of the skull with temporal bone involvement (A) and elevation of the middle fossa, (B) as arrowed.

Vascular accidents

Elderly patients may suffer vascular accidents involving the labyrinthine blood supply (see vertebrobasilar insufficiency, p. 414). In these cases, there is acute vertigo, with associated sudden deafness. The absence of other abnormal physical signs in the central nervous system, together with the history, points to the diagnosis.

Tumours

As in all situations in the body, tumours may be divided into those which are benign and those which are malignant. Aural tumours are, in general, rare, but in the benign category in the elderly, cholesteatomas (see Infection, p. 433), glomus tumours, haemangioma, schwannomas from not only the acoustic nerve sheath (see: Neurological Causes—Infra-tentorial Lesions—Tumours, p. 421), but also arising from other cranial nerves, e.g. the facial and glossopharyngeal, should be considered.

Cancer of the temporal bone is an exceedingly rare condition (Lodge et al, 1955), but, Broders (1921) found the median age for cancer of the ear to be 61 years, and it should, therefore, be considered in the elderly.

In this age group, secondary tumour involvement is important and may be a result of direct extension or distant metastases. Direct extension arises from the nasal part of pharynx, external ear, parotid gland or the temporomandibular joint, or from a meningioma. The most common malignancy to metastasise by the blood stream is a hypernephroma, but other sites of origin, include the lung, prostate, breast and uterus.

A non-metastatic complication of malignant tumours is involvement of the vestibular nerve in the progressive degeneration of carcinomatous encephalomyelitis, i.e. the motor and sensory neuropathy associated with a malignant tumour.

Auto-immune disorders

Auto-immune disorders result in immunological destruction of the body's own tissue, following a breakdown of the body's auto-tolerance. Although the majority of these conditions are rare, the following should be considered in an elderly, vertiginous patient: Wegener's granulomatosis (1963); temporal arteritis, in which vertigo has been reported as a prodromal symptom in 18 per cent (Kinmont and McCullum, 1965); Cogan's syndrome (1945); Behcet's syndrome, in which vertigo and nystagmus have recently been reported (Hughes and Learner, 1979); relapsing polychondritis (McAdam et al, 1976); polyarteritis nodosa (Gussen, 1979) and systemic lupus erythematosis (McRae and O'Reilly, 1957).

The clinician should be aware of the possibility of auto-immune disease presenting with vestibular disturbances, as early diagnosis is important in these potentially lethal, systemic conditions (Stephens, Luxon and Hinchcliffe, 1981). An elevated sedementation rate, disproportionate to the apparent general condition, may be a valuable pointer to an auto-immune pathology. Immunosuppressive drugs and steroids are the mainstays of treatment.

Drug intoxications

The number of drugs and chemical agents, with a documented ototoxic action is legion (Worthington el al, 1973). The most important include antibiotics (particularly the aminoglycosides), salicylates (and other analgesics), antimalarials and diuretics, but other categories of drugs, which may produce dizziness include analeptics, anaesthetic agents, anticonvulsants, antidepressants, antidiabetic agents, antihistamines, antiinflammatory drugs, cytotoxic agents, antituberculous drugs, cardiovascular drugs, hormone therapy, sedatives, tranquillisers and some chemical agents, such as heavy metals, nicotine and tobacco.

Many elderly patients, as has already been discussed, require many drugs and are, therefore, particularly susceptible to vertigo and dizziness on an iatrogenic basis (Alberti and Black, 1968). Cardiovascular drugs are commonly implicated, as they may cause a reduced cardiac output (e.g. betablockers), dysrhythmias (e.g. digoxin) or orthostatic hypotension (e.g. ganglionic blockers). Psychotropic drugs are also frequently prescribed and may result in hallucinations, with distortion of visual and auditory input, or may impair psychomotor and co-ordination functions (Goodman and Gilman, 1975). Furthermore, overdosage with anticonvulsants may result in severe imbalance and nystagmus, indistinguishable from a posterior fossa syndrome (Nozue et al, 1973).

The majority of drugs causing vertigo affect the internal ear. In the elderly, aspirin, which may be taken as a cure for all sorts of ailments, diuretics and the aminoglycoside antibiotics are particularly troublesome. The vestibulotoxic effect of the latter group (streptomycin, kanamycin and neomycin) has been shown to be mainly confined to the labyrinth (Cawthorne and Ranger, 1957). The effect on the vestibular system may be unilateral (Dayal, Smith and McCain, 1974), which results in an imbalance of vestibular tonus and thereby produces vertigo. The aminoglycoside antibiotics are particularly hazardous, especially with concurrent diuretic therapy and/or in the presence of renal failure. It has been emphasised that, especially in the elderly, they should only be used as a lifesaving measure (Ballantyne, 1979).

MISCELLANEOUS CAUSES OF VERTIGO

Ocular vertigo

In 1794, Erasmus Darwin wrote 'many people, when they arrive at 50 or 60 years of age, are affected by slight vertigo; which is generally ascribed to indigestion, but in reality arises from the beginning defect of their sight . . . . These people do not see objects so distinctly as formerly, and by exerting their eyes more than usual they perceive the apparent motions of objects, and confound them with the real motions of them; and, therefore, cannot accurately balance themselves so as easily to preserve their perpendicularity by them.' Ocular vertigo is usually a sense of unsteadiness, or disorientation, caused by mismatch of information gathered from the visual system, the labyrinths and the somatosensory system. The role of these senses in the maintenance of equilibrium has been discussed, and when visual input is defective, such that there is a contradiction between the true visual input, and the expected visual input, pathological visual vertigo results (Brandt, 1981).

Vision plays a major role in postural stabilisation and attenuates body sway by 50 to 100 per cent (Travis, 1945; Edwards, 1946). In the elderly, defective vision may be superimposed upon other defective sensory modalities to result in dizziness, or imbalance, as described by Drachman and Hart (1972). It is well documented that vertigo may be associated with heights, acrophobia, (Adler, 1942) and wide open spaces, agoraphobia. It is of particular interest that Takeya and his colleagues (1978) have reported that the occasional development of acrophobia in the elderly following head or whiplash injury may be attributed to opthalmological abnormalities, e.g. ocular muscle palsies. However, it is possible that this is the result of a post-traumatic neurotic reaction, initiated by damage to the otoliths.

In an elderly population, disturbed orientation in space arising from the use of spectacle lenses is probably the commonest ocular disturbance giving rise to this complaint of dizziness. Spectacles may disturb an individual's meridional magnification and aniseikonia (inequality in size of retinal images) (Belmont, 1967).

Much more rarely, nuclear and supranuclear disorders of eye movement may give rise to oscillopsia, which may be interpreted as dizziness. This disorder is characteristically seen in demyelination involving the cerebellar nuclei (Aschoff, 1974) and in floccular or medullary brainstem lesions, producing down beat nystagmus (Cogan, 1968). Infra-nuclear oculomotor disturbances, e.g. acute ocular muscle paresis, secondary to ocular myaesthenia or vascular insult, may give rise to discrepancies between the expected, and the actual, visual input, which result in difficulties of locomotion and posture. Head exercises promote sensory readjustment, with disappearance of balance disturbances, despite the persistence of the ocular defect.

Odontogenic vertigo

Goodfriend (1967) has written extensively on the aetiological role of dental malocclusion and temporomandibular joint abnormalities in dizziness and vertigo. Both dental malocclusion and temporomandibular joint dysfunction are very common in the elderly population, but the exact pathophysiological mechanism by which they produce vestibular symptoms is not clear. It would seem probable that this postulated relationship is, in fact, merely a reflection of the frequent coincidental occurrence of two very common conditions.

Cervical vertigo

Cervical vertigo is the term used to describe positional dizziness which is induced by changes of the neck with relation to the body. For many years it has been known that movements of the neck can provoke attacks of dizziness and induce nystagmus (Bárány, 1918; Voŝs, 1925; de Kleijn and Nieuwenhuyse, 1927). In normal subjects, rotations of less than 90° will usually suffice to produce these findings. Furthermore, the labyrinths are not essential for the provocation of this type of nystagmus (Bos, 1962).

With this knowledge, many cervical lesions have been implicated as causes of vertigo (cervical spondylosis—Davis, 1953; trauma to the vertebrae—Rebattu and Lesne, 1962; avulsed nerve roots—Decher, Rohr, Unterharnscheidt, 1958; trauma to the joints—Stoddard, 1952; lesions of the neck muscles—Gray, 1956; cervical adenopathy—Mayoux, 1953; involvement of the vertebral artery— Sandstrom, 1962 and brachial radiculitis or neuritis—Biemond, 1940). Twenty-five years ago, Ryan and Cope (1955) highlighted the problem: 'We are convinced that the neck plays a larger part in the mechanism of vertigo than is generally thought,' and it has been re-emphasised more recently by Wyke (1979). 'One such influence which, however, is often not considered in relation to this important clinical problem (senile dysequilibrium) is that arising from alterations in the perceptual and reflexogenic contributions normally made to posture and gait by the mechanoreceptors located in the apophyseal joints of the cervical spine'.

The literature reveals a considerable divergence of opinion as to the underlying pathophysiological mechanisms responsible for dizziness and vertigo in neck disorders. Three theories have been postulated to explain cervical vertigo; (i) sympathetic irritation resulting in circulatory disorders of the vertebro-basilar system (Barré, 1926); (ii) episodic ischaemia of the brainstem as a result of intermittent vertebral artery compression by osteophytes due to cervical spondylosis (Sheehan et al, 1960) and (iii) deranged somatosensory input from the kinaesthetic receptors located within the cervical spine (de Jong, 1967). It would, however, seem probable that vertigo resulting from disorders of the neck is most probably not provoked by one single factor, but is the combined effect of probably all of the above pathogenic factors (Pfaltz and Richter, 1958), especially in the elderly (Fig. 16.17).

Many authors writing on vertigo and nystagmus complicating disorders of the neck, especially in the elderly, have tended to attribute the underlying pathological process to vertebrobasilar insufficiency. Wyke (1979) has emphasised the problems

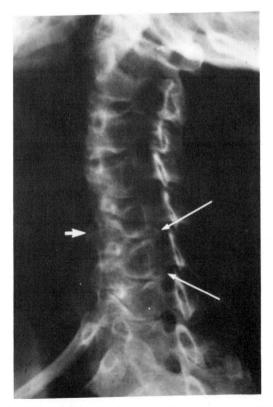

Fig. 16.17 Oblique view of the cervical spine showing degenerative changes at C5/6, C6/7 and C7/8 levels with disc space narrowing and osteophyte encroachment on the exit foramina.

of disturbances of equilibrium faced by many elderly people in their everyday lives, and has drawn attention to the role of the cervical articular mechanoreceptors in this context. Some experimental data (Cohen, 1961; Igarashi et al, 1969) and a number of clinical observations (de Jong, 1967; Jongkees, 1969) have suggested that these receptors are vital for both the sense of balance and cervical kinaesthesis (i.e. awareness of head and neck movement). It has been clearly documented that there is an age-dependent, degenerative loss of mechanoreceptor afferent systems (Arnold and Harriman, 1970), which may partly explain abnormalities of balance in the elderly. It is clear that any additional disease, e.g. arthritis of the cervical spine joints will exacerbate this dysfunction.

In attempting to differentiate the symptomatology of cervical vertigo from vertebrobasilar insufficiency, both Jongkees (1969) and Pfaltz (1981) emphasise the entirely different clinical picture suggesting a peripheral, rather than a central lesion. Furthermore, both Arslan (1952) and Aschan and Hugosson (1966) have drawn attention to the fact that unilateral, or even bilateral, compression of the vertebral arteries will hardly cause any brainstem ischaemia, provided that the internal carotid arteries and the circulus arteriosus (Circle of Willis) are functioning normally.

The symptomatology of vertebrobasilar insufficiency has been fully described above, and at this point, it is perhaps sufficient to emphasise that although vertigo or dizziness is common in vertebrobasilar arterial disease, it is important to seek additional signs of brainstem involvement before making this diagnosis (Troost, 1980). The symptomatology associated with cervical vertigo has been clearly outlined by Kuilman (1959), Jongkees (1969), and Pfaltz (1981). Essentially, the features consist of the classical symptoms of neck and occipital pain, especially in the morning, associated with paraesthesiae in the arms, affecting the involved cervical roots. There may be muscle weakness and wasting, with depression of the reflexes of the corresponding nerve roots, together with depression of posterior column sensation. Often there are also symptoms of both auditory and vestibular dysfunction. Unilateral sensorineural hearing loss, with evidence of recruitment, may progress to bilateral symmetrical involvement. Approximately one third of Kuilman's (1959) patients complained of tinnitus, and approximately one fifth of disturbances of equilibrium. Jongkees (1969) described a number of patients with cervical vertigo as presenting with a classical Ménière's syndrome, but vestibular symptoms tended to be more prominent than cochlear symptoms.

In distinguishing cervical vertigo from vertebrobasilar insufficiency, the symptomatology, especially the presence of auditory symptoms and pain in the neck or base of skull, together with normal optokinetic responses, and a positive, passive neck torsion test (Jongkees, 1969; Toglia, 1975) help to confirm the diagnosis. It should be emphasised that radiographs may not be helpful, as many persons over sixty years of age show osteo-arthritic spurs or other degenerative changes of the cervical vertebrae.

Vestibulocochlear symptoms associated with cervical spondylosis, but without evidence of a circulatory disorder, may be explained on the basis of a disturbance of the mechanoreceptors of the cervical spine apophyseal joints and/or, by chronic irritation of the sympathetic plexus. Rotation and/or hyperextension of the neck may lead to erroneous information regarding the position of the head in space, caused by pathological sensory input from the kinaesthetic receptors in the cervical spine. This, in turn, leads to spatial disorientation and subjective vertigo. Irritation of the sympathetic chain may lead to alterations in the blood circulation of the internal ear, causing tinnitus, hearing loss, vertigo and nystagmus.

Local treatment in the form of heat, massage, correction of posture, immobilisation of the neck in a cervical collar, cervical contour pillow, neck traction, neck exercises, muscle relaxant drugs and psychotherapy all have a place in the treatment of this disorder (Jackson, 1958). If these simple measures fail, local anaesthetic infiltration may be of value in an acutely painful situation with severe symptoms. The need for judicious, gentle traction must be underlined in view of Ryan and Cope's (1955) experience of severe cervical vertigo as a result of more vigorous traction.

MANAGEMENT AND TREATMENT

The foregoing discussion underlines the observation that dizziness is a very common problem for many elderly people, and difficulties in treatment, undoubtedly, arise as a result of the many different and varied pathologies, which may result in this symptom. The initial management of the new patient must be directed at establishing the underlying diagnosis of the condition (or conditions) giving rise to vertigo, and instituting the correct therapy for each general medical, neurological or otological condition. The specific treatment of disorders responsible for dizziness is beyond the scope of this presentation but a brief outline of therapeutic options has been mentioned under each disease heading. The following discussion is centred around the symptomatic treatment of dizziness, when all treatable conditions have been excluded and/or appropriately treated, with persistent symptoms.

In reviewing the treatment of dizziness, it is perhaps valuable to recall certain facts regarding the underlying mechanisms of this symptom. In general, the pathophysiology of most vestibular disorders is poorly understood, and it is therefore impossible to consider specific therapy. The literature abounds with reports of 'successes' with different modes of treatment. However, many of these reports are based on insufficient data obtained from uncontrolled and/or poorly designed clinical trials. The reasons for this are multiple: the differential diagnosis of vestibular disorders may be difficult; difficulty may be experienced in evaluating therapeutic results in conditions with natural remissions, (in Ménière's disease, a 60–80 per cent 'success rate' has been reported regardless of the treatment modalities-Torok, 1977). Moreover, there is difficulty in objectively evaluating a subjective symptom such as dizziness or vertigo. Furthermore, it can hardly be expected that this symptom, which may arise by means of a number of pathological processes, will respond to a single particular drug.

The symptomatic treatment of dizziness may be divided into medical and surgical aspects.

1. Medical treatment
    a. Counselling
    b. Drug therapy
    c. Head and balance exercises
2. Surgical treatment

Medical

Counselling

There are many reports of the anxiety experienced by patients suffering from episodes of dizziness or vertigo (Cawthorne 1957; Rubin, 1973). This is especially important in the elderly, who may not only be fearful that they are suffering from a brain tumour, or some other incurable illness, but who also, because of their circumstances, e.g. living alone, crippled by arthritis, may be terrified of the consequences of repeated severe attacks of vertigo, during which they are unable to summon outside assistance. For these reasons it is especially important in the elderly to listen to the patient's complaints and anxieties, to perform a full examination with particular attention to the neurological and otological systems and to institute the most appropriate system of investigation. By these means, it is possible to provide the patient with a simple and clear explanation of their problem and the therapeutic measures, which will be undertaken. Conscientious evaluation of the elderly patient results in a good doctor-patient rapport, which is essential if any progress is to be made in the management of this problem. Furthermore, it ensures that the patient does not feel that he himself, or his problem, is being dismissed, purely because of his age.

Drug therapy

Many different pharmacological agents have been used in an attempt to alleviate the symptoms of dizziness and vertigo.

Psychotherapeutic drugs.   Sedatives and tranquillisers are used on the assumption that they may change the threshold of response of the vestibular receptors, or of the synaptic connections in the vestibular pathways (Goodman and Gilman, 1970). Simple sedatives, such as diazepam are to be preferred, but barbiturates may be used (Hinchcliffe, 1972), although the problems of addiction, drug interaction, and overdose, must be borne in mind. Tranquillisers of the phenothiazine type should be avoided, especially in the elderly, because of their autonomic and, particularly, extrapyramidal side effects (Ekbom and Ekstrand, 1972). Thiethylperazine, a phenothiazine derivative, has been reported to accumulate in the vestibular nuclear areas of the cerebellum and it has, therefore, been advocated in the treatment of vertigo of central origin. There is, however, no good evidence of its efficacy (Jungert, 1978). After careful evaluation, antidepressants may on occasions be valuable in the treatment of vertigo (Hinchcliffe, 1972). However, it must be borne in mind that, in the elderly, with reduced cerebral reserve, all these categories of drugs may result in toxic confusional states and/or chronic intoxication, including dizziness, weakness, slurred speech and nystagmus.

Antihistamines.   This group of drugs has been extensively used in the treatment of dizziness, both because of their effects of lowering the threshold of reactivity of the vestibular system, and also because of an assumed central affect on the reticular formation and thalamus (Dolowitz et al, 1967). In the elderly, their anticholinergic side effects may be especially troublesome, as may be the potential hazard of accidents associated with sedation and somnolence. Difenidol is an atypical member of this group (Katz et al, 1969). It has been found to have a markedly suppressive action on the vestibular end organ. The major drawback is the reported side effect of hallucinations. Initial administration of this drug should, therefore, be confined to hospital practice. Despite the initial excellent reports of cinnarizine, (Jongkees, 1964) in the control of dizziness, no unequivocal controlled data has emerged to support this view (Drug and Therapeutics Bulletin, 1981).

Antiemetics. Prochlorperazine is a phenothiazine derivative with stong antihistaminic properties, which is thought to act directly on the brainstem. It is advocated for the treatment of vertigo caused by Ménière's disease, labyrinthitis and many other causes, but there is no definite clinical evidence of its efficacy.

Trimethobenzamide, an ethanol substituted antihistamine, is assumed to have a similar mode of action without the undesirable extrapyramidal and sedative side effects. Rubin (1973) strongly recommends this drug for the control of the vegetative symptoms in patients with dizziness and vertigo.

Anticholinergics. Numerous animal studies indicate that drugs with anticholinergic activity diminish the excitability of the vestibular nucleus neurones. These drugs suppress both the spontaneous firing rate and response to vestibular nerve stimulation, suggesting a cholinergic transmission from the primary to the secondary vestibular neurones. The antivertiginous properties of antihistamines may in part, be due to their weak anticholinergic activity. Both atropine and scopolamine may produce excellent symptomatic improvement when used in the treatment of acute vertigo of labyrinthine origin.

Vasodilators. Vasodilators have been used in the treatment of dizziness ascribed to neurovascular or vascular pathology, e.g. endolymphatic hydrops, sudden vestibular failure, whiplash injuries and head trauma. Nicotinic acid has been widely used, but experimental work has shown that with respect to cerebral vessels, buphenine is more effective.

Histamine is a potent vasodilator and has been used in Ménière's disease on the assumption that arteriolar spasm of the stria vascularis is a cause of endolymphatic hydrops. In view of the difficulty in administration of histamine (sublingual or parenteral), betahistine, an orally active histamine analogue, has been introduced. This drug has been shown to increase the capillary blood flow of the stria vascularis in animals (Snow and Suga, 1973), and postulated therefore to reduce endolymphatic pressure. There have been many unsatisfactory, uncontrolled longitudinal studies supporting the value of this drug in the treatment of vertigo, but only in the case of Ménière's disease has a randomised, double-blind, cross-over trial (Frew and Menon, 1976), supported this claim.

Diuretics. In the treatment of Ménière's disease, hydrochlorothiazide has been convincingly demonstrated (Klockhoff and Lindblom, 1967) to improve symptoms (hearing loss, vertigo and general condition). Similar results have also been reported for chlortalidone (Klockoff et al, 1974). There is no evidence that these drugs are generally helpful in the treatment of vertigo. It should be emphasised that certain diuretics (furosemide and etacrynic acid) are ototoxic and should not be used as diuretics in the prescence of any otological condition.

Anticoagulants. These drugs have been used in the case of sudden vestibular failure and vertigo associated with vertebrobasilar ischaemia. The dangers of cerebral haemorrhage and drug interactions must be weighed against their possible value, especially in the elderly.

Head and balance exercises

With the head erect, vestibular tonus in the normal subject is equal and opposite from the left and right ears. When injury results in an inequality, vertigo is experienced. Initially, the central nervous system may compensate by cerebellar and visual mechanisms, which suppress the undamaged and therefore overactive vestibular nuclei (Courjon et al, 1977; Putkonen et al, 1977). Later, intrinsic activity develops in the depressed vestibular nuclei as a direct result of the imbalance itself (McCabe, 1970). In Lacour's (1976) elegant experiments with baboons, it was clearly shown that promotion of movement following a unilateral vestibular neurectomy resulted in more rapid recovery. Thus the rationale of head and balance exercises in vestibular disorders is to deliberately and systematically provoke episodes of vertigo such that compensations may more rapidly develop.

A system of such exercises was initially described by the late Sir Terence Cawthorne (Cawthorne, 1945) and Dr Cooksey (1945) at King's College Hospital, London. These exercises have been found of particular value in peripheral vestibular lesions, but are of limited value in the treatment of central causes of vertigo. The exercises are particularly valuable in cases of head injury, imbalance following streptomycin intoxication, and in psychogenic disorders. An excellent review of the exact procedure is given by Dix (1979).

SURGICAL TREATMENT

Surgical intervention in the treatment of vertigo is indicated in three situations:

1. To secure the safety of the patient, e.g. complications of otitis media, chronic middle ear disease.
2. To improve the quality of life of a patient suffering from severe, recurrent vertigo, and in whom other measures have failed.
3. To exclude a perilymph fistula.

In the elderly, the indications for surgery must be carefully weighed against the general medical state of the patient. It cannot be over-emphasised that before destructive surgery is undertaken, there must be no doubt as to the exact site and side of the lesion. Furthermore, as has already been noted in the elderly, compensation may be prolonged, or indeed, incomplete as a result of dysfunction of the integrating ability of the central nervous system or other sensory modalities. The risk of persisting imbalance, must, therefore, be carefully considered when advising older patients.

Ludman's (1981) excellent review of the surgical treatment of vertigo, covers, in detail, the indications and alternative procedures available in the management of vertigo. The most pertinent of these are briefly reviewed.

Exploration of the middle ear is mandatory in a vertiginous patient with any evidence whatsoever of middle ear disease. If cholesteatoma is encountered, a labyrinthine fistula should always be sought. The exact operative management of this problem depends, to a large extent, on the type of operation in progress, and the state of auditory and vestibular function in both the operated ear and the other ear. Accidental destruction of the labyrinth, with total cochlear and/or vestibular failure, following a middle ear operation may occur. Following mastoid surgery, vertigo may develop for a number of reasons, as has already been explained under the heading of Infection (see: Otologic Causes of Vertigo, 5).

Intractable, positional vertigo of the benign, paroxysmal type, is probably the commonest cause of vertigo which may necessitate destructive surgery. Again, the surgical alternatives for treatment of this disorder have been mentioned earlier in this Chapter. More rarely in the elderly, Ménière's disease may require operative intervention. Surgical management of this condition may be divided into those procedures which are aimed at improvement of the underlying pathophysiological process, and those aimed at alleviating symptoms, by disconnection of the brain from the diseased labyrinth. A discussion of the rationale behind these different forms of treatment, is beyond the scope of this presentation, but, it should be mentioned that the first group of operations include endolymphatic sac operations (House, 1962), sacculotomy (Cody, 1967), cervical sympathectomy (Wilmot, 1969) and the insertion of a tympanostomy tube ('grommet') (Tumarkin, 1966), while destructive operations include surgical labyrinthectomy (Cawthorne, 1956), ultrasonic vestibular destruction (Angell-James, 1969) and vestibular nerve section (Glasscock et al, 1980). Following labyrinthine destruction, vertigo may persist, and the explanations proposed for this phenomenon are compensation breakdown, persisting vestibular dysfunction and vestibular nerve ending stimulation.

Labyrinthine membrane ruptures, giving rise to perilymph fistulae through the oval or round windows, should be considered following trauma in the elderly. Vestibular symptoms, accompanying typically sudden, severe sensorineural hearing loss, may suggest the diagnosis, and a positive fistula sign may be helpful confirmatory evidence. An exploratory tympanotomy is the only means of effectively demonstrating a perilymph leak; even then, the findings are frequently not clear-cut. It should be noted that surgical repair of a fistula results in excellent improvement of vestibular symptoms, but the results for the restoration of hearing are poor (Althaus, 1977).

REFERENCES

Agate J 1963 The practice of geriatrics. Heinemann, London, p 91
Alberti P W R M, Black J I M 1968 Iatrogenic symptoms in otolaryngology. Journal of Laryngology and Otology 82:731–737
Alder F H 1942 Ocular vertigo. Transactions of the American Academy of Ophthalmology 46:27–32
Alpers B J 1960 Vertiginous epilepsy. Laryngoscope 70:631–637
Althaus S R 1977 Spontaneous and traumatic perilymph fistulas. Laryngoscope 87:364–371
Angell-James J 1969 Ménière's disease: treatment with ultrasound. Journal of Laryngology 83:771–785
Arenburg I K, Bayer R F 1977 Therapeutic options in Ménière's disease. Archives of Otolaryngology 103:589–593
Arnold N, Harriman D G 1970 The incidence of abnormality in control of human peripheral nerves, studied by single axon dissection. Journal of Neurology, Neurosurgery and Psychiatry 33:55–61
Arslan M 1952 La pathogénie du syndrome sympathique postérieur Revue Oto-Neuro-Ophthalmologie 24:1–6
Arslan M 1957 The senescence of the vestibular apparatus Practical Otorhinolaryngology 19:475–483
Aschan G 1961 The pathogenesis of positional nystagmus. Acta Otolaryngologica — Supplement 159
Aschan G 1964 Positional alcohol nystagmus. Confinia Neurologica 24:80–102
Aschan G, Hugosson R B 1966 Vestibular symptoms provoked by head and neck rotations after bilateral carotid ligation. Acta Oto-Laryngologica 61:49–54

Aschoff J C, Conrad B, Kornhuber H H 1974 Acquired pendular nystagmus with oscillopsia in multiple sclerosis: a sign of cerebellar nuclei disease. Journal of Neurology, Neurosurgery and Psychiatry 37:570–577

Backlund L, Celestino D, Eriksson K, Johnson L, Nylnder G, Stahle J 1969 Impedance plethysmography on the vertebral artery. Acta Otolaryngologica 68:303–316

Ballantyne J 1979 Ototoxicity in: Scott-Brown's diseases of the ear, nose and throat. Butterworth & Co Ltd (Publishers): London

Bannister R 1971 Degeneration of the autonomic nervous system. Lancet 2:175–179

Bárány R 1918–1919 Ueber einige augen und Halsmuskelreflexe bei neugeborenen. Acta Otolaryngologica, (Stockholm) 1:97–102

Barber H O, Dionne J 1971 Vestibular findings in vertebro-basilar ischaemia. Annals of Otology 80:805–812

Barber H O 1964 Positional nystagmus, especially after head injury. Laryngoscope 74:891–944

Barnett H J, Hyland H H 1952 Tumours involving the brainstem. A study of 90 cases arising in the brainstem, fourth ventricle and pineal tissue. Quarterly Journal of Medicine 21:265–284

Barré J A 1926 Sur un syndrome sympathique cervical postérieure et sa cause fréquente l'arthrite cervicale. Revue de Neurologie 33:1246–1252

Behrman S 1955 Vestibular epilepsy. Brain 78:471–486

Belmont O 1967 Ocular causes of vertigo. In: Spector M (ed) in dizziness and vertigo. Grune and Stratton, New York

Bender M 1975 The incidence and type of perceptual deficiencies in the aged. Neurological and sensory disorders in the elderly. Stratton, New York, pp 15–31

Bergan J J, Levy J S, Trippel O H, Jurayi M 1967 Vascular implications of vertigo. Archives of Otolaryngology 85:78–83

Bergstrom B 1973 Morphology of the vestibular nerve. Acta Otolaryngologica (Stockholm) 76:173–179, 331–338

Beveridge B R, Bannerman R M, Evason J M, Witts L J 1965 Hypochromia anaemia: a retrospective study and follow-up of 378 in-patients. Quarterly Journal of Medicine 34:145–161

Biemond A 1939 On a new form of experimental position nystagmus in the rabbit and its clinical value. Proceedings Konineijke Nederlandse Akademie van Wetenschappen te Amsterdam 42:370–398

Biemond A 1940 On a new form of experimental positional nystagmus in the rabbit and its clinical value. Proceedings Konineijke Nederlandse Akademie van Wetenschappan te Amsterdam 43:3–31

Bloch K J, Maki D G 1973 Hyperviscosity syndromes associated with immunoglobulin abnormalities. Seminars in Haematology 10:113–124

Boudin G, Barbizet J, Masson S 1959 Vertiges et pertes de connaissance. Revue Neurologique 101:742–750

Bos J H 1962 On vestibular nystagmus without causative endolymphatic displacement. (Thesis) Drukkerij Cloeck en Moedigh NV, Amsterdam, Netherlands

Bradshaw P, McQuaid P 1963 The syndrome of vertebro-basilar insufficiency. Quarterly Journal of Medicine 128:279–295

Brandt T (In Press) Visual vertigo and acrophobia. In: Dix M R, Hood J D (eds). Vertigo Wiley, London

Borders A C 1921 Epitheliomas of the ear: a study of 63 cases. Surgical Clinics of North America 1:1401–1424

Brody H 1955 Organisation of the cerebral cortex. III. A study of ageing in the human cerebral cortex. Journal of Comparative Neurology 102:511–556

Burns R A 1973 Basilar-vertebral artery insufficiency as a cause of vertigo. The Otolaryngologic Clinics of North America 6:287–300

Carmichael E A, Dix M R, Hallipike C S 1954 Lesions of the cerebral hemispheres and their effects upon optokinetic and caloric nystagmus. Brain 77 (3):345–372

Cawthorne T, Hinchcliffe R 1961 Positional nystagmus of the central type as evidence of subtentorial metastases. Brain 84:415–426

Cawthorne T, Dix M R, Hood J D, Spencer-Harrison M 1969 Vestibular syndromes and vertigo. In: Handbook of clinical neurology. North Holland Publishing Co. Amsterdam, vol 2, Ch 14, pp 358–391

Cawthorne T E 1945 Vestibular injuries. Proceedings of the royal Society of Medicine 39:270–273

Cawthorne T 1957a Functional disorders of the ear. Medical Press 237:560–563

Cawthorne T 1959 Vertigo. President's Address. Proceedings of the Royal Society of Medicine 52:529–536

Cawthorne T E 1952 Vertigo. British Medical Journal ii 931–933

Cawthorne T, Hewlett A B 1954 Ménière's disease. Proceedings of the Royal Society of Medicine 47:663–670

Cawthorne T, Dix M R, Hallpike C S, Hood J D 1956 The investigation of vestibular function. British Medical Bulletin 12:131–142

Cawthorne T E, Ranger D 1957 The toxic effect of streptomycin upon balance and hearing. British Medical Journal 1:1444–1446

Cawthorne T E 1956 Ménière's disease. Journal of Laryngology 70:695–700

Cawthorne T 1957b Perilabyrinthitis. Laryngoscope 67:1233–1236

Clemis J D, Becker G W 1973 Vestibular neuronitis. The Otolaryngologic Clinics of North America 6:139–155

Cody D T 1973 The tack operation. Archives of Otolaryngology 97:109–111

Cogan D C 1945 Syndrome of nonsyphilitic interstitial keratitis and vestibulo-auditory symptoms. Archives of Opthalmology and Otolaryngology 33:144–149

Cogan D C 1968 Down-beat nystagmus. Archives of Ophthalmology (Chicago) 80:657–663

Cohen L A 1961 Role of eye and neck proprioceptive mechanisms in body orientation and motor co-ordination. Journal of Neurophysiology 24:1–11!

Contorni L 1960 II Circolo collaterale vertebro-vertebrale nella obliterazione dell'arteria succlavia alle sue origin. Minerva Chirurgica 15:268–275

Cooksey F S 1945 Rehabilitation of vestibular injuries. Proceedings of the Royal Society of Medicine 39:273–278

Corday E, Irving D W 1960 Effect of cardiac arrhythmia on the cerebral circulation. American Journal of Cardiology 6:803–808

Corvera J, Benitez L D, Lopez-Rios G, Rabiela M T 1980 Vestibular and oculomotor abnormalities in vertebrobasilar insufficiency. Annals of Otology 89:370–376

Courjon J H, Jeannerod M, Ossuzio I, Schmid R 1977 The role of vision in compensation of vestibulo-ocular reflex after hemilabyrinthectomy in the cat. Experimental Brain Research 28:235–248

Crain E L, Thorn G W 1949 Functioning pancreatic islet cell adenomas. Medicine 28:427–441

Currier W D 1971 Dizziness related to hypoglycaemia: role of adrenal steroids and nutrition. Laryngoscope 81:18–35

Darwin E 1794 Zoonomia; or the Laws of Organic Life Vol I of Vertigo. Johnson J, London

Davies D G 1968 Paget's disease of the temporal bone. Acta Otolaryngologica Supplement 242

Davis D 1953 A common type of vertigo relieved by traction of the cervical spine. Annals of Internal Medicine 38:778–786

Dayal V S, Smith E L, McCain W G 1974 Cochlear and vestibular gentamicin toxicity: A clinical study of systemic and topical usage. Archives of Otolaryngoloy 100:338–343

De Bakey M E, Crawford E S, Morris J C Jr, Cooley D A 1962 Arterial reconstructive operations for cerebrovascular insufficiency due to extracranial arterial occlusive disease. Journal of Cardiovascular Surgery 3:12–25

Decher H, Rohr H, Unteharnscheidt F 1958–1959 Der Einfluss von traumatische cervicalen Wurzelbaurissen aud den Hor und gleichgewichtsapparat. HNO 7:365–372

Denny-Brown D 1951 Treatment of recurrent cerebrovascular symptoms and the question of vasospasm. Medical Clinics of North America 35:1457–1474

Dix M R 1973 Vertigo The Practitioner 211:295–303

Dix M R 1979 The rationale and technique of head exercises in the treatment of vertigo. Acta Oto-Rhino-Laryngologica 33:370–384

Dix M R, Hallpike C S, (1952) The pathology, symptomatology and diagnosis of certain common disorders of the vestibular system. Annals of Otology, Rhinology and Laryngology 61:987–1016

Dix M R, Hallpike C S 1966 Observations on the clinical features and neurological mechanism of spontaneous nystagmus resulting from unilateral acoustic neurofibromata. Acta Otolaryngologica (Stockholm) 61:1–22

Dix M R, Hallpike C S, Hood J D 1948 Observations upon the loudness recruitment phenomenon with especial reference to the differential diagnosis of disorders of the internal ear and viii nerve. Proceedings of the Royal Society of Medicine 16:516–526

Dolowitz D, Hecker H C, Keller B W 1967 A concept of otolaryngologic allergy Archives of Otolaryngology 86:568–578

Donaldson I 1976 Stapedectomy. Journal of Laryngology and Otology 90:915–918

Drachman D A, Hart C 1972 An approach to the dizzy patient. Neurology, 22:323–334

Droller H, Pemberton J 1953 Vertigo in a random sample of elderly people living in their homes. Journal of Laryngology and Otology 67:689–695

Drugs and Therapeutics Bulletin 1981 Cinnarizine and betahistine in vestibular disorders and Ménière's syndrome. Vol. 19 p 17

Edwards A S 1946 Body sway and vision. Journal of Experimental Psychology 36:526–535

Eggston A A, Wolff D 1947 Histopathology of the ear, nose and throat. Williams and Wilkins Co., Baltimore, p 436

Ekbom K, Ekstrand T 1972 Kroniska dyskinesier vid behandling med tietylperazin. Lakartidningen 69:271–273

Fee G 1968 Traumatic perilymphatic fistula. Archives of Otolaryngology 88:477–480

Ferguson Anderson W 1978 Involution and senescence. Price's Textbook of the Practice of Medicine Oxford University Press Oxford

Ferrer M I 1973 The sick sinus syndrome. Circulation 47:635–641

Fields W S, Weibel J 1964 Effects of vascular disorders on the vestibular system. Neurological aspects of auditory and vestibular disorders, Springfield, Illinois, pp 305–340

Fields W S 1966 Vertigo related to alteration in arterial blood flow. The vestibular system and its diseases. University of Pennsylvania Press, Philadelphia, pp 472–485

Fisher C M 1967 Vertigo in Cerebrovascular Disease. Archives of Otolaryngology (Chicago) 85:529–534

Fisher C M 1970 Occlusion of the vertebral arteries causing transient basilar symptoms. Archives of Neurology 22:13–19

Fleischer K 1972 Morphological aspects of the Aging Ear. HNO Berlin 20(4):103–107

Flemming B 1960 The psychiatric aspects of dizziness and vertigo. Thesis, Temple Medical School, Philadelphia

Forgacs P 1957 The cochlea and vestibular function at advanced age. Ful-Orr-Gegegyogyaszat 1:5–10

Fowler E P, Zeckel A 1952 Psychosomatic aspects of Ménière's disease. Journal of the American Medical Association 148:1265–1268

Frew I J C, Menon G N 1976 Betahistine hydrochloride in Ménière's disease. Postgraduate Medical Journal 52:501–503

Gacek R 1978 Further observations of posterior ampullary nerve transection for positional vertigo. Annals of Otology, Rhinology and Laryngology 87:300–305

Gillilan L A 1964 The correlation of the blood supply to the human brainstem with clinical brainstem lesions. Journal of Neuropathology and Experimental Neurology 23:78–108

Glasscock M E, Davis W E, Hughes G B, Jackson C G 1980 Labyrinthectomy versus middle fossa vestibular nerve section in Ménière's disease. Annals of Otology, Rhinology an Laryngology 89:318–324

Goldberg A D, Raftery E B, Cashman P M M 1975 Ambulatory electrocardiographic records in patients with transient cerebral attacks or palpitation. British Medical Journal ii:569–571

Goodfriend D J 1967 Odontogenic dizziness and related symptoms. In: Dizziness and Related Symptoms Grune and Stratton, New York

Goodman L S, Gilman A 1975 The pharmacological basis of therapeutics, 5th edn. MacMillan, New York

Gowers W 1886–1888 Manual of diseases of the nervous system, 2nd edn. Churchill, London

Gowers W R 1964 Epilepsy and other chronic convulsive disease: their causes, symptoms and treatment. Dover, New York

Gray L B 1956 Extra-Labyrinthine vertigo due to cervical muscle lesions. Journal of Laryngology 70:352–361

Gribben B, Pickering T G, Sleight P, Peto R 1971 Effect of age and high blood pressure on baroreflex sensitivity in man. Circulation Research 29:424–431

Gussen R 1979 Polyarteritis nodosa and deafness. A human temporal bone study. Archives of Oto-Rhino-Laryngology 217:263–271

Hallpike C S 1967 Some types of ocular nystagmus and their neurological mechanism. Proceedings of the Royal Society of Medicine 60:1043–1054

Hallpike C S, Spencer Harrison M 1950 Clinical and pathological observations on a case of leukaemia with deafness and vertigo. Journal of Laryngology and Otology 64:427–430

Hallpike C S, Spencer Harrison M, Slater E 1951 Abnormalities of the caloric test results in certain varieties of mental disorder. Acta Otolaryngologica (Stockholm) 39:151–159

Harrison D C, Fitzgerald J W, Winkle R A 1976 Ambulatory eletrocardiography for diagnosis and treatment of cardiac arrhythmias. New England Journal of Medicine 294:373–380

Hart C W 1973 Evaluation of Post-Traumatic vertigo. The Otolaryngologic Clinics of North America 6.1:157–168

Henriksson N, Rubin W, Janeke J, Claussen C 1970 A synopsis of the vestibular system. Barany Society, Sandoz, Lund, Sweden

Henriksson N G, Afzelius L E, Wahlgren L 1976 Vertigo and rocking sensation. A clinical analysis. ORL: Journal for Oto-Rhinolaryngology and its Borderlands 38:206–217

Herbert G 1954 Post-Infectious meningo-encephalitis as an aetiologic factor in certain cases of vertigo. Acta Otolaryngologica (Stockholm) Supplement 118:109–113

Hinchcliffe R 1972 Vestibular function and its disorders. In: Ellis M P (ed) Modern trends in diseases of the ear. Butterworth, London

Hinchcliffe R 1978 Dizziness. British Journal of Hospital Medicine 20: 202–203

House W F 1962 Subarachnoid shunt for drainage of endolymphatic hydrops. Laryngoscope 72: 713–729

House W F 1978 Acoustic neuroma perspective. Laryngoscope 88: 816–818

Hughes R A C, Lehner T 1979 Neurological aspects of Behcet's syndrome. In: Lehner T, Barnes P (eds) Behçet's Syndrome. Academic Press, London

Humphries A W 1965 Relief of vertebro-basilar symptoms by carotid endarterectomy. Surgery 57: 48–52

Igarashi M, Alford B, Watanabe T, Maxian P M 1969 Role of neck proprioceptors for the maintenance of dynamic bodily equilibrium in the squirrel monkey. Laryngoscope 79: 1713–1727

Irvine W T, Luck R J, Jacobey J A 1965 Reversed blood flow in vertebral arteries causing recurrent brainstem ischaemia. Lancet i: 994–996

Jackson R 1958 The cervical syndrome. Thomas, Springfield, Illinois

Johnson E W 1968 Auditory findings in 200 cases of acoustic neuromas. Archives of Otolaryngology 88: 598–603

Johnsson L G, Hawkins J E 1972 Sensory and neural degeneration with aging as seen in microdissections of the human inner ear. Annals of Oto-Rhino-Laryngology 81: 179–193

Jongkees L B W 1964 Medical treatment of Ménière's disease. Acta Otolaryngologica Supplement 192: 109–112

Jongkees L B W 1969 Cervical vertigo. Laryngoscope 79: 1473–1484

De Jong J M V B 1967 Over cervicale nystagmus en aanverwante verschijnselen. Academic Thesis, Amsterdam

Jorgenson M B 1961 Changes of aging in the inner ear. Archives Otolaryngology 74: 56–62

Jungert S 1978 Comparative investigation between thiethylperazine and meclizine in vertigo of different genesis. Acta Oto-Rhino-Laryngologica Belgica 32: 264–272

Kanejama M 1965 Vertigo and drop attack. Geriatrics 20: 892–900

Kaplan B M, Langendorf R, Lev M, Pick A 1973 Tachycardia-bradycardia syndrome (so-called 'sick sinus syndrome'). Pathology, mechanisms and treatment. The American Journal of Cardiology 31: 497–508

Katz R D, Eviatar A, Goodhill V 1969 Diphenidol and vestibular function. Archives of Otolaryngology 89: 488–493

Kinmont P D C, McCallum D I 1965 The aetiology, pathology and course of giant cell arteritis. British Journal of Dermatology 77: 193–202

Kleijn A de, Nieuwenhuyse A C 1927 Schwindelanfalle und nystagmus bei einer bestimmten lage des kopfes. Acta Otolaryngologica (Stockholm) 11: 155–167

Klockhoff I, Lindblom U 1967 Ménière's disease and hydrochlorthiazide: A critical analysis of symptoms and therapeutic effects. Acta Otolaryngologica 63: 347–365

Klockhoff I, Lindblom U, Stahle J 1974 Diuretic treatment of Ménière's disease: Long-term results with chlorthalidone. Archives of Otolaryngology 100: 262–265

Kristensen H K 1963 Ménière's disease, pathology and pathogenesis. Acta Otolaryngologica Supplement 188: 149

Kuilman J 1959 The importance of the cervical syndrome in otology. Practical Oto-Rhino-Laryngology 21: 174–185

Lacour M, Roll J R, Appaix M 1976 Modifications and development of spinal reflexes in the alert baboon following an unilateral vestibular neurotomy. Brain Research 113: 255–269

Lennox L G 1960 Epilepsy and related disorders. Little, Brown and Co, Boston

Lindsay J R, Hemenway W G 1956 Postural vertigo due to unilateral sudden partial loss of vestibular function. Annals of Otology 65: 692–708

Lodge W O, Jones H W, Smith M N 1955 Malignant tumours of the temporal bone. Archives of Otolaryngology 61: 535–541

Loeb C, Meyer J S 1965 Strokes due to vertebro-basilar disease. Thomas, Springfield, Illinois

Ludman H 1981 Surgical treatment of vertigo. In: Dix, M R Hood J D (eds) Vertigo. Wiley, London

Luxon L M, Lees A J, Greenwood R J 1979 Neurosyphilis Today. Lancet i: 90–93

Luxon L M, Crowther A, Harrison M J G, Coltart D J 1980 Controlled study of 24-hour ambulatory electrocardiographic monitoring in patients with transient neurological symptoms. Journal of Neurology, Neurosurgery and Psychiatry 43: 37–41

McAdam L P, O'Hanlan M A, Bluestone R, Pearson C M 1976 Relapsing Polychondritis. Medicine 55: 193–215

McCabe B S 1970 Labyrinthine exercises in the treatment of diseases characterised by vertigo: Their physiologic basic and methodology. Laryngoscope 80: 1429–1433

MaCrae D, O'Reilly S 1957 On some neuro-oto-ophthalmological manifestations of systemic lupus erythematous and polyarteritis nodosa. Eye, Ear, Nose and Throat Monthly 36: 721–726

Matthews W B 1978 Demyelinating disease. Price's textbook of the practice of medicine. Oxford University Press, Oxford, p 1356–1359

Mayoux R 1953 Quelques notions nouvelles sur le vertige. Methodes d'exploration de l'appareil vestibulaire. Masson, Paris

Ménière P 1861 Memoire sur des lesions de l'oreille interne don.   . lieu a des symptoms de congestion cerebrale apoplectiforme. Gazette Medicale Paris 16: 597–601

Merritt H H, Adams R D, Soloman H C 1946 Neurosyphilis. Oxford University Press, New York pp 40 and 91.

Millikan C H, Siekert R G 1955 The syndrome of intermittent insufficiency of the basilar arterial system. Proceedings of the Staff Meetings of the Mayo Clinic 30: 61–68

Money R A 1968 Some neurosurgical aspects of vertigo. Medical Journal of Australia 1: 1040–1043

Morrison A W 1975 Management of sensori-neural deafness. Butterworth, London

Morrison A W 1978 Translabyrinthine surgical approach to the internal acoustic meatus. Journal of the Royal Society of Medicine 71: 269–273

Morrison A W 1979 Diseases of the otic capsule i and ii. In: Scott-Brown's diseases of the ear, nose and throat. Butterworth, London

Mulch G, Petermann W 1979 Influence of age on results of vestibular function tests. Annals of Otology, Rhinology and Laryngology. Vol 88 Supplement 56 1–17

Nadol J, Weiss A, Parker S 1975 Vertigo of delayed onset after sudden deafness. Annals of Otology, Rhinology and Laryngology 84: 841–846

Nielson J M 1959 Tornado epilepsy simulating Ménière's syndrome. Neurology 9: 294–296

Noffsinger D, Olsen W O, Carhart R, Hart, C W, Sahgal V 1972 Auditory and vestibular aberrations in multiple sclerosis. Acta Otolaryngologica Supplement 303

Nozue N, Mizuno M, Kaga K 1973 Neuro-otological findings in diphenylhydantoine intoxications. Annals of Otology 82: 389–394

Nylen C O 1939 The otoneurological diagnosis of tumours of the brain. Acta Otolaryngologica (Stockholm) Supplement 33

Nylen C O 1950 Positional nystagmus. A review and future propects. Journal of Laryngoscopy and Otology 64: 295–318

Ommaya A K, Fass F, Yarnell P 1968 Whiplash injury and brain damage: An experimental study. Journal of the American Medical Association 204: 285–289

Paparella M M, Chasin W D 1966 Otosclerosis and vertigo. Journal of Laryngology and Otology 80: 511–519

Pearson B W, Barber H O 1973 Head injury. Some otoneurologic sequelae. Archives of Otolaryngology 97: 81–84

Pfaltz C R, Richter H 1958 Die cochleo-vestibulare symptomatologie des cervicalsyndrome. Archiv fur Ohren-' Nasen- und Kehlkopfheilkunde 172: 519–534

Pfaltz C R 1982 Vertigo in disorders of the neck. In: Dix M R, Hood J D (eds) Vertigo. Wiley, London

Pincus J 1978 Hyperventilation syndrome. British Journal of Hospital Medicine 19: 312–313

Pirozzi D J 1973 Syphilis and penicillin. Annals of Internal Medicine 79: 447–449

Powers S R, Dirslane T M, Nevins S 1961 Intermittent vertebral artery compression: A new syndrome. Surgery 49: 257–264

Pulec J L, House W F, Britton G H, Hitselberger W E 1971 A system of management based on 364 Cases. Transactions of the American Academy of Ophthalmology and Otolaryngology 75: 48–55

Pulec J L 1972 Symposium on Ménière's disease. I Ménière's disease: Results of a two and one-half year study of etiology, natural history and results of treatment. Laryngoscope 82: 1703–1715

Pulec J L 1973 Ménière's disease. The Otolaryngologic Clinics of North America 6(1): 25–39

Putkonnen P T S, Courjon J H, Jeannerod M 1977 Compensation of postural effects of hemilabyrinthectomy in the Cat. Experimental Brain Research 28: 249–257

Rasmussen A F 1940 Studies of the viii cranial nerve in man. Laryngoscope 50: 67–83

Rebattu J P, Lesne G 1962 Syndrome cochleovestibulaire en rapport avec une subluxation cervicale par mise en traction. Journal Francais d'Otorhinolaryngologie et Chirurgie Maxillo-Faciale 11: 1091–1098

Reivich M, Holling H E, Roberts B, Toole J F 1961 Reversal of blood flow through the vertebral artery and its effect on cerebral circulation. New England Journal of Medicine 265: 878–885

Rosenhall U 1973 Degenerative patterns in the ageing human vestibular neuro-epithelia. Acta Otolaryngologica (Stockholm) 76: 208–220

Rosenhall U 1974 Epithelial cysts in the human vestibular apparatus. Journal of Laryngology and Otology 88: 105–112

Rosenhall U, Rubin W 1975 Degenerative changes in the human vestibular sensory epithelium. Acta Otolaryngologica (Stockholm) 79:67–85

Rubin W 1973 Whiplash with vestibular involvement. Archives of Otolaryngology 97:85–87

Rubin W 1973 Vestibular suppressant drugs. Archives of Otolaryngology 97:135–138

Ryan G M S, Cope S 1955 Cervical vertigo. Lancet 2:1355–1358

Samet P 1973 Haemodynamic sequelae of cardiac arrhythmias. Circulation 47:399–407

Sandstrom J 1962 Cervical syndrome with vestibular symptoms. Acta Otolaryngologica 54:207–226

Saxén A, Von Fieandt H 1937 Pathologie und klinik der altersschnerhorigkeit. Acta Otolaryngologica Supplement 23:1–85

Schiller F, Hedberg W C 1960 An appraisal of positional nystagmus. Archives of Neurology 2:309–316

Schoder H J 1973 Zur reaktionsweise des vestibularsystems im alter. Verkehrsmedizin lhre. Grenzgebiete 20:108–183

Schuknecht H F 1964 Further observations on the pathology of presbyacusis. Archives of Otolaryngology 80:369–382

Schuknecht H F 1969 Cupulolithiasis. Archives of Otolaryngology 90:113–126

Schuknecht H F 1978 Delayed endolymphatic hydrops. Annals of Otology, Rhinology and Laryngology 87:743–748

Schuknecht H F, Igarashi M, Gacek R 1965 The pathological types of cochleo-saccular degeneration. Acta Otolaryngologica 59:154–170

Sheehan S, Bauer R B, Meyer J S 1960 Vertebral artery compression in cervical spondylosis. Neurology 10:968–986

Shneider R C, Calhoun H D, Crosby E C 1968 Vertigo and rotational movement in cortical and subcortical lesions. Journal of Neurological Sciences 6:493–516

Shy G M, Drager G A 1960 A neurological syndrome associated with orthostatic hypotension: A clinical pathologic study. Archives of Neurology 2:511–527

Silverside J L 1954 Basilar artery stenosis and thrombosis. Proceedings of the Royal Society of Medicine 47:290–293

Slater R 1979 Benign recurrent vertigo. Journal of Neurology, Neurosurgery and Psychiatry 42:363–367

Sleight P 1978 Hypertension. Price's textbook of the practice of medicine. Oxford University Press, Oxford

Sloane P 1967 In: Spector M (ed) Psychiatric aspects of vertigo, dizziness and vertigo. Grune and Stratton, New York, pp 258–262

Snow J B, Suga F 1973 Labyrinthine Vasodilators. Archives of Otolaryngology 97:365–370

Spector M 1967 Dizziness and vertigo. Grune and Stratton, New York

Spencer-Harrison M, Ozsahinoglu C 1972 Positional vertigo: Aetiology and clinical significance. Brain 95:369–372

Spencer-Harrison M, Ozsahinoglu C 1975 Positional vertigo. Archives of Otolaryngology 101:675–678

Stahle J 1968 Electronystagmographic results in Ménière's disease. Otolaryngologic Clinics of North America 1:509–518

Stebbins R, Bertino J R 1976 The Anti-Folate Drugs Clinical Haematology 5:619–630

Stephens S D G, Luxon L M, Hinchcliffe, R. (1982) Immunological disorders and auditory lesions. Audiology 21:128–148

Stewart T G, Holmes G 1904 Symtomatology of cerebellar tumours. A study of 40 cases. Brain 27:522–591

Stoddard A 1952 Letter to editor regarding vertigo. British Medical Journal 2:1043

Sunderland S 1945 The arterial relations of the internal auditory meatus. Brain 68:23–27

Takeya T, Baron J B, Ohno Y, Agathon M, Anderson J C, Ushio N, Bessineton J C, Pacifici M, Lemaire V, Chavannes N, Noto R 1978 Comparative study of post-traumatic and psychogenic acrophobia. Agressologie 19:92–92

Toglia J U 1975 Dizziness in the elderly. In: Fields WS (ed) Neurological and sensory disorders in the elderly. Stratton Intercontinental Medical Book Corporation, New York

Toglia J U, Rosenberg P E, Romis M L 1970 Post-Traumatic dizziness. Archives of Otolaryngology 92:485–492

Torok N 1964 Classification of pathologic conditions responsible for vertigo and neuro-otologic diseases. Laryngoscope 74:528–535

Torok N 1977 Old and new in Ménière's disease. Laryngoscope 87:1870–1877

Travis R C 1945 An experimental analysis of dynamic equilibrium. Journal of Experimental Psychology 35:216–234

Troost B T 1980 Dizziness and vertigo in vertebrobasilar disease. Stroke 11:301–303, 413–415

Tumarkin A 1966 Thoughts on the treatment of labyrinthopathy. Journal of Laryngology 80:1041–1053

Tzivoni D, Stern S 1975 Pacemaker implantation based on ambulatory ECG monitoring in patients with cerebral symptoms. Chest 67: 274–278

Uesu C T, Eisenman J I, Stemmer E A 1976 The problem of dizziness and syncope in old age: Transient ischaemic attacks versus hypersensitive carotid sinus reflex. Journal of the American Geriatrics Society 24(3): 126–135

Valvassori G, Dobben G D 1979 Vertebrobasilar insufficiency. Annals of Otology, Rhinology and Laryngology 88: 689–692

Van Der Laan F L, Oosterveld W J 1974 Age and vestibular function. Aerospace Medicine 45: 540–547

Voss O 1925 Geburtstrauma und gehororgan. Internationale Zeitschrift fur Ohrenheilkunde 24: 16–19

Voss O 1934 Foreign letters. Journal of the American Medical Association 103: 1721–1722

Wayne H H 1961 Syncope. American Journal of Medicine 30: 418–438

Wegener F 1936 Uber generalisierte, septische gefasserkrankungen. Verhandlungen der Deutsche Gesellschaft fur Pathologie 29: 202–210

Weiss E, English O S 1957 Psychosomatic medicine, 3rd edn. Saunders, Philadelphia

Wickstrom J, Martinez J, Rodriguez R 1960 Cervical sprain syndrome. Experimental acceleration of the head and neck. The Prevention of Highway Injury, University of Michigan, Highway Safety Institute, Ann Arbour

Williams D, Wilson G 1964 Vertebro-basilar ischaemia. British Medical Journal 1: 84–86

Williams H L 1952 Allergy of the inner ear. Archives of Otolaryngology 56: 24–44

Wilmot T J 1969 Sympathectomy for Ménière's disease—a long term review. Journal of Laryngology 83: 323–331

Worthington E L, Lunen L F, Heath M, Catlin F I 1973 Index handbook of oto-toxic agents 1966–1971. Johns-Hopkins University Press, Baltimore and London

Wyke B 1979 Cervical articular contributions to posture and gait: Their relation to senile dysequilibrium. Age and Ageing 8: 251–258

Yasargil M G, Fox J L 1974 The microsurgical approach to acoustic neurinoma. Surgical Neurology 2: 393–398

Psychological and sociological facets of balance disorders

PSYCHOLOGICAL ASPECTS

Epidemiological studies in Britain by Kay, Beamish and Roth (1964) and by Williamson and his colleagues (1964) indicate that, amongst the elderly, about 14 per cent suffer from neurotic disorders, 10 per cent from depressive disorders and 6 to 27 per cent (depending on whether or not 'mild' cases are included) from dementia. There is thus a high likelihood that an older person afflicted with a balance disorder will also have a psychological disorder. In such a case, the latter can only serve to colour the way that the balance disorder presents, the manner in which it affects the subject, his family and his friends and the response to management. Moreover, there is the possibility of a more direct involvement of a psychological condition in generating, or precipitating, an organic disorder, i.e. in the concept of psychosomatic disease. Furthermore, the physical illness itself may generate psychological disorders (somatopsychic effect). It is thus not surprising that epidemiological studies show a positive association between physical and mental disorders (Eastwood and Trevelyan, 1972).

In the context of balance disorders and their investigations which may also be relevant to older subjects, six topics merit more detailed consideration, i.e. vestibulogenic anxiety states, psychogenic dizziness, post-traumatic dizziness, Ménière's disorder, dizziness and falling in elderly psychiatric patients, and iatrogenic psychological effects.

Vestibulogenic anxiety states

None can doubt that the sudden loss of balance, without any warning whatsoever, could have a profound psychological impact on the affected individual. Indeed one could formulate a hypothesis that the somatopsychic effect would be a function of the rate of development of the balance dysfunction, its severity and the psychological constitution of the affected individual. With recurrent episodes of balance malfunction, the probable determinants could be extended to incorporate the frequency of attacks and their randomness. Although there have not yet been any attempts to quantify this somatopsychic effect, there are a number of reports in the literature (Gowers, 1893; Cawthorne, 1947; Roth and Kay, 1956; Pratt and McKenzie, 1958; Martin, 1970) attesting to it.

Pratt and McKenzie reported a series of twelve patients with anxiety states which they considered were the result of a vestibular disorder. Eight of these patients had 'episodes of frank rotatory vertigo, usually of brief duration'. The most common psychological symptoms in their series were: panic attacks (seven patients), fear of travelling (five patients), reactive depression (five patients), feelings of tension (three patients, in two of whom it was particularly severe in the barber's chair) and exhaustion (two patients). The fear of travelling, or even going out of the house, is such a conspicuous feature of the somatopsychic effect of balance disorders that Levy and O'Leary (1947) referred to the condition as a 'street neurosis'.

Psychogenic dizziness

Pratt and McKenzie provided three case reports to illustrate their evidence for the existence of somatopsychic effects of vestibular disorders. They reported that 'no otological diagnosis was made' in any of the three illustrative cases, but the caloric testing reproduced the vestibular symptoms. The first illustrative case initially complained of feelings, 'as if mildly drunk', which were increasingly accompanied by panic attacks and fears of dying; rotatory vertigo did not develop until six months after the onset of the illness. The patient of the second illustrative case report 'was adopted, had an unhappy childhood, walked once in his sleep, wet the bed until the age of six years, and occasionally stammered when flustered'. The initial symptoms in the third case were 'a muzzy feeling with continuous headaches and depression, and three months later spent three weeks in bed feeling exhausted'. One might therefore wonder as to whether or not vestibular symptoms might be precipitated by psychological factors and/or the psychological characteristics of an individual and/or the stresses to which he is exposed may play a part in the genesis of these vestibular symptoms. There is of course no reason to assume that a patient who has previously suffered from a psychological disorder should not subsequently be afflicted by an organic disorder.

As Magnusson, Nilsson and Henriksson (1977) point out, the close connection between anxiety and dizziness in psychopathological functioning has previously been emphasized by many workers. Amongst them have been Freud (1895), Bauer and Schilder (1919), Schilder (1933, 1939), Moore and Atkinson (1958), Sloane (1967) and Rallo (1972).

Magnusson and his colleagues studied 23 vertigo patients who had been drawn from a neuro-otological clinic and who had been shown, on examination, to have no vestibular abnormality. A control group comprised the same number of patients who had been matched for sex, age, education and occupation. The instruments used in the study included questionnaires and two techniques of percept-genetic analysis, i.e. Kragh's (1969) defence mechanism test and the meta-contrast technique of Smith, Johnson, Ljunghill-Andersson and Almgren (1970). One of the questionnaires was completed by the patient before his clinical examination; the other questionnaire was sent out about two years after the initial investigation. The percept-genetic technique enabled the authors not only to measure anxiety but also to recognise a 'primitive hysteroid' subgroup and an 'obsessive-compulsive' subgroup. A third subgroup comprised those patients who had neither signs of 'primitive-hysteroid' functioning nor signs of 'obsessive-compulsive' functioning. The primitive-hysteroid subgroup was characterised by the absence of the history of anxiety before the first vertigo attack, which was 'diffuse and lingering'. Anxiety appeared late, if at all, in the percept-genetic test. This subgroup had the best prognosis. The other two subgroups gave a history of anxiety before the first vertigo attack, which was sudden and linked to a precise event. Anxiety appeared early in the percept-genetic tests. It may be hypothesised that, in terms of Schur's (1955) thesis, the vestibular symptoms in the 'primitive-hysteroid' subgroup may be considered as an anxiety equivalent and that, in the obsessive-compulsive subgroup, an anxiety concomitant. Anxiety equivalents are held to be discharge phenomena in which the conscious experience is limited to the discharge phenomenon itself and the experience of anxiety either does not exist or, at most, is of secondary importance. Anxiety concomitants comprise a set of discharge phenomena (perspiration, respiratory distress and tachycardia) associated with a conscious feeling of anxiety.

Although none of the patients in the study conducted by Magnusson and his colleagues were older than 55 years of age, psychogenic vertigo and other balance disorders may also occur in older people. In Chapter 10, reference is made to the epidemiological study conducted by Tanja and his colleagues (1979) on people over the age of 64 years. The study showed a 'strong positive association between complaints about dizziness and the results of a psychosomatic questionnaire'. In clinical practice, imbalance symptoms unassociated with other symptoms or signs in older subjects are more likely to be ascribed to transient ischaemic attacks. In many cases there is no corroborative evidence for this. Cerebrovascular degenerative disorder increases with increasing age, as does organic disease in general. There are reports that psychosomatic disorders do likewise (Leighton, 1959; Srole, Langner and Michael, 1962).

Post-traumatic dizziness

Dizziness, together with headache, sleeplessness, irritability, fatigue and loss of memory, is a component of the post-concussional syndrome (Verjaal and Van 'T Hooft, 1975). Hill (1914) argued that the post-concussional syndrome was psychogenic in origin. This view was supported by Lewis (1942) and by Guttman (1943) who showed that early mobilisation and reactivation of patients who had sustained a head injury had much to recommend it. Subsequently, Lidvall, Linderoth and Norlin (1974), after an extensive study, concluded that not only the post-concussional, but also the post-contusional, syndrome should, in most cases, be regarded as a psychoneurosis with a multifactorial aetiology.

However, increasing evidence has accumulated over the past thirty years that there is an organic basis to many cases of post-traumatic dizziness, especially when the anamnesis clearly indicates that the patient suffers from a hallucination of movement, i.e. a true vertigo (rotational or non-rotational, subjective or objective), but particularly when objective, rotatory vertigo is experienced. Dix and Hallpike (1952), Cawthorne (1954) and Gordon (1954) showed that much of post-traumatic dizziness was in the nature of a positional vertigo which was due to a positioning (benign paroxysmal) nystagmus. The pathological basis advanced for this by Schuknecht (1974) is that the head injury produces disruption of the utricular otolithic membrane and release of otoliths (otoconia) into the endolymph of the pars superior of the labyrinth. These otoliths, or their degradation products, are then deposited on the cupula of the posterior semicircular canal so rendering it particularly sensitive to gravitational forces. This pathological process, which Schuknecht refers to as cupulolithiasis, is therefore claimed to be the basis for the observed positioning nystagmus.

The pathology of organic post-traumatic vestibular disorders is, however, not restricted to cupulolithiasis. The trauma may have produced symptoms of imbalance by damaging other parts of the vestibular labyrinth, nerve or central pathways. Increasing recognition is being accorded to the possibility that the injury has produced a labyrinthine window rupture. Fee (1968) has described a Ménièreiform syndrome arising after head injury and being due to a perilymph leak at the anterior end of the stapes base.

Hinoki, Nakanishi, Ito, Ushio and Ichibangase (1978) have however, distinguished a neurotic vertigo from the organic post-traumatic vertigos. In such cases, the injection of normal saline in association with suggestion accentuates, or precipitates, the vertigo and/or ataxia. The patients with post-traumatic neurotic vertigo were also differentiated from other post-traumatic vertigos on psychological tests and by the response (better) to a benzodiazepine drug, cloxazolam.

It is yet to be ascertained to what extent post-traumatic neurotic vertigo represents a nosologically distinct entity. The question arises as to whether or not the neurotic post-traumatic vertigos are merely those organic post-traumatic vertigos who show a marked functional overlay.

Ménière's disorder

Ménière's disorder is not uncommon in older people. The percentage of patients who are over the age of 60 years has been reported as 8.4 per cent (Green and Douglass, 1951), 15·3 per cent (Cawthorne, 1947), 17·3 per cent (Harrison and Naftalin, 1968) and 36·7 per cent (Brain, 1938). Green and Douglass' proportion is lower than that of the other since it refers to the age at onset of symptoms and not the age at the first visit to the physician.

A number of authors have commented on the psychological disturbances which have been associated with Ménière's disorder. 'A variable and sometimes distressing feature of the complaint was the depressing influence that the sudden attacks exerted upon the general well-being and everyday life of the patient. . . . Obviously to withstand these attacks with equanimity calls for a stout heart, and it is not surprising that one encounters a variety of psychological disturbances as the result of previous attacks' (Cawthorne, 1947). At least three papers (Bystrzanowska and Jablonska, 1972; Watson, Barnes, Donaldson and Klett, 1967; Crary and Wexler, 1977) attribute the psychological features of Ménière's disorder entirely to somatopsychic effects.

There have, however, been a number of reports, e.g. by Parrisius (1924), Koch (1932), Portmann (1937), Fowler and Zeckel (1952, 1953), Ceroni and Franzoni (1963), Jongkees (1964), Siirala, Siltala and Lumio (1965), Hinchcliffe (1967abc, 1970), Williamson and Gifford (1971), Stephens (1975) and Czubalski, Bochenek and Zawiska (1976), providing evidence in support of the thesis that Ménière's disorder is, at least in part, a psychosomatic one. In the most recent study (Czubalski et al, 1976), a psychological and psychiatric assessment was made on a random sample of 30 patients with Ménière's disorder. The ages ranged from 18 to 65 years of age. Various psychic stresses experienced in childhood were found to have been more common in the Ménière's group than in the control group.

Crary and Wexler point out that the relevant questions are extremely complicated. Nevertheless they proceed to analyse systematically the methodological problems facing an appropriate investigation. The shortcomings in previous reports are also distinguished. An analysis of the methodology adopted in published reports is presented succinctly in tabular form. Crary and Wexler were particularly concerned to control for the episodes of vertigo which may have profound somatopsychic effects, and which, in their own words is 'the disease's most devastating symptom'. After citing the criteria adopted for identifying a psychosomatic disease (Halliday, 1948; Crary, Wexler and Foreman, 1976), the authors proceed to discuss their experimental design. Four groups of patients were studied. Two of these groups had been diagnosed as having Ménière's disease (one group did not participate in the study). The other two groups were composed of 'patients with otological problems other than Ménière's disease'; one of these groups was vertiginous, the other was not. The test instruments used in this study were; (1) a general biomedical questionnaire, (2) a Scaled Dizziness Questionnaire (3) the MMPI (Minnesota Multiphasic Personality Inventory), (4) Spiegelberger's State Anxiety Scale, (5) Psychosomatic Check Lists for both the patient and his family, (6) a Self-esteem Scale, (7) Doctor-patient Relationship Scale, (8) the Recent Life Changes Questionnaire (Holmes and Matsuda, 1972; Rahe, Floistad, Bergan, Ringdal, Gerhardt, Gunderson and Arthur, 1974), which surveys the occurrence of stressful events within a prior 2-year period, and (9) an Improvement Scale.

The results of Crary and Wexler's study showed that all three vertigo groups had a history of significantly more psychosomatic symptoms than the non-vertigo control group. Although both male and female Ménière's patients gave a history of more psychosomatic symptoms in the family than the non-vertiginous control group, this did not attain significance level in Crary and Wexler's study. All three vertigo groups had a significantly higher score on the MMPI hypochondriasis scale than the non-vertigo control group. Moreover, the non-vertigo control group reported significantly less life stress over the 2-year period preceding the onset of the illness than did either the Ménière's group or the control vertigo group. Furthermore, the daily diary sheets of a random sample of the Ménière's group were studied. Crary and Wexler reported that there was no significant difference between the frequency of emotional stress occurring before an attack of vertigo and that occurring after an attack.

Crary and Wexler summarised their findings by saying that there seemed to be no evidence to support the contention that Ménière's patients are any different from other vertiginous patients on measures of personality, anxiety, self-esteem, appearance of psychosomatic symptoms and the like. The conclusions that they drew were that the psychological features of Ménière's disorder were best explained on a somatopsychic hypothesis.

However, it is possible to advance an alternative explanation for Crary and Wexler's findings. The inability to effectively distinguish the Ménière's group from the 'organic' vertigo control group could be held to imply that this is because they both belonged to one and the same group of conditions. It is noted that the most common diagnosis in the control vertigo group was 'cause unknown' (29 per cent of the group) with 'sensory neural' (27 per cent) as the next most common cause. The other diagnoses amongst the remaining 42 cases were labyrinthine ischaemia (10 cases), postural vertigo (7 cases), otosclerosis (7 cases), otitis media (6 cases), stenosis of the internal acoustic meatus (3 cases), CNS (2 cases) and acoustic neuroma (2 cases) with one case each of cervical vertigo, metabolic vertigo, ossicular dislocation, temporomandibular joint dysfunction and vascular accident.

Previous attempts (Hinchcliffe, 1967d) to classify vertigos using quantitative methods indicated that an essentially homogeneous population was obtained after the exclusion of patients with a history of head injury, ototoxic drug administration, other neurological symptoms or signs, evidence for middle ear disease or positive treponemal serology. Some of these patients had vertigo as a sole symptom; others had auditory symptoms but without measurable hearing loss; finally, there were those with the full blown syndrome of recurrent episodes of objective rotatory vertigo associated with a sensation of fullness in the ears, tinnitus and hearing loss. It was concluded that those cases which would not meet the criteria for a diagnosis of Ménière's disease were nevertheless *formes frustes* of this disorder, or variants.

The acceptance that many non-Ménière's vertigo patients belong, together with Ménière's patients, to a single nosological group of 'psychosomatic disorders' would also explain Crary and Wexler's finding that their three vertiginous groups reported more life stressing events than did the non-vertigo control group prior to the onset of the disorder. There would thus not be the need to postulate that 'individuals who are currently stressed by their disorder recall, or project, more stress into the period preceding the onset of symptoms'.

It has previously been reported that elevation of the neurotic triad of the MMPI is an inverse function of the severity of the organic dysfunction in Ménière's disorder (Hinchcliffe, 1970). This is compatible with Crary and Wexler's finding that the control vertigo group showed higher scores on some of these neurotic triad scales than did the Ménière's group.

The findings, from Crary and Wexler's diary study, that psychological events were as common after a vertiginous episode as before could be considered to indicate merely that the somatopsychic and psychosomatic effects were equipollent. Indeed the balance of the evidence available to date on Ménière's disorder would be compatible with the thesis that there are both psychosomatic and somatopsychic effects. In this concept, the histopathological picture of endolymphatic hydrops (Hallpike and Cairns, 1938) would be considered as the result, and not the cause, of the basic disorder. Structural anomalies which have been reported in the internal ear (Black, 1969; Gussen, 1971), including the endolymphatic duct (Yuen and Schuknecht, 1972), of Ménière's patients would be construed as being the basis for the *locus minoris resistentiae* which, on classical theory, accounts for organ selection in psychosomatic disease (Cobb, 1947).

Perhaps the acquisition of a sizeable and unselected vertigo control group that is aetiologically distinct from Ménière's disorder is an unattainable ideal. Nevertheless, further studies should seek to do this when the experimental design is contemplated. Moreover, future studies should encompass criteria additional to those given by Crary and Wexler. Since the concept not only of Ménière's disorder but also of vertigo in general is bristling with many semantic difficulties, strict definitions of the terms used should be provided, together with methods of sampling, statistical parameters of the population studied and specifications of the taxonometric procedures used in the classification of the disorder studied (Hinchcliffe and Prasansuk, 1973).

Future studies should bear in mind the changing concept of psychosomatic medicine. Previously workers have used the concept of a linear psychosomatic model. As Reiser (1975) has pointed out, the broadened understanding over the past quarter of a century has made it clearer than ever that mind and body can no longer be regarded, or dealt with, as separate despite our bondage to Cartesian dualism. The corollary of this is that the distinction of psychosomatic from other disorders is rapidly losing its meaning and utility. Indeed, it is now reasonable to think of man as existing as a 'biopsychosocial' field (Fig. 17.1).

Dizziness and falling in elderly psychiatric patients

Monica Blumenthal and Davie (1980) studied 100 psychiatric out-patients who were 60 years of age of over in respect of symptoms of dizziness or falling. *Inter alia* an examination for orthostatic hypotension was also done. Almost 40 per cent of the sample complained of dizziness and falling, although only 27 per cent had

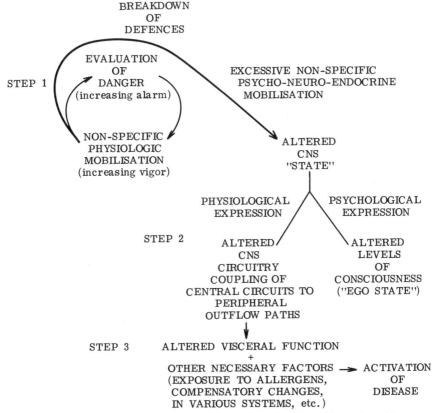

Fig. 17.1 Hypothesised steps in precipitation of disease in conjunction with psychosocial stress (Reiser, 1975).

systolic orthostatic hypotension. Drug treatment, especially in a combination of tricyclic antidepressants with other orthostatic hypotension producing drugs, was considered as the most important factor accounting for the dizziness and falling. Organic disease was also a factor. Patients who suffered from two or more diseases, e.g. cervical arthritis and cardiac disorder leading to low cardiac output, appeared to be especially vulnerable. Amongst patients suffering from only one illness, those with cervical arthritis showed the greatest proportion of imbalance symptoms.

Iatrogenic psychological effects

As Wahl (1962) has pointed out, the physician can both magically heal as well as magically afflict. There are thus both beneficent and maleficent psychological effects. These effects can stem not only from the physician himself but also from the whole team of health care personnel, together with the investigative process. Because of the complex and symbolic significance of the role of the physician in society, small acts of commission or omission on his part can have profound effects (for good or ill) on the patient. The complexity of the effect is also added to by the physician subsuming a parental figure, which may have a particular relevance to the patient.

Beneficent

Beneficent iatrogenic psychological effects comprise the effects of 'therapeutic listening', 'being properly investigated', explanation, reassurance, 'short-term' psychotherapy and 'placebo response'. However, there is a danger, as Frank (1973) has pointed out, in the potential power of these effects. Distress due to serious disease may be relieved. This may result in the neglect of investigations that would have revealed an organic aetiology which could well be of serious nature.

Maleficent

Maleficent iatrogenic psychological effects comprise a whole corpus of psychological disorders. In 1950 Ebaugh coined the term iatrogenic anxiety to describe the commonest maleficent psychological effect; indeed there are some who would claim that this is the most common iatrogenic disorder, far surpassing that of drugs. Wahl refers to the iatrogenic neuroses which he defined as 'those neurotic diseases produced, augmented, reinforced, or intensified by the physician.'

The factors contributing to the production of iatrogenic psychological disorders have been discussed by Burgess and Burgess (1966), Ebaugh (1950), Echikson and Bazilian (1959), Shey (1971) and Wahl (1962). Burgess and Burgess considered that discussion of symptoms and signs within the patient's hearing is particularly important in the generation of iatrogenic anxiety. Hospital ward rounds are particularly implicated in this respect (Echikson and Bazilian, 1959; Wahl, 1962). A concerned look during testing is particularly liable to generate anxiety (Shey, 1971). Ebaugh considered that multiple specialty consultations, in association with what he termed the 'total examination technique', might be a factor. Similar views were expressed by Wahl in referring to what he termed the 'diagnostic over-study'. However, the first factor in generating iatrogenic anxiety mentioned by Wahl was the use of technical terms in explanations. Severe anxiety states had been precipitated by the patient misinterpreting explanations couched in such terms. Even if the explanation is simple and comprehensible, anxiety may be generated because it is inadequate; the patient may suspect that the physician is withholding something, and such a thing bodes ill.

There is thus the need not only to explain every test procedure to the patient, but to do so in simple and adequate terms. Explanations should also be accompanied by reassurance. Differences in the nature and degree of explanation and reassurance must account, partially or wholly, for differences in the nature and degree of adverse effects reported, for example, from investigations such as the caloric test.

Although the need for the physician to adopt an optimistic attitude has frequently been taught (Alvarez, 1951), McNeill (1951) has cogently argued that imperturbability and a poker face are the absolute essentials to good medical practice.

Finally there is the need to explain the condition to the patient and reassure him after investigations have been completed. As Mears (1963) and others have pointed out, a thorough investigation itself frequently provides the necessary reassurance.

Unfortunately, the whole topic of iatrogenic anxiety, which is being increasingly publicised, rests so much at the anecdotal level. There is no good evidence as yet that the extent of the medical investigation *per se* is a significant factor. It is much more likely that any anxiety generated, or perpetuated, by an investigation has been unwittingly generated by the health care personnel involved in the testing. Clearly, the chance of this happening will be a function of the number of health care personnel involved in the investigatory process, their degree of training and the duration of contact with the patient. Multiple consultations may not be hazardous *per se*; the increased risk of generating iatrogenic psychological disorders in such cases may well be due to the increased risk of different explanations and recommendations for treatment being given to the patient. Inevitably this can only produce loss of confidence in the health care personnel involved. It is thus important that appropriate training of personnel and the ensurance of adequate, yet simple and single explanations with reassurance, together with the constant awareness of the existence of the phenomenon of iatrogenic anxiety should go a long way to containing adverse psychological effects.

SOCIOLOGICAL ASPECTS

The cultural setting and linguistic factors influence the way in which symptoms of imbalance, like many other symptoms, present. For example, in Thailand, the patient will use an umbrella term to cover general malaise, headache, light-headedness, unsteadiness and vertigo.

Social factors are relevant to the development and severity of both physical and psychological symptoms as Miller and Ingham (1976) and others have pointed out. Indeed, as Livsey (1972) has argued, the evaluation of any patient is incomplete without a detailed inquiry into his family interactions and the ways and degrees in which they are affected by the patient's illness, and, in turn, have affected him.

As Capildeo, Court and Rose (1976) point out, doctors have become increasingly aware that they cannot treat a patient's illness without regard to his social environment. The problems of discharge from hospital are often social and if information regarding these is obtained as soon as possible, plans may be made well in advance of discharge.

SOCIO-ENVIRONMENTAL NETWORK DIAGRAM

Name: .....Mrs. Coles....

Case No.: ....

Serial No.: .....1.........

Date: ....

FAMILY

NON-FAMILY

Non-modernised
2-storey terraced house

1d (70y) ──────►

| 96F |
| (ht; −16) |

HAZARDS: Loose mats; trailing flex; poor lighting

ENVIRONMENTAL AIDS: Acoustic: Nil

Locomotor: Nil

a

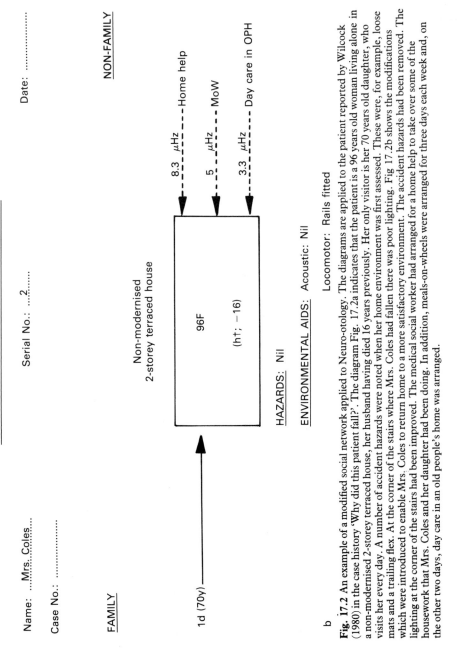

Fig. 17.2 An example of a modified social network applied to Neuro-otology. The diagrams are applied to the patient reported by Wilcock (1980) in the case history 'Why did this patient fall?'. The diagram Fig. 17.2a indicates that the patient is a 96 years old woman living alone in a non-modernised 2-storey terraced house, her husband having died 16 years previously. Her only visitor is her 70 years old daughter, who visits her every day. A number of accident hazards were noted when her home environment was first assessed. These were, for example, loose mats and a trailing flex. At the corner of the stairs where Mrs. Coles had fallen there was poor lighting. Fig 17.2b shows the modifications which were introduced to enable Mrs. Coles to return home to a more satisfactory environment. The accident hazards had been removed. The lighting at the corner of the stairs had been improved. The medical social worker had arranged for a home help to take over some of the housework that Mrs. Coles and her daughter had been doing. In addition, meals-on-wheels were arranged for three days each week and, on the other two days, day care in an old people's home was arranged.

The inadequacy of the socioeconomic background of the elderly with imbalance disorders may be just as important as the psychological background in influencing the genesis, course and management of the disorder. The study conducted by Williamson and his colleagues (1964) showed that housing was unsatisfactory for 24 per cent of the elderly living at home, basic financial needs were not being met in 18 per cent and about 30 per cent of city patients and 10 per cent of small town patients lacked adequate human contacts.

The nature of the home situation is particularly important in respect of falls in older people. Deidre Wild, Nayak and Isaacs (1981) found that half of their fallers lived alone and 40 per cent of the remainder lived with an aged spouse only. Falls made more use than did controls of home helps and community nurses; and more fallers lived in residential homes. One half of the fallers and a similar proportion of the controls lived in houses that were equipped with a telephone, but only ten (nine of them in sheltered housing) of the 125 fallers had an alarm system. No faller used the telephone after falling, but one received an incoming call and was able to indicate her plight. Of the nine callers with a call-system, two used it successfully, one attempted unsuccessfully to use it, and the other six made no attempt to use it. However, Wild and her colleagues said that those at risk could be readily identified. They probably constitute not more than 1 per cent of any practice list and are in touch with the family doctor. Organising a preventive visiting service for them should not be beyond the resources of the average general practice. The visit should include a review of medication, a check of blood pressure, a general physical examination, a search for environmental hazards and a review of arrangements for surveillance, especially in the event of a further fall. The more elaborate system, practised in Stockport (Northwest England) and elsewhere, in which radio-controlled home helps are summoned to the homes of older people who have fallen, is pointed to as an imaginative technical advance.

Capildeo and his colleagues recommended summarising a patient's relevant socioenvironmental factors in a diagram which they term the social network diagram. This is constructed by drawing a rectangle on a sheet of paper to represent the patient's home (Fig. 17.2). All individuals living in this home are listed in the rectangle. Other relatives, friends and neighbours are listed outside the rectangle. Lines of communication are drawn to indicate contact with the patient, and also the direction of contact. A solid line is drawn when a relative or friend visits the patient daily, but when visits are less frequent, the line is dotted, with abbreviations above the line to indicate the frequency of visits, e.g. 3/7 indicates three visits per week; 2/52 indicates a visit every two weeks.[†] Other lines of support, e.g. meals-on-wheels, are also indicated. Means of support that have been lost are shown by a cross through the appropriate line.

Capildeo and his colleagues point out that the particular value of this diagram is that the patient's social environment may be seen in comparative detail at a glance. This lessens the need for lengthy social reports and reduces the pressures on the

---

[†] This system of indicating frequency can be confusing. It might be less confounding, and more helpful, especially when data are being analysed, to express frequency according to the Système International d'Unités, i.e. in hertz. Thus 5 μHz would denote a frequency corresponding to three visits a week and 0·8 μHz would indicate the frequency corresponding to a visit every two weeks. A simple conversion table could be used to convert periods expressed colloquially to frequencies in SI units.

medical social work department. It is applicable to any patient admitted to hospital who is potentially at risk as well as to disabled or elderly patients at home. Any breakdown in the home environment may be identified easily and appropriate support given thereby avoiding unnecessary admission.

CONCLUSIONS

As Goldie (1978) has pointed out, there is a rich seam of psychopathology running through the whole of otolaryngology. Indeed Tello (1971) considers the area of clinical neuro-otology to be more appropriately designated 'otoneuropsychiatry'. There are, however, problems in ascertaining the extent to which psychological disturbances are the consequence, and not the cause, of the disorder. As Lipowski (1975a) says, physical illness itself is a major cause of psychiatric morbidity, but the mechanisms are still imperfectly understood. Moreover, as Lipowski (1975b) has also indicated, no disease is caused by a single factor, although one factor may outweigh all the others. These causal factors vary in their respective contribution to a patient's malfunction and their assessment constitutes the process of comprehensive diagnosis (Susser, 1973). This remark applies equally well to neuro-otology. The patient must be viewed as existing in a biopsychosocial field. However, there is much yet to learn. One can only echo the concluding remarks of Crary and Wexler following their study in this area: 'If we learn anything from the history of science, it is that final results are never final.'

REFERENCES

Alvarez W C 1951 The neuroses. Saunders, Philadelphia
Bauer J , Schilder P 1919 Über einige psychophysiologische Mechanismen funktioneller Neurosen. Deutsche Zeitschrift für Nervenheilkunde 64 : 279–299
Black F O, Sando I, Hildyard V H, Hemenway W G 1969 Bilateral multiple otosclerotic foci and endolymphatic hydrops. Histopathological case report. Annals of Otology, Rhinology and Laryngology 78 : 1062–1073
Blumenthal M, Davie J W 1980 Dizziness and falling in elderly psychiatric outpatients. American Journal of Psychiatry 137 : 203–206
Brain W R 1938 Vertigo: its neurological, otological, circulatory and surgical aspects. British Medical Journal 2 : 605–608
Burgess A M, Burgess A M Jr 1966 Caring for the patient—A thrice told tale. New England Journal of Medicine 274 : 1241–1244
Bystrzanowska T, Jablonska K 1972 Badania psychologic zne u chorych z zaburzeniami blednikowymi. Otolaryngologia Polska 26 : 695–700
Capildeo R, Court C, Rose F C 1976 Social network Diagram. British Medical Journal 1 : 143–144
Cawthorne T E 1947 Ménière's disease. Annals of Otology, Rhinology and Laryngology 56 : 18–38
Cawthorne T E 1954 Positional nystagmus. Annals of Otology, Rhinology and Rhinology 63 : 481–490
Ceroni T, Franzoni M 1963 Aspetti psicosomatici della malatti di Ménière. Annuali Laringologia 62 : 352–358
Cobb S 1947 Psychosomatic medicine. In: Cecil R L (ed) Textbook of medicine. Saunders, Philadelphia
Crary W G, Wexler M 1977 Ménière's disease: A psychosomatic disorder? Psychological Reports 41 : 603–645
Crary W G, Wexler M, Forman R 1976 A psychological investigation of Ménière's disease: background, design, and preliminary results. Journal Supplements and Abstracting Service 6, No 112
Czubalski K, Bochenek W, Zawisza E 1976 Psychological stress and personality. Journal of Psychosomatic Research 20 : 187–191

Dix M R, Hallpike C S 1952 The pathology, symptomatology and diagnosis of certain common disorders of the vestibular system. Proceedings of the Royal Society of Medicine 45: 341–354

Eastwood M R, Trevelyan M H 1972 Relationship between physical and psychiatric disorder. Psychological Medicine 2: 363–366

Ebaugh F G 1950 Iatrogenicity in medicine. Journal of the Michigan State Medical Society 49: 79–84

Echikson E E, Bazilian S E 1959 Iatrogenic emotional problems associated with ward rounds. Journal of the Einstein Medical Center 7: 262–286

Fee G A 1968 Traumatic perilymphatic fistulas. Archives of Otolaryngology 88: 477–480

Fowler E P, Zeckel A 1952 Psychosomatic aspects of Ménière's disease. Journal of the American Medical Association 148: 1265–1268

Fowler E P, Zeckel A 1953 Psychophysiological factors in Ménière's disease. Psychosomatic Medicine 15: 127–139

Frank J D 1973 Persuasion and healing. Johns Hopkins Press, Baltimore

Goldie E L 1978 Psychiatric aspects of otolaryngology. Practioner 221: 701–702

Gordon N 1954 Post-traumatic vertigo, with special reference to positional nystagmus. Lancet 1: 1216–1218

Gowers W R 1893 A manual of disease of the nervous system. London, vol 2, p 78

Green R E, Douglass C C 1951 Intracranial section of the eight nerve for Ménière's disease. Annals of Otology, Rhinology and Laryngology 60: 610–621

Gussen R 1971 Ménière's disease: New temporal bone findings in two cases. Laryngoscope 81: 1695–1707

Guttman E 1943 The prognosis in civilian head injuries. British Medical Journal 1: 94–106

Halliday J L 1948 Psychosocial medicine. Heinemann, London

Hallpike C S, Cairns H 1938 Observations on the pathology of Ménière's syndrome. Journal of Laryngology and Otology 53: 625–655

Harrison M S, Naftalin L 1968 Ménière's disease. Chas C Thomas, Springfield, Ill

Hill D 1941 Head injuries and war neurosis. Medical Press 205: 140–144

Hinchcliffe R C 1967a Emotion as a precipitating factor in Ménière's disease. Journal of Laryngology and Otology 81: 471–475

Hinchcliffe R 1967b Personality profile in Ménière's disease. Journal of Laryngology and Otology 81: 477–481

Hinchcliffe R 1967c Personal and Family Medical History in Ménière's disease. Journal of Laryngology and Otology 81: 661–668

Hinchcliffe R 1967d An attempt to classify the primary vertigos. Journal of Laryngology and Otology 81: 849–859

Hinchcliffe R 1967e Headache and Ménière's disease. Acta Otolaryngologica 64: 384–390

Hinchcliffe R 1970 La maladie de Ménière. Cahiers d'Otorhinolaryngologie 5: 725–732

Hinchcliffe R, Prasansuk S 1973 Ménière's disorder. Siriraj Hospital Gazette 25: 1802–1805

Hinoki M, Nakanishi K, Ito S, Ushio N, Ichibangase T 1978 "Neurotic vertigo" from the standpoint of neurotology. Agressologie 19: 269

Holmes T H, Masuda M 1972 Psychosomatic syndrome. Psychology Today 5: 106–107

Jongkees L B W 1964 Medical treatment of Ménière's disease. Acta Otolaryngologica (Stockholm) 192: 109–112

Kay D W, Beamish P, Roth M 1964 Old age mental disorders in Newcastle-upon Tyne. Part I: A study of prevalence. British Journal of Psychiatry 110: 146–158

Koch J 1932 Betrachtungen über die beziechungen Ménière artigen Krankheitsbilder zum mechanischen und psychischen trauma. Archiv für Ohrenkrankheiten 132: 29–41

Kragh V 1969 Defence Mechanism Test Manual. Skand. Testforlaget, Stockholm

Leighton A N 1959 The Stirling County Study of Psychiatric Disorder and Sociocultural Environment. In: My Name is Legion: Foundations for a Theory of Man in Relation to Culture. Basic Books, New York

Levy I, O'Leary J L 1947 Incidence of vertigo in neurologic conditions. Transactions of the American Otologic Society 35: 329–347

Lewis E 1942 Discussion of differential diagnosis and treatment of post-concussional states. Proceeding of the Royal Society of Medicine 35: 607–634

Lidvall H F, Linderoth B, Norlin B 1974 Causes of the post-concussional syndrome. Acta neurologica Scandinavica Suppl 56 p 128

Lipkowski Z J 1975a Psychiatry of somatic diseases: Epidemiology, Pathogenesis, Classification. Comprehensive Psychiatry 16: 105–124

Lipowski Z J 1975b Physical Illness, the patient and his environment: Psychosocial Foundations of Medicine. In: American Handbook of Psychiatry. Basic Books, New York, vol 4

Livsey C G 1972 Physical illness and Family Dynamics. In: Lipowski 25 (ed) Psychosocial Aspects of

Physical illness. Advances in Psychosomatic Medicine. Karger, Basel, vol 8

McNeill J H 1951 Iatrogenic disease. North Carolina Medical Journal 12:231–233

Magnusson P-A, Nilsson A, Henriksson N-G 1977 Psychogenic vertigo within an anxiety frame of reference: An experimental study. British Journal of Medical Psychology 50:187–201

Martin M J 1970 Functional disorders in otolaryngology. Archives of Otolaryngology 91:457–459

Mears A 1963 The Management of the Anxious Patient. Saunders, Philadelphia

Miller P McC, Ingham J G 1976 Friends, Confidants, and Symptoms. Social Psychiatry 11:51–58

Moore E, Atkinson M 1958 Psychogenic vertigo. The importance of its recognition. Archives of Otolaryngology 67:347–353

Parrisius W 1924 Anomalien des periphersten Gefässsystems als Krankheitsursache speziell bei Ménière und Glaukom. München Medizinische Wochenschrift 71:224–225

Portmann G 1931 L'angiospasme labyrinthique. Revue de Laryngologie 52:467

Pratt R T C, McKenzie W 1958 Anxiety states following Vestibular Disorders. Lancet 2:347–349

Rahe R H, Floistad I, Bergan T, Ringdal R, Gerhardt R, Gunderson E K E, Arthur R J 1974 A model for life changes and illness research. Archives of General Psychiatry 31:172–177

Rallo J 1972 Aggressiveness, feelings of giddiness and muscular tension. International Journal of Psycho-Analysis 53:265–269

Reiser M F 1975 Changing theoretical concepts in Psychosomatic Medicine. In: American Handbook of Psychiatry. Basic Books, New York

Roth M, Kay D W K 1956 Affective disorder arising in the senium. II Physical disability as an aetiological factor. Journal of Mental Science 102:141–150

Shey H H 1971 Iatrogenic Anxiety. Psychiatric Quarterly 45:344–356

Schilder P 1933 The vestibular apparatus in neurosis and psychosis. Journal of Nervous and Mental Diseases 78:1–23, 137–164

Schilder P 1939 The relations between clinging and equilibrium. International Journal of PscyhoAnalysis 20:58–64

Schur M 1953 The ego in anxiety. In: Lowenstein R M (ed) Drives, Affects, Behavior. International Universities Press. New York

Shrala U, Siltala P, Lumio J S 1965 Psychological aspects of Ménière's disease. Preliminary report. Acta Otolaryngologica (Stockholm) 59:350–357

Sloane P 1967 Psychiatric aspects of vertigo. In: Spector M (ed) Dizziness and Vertigo, Grune and Stratton, New York

Smith G J W, Johnson G, Ljunghill-Anderson J, Almgren E 1970 MCT—metakontrast tekniken. Skand. Testförlaget. Stockholm

Srole L, Langner T S, Michaels S T 1962 The Midtown Manhattan study. In: Mental Health in the Metropolis. McGraw-Hill, New York, vol I

Stephens S D G 1975 Personality tests in Ménière's disorder. Journal of Laryngology and Otology 89:479–490

Susser M 1973 Causal Thinking in the Health Services. Oxford University Press, Oxford

Tanja T A, Hofman A, Valkenburg H A 1979 Een epidemiologisch onderzoek onder bejaarden (EPOZ). II Duizeligheid bij bejaarden; mogelijke oorzaken en gevolgen. Nederlandsch tijdschift voor Gerontologie 10:195–201

Tello A 1971 Otoneuropsiquiatria: Andres Bello. Santiago, Chile

Wahl C W 1962 Iatrogenic neuroses, their production and presentation. Psychosomatics 3:450–453

Watson C C, Barnes C M, Donaldson J A, Klett W G 1967 Psychosomatic aspects of Ménière's disease. Archives of Otolaryngology 86:543–549

Wilcock G 1980 Why did this patient fall? Geriatric Medicine 26:17–18

Wild D, Nayak U S L, Isaacs B 1981 How dangerous are falls in old people at home? British Medical Journal 282:266–268

Williamson D G, Gifford F 1971 Psychosomatic aspects of Ménière's disease. Acta Otolaryngologica (Stockholm) 72:118–120

Williamson J, Stokoe I H, Gray S, Fisher M, Smith A, McGhee A, Stephenson E 1964 Old people at home. Their unreported needs. Lancet 1:1117–1120

Yuen S S, Schuknecht H F 1972 Vestibular aqueduct and endolymphatic duct in Ménière's disease. Archives of Otolaryngology 96:553–555

Rehabilitation of elderly patients with disorders of balance

There is no field so well suited to the person with optimism, energy and curiosity as that of rehabilitation of the elderly. The initial goal is never less than a full recovery of function and a return to an independent life at home, although this aim may have to be modified according to the patient's progress. Despite the feeling of helplessness or hopelessness that so often surrounds an ill old person and his attendants the principles of treatment are well established and it has been repeatedly shown that if a team applies them with enthusiasm and skill then satisfactory results are obtained surprisingly often. However, it is remarkable that fundamental questions about the nature of the decline in function with increasing age and the basis on which treatment may be applied have rarely been asked.

ASSESSMENT

Most elderly persons who fall do not seek medical advice and those that are taken to a hospital casualty department are usually sent home straightaway unless they have sufficient injury to require admission. No precise figures are available but there is a strong clinical impression that many of these patients have repeated falls and suffer a rapid, catastrophic loss of confidence and become fearful, immobile and housebound. Rather than delay admission until the person is no longer able to manage independently it is better to make a full assessment, which can often be done in the day hospital, when the falls first begin.

The team approach is essential for successful rehabilitation of an elderly patient. Murphy (1977) identified improved team work and early assessment by a social worker as two of the key factors in preventing the 'blocked bed' syndrome. That geriatricians and their teams are effective in improving the discharge rate from general medical wards was clearly shown by Burley and her colleagues (1979).

Functional assessment (Fig. 18.1) must be made of every patient in order to understand his illness and to formulate a plan of rehabilitation. His disability usually has physical, psychological and social consequences and each of these must be examined (Exton-Smith, 1977).

Physical state
In addition to a full list of medical diagnoses the doctor should try to determine the cause of the balance disorder and the treatment which is likely to be most effective.

PHYSIOTHERAPY DEPARTMENT (GERIATRIC UNIT)

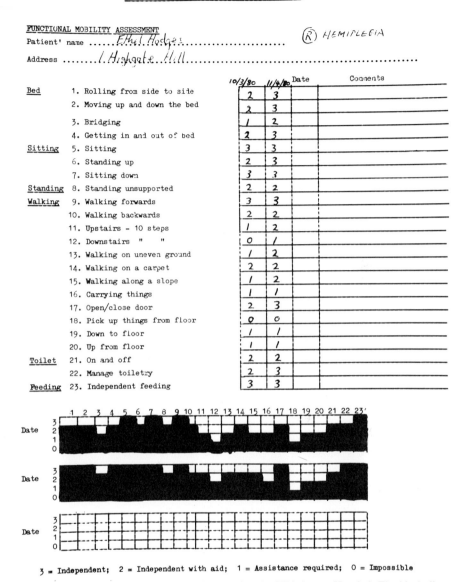

FUNCTIONAL MOBILITY ASSESSMENT

Patient' name ......*Ethyl Hodges*...................... ®) HEMIPLEGIA

Address ....*1. Highgate Hill*...

			10/3/80	11/4/80	Date	Comments
Bed	1.	Rolling from side to side	2	3		
	2.	Moving up and down the bed	2	3		
	3.	Bridging	1	2		
	4.	Getting in and out of bed	2	3		
Sitting	5.	Sitting	3	3		
	6.	Standing up	2	3		
	7.	Sitting down	3	3		
Standing	8.	Standing unsupported	2	2		
Walking	9.	Walking forwards	3	3		
	10.	Walking backwards	2	2		
	11.	Upstairs - 10 steps	1	2		
	12.	Downstairs " "	0	1		
	13.	Walking on uneven ground	1	2		
	14.	Walking on a carpet	2	2		
	15.	Walking along a slope	1	2		
	16.	Carrying things	1	1		
	17.	Open/close door	2	3		
	18.	Pick up things from floor	0	0		
	19.	Down to floor	1	1		
	20.	Up from floor	1	1		
Toilet	21.	On and off	2	2		
	22.	Manage toiletry	2	3		
Feeding	23.	Independent feeding	3	3		

3 = Independent; 2 = Independent with aid; 1 = Assistance required; 0 = Impossible

Fig. 18.1 Example of simple assessment chart used at the Whittington Hospital. The block diagram shows at a glance which activities the patient is having difficulties with so that treatment can be directed at them.

Postural control depends on four inter-related variables: somatic proprioception, vision, vestibular mechanisms and the supporting base. Some of these are more important that others and Magnus (1926) noted that higher animals were less dependent on vestibular function than those lower down the evolutionary scale.

It may be possible to place a patient's disability directly into one of these categories because, for example, he is known to have Ménière's disease, but it is still instructive to examine his normal balance and standing reflexes. The postural

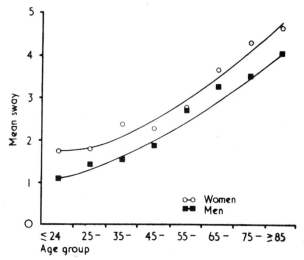

Fig. 18.2 Postural sway increases with age and is significantly (p < 0·01) higher in women. (after Overstall, 1977. Reproduced by permission of the Editor of the British Medical Journal.)

reflexes that are concerned with the upright posture and locomotion have been described by Martin (1967). How far these reflexes are altered in normal old age is largely unknown although it has been observed (Overstall et al, 1977) that sway in the anter-posterior plane, which reflects the integrity of the anti-gravity mechanism when standing, increases with advancing age (Fig. 18.2).

The clinician is most concerned with the normal reflex reactions which occur when body weight is displaced or when the support is moved. These are the lateral sway, propping, stepping and hopping reactions with appropriate movements of the head, trunk and upper limbs which occur both in normal movements and in response to lateral displacement. In practice the need is to assess what the patient is required to do in the course of his normal daily activities and his ability to do it. This means looking at:

1. The support required to maintain balance.
   Can the patient sit unassisted and if so for how long? How much support does he require? Does he require more support with his eyes shut? Does he require less support with additional visual information?
2. The response to a disturbing force.
   Does the patient respond to disturbance of balance? How does he respond: with support reaction from his arms, correction or establishment of a new stable position? Can be maintain balance whilst his attention is directed elsewhere and, if so, for how long?
3. The degree of independent activity attainable.
   Can the patient maintain balance whilst moving his head, his trunk, his arms and trunk? In each case can he regain the original position exactly? Is he stable throughout the movement? Can he vary the speed of movement? Can he perform the movement with his eyes shut? Can he get up from the floor unaided? (Lane, 1969)

In addition the patient's joint mobility (including the cervical spine), muscle strength and co-ordination must be tested. Osteoarthritis of knees, hips and lumbar-sacràl spine is a common problem in the elderly and can so reduce the normal suppleness of movement that despite an intact neurological system righting reactions are ineffective. The patient's feet and his footwear should also be inspected since loose fitting slippers may cause falls (Svanström, 1974).

When assessing the patient it is important to be able to establish the degree of disability, record progress and assess the point at which treatment ceases to be of value. Many ways of measuring the patient's progress have been devised (Katz et al, 1970; Fugl-Meyer et al, 1975) but so far none can be said to be ideal. A system may be simple and quick to use based on, say, a 0–5 grading scale of various movements and displayed on a block diagram (Stichbury, 1975). However, it suffers from a lack of qualitative information on the manner in which the patient moves or the effort required. On the other hand, videotapes made of walking and balancing exercises provide a wealth of qualitative detail and it can usually be seen at a glance whether there is an improvement. Another advantage is that the patient enjoys seeing himself on television and may gain encouragement from watching his own progress (Graham, 1975). Even with a filmed record there is still the problem of accurately defining the exact nature of gait and balance deficiencies and their response to treatment.

One method which provides comprehensive results in an easily understandable form uses a walkway for gait analysis. Conducting rods are set into the ribbing of the walkway and when two of these rods are shorted out by an aluminium tape on the patient's shoes a current flows, which is measured on a U-Vrecorder. The recorder provides a graph of current against time and from this can be calculated factors such as stride time, swingtime, stride length, step length, velocity and double support-time (Wall and Ashburn, 1979).

Among patients who have had a stroke the mental barriers to recovery (Adams and Hurwitz, 1963) must be recognised at the outset since visual neglect, in particular, will have an adverse effect on balance.

Drugs must be reviewed for any possible harmful effects on balance. This may involve stopping certain hypnotics such as barbiturates (Macdonald and Macdonald, 1977) or substituting one with a shorter plasma half-line so that hangover effects the next morning are reduced (Nayal et al, 1978).

Finally the activities of daily living are assessed to find out if the patient can get in and out of bed, transfer from bed to chair, stand up from the chair, use the lavatory, manage stairs and so on. Clearly it is important to know what the patient was capable of in the past so that realistic goals may be set.

Psychological state

The value of routine assessment of mental function (Table 18.1) is that it very often brings to light a previously unrecognised depression or mild dementia. If short term memory and concentration are poor then all the rehabilitation staff need to be told since allowances can then be made for the patient's poor response to instructions and his apparent refusal to co-operate. Suitable tests have been described by Isaacs and Marks (1973) and Strub and Black (1977).

Table 18.1 Simple assessment of mental function.

1. *Concentration and short-term memory*
   Test by asking the patient to repeat a number of digits. Start with three and work up. A normal person should be able to repeat at least seven digits (∓ 2).

2. *Long-term memory*
   Use the set test: the patient is asked to tell the examiner all the colours he can think of. One point is scored for each correct answer to a maximum of 10. Similarly for animals, fruits and towns, making a maximum of 40.

3. *Orientation*
   Ask patient his name, age and date of birth; his address; where he is now; time, day, month and year.

4. *Constructional ability*
   Ask patient to draw a clock or a house and copy simple shapes. This ability is usually lost early in the course of dementia, as well as in stroke patients with parietal lobe damage.

Social

The role of the hospital social worker is to prepare the patient, his relatives and the community for discharge. Unless plans are made soon after admission much hard work may come to nothing when it is discovered, on the eve of discharge, that home circumstances are unsuitable and the key supporter at home is no longer available. Putting matters right may take weeks and the frustrated patient loses heart, his mobility declines and it may be very difficult for him to regain the ground that he has lost.

ACTIVITY IN OLD AGE

Spontaneous activity in animals reaches a peak in early life and thereafter declines with increasing age (Smith and Dugal, 1965). In man high motor drive appears in childhood at an age when control of postural reflexes is not fully developed and although their motor drives are quite dissimilar both young and old have increased body sway (Sheldon, 1963). It may be that the great activity of children is a necessary part of acquiring the fine skills of balance. As we age some of this skill is lost although special training, such as gymnastics, may increase it. Active elderly people generally sway less than the inactive but it is not clear whether maintenance of balance is a consequence of activity or simply an absence of ill health. Poor health seems to be a major factor in those who fall so it is difficult to determine the importance of inactivity in these patients. Even though postural balance can be improved during convalescence this may be due as much to improvements in health as to increased activity.

　Malnutrition is an important factor in reducing activity. Although an inadequate diet, particularly if it is deficient in vitamins, may cause clearly recognised clinical syndromes, this is not such a common problem as the other form of malnutrition, obesity. Obese persons are significantly less active than the non-obese and this difference is most marked in women (Chirico and Stunkard, 1960). Other things being equal we might expect the obese person with balance problems to fall more frequently than his non-obese counterpart because his inertia is that much greater.

Even a modest 5 per cent increase in a person's activity can produce a 10 kg loss of weight over three months (Shephard, 1969).

At any age it is not always possible to separate the mental effects of physical fitness from the effects on the body. Although it is generally assumed that physical fitness has a beneficial influence on many psychological factors, including anxiety and wellbeing, it is possible that persons with certain psychological characteristics are attracted to keep-fit programmes (Hammett, 1967).

The question remains as to whether physical activity in old age will improve balance. Longitudinal studies have shown that maintenance of activity is important for successful ageing (Palmore and Maddox, 1977) and despite the decline in neuromuscular function with age (Gutman and Hanzíková, 1972) it seems reasonable to expect that an improvement in performance will follow suitable training. The theory behind this postulates that the beneficial effect of exercise depends on the repeated activation of nervous pathways from brain to muscle. Skills that are lost have to be relearnt by establishing new pathways in the central nervous system and to be successful training must involve constant repetition. In short, neuromuscular education depends on maximal activity, induced by maximal voluntary effort and repeated the maximal number of times (Kabat, 1947).

MANAGEMENT AT HOME

The problem with many old people who fall is that as their confidence declines so does their mobility and the frequency of falling often increases. It is necessary to help restore confidence and this is best done by a physiotherapist working in a day hospital or in the patient's home.

Apart from the therapeutic benefit from prescribed exercises a visit to the day hospital two or three times a week has a valuable stimulant effect, particularly for patients who may not have been out of doors for months or even years. Given a chance to take part in group activities within an encouraging environment many patients exert themselves to an extent which they would never consider at home.

Building up a person's confidence depends on improving his feeling of wellbeing although it has been already noted that the relationship between activity and psychological states is unclear. In eastern Europe studies have claimed to show the benefit to workers of having physical training instead of a coffee break. A group of radiotelegraph operators who exercised for four hours a week improved both their working performance and their score on objective tests of attention and concentration. These changes were attributed to a lessening of anxiety but as Shephard (1969) points out the improvements could just as well be due to relief of boredom and greater cortical arousal resulting from a fresh type of activity. This is likely to be at least part of the explanation for the improvement seen in old people. Boredom and lack of concentration appear to be relevant factors in many falls and raising the level of attention is likely to be beneficial.

At home a similar effect can be produced by a visiting physiotherapist who, in addition to specific exercises, can walk with the patient to the shops and encourage a return to normal activities. The availability of this type of service is being gradually extended and there is usually direct access for general practitioners and hospital consultants. For it to be effective the doctor must give adequate information to the physiotherapist on referral and there should be feedback on the patient's progress (Partridge and Warren, 1977)

Activities of daily living

Whether the patient is in hospital or still at home it is helpful if the therapist makes a home visit and views the patient's daily routine. It may be found that balance difficulties are limited to certain activities such as getting on and off the lavatory and a raised seat or rail around the lavatory may substantially reduce the risk.

The hazardous home environment of some elderly persons has been described by Agate (1970) but it is common to find that many of them are able to cope successfully with the dangers for years. Only when ill health reduces mobility and attention does the trailing wire or loose rug present a real problem. Even then too much emphasis on potential hazards is not the best way to restore confidence. Indeed, the therapist who insists on clearing a cluttered room of excess furniture may find that the patient, lost without his familiar props and handholds falls more frequently. It is important that the patient is taught how to get up from the floor (Fig. 18.3) if he does have a fall and fitting an alarm bell so that he can summon help if needed may help his morale.

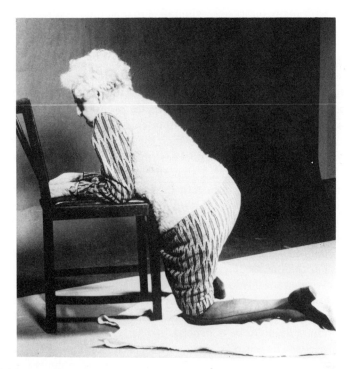

Fig. 18.3 Advice to patients for getting up from the floor. (1) Gain composure. (Many patients fail in their attempts because of panic.) (2) Find your way to a stool or chair. (3) Using the stool or chair come up on to your knees. (4) Place one foot flat on the floor. (5) Press on stool or seat of the chair and stand up.

RESIDENTIAL HOMES

Physiotherapy in residential (Part III) homes is still something of a novelty. Some superintendents are unenthusiastic because of a misunderstanding of what the physiotherapist can offer in the way of help. Yet in an 'average' 55 place home it was found that 36 per cent of residents needed rehabilitation and 45 per cent needed training in functional activities (Ransome, 1978). Functionally nearly all the residents were independent but they still spent most of the day sitting in chairs lined up against the walls. This lack of exercise was blamed for the deleterious effect on joints and balance and Ransome advised that keep fit classes should be routine in all residential homes. Suitable exercises for such a class, which could be led by any of the staff members, have been described by Davies (1975).

Homes where there was a high level of activity and where staff expected residents to carry out domestic tasks, such as making their own beds, were, as might be expected, more lively. Whether the residents in these homes had fewer falls is not mentioned although it is quite possible that falls were more common than in the low activity 'they are too old to do anything much' homes. Activity increases the opportunity for falling but there is a considerable difference between an old person bustling about and not paying too much attention to the occasional fall and a chairfast resident whose mobility is totally dependent on a helping arm and is constantly worrying about falling.

STROKE REHABILITATION

The principles of stroke rehabilitation in the elderly are already well described (Garraway and Akhtar, 1978). Many years ago it was recognised that active rehabilitation by trained personnel was likely to influence the degree of recovery (Lowenthal et al, 1959) and that, in general, the prognosis was better under the 'prolonged supervised convalescence' of a geriatric unit than in the average medical ward (Adams and McComb, 1953). However, deciding who is most likely to benefit from intensive treatment is still not resolved and depends first on developing a method of predicting prognosis and secondly on a clearer understanding of the role of physiotherapists and possible long term treatment alternatives. For the patient with a severe stroke whose disability is great and recovery is poor Brocklehurst and his colleagues (1978) have suggested the use of volunteers and simply trained personnel working with groups and stroke clubs.

A physiotherapist no longer simply talks to her patient but constantly handles his body so as to acquire directly an awareness of his motor condition. This allows her to feel even minor changes in posture and to prevent undesirable reactions. The main problem with most hemiplegic patients is not muscle weakness but a lack of power caused by opposition of spastic antagonists. We normally maintain posture by continuous movement and are dependent on this integrated activity of reflex mechanisms. Spasticity, however, produces abnormal patterns of posture which prevent movement and is the result of both an increased and an abnormal distribution of tone (Bobath, 1978). The therapist's long term aim therefore is to inhibit or control spasticity and introduce the normal movements necessary for skilled, co-ordinated movement.

In patients with flaccidity, postural activity has to be increased by using tactile and proprioceptive stimulation. This must be done with care since excessive stimulation may result in abnormal tonic reflex activity instead of the desired normal increase of tone. Many patients have a mixture of flaccidity and spasticity: a flaccid arm with loss of postural tone and reflexes and a spastic leg due to the release of abnormal reflexes. Thus it is essential to assess each patient in terms of his postural tone and how it changes with position and movement.

There is little place in physiotherapy for a dogmatic adherence to any particular system of treatment. All systems can give good results in skilled hands and so far no controlled trial has shown unequivocally that one approach is superior to another. This is hardly surprising when one considers the enormous number of variables and the difficulty in finding untreated controls. The most that can be asked at present is that therapists constantly examine the assumptions on which treatment is based.

Three commonly used techniques are briefly described here although this certainly does not cover all the available methods. At first sight it might appear that these different approaches are contradictory. Bobath (1978) specifically warns against the use of gross limb synergies in case repeated use makes it more difficult for the patient to learn other movement combinations. Whereas Brunnstrom (1970) encourages the training of these primitive patterns since they can be brought under voluntary control and used to good effect. Much depends on a full assessment by an experienced physiotherapist who can then decide on the appropriate method.

Bobath technique

The emphasis here is on reduction of spasticity and the introduction of more selective movement patterns in preparation for the return of function (Bobath, 1978). Knowledge of the normal childhood development of postural reflexes is important since these automatic reflexes are the background for all voluntary activity (Bobath, 1971). The Bobath approach is particularly useful in treating elderly patients with balance disorders, both those with minor cerebrovascular disease and those with a normal central nervous system but who still have problems of co-ordination. This latter group, either because of painful joints or because of a fear of falling may have developed widespread protective muscle spasm. This may be very similar to spastic patterns. Thus techniques to reduce hypertonus combined with treatments aimed at increasing muscle power can be very helpful.

Standing balance

In many patients who have only mild cerebrovascular disease or who have largely recovered from a hemiparesis, spasticity is slight and does not impair movement. There may be a transient increase in spasticity when the patient becomes excited, moves too quickly or makes too much of an effort. Co-ordination then deteriorates and the knee and foot stiffen. The aim is to produce more selective movements of the knee, ankle and toes independent of the position and movement of the hip. Full dorsiflexion of ankles and toes is essential for a normal gait and for the postural reflex which prevents falling backwards. How far this reflex is impaired can be seen by standing behind the patient and with hands on his waist, pulling backwards. A normal person will move his head and arms forwards and dorsiflex his ankles and toes. A patient with a spastic leg will, instead, push the sole of his foot against the ground.

The patient starts by practising dorsiflexion in the step position with the sound foot forward and his hip well over it. He then bends his knee on the affected side but keeps his toes on the ground so that they became fully dorsiflexed. The movement is reversed and repeated until there is no extensor spasticity. The affected foot can be placed on a small trolley on castors and moved backwards and forwards to improve control of the swing phase.

To improve balance on the affected leg the therapist helps the patient to weightbear on that leg and encourages him to flex his head to the sound side. When he has mastered this he should do small bending and straightening movements at the knee. Balance and hip control can be further improved by standing with legs crossed and externally rotated. Rotation of the pelvis and shoulder girdle is important practice to improve co-ordination in walking.

Proprioceptive neuromuscular facilitation (PNF)

This approach is based on the work of Kabat (1947) who emphasised the use of maximal resistance throughout the range of movement. He explained subsequent recovery on the formation of new pathways within the central nervous system. He recommended the development, not of individual muscles but of movements related to primitive patterns. He used postural and righting reflexes. The movements are related to functions such as standing up and walking. It was found that they were most effective when they were diagonal and spiral in character since this allowed maximal elongation of related muscle groups and produced a stretch reflex pattern. Sensory stimuli, particularly stretch, is used for greater proprioceptive stimulation since this facilitates motion. Other techniques include repeated contraction to improve range and endurance and 'rhythmic stabilisation' where the patient contracts isometrically the agonist and then the antagonist.

Support for these facilitatory exercises came from Twitchell (1951) who described the motor recovery following hemiplegia as beginning with a simple proprioceptive reflex which then became more complex until the patient learned to utilise first the flexor synergy and then the extensor synergy. As spasticity declined, willed movements improved and these could be facilitated and modified by tactile stimuli.

PNF is particularly good for improving muscle strength and motor skills, although it is probably less useful than Bobath for reducing spasticity.

Standing balance

To stimulate postural reflexes and improve the response of specific groups of muscles, maximal pressure and resistance are applied. The therapist disturbs the patient's balance in a diagonal direction by applying pressure at the head, shoulder or pelvis from left anterior to right posterior and in the reverse direction. In this way diagonal and antagonist patterns, which maintain normal posture are stimulated (Knott and Voss, 1968).

For example, in one exercise the therapist stands facing the patient and holds the back of his head with her left hand and places her right hand on his left hip. The patient extends his head with rotation to the right and also rotates his lower trunk to the right. The therapist then applies pressure and instructs him not to let his head be pulled forward or his hip pushed back.

Brunnstrom technique

This technique has been developed almost entirely on stroke patients and is based on Magnus' (1926) neurophysiological research and the primitive patterns of movements and reflexes described by Fay (1954). No two stroke patients are the same but there are some common elements of motor behaviour and Brunnstrom uses these in her treatment.

When the hemiplegic patient is regaining motor control it is often observed that muscles will respond only with certain combinations. For example, a patient with a left sided flaccid paralysis may be unable to move his left arm voluntarily. Yet if he attempts to extend his right elbow against resistance, with increasing effort an associated flexor synergy appears in the left arm. The left elbow flexes, the shoulder abducts and externally rotates, and the forearm supinates.

The aim is to use and modify these basic movement synergies for functional activities. Advantage is taken of various facilitatory influences which affect the tone on the affected side. For instance, when the patient turns his head the asymmetrical tonic neck reflex will produce an increase of flexor tone in the 'skull' limbs and an increase of extensor tone in the 'jaw' limbs.

Standing balance

The patient stands with arms by his side and rotates his trunk. As the trunk rotates to the left his left arm swings behind the body until the hand reaches the buttock, while the right arm swings in front of the body, the palm reaching for the hip. The arms should move as a result of the trunk rotation and not by forceful effort.

The next step is slow walking with exaggerated trunk rotation but without the arms moving to the full wrap-around position. As the left foot swings forward the trunk rotates to the left and the right arm swings forwards. The aim is a steady rhythmic motion with the therapists avoiding manual correction in case this increases spasticity (Brunnstrom, 1970).

PARKINSONISM

In the early stages of the disease, where there may be little disruption to the patient's life other than a tendency to fall, drugs are often withheld since it is felt that unwanted side effects may outweigh any benefit. However, there is no need to deny the patient physiotherapy. In general, the earlier the patient is seen by a physiotherapist the better, since it is easier to prevent loss of normal movement patterns than to regain them later.

The positive and negative symptoms which characterise disease of the basal ganglia (Martin, 1967) affect balance in a number of ways. Rigidity can cause foot deformities; postural adjustments which maintain the stability of the body during normal activities may be lost; protective reactions when there is a loss of equilibrium (such as staggering) are inadequate or absent altogether; and the loss of the rotational element in movement means that the patient may not turn sufficiently when he goes to sit down and falls off the edge of the chair. Martin noted that these patients frequently fail to make voluntary adjustments to overcome their disability and thought that this may be due to diminished awareness or neglect of the changes in posture.

Rigidity

The aims of treatment are threefold (Atkinson, 1977). First the therapist tries to reduce the sensitivity of the stretch reflex by teaching general relaxation and using rhythmical passive and assisted active movements. Trunk rotation is important as are exercises where the trunk is first flexed and rotated to one side and then extended with rotation to the other side.

Secondly, as muscle tone subsides, the patient is helped to experience more normal reactions. Trunk rotation with rhythmic arm swinging and, when sitting, trunk rotation with hand support forwards or sideways encourages normal protective balance reactions.

Thirdly, movements are developed which follow the normal pattern in as wide a range and as freely as possible. Again, the emphasis is on trunk rotation, rhythmical swaying and standing up with hand support to alternate sides. Walking practice should include turning, arm swinging, stepping backwards and stepping across the other leg.

Tendency to fall backwards

This is a common problem and shows a failure of the antero-posterior control of balance. Martin described how one patient could be induced to walk almost normally by carrying a 14 pound metal framed chair in front of her, which had the effect of bringing forward the centre of gravity. Other ways of overcoming this difficulty include a waistcoat with specially adapted pockets at the front in which weights are placed and, if a walking frame is used, lowering the front two legs so that the patient tilts forwards.

Locomotion

Although rigidity plays a part in Parkinsonian gait disorders Martin showed that normal stepping could be elicited in some patients and that the main defect was in the ability to initiate and control stepping. Patients who cannot walk at all or who walk only in short shuffling steps can be helped by the therapist standing behind, tilting the patient slightly forwards and rocking the trunk from side to side. This can produce a nearly normal gait. The explanation is that because the patient is unable to sway laterally his weight cannot be shifted to one side to allow the other foot freedom to move.

These same patients can be helped to initiate a step if suitable visual cues are provided. These may be transverse lines painted on the floor at eighteen inch intervals or a small obstacle placed in front of the foot. By lifting his foot to step over it the patient tilts his body to the opposite side and the raised foot is then freed to swing forward. Occasionally once started he can carry on but repeated lines or obstacles are usually necessary to keep him walking. Frequently it is found that using stairs is easier than walking along level ground.

General measures

Problems with balance can be reduced by keeping the patient as active and independent as possible. Relatives should be taught how to use rotational movements, particularly in the morning, to lessen rigidity and help the patient loosen up. The patient himself may find it useful to turn over a few times upon wakening before getting out of bed. Whilst sitting he should sway in different directions before standing or walking. Periods of intensive physiotherapy together with routine daily exercises at home will help to maintain the memory of normal activity and delay the onset of rigidity and the accompanying joint stiffness.

CEREBELLAR LESIONS

The main problems are hypotonia and ataxia. Because of loss of tone in the muscles around joints it is difficult for the patient to move precisely or to maintain a stable posture. Normal balance reactions are slowed. The therapist has to teach normal movements and stimulate awareness of balance and posture. Initially the patient will have to use voluntary control, which may well hinder his movements, but with constant repetition a normal pattern of movement can be achieved.

The patient is started in a position where his centre of gravity is low and his base wide (Atkinson, 1977). If the therapist applies pressure (approximation) in the direction of weight bearing the stimulus already supplied by gravity is reinforced. This stimulates the extrapyramidal system and increases co-contraction of muscles around the weight bearing joints. Gentle swaying at the same time will elicit postural reactions. The patient is instructed to resist when rhythmic pressure is applied in various directions. As his confidence and postural control increase he is discouraged from relying on hand support when sitting and standing and his response is tested to gentle and unexpected disturbances of balance.

VISUAL DISTURBANCES

Vision is important for precise postural control (Smith and Ramana, 1970) but is not essential for maintenance of balance under normal circumstances provided that the other afferent systems are intact. However, even normal subjects may lose their balance if they are given false visual information in experiments which provide conflicting visual and somatic proprioceptive information. In 'moving room' experiments toddlers can be induced to fall, forwards or backwards, in the same direction as the surrounding 'room' moves. Presumably this is because the child's somatic proprioceptive information is poor, since young adults do not fall but do sway more (Lee and Lishman, 1975). It has been suggested that the elderly place greater reliance on vision to compensate for impaired function in the other afferent systems and that falls may occur when visual information is minimal, ambiguous or misleading (Over, 1966). Suitable spectacles, cataract extraction and brighter illumination might be expected to help. There is anecdotal evidence to suggest that some patients' balance improves with a walking stick. This is not used to bear weight but seems to serve as a visual cue.

Complaints of dizziness or imbalance in some stroke patients appear to be due to a directional rotation of the entire subjective visual field (Birch et al, 1960a). Both right and left hemiplegics perceive the median plane to be displaced to the affected side (Birch et al, 1960b) and this may be the explanation for the tendency of hemiplegics to lean towards the affected side. Sitting and standing practice in front of a mirror or using biofeedback techniques (q.v.) may be effective in correcting posture.

Visual neglect in stroke patients is a serious problem that occurs almost as often with left cerebral lesions as with right. However the severity of the neglect is greater when the right hemisphere is affected (Alberti, 1973). The patient should learn to recognise his visual deficit and compensate by turning his head. Activities which encourage this include reading aloud, making puzzles with the pieces scattered to the affected side and ensuring that staff and visitors approach from the affected side.

SENSORY DISTURBANCES

Limb sensation is essential for normal movement and the devastating effect of afferent neural loss was shown by Twitchell (1954). Where the loss is partial the limbs will be ataxic and the patient should be taught to compensate visually. If this is not possible a noisy bracelet or weighted cuff on the affected limb may act as a reminder (Trombly and Scott, 1977). Constant handling of the affected side may help as may heavy pressure applied by the therapist to the leg when it is weight bearing.

CERVICAL SPONDYLOSIS

This can cause imbalance in three ways, i.e by producing spastic ataxia, vascular constriction or impaired mechanoreceptor function.

Spastic ataxia

Although an important remediable cause of combined sensory ataxia or spasticity in old age is Vitamin B_{12} deficiency, this disorder is most commonly due to the effect on the spinal cord of cervical spondylosis.

It is often found that the patient's confidence and balance improve following simple walking exercises with a frame, even though the neurological signs remain unchanged. Frenkel's precision exercises (Table 18.2) which teach the patient to associate movements of the upper body with that of the legs may be helpful.

Table 18.2 Frenkel's exercises for the treatment of ataxia

The principles are:
1. Precision
2. Repetition
3. Patient's full attention on movements

Suitable exercises using floor markings:
1. Stand on traced footprints, raise each foot alternately and replace firmly and precisely on ground.
2. Walk and turn, placing feet on traced footprints.
3. Practice change of direction by walking along zigzag strip.
4. Group work to teach movement in the presence of others and increase confidence for walking in the street.

Movements in pattern are done rhythmically to counting and the patient is encouraged to use his eyes and ears as substitutes for other afferent information (Atkinson, 1977). Hard surfaces help more than soft ones and the stimuli applied by the therapist may have to be exaggerated.

If the patient has pain due to nerve root irritation exercises are best avoided in the acute stage, although massage sometimes offers relief. Advice should be given on resting and working conditions, including dressing and getting in and out of bed, to minimise stretch or constriction of the affected roots. During the recovery stage the aim is to strengthen all the muscles controlling the neck, especially the deep flexors and the patient should be warned to avoid sudden movements, particularly of flexion and extension. This regime seems to minimise the frequency of episodes (Gabell, 1979).

If the symptoms of cervical cord compression are rapidly progressive, operation is indicated irrespective of the age (Symon, 1971).

Vascular constriction
Undoubtedly this is a cause of vertebrobasilar ischaemia and its associated symptoms but it seems to have been used all too often in the past as a convenient explanation for any kind of vertiginous episode in an elderly person.

Neck exercises are probably unwise because of the risk of increasing the constriction. However, breathing exercises may help considerably, especially if they are given with abdominally assisted expiration. The rationale is that increased venous return improves cardiac output and leads to a greater flow rate through the narrowed arteries. The exercises should be used before moving from lying to sitting or sitting to standing; whenever one position has been maintained for any length of time, and whenever a feeling of unsteadiness occurs. Frequent changes of position should be encouraged and as much general activity as possible to stimulate deeper breathing (Gabell, 1979).

Impaired mechanoreceptor function
The contributions made to normal posture and gait by mechanoreceptors in the apophyseal joints of the cervical spine have been described by Wyke (1979). The loss of afferent information from these receptors with advancing age is probably due largely to degenerative disease, which is almost universal (at least on X-ray) after the age of 60 years. The consequences include impairment of the precise control of movement and symptoms which closely resemble those produced by vertebro-basilar insufficiency: vertigo, nystagmus and ataxia.

Because of diagnostic difficulties in distinguishing between vertigo caused by disease of the labyrinths, cervical receptors or the vertebro-basilar system (indeed all three may be affected) it is not surprising that there is a lack of information on treatment aimed specifically at patients with cervical receptor dysfunction. However, it seems reasonable to encourage a greater reliance on vision and to follow the regime described in the treatment of vertigo (q.v.). Gentle exercises to improve the range of neck movements may be helpful since Wyke noted that restriction of movements by a cervical collar made the wearer feel unsteady in the dark. A walking frame improves stability and general balance exercises, such as those described at the end of the chapter, help build up confidence.

POSTURAL HYPOTENSION

This is a well recognised problem in the elderly (Exton-Smith, 1978) and is often aggravated by drugs such as diuretics, antihypertensive agents and tranquillisers. Inactivity, especially bedrest, is a contributory factor and symptoms often subside as mobility increases.

For difficult cases it is usually necessary to start with the patient semi-reclining in a tilting chair which is brought to the vertical for longer and longer periods each day as his tolerance improves. Elastic stockings are often ineffective on their own unless accompanied by an abdominal binder. Before attempting to get out of bed or a chair the patient should try to raise his blood pressure by spending a few minutes doing isometric muscle exercises and dorsiflexing his feet; breathing exercises (see under cervical spondylosis) may also be helpful. Fludrocortisone 0.5 to 2.0 mg daily will usually raise the blood pressure for a week or two (there is a danger of it precipitationg congestive cardiac failure) and this may allow time for the patient to be successfully mobilised.

VERTIGO

Drugs can cause or relieve vertigo and so must be used with care in the elderly. Tranquillisers, especially the phenothiazines with their powerful sedative action, often aggravate the symptoms of a central vestibular lesion but are most effective in labyrinthine disorders. However, even here, the drugs of first choice are either betahistine 8 mg three times a day or cinnarizine 15 mg three times a day. Betahistine is an orally active histamine analogue which is capable, in animals of producing vasodilatation of capillaries and arterioles in the stria vascularis (Martinez, 1972). Cinnarizine has antihistaminic properties which probably account for its vestibular sedative action. It is also a calcium antagonist and may normalise endolymph flow by preventing vasoconstriction of the stria vascularis. Both drugs can relieve vertigo due to labyrinthine disease (Frew and Menon, 1976; Philipszoon, 1962).

The Cawthorne and Cooksey exercises were developed at King's College Hospital specifically for peripheral vestibular lesions but are valuable in any case of vertigo. They aim to increase the patient's tolerance of unequal balance between the two ears and should be performed for at least five minutes three times daily. The patient is advised to seek out head positions and movements that cause vertigo, as far as can be tolerated, because the more frequently vertigo is induced the more rapidly tolerance develops.

Eye movements: up and down; from side to side; focus on finger moving from three feet to one foot away from the face.

Head movements: bend forwards and backwards; turn from side to side. These should be done initially with eyes closed, later with eyes open. At first the movements are done in bed, later when sitting and standing. They should begin slowly and gradually speed up.

Additional movements when sitting: shrug shoulders and move upper body in circles; bend forwards and pick up objects from the ground.

When standing: stand up with eyes open and closed; throw a small ball from hand to hand above eye level and then under the knees; change from sitting to standing and turn round in between.

When moving about: walk across the room, up and down a slope and up and down stairs with eyes open and then closed; group games involving throwing and catching a ball.

Tilting reactions in normal people only occur when the body is unstable and of all the postural reflexes this is the only one for which labyrinthine activity is essential (Martin, 1965). If labyrinthine function is completely absent, vision and proprioception usually provide adequate compensation, but if the light is poor and the ground uneven falls are very common. Patients are often aware of these dangerous situations but may need to be warned to turn on the light before getting out of bed at night and to ensure that their stairs are well lit.

BIOFEEDBACK

Biofeedback training depends on providing the patient with additional, immediate information of some biological function which is normally poorly perceived: the aim is to use this extra information to improve performance. The systems used in rehabilitation provide indirect feedback of motor performance compared with the direct feedback derived from movement, vision and proprioception.

It was shown early on using a needle electrode EMG that individual motor units could be controlled. After training, and even in the absence of auditory and visual feedback, some subjects were able to recall into activity different single motor units while inhibiting the activity of neighbouring units (Basmajian, 1963). Training improves a person's ability to control single motor units and there is some evidence that men are rather better at it than women (Zappalá, 1970).

In a critical review Blanchard and Young (1974) concluded that biofeedback probably had a clinical use in muscle retraining. Using auditory feedback from an EMG electrode on the paralysed limb hemiplegic patients, who still had no return of function many months after their stroke, could rapidly regain limb movement. Some learnt to dorsiflex the foot and walk without a leg brace.

Another study of chronic, resistant post-stroke cases used both an auditory and a visual signal from a surface EMG electrode. Half hour sessions were given three times a week. Some voluntary control of movement and even a reduction in spasticity appeared after one to three sessions. If the patient could maintain his control and functional improvement over several sessions the biofeedback treatment was gradually withdrawn and replaced by observation of the moving limb. Even several months after indirect feedback was stopped motor control was maintained in some patients and had 'become incorporated into the system of patterned volitional movements' (Brudny et al, 1974).

Some instruments which were developed to investigate and measure movement can be modified to provide feedback. One example is the polarised light goniometer which uses small lightweight optical sensors attached to the limbs and illuminated by polarised light from a projector. This can provide both visual and auditory feedback of posture and movement (Mitchelson, 1978). Mitchelson has recently developed a device which is attached to the patients waist and shows him how far he is leaning from the vertical. Stroke patients can improve their balance using this technique but it is not yet known whether the benefit is longlasting nor have these patients been compared with controls (Ashburn, 1979). Visual feedback makes little difference to a normal person's balance when illumination is good but patients with vestibular lesions improve significantly, even in full illumination (Begbie, 1967).

Videorecording can be used to help the stroke patient relearn his body image and improve gait and balance, particularly if he finds mirrors confusing. The film is immediately played back to show him his mistakes (van Gestel, 1971).

It is difficult to assess the value of biofeedback because most of the reported studies are uncontrolled. The results often look impressive because there is usually a long baseline of failure to respond to conventional treatment. However, the one controlled trial included in a recent review (Miller, 1978) showed that controls who were only given physical therapy improved considerably and by an amount that was probably not statistically significant from the experimental group who also had EMG feedback. A more promising study is one which examined elderly chronic hemiplegics in a residential home. Twenty patients with an average age of 72 were assessed for strength and range of leg movements and gait. They all had 15 minutes' treatment twice a week for six weeks but ten of them had feedback from EMG surface electrodes on the tibialis anterior and gastrocnemius muscles. All of the group who had biofeedback improved their gait, strength and range of leg movements but only two out of the 10 controls improved (Burnside, 1981).

MOTIVATION

We have all met the patient who appears not to want to get better and resists any attempts at mobilisation. Reasons for this include pain, or the prospect of pain, fear of failure, low morale of the therapist, mental illness (including dementia) and reluctance to surrender to another's will (O'Gorman, 1975). Some elderly patients are liable to be labelled as 'difficult', 'senile' or 'bed-blockers' and come to accept these negative attitudes (Stewart, 1975).

Finding a suitable incentive is usually necessary and for hospital patients a home visit may kindle enough enthusiasm for them to start walking. Relatives can sometimes give a clue about past interests or hobbies which can be used as a starting point to gain the patient's attention. Satisfaction from exercising an acquired skill is an important motivating factor and patients have to be persuaded by any means available to take the first step towards relearning that skill.

Positive incentives should be used to reinforce the desired activities. This means setting realistic goals which the patient is capable of achieving in the short term. Full walking independence and a return home may be the ultimate goal but can seem such a distant prospect to the patient that he becomes disheartened. However, simply to be able to stand upright, at first with help and then independently for increasing lengths of time, is a more realistic goal which, once achieved, encourages progress. Teaching simple daily living activities so that the patient can be in control of one small area of movement increases self respect and shows that the seemingly impossible can be achieved (Ibbotson, 1975). Above all the therapist must be sympathetic, patient and friendly. Enthusiasm is necessary but she must not be too demanding and should be careful not to unwittingly 'reward' unsatifactory behaviour by getting upset.

The attention span of demented patients may be improved by reality orientation (Holden and Sinebruchow, 1978) and the motivation of other disabled elderly persons may respond to sensory stimulation. The techniques are simple, are suitable for group work and are designed to overcome such problems as loneliness, alienation, fear of getting lost and boredom (Burnside, 1969).

The 'poor motivation syndrome' is much commoner in women and may respond satisfactorily to amphetamines. Over a two year period Clark and Mankikar (1977) saw 88 cases: more than half the treated patients showed definite improvement and more than a quarter could be discharged home. They used dexamphetamine in a starting dose of 2·5 mg at 8 a.m. and 12 noon increasing, if necessary to 5 mg in the second week and 10 mg in the third week. The commonest side effects were confusion and restless behaviour and usually occurred during the first week. The drug was stopped after three weeks and was only used on in-patients to avoid the risk of widespread or indiscriminate use.

CONCLUSIONS

Rehabilitation is likely to be most successful where the cause of the imbalance has been accurately diagnosed and a specific programme is prescribed as part of a team approach to the patient as a whole. General balancing exercises may be useful not only for patients who have had falls but for any elderly person whose activity is low. They should be done daily and could form part of group keep-fit classes in residential homes or day centres. A suitable programme (Kinsman 1979) might include:

1. Standing, with finger support, first on one leg and then the other. Gradually build up the time that this position can be held.
2. Whilst sitting on a dining chair turn and look to left and right. Repeat with arms abducted. Repeat, touching the left foot with the right hand and then the right foot with the left hand.
3. Again, whilst sitting pick up an object from the floor, straighten up and then replace it on the floor.
4. Whilst standing pick up an object from a table place it on a chair and then back on the table. Repeat, but this time place the object on the floor.
5. Heel-to-toe walking along a straight line.

Falls should not be accepted as an inevitable part of ageing. If the problems of low activity and loss of confidence are recognised and treated the patient can be helped to regain his independence. Day centres, day hospitals and community physiotherapists should be used to maintain the patient's interest and to keep up his morale.

REFERENCES

Adams G F, Hurwitz L J 1963 Mental barriers to recovery after strokes. Lancet ii: 533
Adams G F, McComb S G 1953 Assessment and prognosis in hemiplegia. Lancet, ii: 266
Agate J 1970 Accidents to old people. Community Health 2: 29

Alberti M L 1973 A simple test of visual neglect. Neurology 23:658

Ashburn A 1979 Personal communicaton

Atkinson H W 1977 Principles of treatment. In: Cash J (ed) Neurology for physiotherapists, 2nd edn. Faber and Faber, London

Basmajian J V 1963 Control and training of individual motor units. Science 141:440

Begbie G H 1967 Some problems of postural sway In: Myotatic, Kinesthetic and Vestibular Mechanisms. Ciba Foundation Symposium. Churchill, London

Birch H G, Proctor F, Bortner M, Lowenthal M 1960a Perception in hemiplegia; judgment of vertical and horizontal by hemiplegic patients. Archives of Physical Medicine and Rehabilitation 41:19

Birch H G, Proctor F, Bortner M, Lowenthal M 1960b Perception in hemiplegia: judgment of the median plane. Archives of Physical Medicine and Rehabilitation 41:71

Blanchard E B, Young L D 1974 Clinical applications of biofeedback training. Archives of general psychiatry 30:573

Bobath B 1971 Abnormal postural reflex activity caused by brain lesions, 2nd edn. Heinemann, London

Bobath B 1978 Adult hemiplegia: evaluation and treatment, 2nd edn. Heinemann, London

Brocklehurst J C, Andrews K, Richards B, Laycock P J 1978 How much physical therapy for patients with stroke? British Medical Journal, 1:1307

Brudny J, Korein J, Levidow L, Grynbaum B B, Lieberman A, Friedmann L W 1974 Sensory feedback therapy as a modality of treatment in central nervous system disorders of voluntary movement. Neurology 24:925

Brunnstrom S 1970 Movement therapy in hemiplegia. Harper and Row, New York

Burley L E, Currie C T, Smith R G, Williamson J 1979 Contribution from geriatric medicine within acute medical wards. British Medical Journal, 2:90

Burnside I G, Tobias H S, Bursill D 1981 Electromyographic feedback in the remobilisation of stroke patients. Research in psychology and medicine. Academic Press, London, vol 2

Burnside I M 1969 Sensory stimulation: an adjunct to group work with the disabled aged. Mental Hygiene 53:(3) 381

Chirico A M, Stunkard A J 1960 Physical activity and human obesity. New England Journal of Medicine 263:935

Clark A N G, Mankikar G D 1977 Amphetamine assisted rehabilitation Paper read to Autumn meeting of British Geriatrics Society, London

Davies E 1975 Lets get moving. Age Concern, England

Exton-Smith A N 1977 Rehabilitation of the elderly In: Mattingly S (ed) Rehabilitation Today. Update, London

Exton-Smith A N 1978 Disturbances of autonomic regulation In: Isaacs B (ed) Recent Advances in Geriatric Medicine Churchill Livingstone, Edinburgh

Fay T 1954 The use of pathological and unlocking reflexes in the rehabilitation of spastics. American Journal of Physical Medicine 33:347

Heinemann, London

Frew I J C, Menon G N 1976 Betahistine hydrochloride in Ménière's disease. Postgraduate Medical Journal 52:501

Fugl-Meyer AR, Jääsko L, Leyman I, Olsson S, Steglind S 1975 The post hemiplegic patient: A method for evaluation of physical performance. Scandinavian Journal of Rehabilitation Medicine 7:13

Gabell A 1979 Personal communication

Garraway M, Akhtar A J 1978 Theory and practice of stroke rehabilitation. In: Isaacs B (ed) Recent Advances in Geriatric Medicine-1 Churchill Livingstone, Edinburgh

Graham O 1975 Closed circuit television in assessment of disability following severe head injury. Physiotherapy 61:272

Gutmann E, Hanzlíková V 1972 Age changes in the neuromuscular system. Scientechnica, Bristol

Hammett V B O 1967 Psychological changes with physical fitness training. Canadian Medical Association Journal 96:764

Holden U P, Sinebruchow A 1978 Reality orientation therapy: a study investigating the value of this therapy in the rehabilitation of elderly people. Age and Ageing 7:83

Ibbotson J 1975 Motivation—the occupational therapist's approach. Physiotherapy 61:189

Isaacs B, Marks R 1973 Determinants of outcome of stroke rehabilitation. Age and Ageing 2:139

Kabat H 1947 Studies on neuromuscular dysfunction. Reprinted 1977 In: Payton O D, Hirt S, Newton R A (eds) Scientific bases for neurophysiologic approaches to therapeutic exercises. Davis, Philadelphia

Katz S, Downs T D, Cash H R, Grotz R C 1970 Progress in development of the index of ADL. The Gerontologist 10:(1) 20

Kinsman R 1979 Personal communication

Knott M, Voss D E 1968 Proprioceptive neuromuscular facilitation, 2nd edn. Harper & Row, New York

Lane R E J 1969 Physiotherapy in the treatment of balance problems. Physiotherapy 55:415

Lee D, Lishman R 1975 Vision in movement and balance. New Scientist, 65:59

Lowenthal M, Tobis J S, Howard I R 1959 An analysis of the rehabilitation needs and prognoses of 232 cases of cerebral vascular accident. Archives of Physical Medicine and Rehabilitation 40:183

MacDonald J B, MacDonald E T 1977 Nocturnal femoral fracture and continuing widespread use of barbiturate hypnotics. British Medical Journal, 2:483   •

Magnus R 1926 Some results of studies in the physiology of posture. Lancet ii:531 and 585

Martin J P 1965 Tilting reactions and disorders of the basal ganglia. Brain 88:855

Martin J P 1967 The basal ganglia and posture. Pitman, London

Martinez D M 1972 The effect of serc (betahistine hydrochloride) on the circulation of the inner ear in experimental animals. Acta Oto-laryngology Supplement 305:29

Miller N E 1978 Biofeedback and visceral learning. Annual Review of Psychology 29:373

Mitchelson D L 1978 Instrumented movement analysis as a means of motor function assessment and therapy. In: Jukes A M (ed) Baclofen: spasticity and cerebral pathology Cambridge Medical Publications, Northampton

Murphy F W 1977 Blocked beds, British Medical Journal 1:1395

Nayal S, Castleden C M, George C F, Marcer D 1978 The effect of an hypnotic with a short half life on hangover effect in old patients. Age and Ageing, 7:Supplement 50

O'Gorman G 1975 Anti-motivation. Physiotherapy 61:176

Over R 1966 Possible visual factors in falls by old people. Gerontologist, 6:212

Overstall P W, Imms F J, Exton-Smith A N, Johnson A L 1977 Falls in the elderly related to postural imbalance. British Medical Journal 1:261

Palmore E, Maddox G L 1977 Sociological aspects of ageing In: Busse E W, Pfeiffer, E (eds) Behaviour and Adaptation in Late Life. Little Brown, Boston

Partridge C J, Warren M D 1977 Physiotherapy in the Community. Health Services Research Unit, Canterbury

Philipszoon A J 1962 Influence of cinnarizine on the labyrinth and on vertigo. Clinical Pharmacology and Therapeutics 3:181

Ransome H 1978 Part III homes: unexpected rehabilitation resource. Modern Geriatrics, Dec. 25

Sheldon J H 1963 The effect of age on the control of sway. Gerontologia Clinica 5:129

Shephard R J 1969 Endurance Fitness. University of Toronto

Smith K U, Ramana D S V 1970 Feedback analysis of posture as a body tracking mechanism. American Journal of Physical Medicine 49:112

Smith L C, Dugal L P 1965 Age and spontaneous running activity of male rats. Canadian Journal of Physiology and Pharmacology 43:852

Stewart M C 1975 Motivation in old age. Physiotherapy 61:180

Stichbury J C 1975 Assessmet of disability following severe head injury. Physiotherapy 61:268

Strub R L, Black F W 1977 The mental status examination in neurology. Davis, Philadelphia

Svanström L 1974 Falls on stairs: an epidemiological accident survey. Scandinavian Journal of Social Medicine 2:113

Symon L 1971 Surgical treatment In: Wilkinson M (ed) Cervical spondylosis Heinemann, London

Trombly C A, Scott A D 1977 Occupational therapy for physical dysfunction. Williams and Wilkins. Baltimore

Twitchell T E 1951 The restoration of motor function following hemiplegia in man. Brain 74:443

Twitchell T E 1954 Sensory factors in purposive movement. Journal of Neurophysiology 17:239

Van Gestel A P M 1971 Television and video-recorder in therapeutic exercise. Scandinavian Journal of Rehabilitation Medicine 3:79

Wall J C, Ashburn A 1979 Assessment of gait disability in hemiplegics. Scandinavian Journal of Rehabilitation Medicine 11:(3) 95

Welford A T 1977 Causes of slowing of performance with age. Interdisciplinary Topics in Gerontology 11:43

Wyke B 1979 Cervical articular contributions to posture and gait: their relation to senile disequilibrium. Age and Ageing 8:251

Zappalá A 1970 Influence of training and sex on the isolation and control of single motor units. American Journal of Physical Medicine 49:348

A glossary of some official and unofficial abbreviations, symbols and terms which may be encountered in neuro-otology*

*compiled by *Susan Bellman, Sava Součková* and *Joanna Zlotnik*

Appendix 1

Abbreviations and symbols

A ampere; if engraved on a tuning fork, it denotes decay rate of fork in air-conduction mode (expressed as time in seconds for sound intensity to fall by 3 dB); argon

A scale The scale on a sound level meter which indicates the sound level after the noise being measured has been attenuated over the lower frequencies to the extent of 10 dB per octave for the range below 250 Hz and 5 dB per octave over the range 250 Hz to 1000 Hz. The level of sounds so measured would be expressed in dB(A)

Å ångstrom (an obsolete unit of length; equivalent to 10^{-1} nm)

AAA Abnormal auditory adaptation

AAF Acute auditory failure

AAOO American Academy of Ophthalmology and Otolaryngology

ABC Absolute bone conduction

ABLB Alternate (alternating) binaural loudness balance test; syn. Fowler test for loudness recruitment

ABLM Alternate binaural loudness matching; syn. Fowler test for loudness recruitment

ABR Auditory brain stem response, i.e. the brain stem AEP

ac Alternating current

AC Air conduction

AD Auris dextra (right ear)

ADC Analog-to-digital converter

ADL Activities of daily living

AEG Air encephalogram

AEP Acoustically evoked potential

AG Angiography

AGC Automatic gain control

AHL Average hearing level

AICA Anterior inferior cerebellar artery

ALF Acute labyrinthine failure

ALS Amyotrophic lateral sclerosis

AM Amplitude modulated

AMR Auditory middle response

ANSI American National Standards Institute

AOE Acute otitis externa

AOM Acute otitis media

AP Action potential
AR Acoustic reflex
ART Acoustic reflex threshold; auditory reaction time
AS Auris sinistra (left ear)
ASHA American Speech and Hearing Association
ASR Acoustic stapedius reflex
ASRD Acoustic stapedial reflex decay
ASRT Acoustic stapedial reflex threshold
AVF Acute vestibular failure

B bel, (a dimensionless unit used to express magnitudes by expressing them in terms of logarithmic ratios, e.g. a sound intensity expressed in bels would be the logarithm of the ratio of that intensity to a reference intensity. If engraved on a tuning fork, B denotes decay rate of fork in bone conduction mode (expressed as time in seconds for sound intensity to fall by 3 dB); boron, binaural (as in 'B-questions' and 'B-type questionnaire')

B scale The scale on a sound level meter which indicates the sound level after the noise being measured has been attenuated over the lower frequencies to the extent of 4 dB per octave for the frequencies below 300 Hz. The level of sounds so measured would be expressed in dB(B)

B_A Acoustic susceptance
B_c Capacitive susceptance
B_L Inductive susceptance
BAAP British Association of Audiological Physicians
BAO British Association of Otolaryngologists
BBN Broad-band noise
BC Bone conduction
BE Behind the ear (usually in reference to type of hearing aid)
BEA Better ear average (hearing threshold levels)
BICROS Bilateral CROS
BINO Bilateral internuclear ophthalmoplegia
bit Binary digit
BPN Benign paroxysmal nystagmus
BPPV Benign paroxysmal positional vertigo
BS British standard
BSER Brain stem electric response
BTHL Bilateral total hearing loss
BW Body worn (usually in respect of hearing aids)
BWt Body weight

C carbon; coulomb (SI unit of electric charge, i.e. quantity of electricity); if engraved on a tuning fork, C denotes *characteristic* of fork (*stem-transmission* factor); this is defined as the number of *half-intensity periods* for which the fork can be heard by air conduction, after hearing by bone conduction has ceased (a half-intensity period is the time required for the sound intensity to fall to a half, i.e. by 3 dB)

C scale The scale on a sound level meter which has an essentially flat response over the frequency range 20 Hz to 10 kHz.

CANS Central auditory nervous system

CAP Compound action potential

CAR Crossed acoustic response (*see* PAM)

CARE Comprehensive assessment and referral evaluation

CAT Computerised axial tomography; Combined approach technique

ccd Charge-coupled device

ccw Counter-clockwise

CERA Cortical evoked response audiometry

CETT Circular eye-tracking test

CF Characteristic frequency

CGS Centimetre-gram-second system of units; now succeeded by the SI

CID Central Institute for the Deaf (St. Louis, Missouri, USA)

CM Cochlear microphonic

CMRR Common mode rejection ratio

CMV Cytomegalovirus

CN Congenital nystagmus

CNV Contingent negative variation

COE Chronic otitis externa

COM Chronic otitis media

CP Canal paresis

CPA Cerebellopontine angle; critical path analysis

CPN Central positional nystagmus

CROS Contralateral routing of signals (a hearing aid system where the microphone is on the side of the poorer ear, but the acoustic signal is fed to the opposite ear)

CSF Cerebrospinal fluid

CSOM Chronic suppurative otitis media

CT Computerised tomography, viz. computerised axial tomography

CTS Compound threshold shift, ie auditory threshold shift that has both temporary and fresh persisting (permanent) components; Contralateral threshold shift.

CV Conversational voice; Curriculum vitae

CVC Consonant-vowel-consonant

cw Clockwise

DAF Delayed auditory feedback

db Diplacusis binauralis

dB decibel, which is one-tenth of a bel, which is the logarithm of the ratio of two sound intensities. Since sound intensity is proportional to the square of the sound pressure, the bel is the logarithm of the square of the ratio of two sound pressures. Thus a decibel is 20 times the logarithm of two pressure ratios. The numerical value of a sound level in decibels will thus depend on the reference sound pressure. Nevertheless, one decibel corresponds to a change in sound pressure of about 12 per cent

dc Direct current

DHSS Department of Health and Social Security (UK)
DL Difference limen; Discrimination loss
DP Directional preponderance
DS Disseminated sclerosis; Discrimination score
D-S Doerfler-Stewart test
DSFB Delayed speech feedback

E exa (as prefix indicating to multiply by 10^{18})
E scale Extraversion-introversion scale of one or other of Eysenck's personality
    inventories (psychological questionnaires)
EAM External acoustic meatus
EC Eyes closed
EC_b Eyes closed (going) backwards (in heel-to-toe test)
EC_f Eyes closed (going) forward (in heel-to-toe test)
ECMR Evoked cochlear mechanical response; syn. Kemp effect
ECochG Electrocochleogram or electrocochleography
ECS Experimental comparative study
EEG Electroencephalography
ENG Electronystagmography or electronystagmogram (a special case of EOG, i.e.
    when recording nystagmus)
EO Eyes open
EO_b Eyes open (going) backwards (in heel-to-toe test)
EO_f Eyes open (going) forward (in heel-to-toe test)
EOG Electro-oculography
EP Evoked potential; Endocochlear potential
Epi Epilepsy
EPI Eysenck personality inventory (a psychological questionnaire)
ERA Electric response audiometry
ETT Eye tracking test

FATB Floor ataxia test battery
FFA Free field audiometry
FFR Frequency following response
FFT Fast Fourier transform; Failure of fixation suppression
FIT Fusion at inferred threshold
FM Frequency modulated
FTA-ABS Fluorescent treponemal antibody absorption test
FTC Frequency tuning curve
FW Forced whisper

g gram
G giga (as prefix to a unit indicating to multiply by 10^9); Gravitational constant
G_A Acoustic conductance (as in acoustic immittance measurements of the ear)
G_E Electric conductance (SI unit is siemens, S)
G_M Mechanical conductance
GMP Graduated masking procedure (as in measurement of the threshold of
    hearing by bone conduction)

Gs gauss (CGS unit for magnetic flux density; 1 Gs corresponds to 10^{-4}T)
Gy gray (SI unit of absorbed dose of ionizing radiation)

H Hydrogen; henry (SI unit of self-inductance); Symbol for high-frequency emphasis, e.g. on hearing aid tone-controls
HA Headache
H/A Hearing aid
HAIC Hearing Aid Industry Conference standard
HANES Health and Nutrition Examination Survey 1971–74
HBX Head and balance exercises
HES Health Examination Survey 1960–61
HHS Hearing handicap scale
HIS Health Interview Survey (1971)
HL Hearing loss; Hearing level
HMS Hearing Measurement Scale
HP High pass
HPF High-pass filter
HSN Head shaking nystagmus
HTL Hearing threshold level
Hz hertz
HZO Herpes zoster oticus

I 'In' operation (international symbol for 'on', especially in respect of hearing aids); Iodine
IAM Internal acoustic meatus
IAPA International Association of Physicians in Audiology
IE Internal ear
IEC International Electrotechnical Commission
IFOS International Federation of Otolaryngological Societies
IHC Inner hair cells (of spiral organ of the cochlea)
IHR Institute of Hearing Research (MRC, Nottingham)
Imp Impression for ear moulds
INO Internuclear ophthalmoplegia
IO Inferior oblique muscle; Inferior olive
IQR Interquartile range, i.e. the range between the upper and lower quartiles
IR Inferior rectus muscle
IRV Infra-red viewer
ISA International Society of Audiology
ISI Interstimulus interval
ISO International organisation for standardisation
ISVR Institute of Sound and Vibration Research (University of Southampton)
IVBAI Intermittent vertebro-basilar artery insufficiency

JCHMT Joint Committee on Higher Medical Training
jnd Just noticeable difference

k kilo (as prefix to a unit, e.g. kg, kilogram, indicating to multiply by 10^3)
K kelvin (SI unit for temperature); Potassium

KEMAR Knowles Experimental Manikin for Acoustic Research
kg kilogram
kHz kilohertz
KN *Kopfschüttelnystagmus* (head shaking nystagmus)

L Left; Symbol for self-inductance; Symbol for low-frequency emphasis, e.g. on hearing aid tone-controls
L scale Lie scale of one or other of Eysenck's personality inventories (psychological questionnaires)
LAP Lateral ampulloneural preponderance
LDL Low-density lipoproteins; Loudness discomfort level (but, of course, there are many loudness discomfort levels for a given individual, but only one TUL, i.e. threshold of uncomfortable loudness)
LED Light-emitting diode
Leq Equivalent continuous sound level, expressed in dB(A)
LGB Lateral geniculate body
LLAP Left lateral ampullo-neural preponderance
LMR Labyrinthine membrane rupture
LP Lumbar puncture; Labyrinthine preponderance; Low-pass
LPF Low-pass filter
LR Loudness recruitment; Lateral rectus muscle
Lt Left
LWR Labyrinthine window rupture
lx lux (SI unit of illuminance)

m milli (as prefix indicating to multiply by 10^{-3})
M mega (as prefix to a unit, e.g. Mm, megametre, indicating to multiply by 10^{6}); Microphone input selection (international symbol on hearing aids); Monaural (as in 'M-questions' and 'M-type questionnaire')
MAF Minimum audible field
MAP Minimum audible pressure
MCL Most comfortable listening level
MCLL Most comfortable loudness level
md Monaural diplacusis
MD Mental defect; Doctor of Medicine
ME Middle ear
MEG Magneto-encephalography
MEGAAER Magneto-encephalographic averaged acoustically evoked response
MEGAVER Magneto-encephalographic averaged visual evoked response
MGB Medial geniculate body
mHz millihertz
MLB Medial longitudinal bundle
MLD Masking level difference
MLF Medial longitudinal fasciculus (*see* MLB)
mm millimetre (10^{-3}m)
MMPI Minnesota Multiphasic Personality Inventory
MO Medulla oblongata

mol mole (SI name for unit of amount of substance)
MR Medial rectus muscle
mrad milliradian
MRC Medical Research Council
ms millisec
mS millisiemens
MS Multiple sclerosis; Motion sickness
MSC Medical Steering Committee
MT Membrana tensa (of tympanic membrane)

n nano (as prefix to a unit, e.g. nm); Symbol for sample size in statistical analyses.
N newton (SI unit of force); nitrogen; Symbol for 'normal' position on hearing
    aid tone-control; Sample or population size in statistical analyses
N scale Neuroticism scale of one or other of Eysenck's personality inventories
          (psychological questionnaires)
N_1 First negative wave in an AEP
N_2 Second negative wave in an AEP
NI, NII, NIII, NIV, NV and NVI First, second, third, fourth, fifth and sixth
                              mastoid negative peaks in brain stem AEP
                              (Jewett classification)
NBN Narrow band noise
NIHL Noise-induced hearing loss
NIL Noise immission level (noise dose). The sum of the Leq and 10 times the
    logarithm of the exposure time in years
NIPTS Noise-induced permanent threshold shift
NITTS Noise-induced temporary threshold shift
nm nanometre $(10^{-9}m)$
NMR Nuclear magnetic resonance
NOHL Non-organic hearing loss
NPL National Physical Laboratory (UK)
NSH National Study of Hearing (UK)
NVC Non-verbal comprehension
Ny Nystagmus

O Out of operation (international symbol for 'off', especially in respect of hearing
    aids); Oxygen
OCR Ocular countertorsion reflex: syn. counter-rolling
OE Otitis externa
OFI Ocular fixation index
OGI Oculogyral illusion
OHC Outer hair cells (of spiral organ of the cochlea)
OKAN Optokinetic after-nystagmus
OKN Optokinetic nystagmus
OME Otitis media with effusion
ONIHL Occupational noise-induced hearing loss
OS Otosclerosis; Otological screening (or screened)
OW Oval window

P Phosphorus; peta (as prefix indicating to multiply by 10^{15})

P_1 First positive wave in an AEP

P_2 Second positive wave in an AEP

Pa Positive peak in AMR occurring at 35 to 50 ms after stimulus onset

PAM Postauricular muscle response

PAN Periodic alternating nystagmus; Positional alcohol nystagmus

PAS Periodic acid Schiff (a staining reaction characteristic of glycoprotein compounds)

Pb Positive peak in adult AMR occurring at 55 to 65 ms after stimulus onset; Lead

PB Phonetically balanced

PC Peak clipping

PEG Pneumo-encephalogram

PENG Photo-electric nystagmography

P̈erf. Perforated tympanic membrane

PETT Pendular eye-tracking test

PHU Partially-hearing unit

PICA Posterior inferior cerebellar artery

PN Pink noise; Positional (or provocation) nystagmus

PNF Proprioceptive neuromuscular facilitation

PP Past-pointing

PPN Paroxysmal positional nystagmus

PPRF Paramedian zone of the pontine reticular formation

PRBS Pseudo-random binary sequence (a form of rotating chair stimulus for testing vestibular system)

PTA Pure tone audiogram

PTC Psychophysical (or psychoacoustical) tuning curve; Phenylthiocarbamide (phenylthiourea); Plasma thromboplastin component (syn. Christmas factor, i.e. blood coagulation factor IX)

PTS Permanent threshold shift

Q Question; Questionnaire; Also a figure of merit of an energy storing system, in which respect it may be used to denote sharpness of resonance (if the bandwidth between the 70·7 per cent response points is denoted as Δf and the resonant frequency i.e. the frequency of the peak response, is fo, then $Q = fo/\Delta f$); Q is also the symbol for quantity of electricity or quantity of heat

Q_1 Lower quartile, i.e. 25th percentile

Q_2 Median, i.e. 50th percentile

Q_3 Upper quartile, i.e. 75th percentile

R Right

R_A Acoustic resistance

rad radian (SI unit of angle, it is defined as the plane angle between two radii of a circle which cut off on the circumference an arc equal in length to the radius); Also formerly a unit to express absorbed dose of ionizing radiations (1 rad = 10^{-2}Gy)

RBN Rebound nystagmus

RD Response decline
rem Obsolescent unit of radiation dose equivalence (1 rem $= 10^{-2}$Sv)
REM Random eye movement
RETSPL Reference equivalent threshold sound pressure level
RETT Random eye-tracking test
RIT Residual inhibition test (for tinnitus)
RLAP Right lateral ampulloneural preponderance
RNID Royal National Institute for the Deaf
RRBN Rebound-rebound nystagmus
Rt Right
RT Reaction time
RW Round window

s second
SAC Specialist Advisory Committee
SAE Spiral after effect; Surgical auditory evaluation (in USA)
SAL Sensorineural acuity level test
SAQ Self-answered questionnaire
SCV Slow component velocity
sd Standard deviation
SDT Speech detection threshold; Square drawing test
SHHI Social Hearing Handicap Index
SI Le Système International d'Unités (International System of Units)
SIN Sentence-in noise test
SISI Small increment sensitivity index
SL Sensation level, i.e. the level of a sound expressed in dB with respect to a
    particular person's threshold of hearing at the frequency in question
SLM Sound level meter
SML Simultaneous midplane lateralisation test
SN Spontaneous nystagmus; sensorineural; Surgical neurology
S/N Signal-to-noise ratio
SNHL Sensorineural hearing loss
SO Superior oblique muscle; Superior olive
SOM Superior oblique myokyonia; superior oblique muscle; (*see* OME)
SP Summation potential
SPIN Speech intelligibility in noise test
SPL Sound pressure level
SPN Stationary positional nystagmus
SPS Slow pursuit system
SR Superior rectus muscle; Stimulus-response
SRT Speech reception threshold
SSW Staggered spondaic word test
Sv sievert (SI unit of radiation dose equivalence)
Sy Syphilis

T tesla (SI unit of magnetic flux density); tera (as prefix to a unit indicating to
    multiply by 10^{12}, e.g. Ts, teraseconds);

TDT Tone decay test
Ti Tinnitus
TD 'Tone decay' (syn. AAA)
TIA Transient ischaemic attacks
TM Tympanic membrane
TSR Tactile stapedius reflex
TTS Temporary threshold shift
TUL Threshold of uncomfortable loudness
TUO Tinnitus of undetermined origin

UCLL Uncomfortable loudness level (but, of course, there are many such levels
     for any one individual, but only one TUL)

V volt(s); Vertigo; Vanadium
V-potential Vertex potential
VBI Vertebrobasilar insufficiency
VC Verbal comprehension
VE Verbal expression
VER Visual evoked response
VOR Vestibulo-ocular reflex
Vtg Vertigo
VUO Vertigo of undetermined origin

W-response Response pattern in intermediate levels of vestibulocochlear nerve
     compound action potential where N_1 and N_2 coexist
WBN Wide band noise
WEA Worse ear average (re hearing threshold levels)
WN White noise; Whole nerve, e.g. as whole nerve AP
WOFEC Walk on floor with eyes closed (a standardised heel-to-toe test)

X_A Acoustic reactance
X_C Capacitive reactance
X_L Inductive reactance

Y_A Acoustic admittance

Z_A Acoustic impedance

θ Symbol for angular displacement, e.g. of semicircular canal cupula
$\dot{\theta}$ First time derivative, i.e. velocity, of, for example, cupular displacement
$\ddot{\theta}$ Second time derivative, i.e. acceleration, of, for example, cupular displacement
μ One millionth, e.g. as μm (10^{-6}m)
Ω ohm
$\star$ not known or not knowable; symbol for multiplying function in computer
  languages
$<$ symbol for 'less than'; ERA symbol for a threshold in the right ear
$>$ symbol for 'greater than'; ERA symbol for a threshold in the left ear

Appendix 2

Glossary of terms

Abasia
Inability to walk, frequently restricted to cases where no neurological or other defect can be demonstrated.

Acoustically evoked potentials
A variety of electric potentials which may be recovered (invariably with computerised signal extraction techniques) from the internal ear, various muscles and the nervous system in response to acoustic stimuli to the ear.

Admittance, acoustic (Y_A)
Defines the ease with which the flow of sound energy can be accomplished.

Anacusis
No hearing, i.e. total hearing loss.

Artery, brachiocephalic
That branch of the arch of the aorta which was formally termed the innominate, and which divides into the right common carotid and the right subclavian arteries.

Artery, innominate
see artery, brachiocephalic.

Artery, internal auditory
see artery, labyrinthine.

Artery, labyrinthine
That branch of the anterior inferior cerebellar artery (or basilar artery) which was formally known as the internal auditory artery and which passes through the internal acoustic meatus to supply the internal ear.

Astasia
The inability to stand, frequently restricted to cases where no neurological or other defects can be demonstrated.

Ataxia
Incoordinated muscular action.

Ataxia of gait
Unsteadiness due to cerebellar disease or sensory losses.

Audiogram
The graphic representation of the results of a hearing test performed with an *audiometer*. If 'an audiogram' is referred to without any other qualification, it usually implies a record of the threshold of hearing for air conduction as a function of frequency.

Audiogram, air conduction
An audiogram which shows the threshold of hearing as measured by air conduction audiometry.

Audiogram, bone conduction
An audiogram which shows the threshold of hearing as measured by bone conduction audiometry.

Audiogram, pure tone
An audiogram which shows the threshold of hearing for pure tones at certain discrete frequencies (usually in an octave relationship); it usually refers to an air conduction threshold but may also include bone conduction threshold measurements; it also usually implies that the threshold(s) has (have) been measured using manual (non-automatic) audiometry.

Audiometer
An electroacoustic instrument with which *audiometry* is performed.

Audiometry
The measurement of hearing using an *audiometer*. The term has been variously subdivided, e.g. into *air conduction* and *bone conduction audiometry*. The term has also been subdivided into *subjective* and *objective audiometry*. However, since hearing is one of the special senses, any tests of hearing must be subjective, and any tests which do not involve the subject judging the sensation of an acoustic stimulus cannot be covered by the term audiometry. Thus the adjective 'subjective' is redundant and the adjective 'objective' is contradictory.

Audiometry, Békésy
A form of automatic, self-recorded audiometry. It has the advantage of providing a graphic recording of the responses and of excluding operator variability. Typically, there are facilities for sweep frequency testing (i.e. covering all of a band of frequencies from 100 Hz to 10 kHz) and for two test tone modes (continuous and intermittent).

Audiometry, objective
A term sometimes used to cover the measurement of auditory function by methods using *acoustically evoked potentials;* see Audiometry.

Audiometry, speech
Measurement of the ability to hear speech using a special type of audiometer designed for this purpose.

Bárány box
A noise-generating instrument which can be applied to an ear so that the ear is unable to pick up any other sounds. The instrument is thus useful in tuning fork tests of the hearing of one ear to ensure that the other ear is not responding to the test sounds.

Base, stapes
That part of the stapes which occupies the fenestra vestibuli (oval window); previously termed the footplate.

bel
The logarithm of the ratio of two sound intensities; since sound intensity is proportional to the square of sound pressure, the bel is also the ratio of the squares of two sound pressures.

Bing test

A tuning fork test used to detect minimal conductive hearing losses which would be undetected by the *Rinne test*. The footpiece of a vibrating tuning fork is applied to the mastoid process and the subject's ability to hear the sound is compared with the external acoustic meatus occluded and with it unoccluded. A subject with an essentially normal sound transmission system (external and middle ears) observes the sound to be louder when the meatus is occluded. This normal response is again, paradoxically, like the Rinne test response, reported as being 'Bing positive'.

Bobbing, ocular

A condition of spontaneous, abrupt, erratic downward jerks of the eyes followed by a return to mid-position.

Caloric test

A test used to examine the functional integrity of the vestibular labyrinth and vestibulo-ocular pathway. By irrigating the external acoustic meatus with air or water at a temperature different to that of body temperature, heat is transferred to the internal ear. With appropriate positions of the head, convection currents may then be set up in one or other (usually the lateral) semi-circular canal fluids. With the caloric test a one-sided rotatory stimulus can be simulated and the resulting endolymph flow provides the appropriate stimulus to the vestibular sensory receptors.

Cephalography

The recording of head movement.

Cholesteatoma

An aural epidermoid cyst (partial or complete).

Command eye movements

Eye movements in response to verbal directions (commands) given by the examiner.

Corneo-retinal potential

The electrical potential generated as a consequence of the eyeball behaving as an electrical dipole. The existence of this potential is made use of in *electro-oculography*.

Cycle

A single complete pattern of events in a recurring series.

Cycles per second

The former unit of frequency: now superseded by the *hertz*.

Deafness

A term which is now restricted to a *hearing loss* which is so severe that the individual is unable to hear any sounds, even with a hearing aid. Synonymous with *anacusis*.

decibel

A tenth of a bel.

degree

1. a unit of temperature in systems other than SI; 2. a non-SI unit of plane angles (1 degree = $\pi/180$ rad, i.e. 17·4533 mrad).

Diplacusis
The perception of two sounds when a single tone only is being delivered to the ear (or ears); the diplacusis may refer to one ear or both ears.

Diplacusis binauralis
The condition in which the two ears of a subject perceive a different pitch for the same sound frequency.

Discrimination loss, speech
The failure of a subject to attain a 100 per cent score when responding to replayed speech material(s).

Dysbasia
Difficulty in walking.

Electric response audiometry
A term used to describe the use of *acoustically evoked potentials* to measure auditory function. (The term is a misnomer since the word 'audiometry' implies the measurement of hearing. Nevertheless the term is deeply rooted among clinicians). Sometimes the term is used in a more restricted sense to refer to the slow cortical AEP.

Electrocochleography
The procedure of recording *acoustically evoked potentials* from the cochlea.

Electronystagmography
The use of *electro-oculography* to record *nystagmus*.

Electro-oculography
The use of the *corneo-retinal potential* to record eye movements.

Exercises, head and balance
A system of physical exercises used in vestibular rehabilitation.

Flutter, ocular
A condition characterised by episodes of three or four rapid pendular oscillations of the eyes in the horizontal plane.

Footplate
see stapes base.

Force platform
A platform equipped with mechanoelectrical transducers for the purpose of recording the sway of a standing subject by detecting displacements of the line of gravity.

Formant
A prominence in the acoustic spectrum of a speech sound: most vowels are characterised by the first two or three formants.

Fowler test
The alternate binaural loudness matching test: the test is used to differentiate between cochlear and retro-cochlear types of sensorineural hearing loss, the former group exhibiting *loudness recruitment*.

Frequency
The number of *cycles* of a repetitive event which occur in unit time, i.e. per *second*.

gauss
The electromagnetic CGS unit of magnetic induction; symbol Gs; now superseded by the *tesla*.

Glasses, Frenzel
Spectacles with biconvex lenses and a source of illumination which are used in clinical vestibulology to abolish optic fixation for the purpose of detecting or enhancing *vestibular nystagmus*.

gray
SI unit of absorbed radiation dose, symbol Gy; now superseded by the *rad*.

Grommet
A colloquial term for *tympanostomy tube*.

Güttich test
A test of balance in which the subject stands with the feet together, the eyes closed and the arms extended.

Hearing loss
Any impairment of hearing which is associated with a pathological elevation of the threshold of hearing at one or more frequencies in one or both ears.

Hearing loss, conductive
Hearing loss due to interference with sound transmission through the outer or middle ear. This type of hearing loss is indicated by a negative *Bing response*, a *true negative Rinne* response and a separation between the *air conduction* and *bone conduction threshold of hearing* ('air-bone gap').

Hearing loss, sensorineural
A hearing loss due to a disorder of the cochlea or of the auditory nervous system. This types of hearing loss is indicated by positive Bing and Rinne responses and essentially similar air conduction and bone conduction threshold of hearing.

Hearing loss, speech
A measure of the degree to which speech sounds are attenuated by the hearing defect. It is measured by the number of decibels which a speech audiogram is shifted to the right.

hertz
The SI unit of frequency.

Hypoacusis
Any impairment of hearing other than a total hearing loss, i.e. other than *anacusis*.

Illusion, oculogyral
The visual sensation that stationary objects in the visual field are exhibiting a recurring linear motion, which illusion has been induced by vestibular stimulation.

Immittance, acoustic
The term used to encompass *acoustic admittance* and *acoustic impedance*.

Impedance, acoustic (Z_A)
Defines the difficulty with which the flow of sound energy can be accomplished.

Index, (optic or ocular) fixation

The ratio of some measure of caloric-induced nystagmus with the eyes open to the same measure with the eyes closed. Used for the topdiagnosis of vestibular lesions.

Internal ear

That anatomical structure which incorporates the cochlea and the vestibular labyrinth.

kelvin

SI unit of temperature, symbol K.

Labyrinth

Synonymous with *internal ear*.

Loudness

The subjective magnitude of sound intensity; unit is the *sone*.

Loudness discomfort level

see threshold of uncomfortable loudness.

Masker

1. A sound applied to an ear for the purpose of elevating the threshold of hearing of that ear over a given frequency band and to a given elevation, synonymous with 'masking sound'; 2. An instrument which superficially resembles a hearing aid and which is used to deliver a masking sound to an ear with a view to ameliorating *tinnitus*.

mel

The unit of *pitch*; it is defined as follows: one thousand mels is the pitch of a 1 kHz tone at a level of 40 dB SL; thus one mel is one thousandth of the pitch of a 1 kHz tone at 40 dB SL; the pitch of any sound that is judged by the average normal listener to be n times that of a one mel tone is n mels.

Membrane, Reissner's

Former term for *vestibular membrane*.

Membrane, vestibular

That membrane in the cochlea that separates the cochlear duct from the scala vestibuli.

mole

The SI unit for amount of substance, symbol: mol.

Morpheme

The next largest linguistic unit to *phoneme*; used to refer to units which have mainly a grammatical function (BS 661, 1969).

Myoclonus, ocular

A condition of sustained bilateral pendular oscillations of the eye which are synchronous with associated rhythmical contractions of other midline muscular systems in the head and neck.

Myokymia, superior oblique

A condition characterised by intermittent, small amplitude, uniocular torsional eye movements in otherwise healthy adults.

Nerve, vestibulocochlear
That cranial nerve which connects the *internal ear* to the brain; synonymous with VIII cranial nerve.

newton
The SI unit of force, symbol: N.

Noise, broad band
Noise whose spectrum covers a broad band of frequencies.

Noise, narrow band
Noise whose spectrum covers a narrow band of frequencies.

Noise, pink
Noise having essentially equal energy per octave band.

Noise, random
Noise due to a large number of disturbances which occur randomly in time.

Noise, white
Broad band noise with essentially equal energy per cycle.

Nystagmus
An oscillatory movement of the eye where the same basic pattern (cycle) of movements is repeated.

Nystagmus, circumductive
Nystagmus in which the centre of the cornea describes a circular or elliptical path.

Nystagmus, dissociated
Nystagmus where features of the nystagmus are different in the two eyes.

Nystagmus, head-shaking
Nystagmus provoked by rapid side-to-side movements of the head. Synonymous with *Kopfschüttelnystagmus*.

Nystagmus, optokinetic
Nystagmus induced by an optical stimulus which is usually provided by a rotating, striped drum.

Nystagmus, paroxysmal positional
see Positioning nystagmus.

Nystagmus, pendular
Nystagmus where a cycle of events does not include a fast and a slow phase but instead, shows a to-and-fro movement of the eyes. The basic cycle of movement is that of a sinusoid or paraboloid.

Nystagmus, positional
Nystagmus produced by maintaining the head in a particular position; such nystagmus is independent of the mode, including speed, of attaining that position.

Nystagmus, positioning
Nystagmus produced by maintaining the head in a particular position; such Synonymous with *(benign) paroxysmal positional nystagmus*.

Nystagmus, retraction
Nystagmus which is characterised by the eyes moving back into the orbit.

Nystagmus, vestibular
Nystagmus in which a single *cycle* consists of a slower phase and, in the opposite direction, a quicker phase, and where the pattern of eye movement in each cycle

shows at least some rotatory component; such nystagmus is also typically accentuated when the subject looks in the direction of the quick phase of movement.

Opsoclonus
Spontaneous, chaotic eye movement.
Oscillopsia
The symptom of experiencing a visual oscillation of a fixed, stationary target. Note that, in contrast to objective vertigo, there is no sensation that the entire surroundings are moving.

pascal
The SI unit of pressure. Symbol; Pa.
Phenomenon, doll's head
see reflex, oculocephalic.
Phoneme
The smallest unit of speech (BS 661, 1969).
Pitch
The subjective experience of sound frequency; unit is the *mel*.
Polytomography
Refers to tomographic techniques wherein both the X-ray tube and the film follow a curved motion, e.g. *zonography, hypocycloidial tomography.*
Polytomography, computerised axial
A radiological imaging system where the X-rays are passed through the body in narrow beams to sensitive crystal detectors whose response is measured and analysed by computers.
Posturography
Measurement of body posture.

Quix test
A test of balance in which the subject stands with the feet apart, eyes closed and the arms extended.

radian
The SI unit of plane angles, symbol: *rad,* now supersedes the *degree.*
Recruitment loudness
The increase in the sensation of loudness at a greater rate than is normally the case; this phenomenon occurs in disorders of hearing where the lesion is located in the cochlea.
Reflex, oculocephalic
Compensatory eye movements in response to passive turning of the head. Synonymous with *Doll's head phenomenon.*
rem
A radiation dose equivalence unit which has now been superseded by the sievert.
REM
Random eye movements.
Rinne test
A tuning fork test which is used to ascertain the nature of a hearing loss in an ear.

The test compares a subject's ability to hear sounds by *air conduction* with his ability to hear it by *bone conduction*. Subjects hear better by air conduction if 1. the hearing is normal, 2. there is not more than a minimal *conductive hearing loss*, 3. there is a *sensorineural hearing loss* which is not severe. Subjects hear better by *bone conduction* if 1. there is a severe sensorineural hearing loss or 2. there is a conductive hearing loss other than a minimal one. Paradoxically, the response which is found in ears with a normal sound transmission mechanism, i.e. air conduction better than bone conduction, is termed a 'Rinne positive response'. If bone conduction is heard better than air conduction, the response is termed 'negative'. Further differentiation of the various categories can be achieved using a *Bárány box*, the *Weber test* and the *Bing test*.

Rinne test response, negative, false
A negative Rinne response which becomes a positive response when the test is repeated with the opposite ear *masked*.

Rinne test response, negative, true
A negative Rinne response which persists when the opposite ear is *masked*.

Romberg test
Compares the subject's ability to stand erect with the eyes closed with his ability to do so with the eyes open. If on closing his eyes, he immediately becomes unstable and falls to the ground, then the test is positive. Such a result indicates a spinal cord posterior column lesion.

röntgen
A non-SI unit of radiation exposure, symbol R, where $R = 2 \cdot 58 \times 10^4$ C. kg^{-1} (coulombs per kilogram).

Saccade
A fast eye movement

Saccadomania
see Opsoclonus.

Score, maximum speech discrimination
The maximum percentage score which a *speech audiogram* attains.

Score, optimum speech discrimination
A misnomer for *maximum speech discrimination score*.

second
The SI unit of time, abbreviation: s.

sievert
The SI unit for a radiation dose equivalent, symbol: Sv, supersedes the *rem*.

Skew deviation
Deviation of gaze of one eye above the other due to lesions other than those involving the muscles, their motoneurons or local mechanical factors in the orbit.

sone
The unit of *loudness*; one sone is the loudness of a 1 kHz tone at a level of 40 dB SPL; the loudness of any sound which is judged by the average normal listener to be n times that of the one sone tone is n sones.

Stabilography
A technique of recording body sway using a *force platform*.

Statokinesimetry
see Stabilography.

Strabismus
The condition of chronically misaligned visual axes.

tesla
The SI unit of magnetic flux density, i.e. of magnetic induction, symbol: T.

Threshold of uncomfortable loudness (TUL)
That level on the scale of increasing sound pressure where the sound is judged by that particular listener to have become uncomfortably loud; may be expressed as dB HL or as dB SPL.

Tinnitus
1. The perception of sound(s) in the absence of a corresponding sound outside the body which can be detected by other observers; 2. the sound(s) so perceived.

Tinnitus masking
1. a technique of describing tinnitus by assessing the level at which it can be abolished by a concurrent external noise; 2. a method of managing tinnitus using a *masker*.

Tinnitus matching
A technique of describing tinnitus by determining, using matching procedures, the particular sound (or sounds) to which it corresponds in terms of loudness, pitch and quality.

Tinnitus, subjective
Tinnitus which is not audible to anyone other than the individual experiencing it.

Tinnitus, objective
Tinnitus where the sound in question is also audible to another individual, with or without special detecting or amplifying equipment.

Tomography
The radiological technique of obtaining an image of a single plane of an anatomical structure (or structures) by moving the X-ray tube and film in opposite directions, but synchronously. The thickness of the anatomical section which is analysed is inversely related to the angle of swing of the tube and film.

Tube, auditory
The channel which connects the tympanic cavity and the nasal part of pharynx. Previously termed the *Eustachian tube*, and then the *pharyngotympanic tube*.

Tube, Eustachian
see auditory tube.

Tube, tympanostomy
A tube which is implanted through the tympanic membrane to provide continuity of the air space between the tympanic cavity and the external acoustic meatus.

Tuning fork
A twin-pronged metal instrument which is connected to a single stem by a common part known as the base; for the purpose of providing bone conducted

sound, the stem should end in a part termed the footpiece. When the prongs are struck appropriately, the fork generates a pure tone.

Tympanogram

A graph showing the change in some acoustic *immittance* value as a function of the pressure in the external acoustic meatus; this will correspond to the pressure in the tympanic cavity; the tympanogram provides information regarding the functional integrity of the middle ear and the *auditory tube*; in relationship to this, the presence or absence of fluid in the middle ear is readily detected.

Unterberger test

A test of balancing function wherein the subject is requested to mark time on the spot with the eyes closed and the fore limbs extended with the hands clasped together. The rotation of the body, if any, and its magnitude is noted.

Vertigo

A hallucination of movement, of the self (subjective vertigo) or of the environment (objective vertigo); it may be rotatory or non-rotatory, e.g. a swaying sensation.

Vertigo, positional

Vertigo associated with the attainment of a particular position of the head; this is frequently associated with a *positioning nystagmus*.

Vertigo, positioning

Vertigo induced by changing the position of the head and/or body; paradoxically, this is frequently *not* associated with a positioning nystagmus.

Viseme

Visual equivalent of a phoneme.

Weber test

A hearing test used to determine whether a unilateral *hearing loss* is *conductive* or *sensorineural*. The bone conduction stimulus, which may be generated by either a tuning fork or the bone conduction vibrator (transducer) of an audiometer, is usually applied to the midline of the skull. The subject is asked to say in which ear (or side of the head) he hears the sound. The sound is lateralised to the affected side of the hearing loss in conductive, and to the opposite side in sensorineural losses.

Zonogram

A narrow angle circular tomogram; it provides a convenient method for screening the internal acoustic meatus for vestibulocochlear schwannomas.

Index